S0-ASE-391

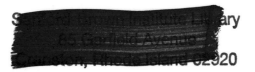

The GALE
ENCYCLOPEDIA of
NURSING &
ALLIED HEALTH

SECOND EDITION

The GALE
ENCYCLOPEDIA *of*
NURSING &
ALLIED HEALTH

SECOND EDITION

VOLUME

5

T-Z

ORGANIZATIONS
GENERAL INDEX
JACQUELINE L. LONGE, EDITOR

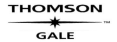

THOMSON

GALE

Detroit • New York • San Francisco • New Haven, Conn. • Waterville, Maine • London • Munich

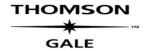

THE GALE ENCYCLOPEDIA OF NURSING & ALLIED HEALTH, SECOND EDITION

Project Editor
Jacqueline L. Longe

Editorial
Donna Batten, Laurie Fundukian, Jeffrey Lehman, Brigham Narins, Shirelle Phelps

Editorial Support Services
Luann Brennan, Grant Eldridge, Andrea Lopeman

Rights Acquisition Management
Margaret Chamberlain-Gaston

Imaging
Randy Bassett, Lezlie Light, Dan Newell, Christine O'Bryan, Robyn Young

Product Design
Tracey Rowens

Composition and Electronic Prepress
Evi Seoud, Mary Beth Trimper

Manufacturing
Wendy Blurton, Dorothy Maki

Indexing
Factiva, a Dow Jones Reuters Business Interactive LLC

LIBRARY OF CONGRESS CATALOGING-IN-PUBLICATION DATA

The Gale encyclopedia of nursing & allied health. – – 2nd ed. / Jacqueline L. Longe, editor.
p. ; cm.
Includes bibliographical references and index.
ISBN 1-4144-0374-7 (set hardcover : alk. paper) – – ISBN 1-4144-0375-5 (v. 1 : alk. paper)
– – ISBN 1-4144-0376-3 (v. 2 : alk. paper) – – ISBN 1-4144-0377-1 (v. 3 : alk. paper) – – ISBN
1-4144-0378-X (v. 4 : alk. paper) – – ISBN 1-4144-0379-8 (v. 5 : alk. paper)
  1. Medicine– –Encyclopedias. 2. Nursing– –Encyclopedias.
  [DNLM: 1. Nursing Care– –Encyclopedias– –English. 2. Allied Health Personnel– –
Encyclopedias– –English. 3. Nursing– –Encyclopedias– –English. WY 13 G151 2007] I. Title:
Encyclopedia of nursing & allied health. II. Title: Gale encyclopedia of nursing and
allied health. III. Longe, Jacqueline L.
  RT21.G353 2007
  610.7303– –dc22
                                                                        2006005012

This title is also available as an e-book
ISBN 1-4144-1044-1 (set)
Contact your Gale sales representative for ordering information.
ISBN 1-4144-0374-7 (set)
1-4144-0375-5 (Vol. 1)
1-4144-0376-3 (Vol. 2)
1-4144-0377-1 (Vol. 3)
1-4144-0378-X (Vol. 4)
1-4144-0379-8 (Vol. 5)

Printed in China
10 9 8 7 6 5 4 3 2 1

CONTENTS

LIST OF ENTRIES

A

Abdominal ultrasound
Abscess
Acid-base balance
Acid-fast culture
Activities of daily living evaluation
Acupressure
Acute kidney failure
Administering medication
Adolescent nutrition
Adrenal gland computed tomography
Adrenal glands
Adrenocortical hormone tests
Adrenomedullary hormone tests
Adult day care
Advanced practice nurses
Aerobic training
Aerosol drug administration
Aging and the aged
AIDS
AIDS counseling
AIDS tests
Airway management
Alcoholic paralysis
Alcoholism
Allergies
Allergy tests
Alzheimer's disease
Ambulatory electrocardiography
American sign language
Americans with Disabilities Act
Amino acid disorders screening
Amniocentesis
Amylase and lipase tests
Anaerobic bacteria culture
Analgesics
Anaphylaxis
Anemias
Anesthesia, general

Anesthesia, local
Angiography
Angioplasty
Antacids
Antepartum testing
Antianxiety drugs
Antibiotics
Anticancer drugs
Antidepressant drugs
Antidiabetic drugs
Antifungal drugs, topical
Antiglobin tests
Antihistamines
Antihypertensive drugs
Antiparkinson drugs
Antipsychotic drugs
Antiretroviral drugs
Antiseptics
Antiulcer drugs
Antiviral drugs
Anxiety
Apgar testing
Aphasia
Appendicitis
Apraxia
Art therapy
Arterial Doppler ultrasound
Arthrography
Arthroscopy
Aseptic technique
Asthma
Astigmatism
Audiology
Audiometry
Auditory integration training
Autoimmune disease tests
Autoimmune disorders
Autopsy

B

Back and neck pain, physical
  therapy for
Bacteria
Balance and coordination tests
Ball and socket joint
Balloon valvuloplasty
Bandages and dressings
Barium enema
Beds and bed preparation techniques
Behavioral optometry
Berg Balance Scale
Bioelectricity
Bioethics
Biological rhythms
Biomechanics
Biomedical engineering
Biomedical equipment technology
Biotin
Bipolar disorder
Birth injuries
Bites and stings
Bladder ultrasound
Bleeding disorders
Blood circulation
Blood coagulation
Blood culture
Blood gas analysis
Blood gases
Blood pressure measurement
Blood pressure
Blood specimen collection
Blood vessels
Blood
Body positioning in x-ray studies
Boils
Bone densitometry
Bone marrow aspiration and biopsy
Bone radionuclide scan

Drug interactions
Drug testing
Drug tests
Dynamic spatial reconstructor
Dysarthria
Dysphagia

E

Ear instillation
Ear irrigation
Echocardiography
Edema
Electroanalgesia
Electrocardiography
Electrocardiography unit
Electroencephalography
Electroencephalography unit
Electrolyte balance
Electrolyte tests
Electromyography
Electromyography biofeedback
Electroneurodiagnostic technology
Electroneurography
Electronic fetal monitoring
Electrophysiology study of the heart
Electrosurgery machines
Electrotherapy
Elimination diet
Emergency medical technicians
Emphysema
Endocarditis
Endocrine system
Endoscope
Endotracheal tube management
Endurance testing
Enema administration
Enemas
Enterostomy
Epidural therapy
Epithelial tissue
Ergonomic assessment
Esophageal function tests
Esophagogastroduodenoscopy
Ethical codes and oaths
Euthanasia
Evidence-based practice
Evoked potential studies
Exercise
Eye examination
Eye glasses
Eyedrop instillation

F

Fad diets
Falls
Family therapy
Fats, dietary
Fecal impaction removal
Fecal incontinence
Fecal occult blood test
Feedback systems
Fertility treatments
Fetal age study
Fetal alcohol syndrome
Fetal biophysical profile
Fetal cell screen
Fetal development
Fetoscopy
Fever
Fibrin degradation products test
Fibromyalgia
Fine motor skills
First aid
First aid kit
Flow cytometry analysis
Fluid balance
Fluoride therapy
Fluoroscope
Fluorosis
Folic acid
Food poisoning
Foot care
Foot orthoses
Foreign bodies
Fractures
Functional Independence
  Measure
Fungal culture
Fungi

G

Gait and balance assessment
Gait and balance problems
Gait training
Gallbladder
Gallbladder x rays
Gallium scan of the body
Gangrene
Gas embolism
Gas exchange
Gas laws
Gases, properties of

Gastric analysis
Gastritis
Gastroesophageal reflux scan
Gene therapy
Genetic counseling
Genetic engineering
Genetic testing
Genital culture
Genital herpes
Geriatric assessment tests
Geriatric nutrition
Gestational diabetes
Gingivitis
Glaucoma
Gliding joint
Glucose tests
Gout
Gram stain
Gross motor skills

H

H. pylori test
Head and neck cancer
Head injury
Health care financing
Health care, quality of
Health history
Health information management
Health promotion and education
Health services administration
Hearing
Hearing aids
Hearing loss
Heart failure
Heart
Heart-lung machines
Heat disorders
Heat treatments
Heimlich maneuver
Hematocrit
Hemodialysis shunt, graft, and fistula
  care
Hemoglobin test
Hemophilia
Henderson theory of nursing
Hepatitis virus tests
Herbalism, Western
Herniated disk
High-risk pregnancy
Hinge joint
Hip fractures rehabilitation
HIPAA

PLEASE READ—IMPORTANT INFORMATION

The *Gale Encyclopedia of Nursing & Allied Health* is a medical reference product designed to inform and educate readers about a wide variety of diseases, treatments, tests and procedures, health issues, human biology, and nursing and allied health professions. Thomson Gale believes the product to be comprehensive, but not necessarily definitive. While Thomson Gale has made substantial efforts to provide information that is accurate, comprehensive, and up-to-date,

Thomson Gale makes no representations or warranties of any kind, including without limitation, warranties of merchantability or fitness for a particular purpose, nor does it guarantee the accuracy, comprehensiveness, or timeliness of the information contained in this product. Readers should be aware that the universe of medical knowledge is constantly growing and changing, and that differences of medical opinion exist among authorities.

INTRODUCTION

The *Gale Encyclopedia of Nursing & Allied Health* is a unique and invaluable source of information for the nursing or allied health student. This collection of over 930 entries provides in-depth coverage of specific diseases and disorders, tests and procedures, equipment and tools, body systems, nursing and allied health professions, and current health issues. This book is designed to fill a gap between health information designed for laypeople and that provided for medical professionals, which may be too complicated for the beginning student to understand. The encyclopedia does use medical terminology, but explains it in a way that students can understand.

SCOPE

The *Gale Encyclopedia of Nursing & Allied Health* covers a wide variety of topics relevant to the nursing or allied health student. Subjects covered include those important to students intending to become biomedical equipment technologists, dental hygienists, dieteticians, health care administrators, medical technologists/clinical laboratory scientists, registered and licensed practical nurses, nurse anesthetists, nurse practitioners, nurse midwives, occupational therapists, optometrists, pharmacy technicians, physical therapists, radiologic technologists, and speech-language therapists. The encyclopedia also coversinformation on related general medical topics, classes of medication, mental health, public health, and human biology. Entries follow a standardized format that provides information at a glance. Rubrics include:

Diseases/Disorders
Definition
Description
Causes and symptoms
Diagnosis
Treatment
Prognosis
Health care team roles

Tests/Procedures
Definition
Purpose
Precautions
Description
Preparation
Aftercare
Complications

Prevention
Resources
Key terms

Results
Health care team roles
Resources
Key terms

Equipment/Tools
Definition
Purpose
Description
Operation
Maintenance
Health care team roles
Training
Resources
Key terms

Human biology/Body systems
Definition
Description
Function
Role in human health
Common diseases and disorders
Resources
Key terms

Nursing and allied health professions
Definition
Description
Work settings
Education and training
Advanced education and training
Future outlook
Resources
Key terms

Current health issues
Definition
Description
Viewpoints
Professional implications
Resources
Key terms

INCLUSION CRITERIA

A preliminary list of topics was compiled from a wide variety of sources, including nursing and allied health textbooks, general medical encyclopedias, and consumer health guides. The advisory board, composed of advanced practice nurses, allied health professionals, health educators, and medical doctors, evaluated the topics and made suggestions for inclusion. Final selection of topics to include was made by the advisory board in conjunction with the Gale editor.

ABOUT THE CONTRIBUTORS

The essays were compiled by experienced medical writers, including physicians, pharmacists, nurses, and allied health care professionals. The advisers reviewed the completed essays to ensure that they are appropriate, up-to-date, and medically accurate.

HOW TO USE THIS BOOK

The *Gale Encyclopedia of Nursing and Allied Health* has been designed with ready reference in mind.

- Straight **alphabetical arrangement** of topics allows users to locate information quickly.

- **Bold-faced terms** within entries direct the reader to related articles.

- **Cross-references** placed throughout the encyclopedia direct readers from alternate names and related topics to entries.

- A list of **Key terms** is provided where appropriate to define terms or concepts that may be unfamiliar to the student.

- The **Resources** section directs readers to additional sources of medical information on a topic.

- Valuable **contact information** for medical, nursing, and allied health organizations is included with each entry. An Appendix of Nursing and Allied Health organizations in the back matter contains an extensive list of organizations arranged by subject.

- A comprehensive **general index** guides readers to significant topics mentioned in the text.

GRAPHICS

The *Gale Encyclopedia of Nursing and Allied Health* is enhanced by over 500 color photos, illustrations, and tables.

ACKNOWLEDGMENTS

The editor would like to express appreciation to all of the nursing and allied health professionals who wrote, reviewed, and copyedited entries for the *Gale Encyclopedia of Nursing & Allied Health*.

Cover photos were reproduced by the permission of Delmar Publishers, Inc., Custom Medical Photos, and Thomson Gale.

ADVISORY BOARD

Several experts in the nursing and allied health community provided invaluable assistance in the formulation of this encyclopedia. The advisory board performed a myriad of duties, from defining the scope of coverage to reviewing individual entries for accuracy and accessibility. The editor would like to express appreciation to them for their time and their expert contributions.

CONTRIBUTORS

Lisa Maria Andres, M.S., C.G.C
San Jose, California

Greg Annussek
New York, New York

Maia Appleby
Boynton Beach, Florida

Bill Asenjo, M.S., C.R.C.
Iowa City, Iowa

William Arthur Atkins, Ph.D.
Pekin, Illinois

Lori Ann Beck, R.N., M.S.N.,
F.N.P.-C.
Berkley, Michigan

Mary Bekker
Willow Grove, Pennsylvania

Linda K. Bennington, R.N.C.,
M.S.N., C.N.S.
Virginia Beach, Virginia

Kenneth J. Berniker, M.D.
El Cerrio, California

Mark A. Best
Cleveland Heights, Ohio

Dean Andrew Bielanowski, R.N.,
B.Nurs.(QUT)
Rochedale S., Brisbane, Australia

Carole Birdsall, R.N. A.N.P. Ed.D.
New York, New York

Bethanne Black
Buford, Georgia

Maggie Boleyn, R.N., B.S.N.
Oak Park, Michigan

Barbara Boughton
El Cerrito, California

Patricia L. Bounds, Ph.D.
Zurich, Switzerland

Mary Boyle, Ph.D.,
C.C.C.-S.L.P.,
B.C.-N.C.D.
Lincoln Park, New Jersey

Rachael Tripi Brandt, M.S.
Gettysburg, Pennsylvania

Peggy Elaine Browning
Olney, Texas

Marilyn Butler
Susan Joanne Cadwallader
Cedarburg, Wisconsin

Barbara M. Chandler
Sacramento, California

Linda Chrisman
Oakland, California

Rhonda Cloos, R.N.
Austin, Texas

L. Lee Culvert
Alna, Massachusetts

Helen Davidson
Chicago, Illinois

Tish Davidson
Fremont, California

Lori De Milto
Sicklerville, New Jersey

Victoria E. DeMoranville
Lakeville, Massachusetts

Janine Diebel, R.N.
Gaylord, Michigan

Stéphanie Islane Dionne
Ann Arbor, Michigan

J. Paul Dow, Jr.
Kansas City, Missouri

Douglas Dupler
Boulder, Colorado

Lorraine K. Ehresman
Northfield, Quebec, Canada

Kim Ensley
L. Fleming Fallon, Jr., M.D.,
Dr.P.H.
Bowling Green, Ohio

Diane Fanucchi-Faulkner,
C.M.T., C.C.R.A.
Oceano, California

Janis O. Flores
Sebastopol, Florida

Paula Ford-Martin
Chaplin, Minnesota

Janie F. Franz
Grand Forks, North Dakota

Sallie Boineau Freeman, Ph.D.
Atlanta, Georgia

Rebecca Frey, Ph.D.
New Haven, Connecticut

Lisa M. Gourley
Bowling Green, Ohio

Meghan M. Gourley
Germantown, Maryland

Jill Ilene Granger, M.S.
Ann Arbor, Michigan

Elliot Greene, M.A.
Silver Spring, Maryland

Stephen John Hage, A.A.A.S.,
R.T.(R), F.A.H.R.A.
Chatsworth, California

Clare Hanrahan
Asheville, North Carolina

Robert Harr
Bowling Green, Ohio

Daniel J. Harvey
Wilmington, Delaware

Katherine Hauswirth, A.P.R.N.
Deep River, Connecticut

David L. Helwig
London, Ontario, Canada

Lisette Hilton
Boca Raton, Florida

René A. Jackson, R.N.
Port Charlotte, Florida

Nadine M. Jacobson, R.N.
Takoma Park, Maryland

Randi B. Jenkins
New York, New York

Michelle L. Johnson, M.S., J.D.
Portland, Oregon

Paul A. Johnson
San Marcos, California

Linda D. Jones, B.A.,
   P.B.T.(A.S.C.P.)
Asheboro, New York

Crystal Heather Kaczkowski,
   M.Sc.
Dorval, Quebec, Canada

Beth Kapes
Bay Village, Ohio

Monique Laberge, Ph.D.
Philadelphia, Pennsylvania

Aliene S. Linwood, B.S.N., R.N.,
   D.P.A., F.A.C.H.E.
Athens, Ohio

Jennifer Lee Losey, R.N.
Madison Heights, Michigan

Liz Marshall
Columbus, Ohio

Mary Elizabeth Martelli, R.N., B.S.
Sebastian, Florida

Jacqueline N. Martin, M.S.
Albrightsville, Pennsylvania

Sally C. McFarlane-Parrott
Mason, Michigan

Beverly G. Miller, M.T.(A.S.C.P.)
Charlotte, North Carolina

Christine Miner Minderovic, B.S.,
   R.T. R.D.M.S.
Ann Arbor, Michigan

Mark A. Mitchell, M.D.
Bothell, Washington

Susan M. Mockus, Ph.D.
Seattle, Washington

Timothy E. Moore, Ph.D.
Toronto, Ontario, Canada

Nancy J. Nordenson
Minneapolis, Minnesota

Erika J. Norris
Oak Harbor, Washington

Debra Novograd, B.S.,
   R.T.(R)(M)
Royal Oak, Michigan

Marianne F. O'Connor, M.T.,
   M.P.H.
Farmington Hills, Michigan

Teresa Odle
Albuquerque, New Mexico

Carole Osborne-Sheets
Poway, California

Cindy F. Ovard, R.D.A
Spring Valley, California

Patience Paradox
Bainbridge Island, Washington

Deborah Eileen Parker, R.N.
Lakewood, Washington

Genevieve Pham-Kanter
Chicago, Illinois

Jane E. Phillips, Ph.D.
Chapel Hill, North Carolina

Pamella A. Phillips
Bowling Green, Ohio

Elaine R. Proseus, M.B.A./T.M.,
   B.S.R.T., R.T.(R)
Farmington Hills, Michigan

Ann Quigley
New York, New York

Esther Csapo Rastegari, R.N.,
   B.S.N., Ed.M.
Holbrook, Massachusetts

Anastasia Marie Raymer, Ph.D.
Norfolk, Virginia

Martha S. Reilly, O.D.
Madison, Wisconsin

Linda Richards, R.D., C.H.E.S.
Flagstaff, Arizona

Toni Rizzo
Salt Lake City, Utah

Nancy Ross-Flanigan
Belleville, Michigan

Mark Damian Rossi, Ph.D, P.T.,
   C.S.C.S.
Pembroke Pines, Florida

Kausalya Santhanam
Branford, Connecticut

Denise L. Schmutte, Ph.D.
Shoreline, Washington

Joan M. Schonbeck
Marlborough, Massachusetts

Kathleen Scogna
Baltimore, Maryland

Cathy Hester Seckman, R.D.H.
Calcutta, Ohio

Jennifer E. Sisk, M.A.
Havertown, Pennsylvania

Patricia Skinner
Amman, Jordan

Genevieve Slomski
New Britain, Connecticut

Bryan Ronain Smith
Cincinnati, Ohio

Allison Joan Spiwak, B.S.,
   C.C.P.
Gahanna, Ohio

Lorraine T. Steefel
Morganville, New Jersey

Margaret A. Stockley,
   R.G.N.
Boxborough, Massachusetts

Amy Loerch Strumolo
Bloomfield Hills, Michigan

Liz Swain
San Diego, California

Deanna M. Swartout-Corbeil, R.N.
Thompsons Station, Tennessee

Peggy Campbell Torpey, M.P.T.
Royal Oak, Michigan

Mai Tran, Pharm.D.
Troy, Michigan

Carol A. Turkington
Lancaster, Pennsylvania

Judith Turner, D.V.M.
Sandy, Utah

Samuel D. Uretsky, Pharm.D.
Wantagh, New York

Michele R. Webb
Overland Park, Kansas

Ken R. Wells
Laguna Hills, California

Barbara Wexler, M.P.H.
Chatsworth, California

Gayle G. Wilkins,
   R.N.,B.S.N.,O.C.N.
Willow Park, Texas

Jennifer F. Wilson
Haddonfield, New Jersey

Angela Woodward
Madison, Wisconsin

Jennifer Wurges
Rochester Hills, Michigan

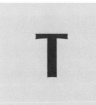

T-cell count *see* **Flow cytometry analysis**

T-uptake test *see* **Thyroid function tests**

T'ai chi

Definition

T'ai chi is an ancient Chinese **exercise** with movements that originate from the martial arts. While used as a type of self-defense in its most advanced form, t'ai chi is practiced widely for its health and **relaxation** benefits. Those in search of well being and a way to combat **stress** have made what has also been called "Chinese shadow boxing" one of the most popular low-intensity workouts around the world.

Origins

Also known as t'ai chi ch'uan (pronounced *tie-jee chu-wan*), the name comes from Chinese characters that translated mean "supreme ultimate force." The concept of t'ai chi, or the "supreme ultimate," is based on the Taoist philosophy of yin and yang, or the nature of when opposites attract. Yin and yang combine opposing, but complementary, forces to create harmony in nature. By using t'ai chi, it is believed that the principal of yin and yang can be achieved. A disturbance in the flow of chi (qi), or the life force, is what traditional Chinese medicine bases all causes of disease in the body. By enhancing the flow of ch'i, practitioners of t'ai chi believe that the exercise can promote physical health. Students of t'ai chi also learn how to use the exercise in the form of **meditation** and mental exercise by understanding how to center and focus their cerebral powers.

The origination of t'ai chi is rooted deep in the martial arts and Chinese folklore, causing its exact beginnings to be based on speculation. The much

disputed founder of t'ai chi is Zhang San-feng (Chang San-feng), a Daoist (Taoist) monk of the Wu Tang Monastery, who, according to records from the Ming-shih (the official records of the Ming dynasty), lived sometime during the period from 1391–1459. Legend states that Zhang happened upon a fight between a snake and a crane, and, impressed with how the snake became victorious over the bird through relaxed, evasive movements and quick counterstrikes, he created a fighting-form that shadowed the snake's strongest attributes. With his experience in the martial arts, Zhang combined strength, balance, flexibility, and speed to bring about the earliest form of t'ai chi.

Historians also link Zhang to joining yin-yang from Taoism and "internal" aspects together into his exercises. This feeling of inner happiness, or as a renowned engineering physicist and t'ai chi master, Dr. Martin Lee, states in his book *The Healing Art of Tai Chi*, "of becoming one with nature," remains a primary goal for those who practice t'ai chi. Although its ancient beginnings started as a martial art, t'ai chi was modified in the 1930s to the relaxing, low-intensity exercise that continues to have the potential to be transformed into a form of self-defense, similar to karate or kung-fu.

Benefits

The art of t'ai chi is many things to the many who practice it. To some, it is a stretching exercise that incorporates a deep-breathing program. To others, it is a martial art—and beyond this, it is often used as a dance or to accompany prayer. While the ways in which it is used may vary, one of the main benefits for those who practice it remains universal—t'ai chi promotes good health. This sense of well being complements t'ai chi's additional benefits of improved coordination, balance, and body awareness, while it also calms the mind and reduces stress. Those in search

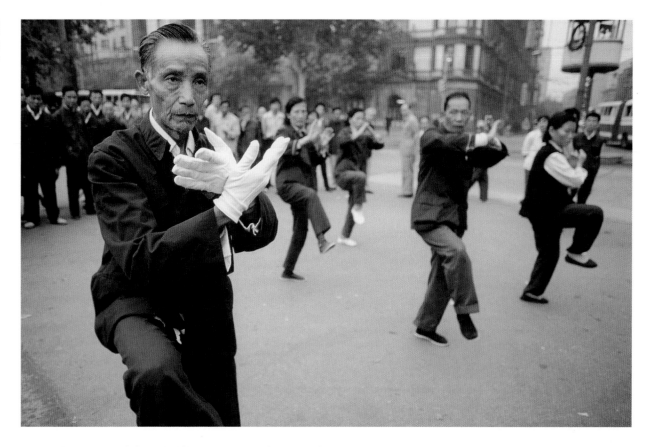

Group of people practicing t'ai chi in the streets of Shanghai, China. *(Kelly-Mooney Photography. Corbis Images. Reproduced by permission.)*

of harmony between the mind and the body practice "dynamic relaxation."

Dr. Martin Lee believes that the ancient art also holds healing powers. In his book, *The Healing Art of Tai Chi,* he states: "By practicing tai chi and understanding chi and its breathing techniques, I was able to heal my **allergies** and other ailments." Lee contends that stress is the culprit of much of the **pain** and suffering that are a part of everyday life. The growing evidence that stress contributes to devastating physical and mental ailments has led Lee to teach a systematic, effective, and manageable way to restore both body and mind to a natural, stress-free state. As of 1996, Lee has been teaching t'ai chi for 20 years to help his students with physical ailments that have been caused by stress. He believes that illness can be overcome through understanding the body as a mental and physical system, which is accomplished through t'ai chi.

While the martial arts are very vigorous and often result in injuries, the practice of t'ai chi is a good alternative to these sports without over-exerting the body. Those with bad backs have also found t'ai chi to ease their discomfort.

Description

Zhang, the notable originator of t'ai chi, created a combination of movements and beliefs that led to the formation of the fundamental "Thirteen Postures" of his art. Over time, these primary actions have transformed into soft, slow, relaxed movements, leading to a series of movements known as the form. Several techniques linked together create a form. Proper posture is a key element when practicing t'ai chi to maintain balance. All of the movements used throughout the exercise are relaxed with the back straight and the head up.

Just as the movements of t'ai chi have evolved, so have the various styles or schools of the art. As the form has grown and developed, the difference in style along with the different emphasis from a variety of teachers has as well. A majority of the different schools or styles of t'ai chi have been given their founder's surnames.

The principal schools of t'ai chi include:

- Chen style
- Hao (or Wu Shi) style

- Hu Lei style
- Sun style
- Wu style
- Yang style
- Zhao Bao style

Many of the most commonly used groupings of forms are based on the Yang style of t'ai chi, developed by Yang Pan-Hou (1837–1892). Each of the forms has a name, such as "Carry the Tiger to the Mountain," and as the progression is made throughout the many forms, the participant ends the exercise almost standing on one leg. While most forms, like "Wind Blows Lotus Leaves," has just one movement or part, others, like "Work the Shuttle in the Clouds," have as many as four. While the form is typically practiced individually, the movement called "Pushing Hands" is a sequence practiced by two people together.

Preparations

Masters of t'ai chi recommend that those who practice the art begin each session by doing a warm-up of gentle rotation exercises for the joints and gentle stretching exercises for the muscles and tendons. Some other suggestions to follow before beginning the exercise include: gaining a sense of body orientation; relaxation of every part of the body; maintaining smooth and regular breaths; gaining attention or feeling; being mindful of each movement; maintaining proper posture; and moving at the same pace throughout each movement. The main requirement for a successful form of t'ai chi is to feel completely comfortable while performing all of the movements.

Precautions

Although t'ai chi is not physically demanding, it can be demanding on the posture. Those who want to practice the exercise should notify their physician before beginning. The physician will know whether the person is taking medications that might interfere with balance, or has a condition that could make a series of t'ai chi movements unwise to attempt.

Research and general acceptance

While the reasons why t'ai chi is practiced vary, research has uncovered several reasons why it may help many medical conditions. For example, people with rheumatoid arthritis (RA) are encouraged to practice t'ai chi for its graceful, slow sweeping movements. Its ability to combine stretching and range-of-motion exercises with relaxation techniques work well to relieve the stiffness and weakness in the joints of RA patients.

In 1999, investigators from Johns Hopkins University in Baltimore, Maryland, studied the effects of t'ai chi on those with elevated **blood pressure**. Sixty-two sedentary adults with high-normal **blood** pressure or stage I **hypertension** who were aged 60 or older began a 12-week aerobic program or a light-intensity t'ai chi program. The exercise sessions both consisted of 30-minute sessions, four days a week. The study revealed that while the aerobics did lower the systolic blood pressure of participants, the t'ai chi group systolic level was also lowered by an average of seven points—only a point less than the aerobics group. Interestingly, t'ai chi hardly raises the **heart** rate while still having the same effects as an intense aerobics class.

In addition to lowering blood pressure, research suggests that t'ai chi improves heart and lung function. The exercise is linked to reducing the body's level of a stress hormone called cortisol, and to the overall effect of higher confidence for those who practice it. As a complementary therapy, t'ai chi is also found to enhance the mainstream medical care of **cancer** patients who use the exercise to help control their symptoms and improve their quality of life.

Physical therapists investigated the effects of t'ai chi among 20 patients during their recovery from coronary artery bypass surgery. The patients were placed into either the t'ai chi group or an unsupervised control group. The t'ai chi group performed classical Yang exercises each morning for one year, while the control group walked three times a week for 50 minutes each session. In 1999, the study reported that after one year of training, the t'ai chi group showed significant improvement in their cardiorespiratory function and their work rate, but the unsupervised control group displayed only a slight decrease in both areas.

T'ai chi has also shown to keep people from falling—something that happens to one in three people over age 65 each year. Researchers from Emory University in Atlanta, Georgia, had dozens of men and women in their 70s and older learn the graceful movements of t'ai chi. The study discovered that those who learned to perform t'ai chi were almost 50% less likely to suffer **falls** within a given time frame than subjects who simply received feedback from a computer screen on how much they swayed as they stood. Those who suffer falls experience greater declines in everyday activities than those who do not fall, and are

KEY TERMS

Coronary artery bypass surgery—A shunt, a surgical passage created between two blood vessels to divert blood from one part to another, is inserted to allow blood to travel from the aorta to a branch of the coronary artery at a point past the obstruction.

Rheumatoid arthritis—A form of arthritis with inflammation of the joints, resulting in stiffness, swelling, and pain.

Taoism—A Chinese religion and philosophy based on the doctrines of Lao-tse that advocates simplicity and selflessness.

also at a greater risk of needing to be placed in a nursing home or another type of assisted living home. Researchers recommend the use of t'ai chi for its ability to help people raise their consciousness of how their bodies are moving in the environment around them. By raising awareness of how the body moves, people can focus on their relationship to their physical environment and situations they encounter everyday.

While the additional benefits of t'ai chi remain to be studied in the United States, it continues to be widely practiced in this and other Western countries. The ancient art maintains its prominence in China, where many people incorporate it into their daily routines at sunrise.

Training and certification

Masters of t'ai chi are trained extensively in the various forms of the art by grandmasters who are extremely skillful of the exercise and its origins. For those who wish to learn t'ai chi from a master, classes are taught throughout the world in health clubs, community centers, senior citizen centers, and official t'ai chi schools. Before entering a class, the instructor's credentials should be reviewed, and they should be questioned about the form of t'ai chi they teach. Some of the more rigorous forms of the art may be too intense for older people, or for those who are not confident of their balance. Participants are encouraged to get a physician's approval before beginning any t'ai chi program.

There is no age limitation for those who learn t'ai chi, and there is no special equipment needed for the exercise. Participants are encouraged to wear loose clothing and soft shoes.

Resources

BOOKS

Lee, Martin, Emily Lee, Melinda Lee, and Joyce Lee. *The Healing Art of Tai Chi*. New York: Sterling Publishing Company, Inc., 1996.

PERIODICALS

Cassileth, B.R. "Complementary Therapies: Overview and State of the Art." *Cancer Nursing* (February 1999).

Filusch Betts, Elaine. "The Effect of Tai Chi on Cardiorespiratory Function in Patients with Coronary Artery Bypass Surgery." *Physical Therapy* (September 1999).

LoBuono, Charlotte, and Mary Desmond Pinkowish. "Moderate Exercise, Tai Chi Improve BP in Older Adults." *Patient Care* (November 1999).

"A No-Sweat Exercise with Multiple Benefits." *Tufts University Health & Nutrition Letter* (December 1999).

Thorne, Peter. "T'ai Chi Ch'uan, A New Form of Exercise." *Fitness Plus* (May 1998).

OTHER

"Yang Style T'ai Chi Ch'uan." <http://www.chebucto. ns.ca/Philosophy/Taichi/styles.html. >.

Beth Kapes

Taste

Definition

Taste is one of the five senses (the others being **smell**, touch, **vision**, and **hearing**) through which all animals interpret the world around them. Specifically, taste is the sense for determining the flavor of food and other substances.

Description

One of the two chemical senses (the other being smell), taste is stimulated through the contact of certain chemicals in substances with clusters of taste bud cells found primarily on the tongue. However, taste is a complex sensing mechanism that is also influenced by the smell and texture of substances. An individual's unique sense of taste is partially inherited, but factors such as culture and familiarity can help determine why one person's favorite food made be hot and spicy while another cannot get enough chocolate.

The primary organ for tasting is the mouth. Clusters of cells called taste buds (because under the **microscope** they look similar to plant buds) cover the tongue and are also found to a lesser extent on

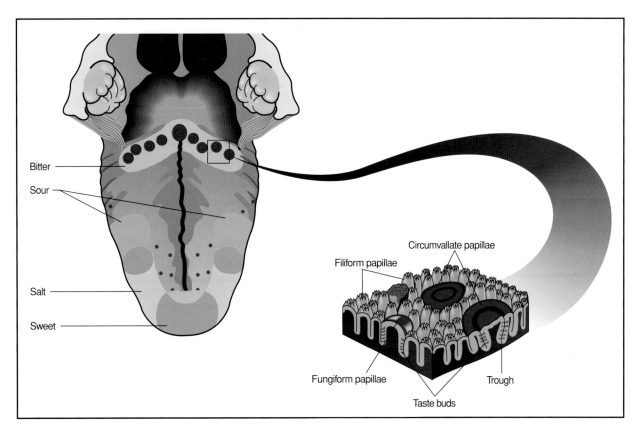

Bitter

Sour

Salt

Sweet

Circumvallate papillae

Filiform papillae

Fungiform papillae

Trough

Taste buds

A simplified illustration of the tongue and taste buds. *(Illustration by Hans & Cassidy. The Gale Group.)*

the cheek, throat, and the roof of the mouth. First discovered in the 19th century by German scientists Georg Meissner and Rudolf Wagner, taste buds lie on the bumps and grooves of the tongue (called the papillae) and have hairlike extensions (microvilli) to increase the receptor surface of the cells. Four different pairs of nerves are involved in the tongue, which helps explain in part why the sense of taste is a robust one, and not easily knocked out by disease or trauma.

Genetic and other factors affecting taste

Scientists have also discovered that genetic makeup partially accounts for individual tasting abilities and preferences for specific foods. According to Yale University researchers, some people are genetically programmed to have more taste buds and, as a result, taste more flavors in a particular food. (The number of taste buds varies in different animal species. For example cows have 25,000 taste buds, rabbits 17,000, and adult people approximately 10,000.) In general, a person's ability to taste can lie anywhere in a spectrum from poor to exceptional, with the ability to sense tastes increasing in proportion to the number of taste buds present. The difference in the number of taste buds can be extreme. Researchers have found

anywhere from 11 to 1,100 taste buds per square inch in various young people tested. They have also found that women tend to have more taste buds than men and, as a result, are often better tasters. How well people taste greatly affects what they like. Studies at Yale, for example, revealed that children with fewer taste buds who are classified as poor tasters liked cheese more often than exceptional tasters, who experienced a more bitter sensation, probably because of increased sensitivity to the combination of **calcium** and the milk protein casein found in cheese.

Despite the important role that taste buds play in recognizing flavors, they do not work alone in providing the experience of taste. For example, the amount of naturally occurring salt in saliva varies; with the result that those with less saliva can better taste the saltiness of certain foods than others, who may end up adding salt to get a similar flavor. The smell and texture of foods are also important contributing factors to how people perceive a food to taste and whether or not they like it. Food in the mouth produces an odor that reaches the nose through the nasopharynx (the opening that links the mouth and the nose). Since smell is much more sensitive to odors than taste is to flavors, people often first experience the flavor of a food by its odor. The texture and temperature of food also influences how it tastes. For example, many people would not think of drinking cold coffee, while others will not eat pears because of a dislike for the fruit's gritty texture.

The predilection for certain foods and tastes is not determined merely by biology. Culture and familiarity with foods greatly influence taste preferences. The Japanese have long considered raw fish, or sushi, to be a savory delicacy. Until the 1990s, few Americans would have enjoyed such a repast. As the number of Japanese restaurants grew along with the sushi bars they often contained, so did Americans' familiarity with this delicacy, resulting in a new taste for it.

Function

Taste's primary function is to react to items placed in the mouth. For most foods and substances, saliva breaks down the chemical components which travel through the pores in the papillae to reach the taste buds. These taste buds specialize primarily in processing one of the four major taste groups: sweet, sour, salty, and bitter. Because the four taste groups may not describe all taste sensations, other proposed tastes include metallic, astringent, and umami. Umami is the oral sensation stimulated by monosodium glutamate.

Taste occurs when specific **proteins** in the food bind to receptors on the taste buds. These receptors, in turn, send messages to the brain's cerebral cortex, which interprets the flavor. The actual chemical processes involved for each major taste group vary and involve various mechanisms. For example, salty and sour flavors occur when saliva breaks down sodium or acids, respectively. The chemical constituents of foods that give bitter and sweet tastes are much more difficult to specify due to the large number of chemical components involved.

Although certain taste buds seemed to have an affinity for one of the four major flavors, continued research into this intricate biological process has revealed a complex neural and chemical network that precludes simple black and white explanations. For example, each taste bud actually has receptors for sweet, sour, salty, and bitter sensations, indicating that taste buds are sensitive to a complex flavor spectrum similar to the way vision is sensitive to a broad color spectrum grouped into the four major colors of red, orange, yellow, and green. Particular proteins of taste are also under study, like gustducin, which may set off the plethora of chemical reactions that causes something to taste bitter and sweet.

Taste buds for all four taste groups can be found throughout the mouth. A common but mistaken tongue diagram shows areas labeled with basic tastes, such as sweet at the tip of the tongue while bitter is at the back. While specific kinds of buds tend to cluster together, the four tastes can be perceived on any part of the tongue and to a lesser extent on the roof of the mouth. Bitterness does appear to be perceived primarily on the back of the tongue because of several mechanisms.

Role in human health

Taste helps people determine whether potential foods are palatable. It also plays a major role in appetite. People constantly regenerate new taste buds every three to 10 days to replace the ones worn out by scalding soup, frozen yogurt, and the like. As people grow older, their taste buds lose their fine tuning because they are replaced at a slower rate. As a result, middle-aged and older people require more of a substance to produce the same sensations of sweetness or spiciness, for example, than would be needed by a child eating the same food.

Common diseases and disorders

The inability to taste is so intricately linked with smell that it is often difficult to tell whether the problem lies in tasting or smelling. An estimated two to four million people in the United States suffer from some sort of taste or smell disorder. The inability to taste or smell not only robs an individual of certain sensory pleasures, it can also be dangerous. Without smell or taste, for example, people cannot determine whether food is spoiled, making them vulnerable to **food poisoning**. Also, some psychiatrists believe that the lack of taste and smell can have a profoundly negative affect on a person's quality of life, leading to depression or other psychological problems.

The reasons for taste and smell disorders range from biological breakdown to the effects of environmental toxins; but a clear precipitating event or underlying pathology is often lacking in taste disorders. Here are some of the more common ones:

- Cold and flu are the most common physical ailments that can assault the sense of taste and smell. **Allergies** and viral or bacterial infections can produce swollen mucous membranes, which diminish the ability to taste. Most of these problems are temporary and treatable.

- Medications, including those used in **chemotherapy** for **cancer** treatments, can also inhibit certain enzymes, affect the body's **metabolism**, and interfere with the neural network and receptors needed to taste and smell.

- Neurological disorders due to **brain** injury or diseases like Parkinson's or Alzheimer's can cause more permanent damage to the intricate neural network that processes the sense of taste and smell.

- Twenty to 30% of head trauma patients suffer some degree of smell disorder, which can in turn affect taste.

- Exposure to environmental toxins like lead, mercury, insecticides, and solvents can also severely hinder the ability to smell and taste by causing damage to taste buds and sensory cells in the nose or brain.

- Aging itself is associated with diminished taste and smell sensitivity.

Resources

BOOKS

Beauchamp, Gary, and Linda Bartoshuk. *Tasting and Smelling: Handbook of Perception and Cognition,* 2nd ed. San Diego: Academic Press 1997.

Goldstein, E. Bruce. *Blackwell Handbook of Perception.* Malden, MA: Blackwell Publishers Ltd, 2001.

Macbeth, Helen. *Food Preference and Taste: Continuity and Change.* Oxford, England: Berghahn Books 1997.

Nagel, Rob. "The Special Senses." In *Body By Design: From the Digestive System to the Skeleton.* Edited by Betz Des Chenes. Farmington Hills, MI: Gale Group, 2000.

PERIODICALS

Smith, David V., and Robert F. Margolskee. "Making Sense of Taste." *Scientific American,* (3 March 2001) <http://www.sciam.com/2001/0301issue/0301smith.html>.

OTHER

BiblioAlerts.com. "NeuroScience-in-Review: The Sense of Taste." Paid subscription service for reports in science and technology. <http://preview.biblioalerts.com/info/com.biblioalerts_biblioalerts_CRE000312.html>.

Kimball's Biology Pages. "The Sense of Taste." <http://www.ultranet.com/~jkimball/BiologyPages/T/Taste.html>.

MEDLINE plus. "Health Information." <http://www.nlm.nih.gov/medplus>.

Linda Richards, R.D.

TB *see* **Tuberculosis**

Technetium heart scan

Definition

The technetium **heart** scan is a non-invasive nuclear scan that uses a radioactive isotope called technetium to evaluate **blood** flow after a heart attack.

Purpose

The technetium heart scan is used to evaluate the heart after a heart attack. It can confirm that a patient had a heart attack when the symptoms and **pain** usually associated with a heart attack were not present, identify the size and location of the heart attack, and provide information useful in determining the patient's post-heart attack prognosis. The scan is most useful when the electrocardiogram and cardiac enzyme studies do not provide definitive results, after heart surgery, for example, or when chest pain occurred more than 48 hours before the patient was examined. It is also used to evaluate the heart before and after heart surgery.

Precautions

Pregnant women and those who are breastfeeding should not be exposed to technetium.

Description

The technetium heart scan is a nuclear heart scan, which means that it involves the use of a radioactive isotope that targets the heart and a radionuclide detector that traces the absorption of the radioactive isotope. The isotope is injected into a vein and absorbed by healthy tissue at a known rate during a certain time period. The radionuclide detector, in this case a gamma scintillation camera, picks up the gamma rays emitted by the isotope.

The technetium heart scan uses technetium Tc-99m stannous pyrophosphate (usually called technetium), a mildly radioactive isotope which binds to **calcium**. After a heart attack, tiny calcium deposits appear on diseased heart valves and damaged heart tissue. These deposits appear within 12 hours of the heart attack. They are generally seen two to three days after the heart attack and are usually gone within one to two weeks. In some patients, they can be seen for several months.

After the technetium is injected into a blood vessel in the arm, it accumulates in heart tissue that has been damaged, leaving "hot spots" that can be detected by the scintillation camera. The technetium heart scan provides better image quality than commonly used radioactive agents such as thallium because it has a shorter half life and can thus be given in larger doses.

During the test, the patient lies motionless on the test table. Electrocardiogram electrodes are placed on the patient's body for continuous monitoring during the test. The test table is rotated so that different views of the heart can be scanned. The camera, which looks like an x-ray machine and is suspended above the table, moves back and forth over the patient. It displays a series of images of technetium's movement through the heart and records them on a computer for later analysis.

The test is usually performed at least 12 hours after a suspected heart attack, but it can also be done during triage of a patient who goes to a hospital emergency room with chest pain but does not appear to have had a heart attack. Recent clinical studies demonstrate that technetium heart scans are very accurate in detecting heart attacks while the patient is experiencing chest pain. They are far more accurate than electrocardiogram findings.

The technetium heart scan is usually performed in a hospital's nuclear medicine department but it can be done at the patient's bedside during a heart attack if the equipment is available. The scan is done two to three hours after the technetium is injected. Scans are usually done with the patient in several positions, with each scan taking 10 minutes. The entire test takes about 30 minutes to an hour. The scan is usually repeated over several weeks to determine if any further

KEY TERMS

Electrocardiogram—A test in which electronic sensors called electrodes are placed on the body to record the heart's electrical activities.

Non-invasive—A procedure that does not penetrate the body.

Radioactive isotope—One of two or more atoms with the same number of protons but a different number of neutrons with a nuclear composition. In nuclear scanning, radioactive isotopes are used as a diagnostic agent.

Technetium—A radioactive isotope frequently used in radionuclide scanning of the heart and other organs. It is produced during nuclear fission reactions.

damage has been done to the heart. The test is also called technetium 99m pyrophosphate scintigraphy, hot-spot myocardial imaging, infarct avid imaging, or **myocardial infarction** scan.

The technetium heart scan is not dangerous. The technetium is completely gone from the body within a few days of the test. The scan itself exposes the patient to about the same amount of radiation as a **chest x ray**. The patient can resume normal activities immediately after the test.

Preparation

Two to three hours before the scan, technetium is injected into a vein in the patient's forearm.

Results

If the technetium heart scan is normal, no technetium will show up in the heart.

In an abnormal technetium heart scan, hot spots reveal damage to the heart. The larger the hot spots, the poorer the patient's prognosis.

Health care team roles

The health care team will need to take a careful history of patient **allergies** and medications, and make sure that necessary **pregnancy** tests are done before the patient is scheduled for the technetium heart scan. The nurse or nurse practitioner will need to educate the patient about the pre-scan regime (not using Viagra 48 hours before the scan and avoiding alcohol, tobacco, **caffeine**, and nonprescription medications). Additional education about the procedure (how the scan is done, what happens during it, what kinds of information the scan can produce for the doctor, etc.) often is necessary to keep the patient informed and to insure cooperation during the procedure.

The technologist will need to verify that the pre-scan protocols have been done and that the patient is not pregnant or allergic to medications used in the scans.

The nuclear heart medicine technologist will also need to reassure the patient before and during the scans in order to keep the patient relaxed and still during the scans.

Resources

BOOKS

DeBakey, Michael E., and Gotto, Antonio M., Jr. "Noninvasive Diagnostic Procedures." In *The New Living Heart.* Holbrook, MA: Adams Media Corporation, 1997, pp.59-70.

Iskandrian, A. S., and Verani, Mario S. "Instrumentation and Technical Considerations in Planar and SPECT Imaging." In *Nuclear Cardiac Imaging: Principles and Applications,* 2nd edition. Philadelphia: F. A. Davis, 1996, pp. 29-44.

Sandler, M. P., et. al. "Radiopharmaceuticals." In *Diagnostic Nuclear Medicine,* 3rd ed., vol. 1. Baltimore, MD: Williams & Wilkins, 1996, pp. 199-208.

PERIODICALS

Kim, Samuel C., et. al. "Role of Nuclear Cardiology in the Evaluation of Acute Coronary Syndromes." *Annals of Emergency Medicine* 30 (2) (August 1997): 210-218.

ORGANIZATIONS

American Heart Association. National Center. 7272 Greenville Avenue, Dallas, TX 75231-4596. (214) 373-6300. <http://www.medsearch.com/pf/profiles/amerh>.

Texas Heart Institute Heart Information Service. P.O. Box 20345, Houston, TX 77225-0345. (800) 292-2221. <http://www.tmc.edu/thi/his.html>.

Lori De Milto

Teeth *see* **Dental anatomy**

Teeth classification *see* **Classification of teeth**

Temperature regulation *see* **Thermoregulation**

Temporomandibular joint disorders

Definition

Temporomandibular joint (TMJ) disorder, also known as TMD, is the name given to a group of symptoms that cause **pain** in the facial muscles and dysfunction in the head, face, and jaw. TMD often has psychological as well as physical causes.

Description

TMD results from pressure on the facial nerves due to muscle tension, injury, or bone abnormalities. Some 70% of adults exhibit at least one sign of TMD, but only 5% seek treatment. Most sufferers are women between ages 20 and 50.

The TMJ connects the temporal bone with the condyle of the mandible anterior to the ear on each side of the **skull**. The jaw pivots on ligaments, tendons, and muscles to allow motion downward and laterally as well as forward. Anything that causes a change in shape or functioning of the TMJ can cause pain and other symptoms.

Causes and symptoms

Causes

TMD has varied causes:

- **Bruxism**, or unconscious clenching or grinding of the teeth, is the most common cause of TMD. Bruxism occurs during periods of **stress** or during sleep. It results in muscle tension and soreness around the jaw joint and in the facial muscles.

- Misalignment of the teeth or displacement of the TMJ disc may contribute to TMD.

- Injury to the jaw or side of the head, either from a direct blow or from repeated and prolonged opening and closing (as in gum chewing) can result in a dislocation of the TMJ and subsequent TMD problems.

- Arthritis in different forms can lead to TMD. Traumatic arthritis from an injury, **osteoarthritis**, and rheumatoid arthritis are all possible causes.

- Hypermobility, a condition in which the ligaments of the TMJ are too loose, may allow the mandible to slip out of position and create TMD.

- Poor posture is another potential cause of TMD. When an individual carries his or her head too far forward and strains the neck muscles, TMD can result. In one research study in Texas, patients who were given posture training along with traditional

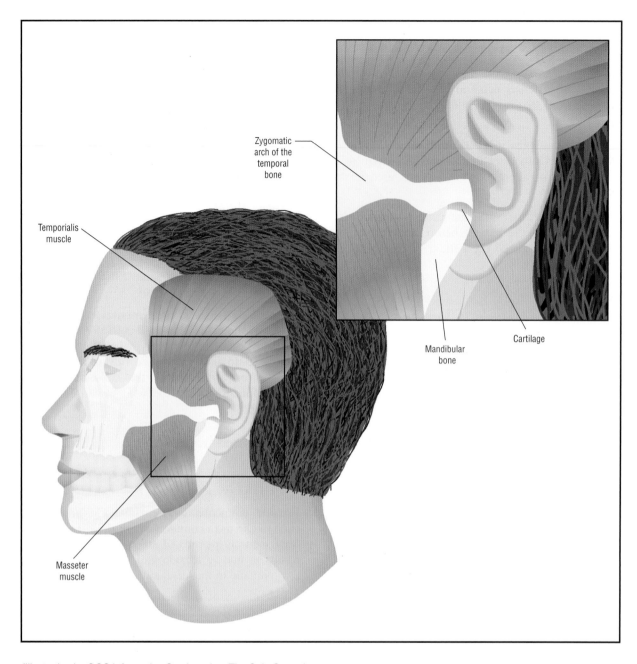

Zygomatic arch of the temporal bone

Temporalis muscle

Mandibular bone

Cartilage

Masseter muscle

(Illustration by GGS Information Services, Inc. The Gale Group.)

treatment had greater improvement than those without posture training.

• Birth abnormalities are the least frequent cause of TMD, but can occur. In some cases, the condyle of the mandible is too large or too small.

Symptoms

The symptoms of TMD depend in part on its cause. They include orofacial pain, restricted jaw function, and clicking or stiffness in the joints. Patients may also suffer from headaches, ear, neck, and shoulder pain, or tinnitus. A classic symptom is pain in front of the ear that spreads to the ear, mandible, cheek, and temple. Pain may be worse in the morning, and may be cyclical. Patients may also report noise in the joint during chewing, and limited mouth opening.

Diagnosis

Physical examination and patient history

TMD is most frequently diagnosed in the dental office based on **physical examination**. As the patient opens, closes, and moves the jaw laterally, palpation (physical examination by feeling with the hands) can detect joint popping and clicking, or a **stethoscope** may be placed in front of the ear to listen to the jaw movements. Jaw and facial muscles are checked for tenderness, and the patient's bite is checked for misalignment.

A careful patient history looks for such clues as recent injury or recent dental work. The patient should be asked about the duration and severity of jaw and face pain. Any history of insomnia, stress, **anxiety**, depression, chronic pain, or **fibromyalgia** should be documented.

Imaging studies

Imaging studies are not usually necessary to diagnose TMD. In most cases, x rays and **magnetic resonance imaging** (MRI) scans of the temporomandibular joint are normal. If the dentist suspects the patient has malpositioning of the TMJ disc, he or she can use **arthrography** to make the diagnosis. Arthrography can be used to evaluate the movement of the jaw and disc as well as their size and shape, and to evaluate the effectiveness of treatment.

Treatment

In 80% of TMD sufferers, symptoms improve in six months without treatment. When treatment is necessary, various modalities are used.

Phase I treatment

Phase I treatment is conservative and non-invasive, with no irreversible changes. Its purpose is to eliminate muscle spasms, swelling, and pain. Initially, a dentist may prescribe moist heat, aspirin, or a **nonsteroidal anti-inflammatory drug**, with a soft diet to alleviate symptoms.

Patients who have difficulty with bruxism are usually treated with splints. A plastic splint called a nightguard or mouthguard is constructed and worn at night. The splint can break the cycle of bruxing and allow sore muscles to relax. Splints can also be used to treat malpositioning by holding the mandible forward and keeping the disc in place until the ligaments tighten. The splint is adjusted over a period of two to four months.

Muscle relaxants can be prescribed if symptoms are related to muscle tension or fibromyalgia. If the TMD is related to rheumatoid arthritis, it may be treated with **corticosteroids**, methotrexate (MTX, Rheumatrex), or gold sodium (Myochrysine).

TMD can also be treated with ultrasound, electromyographic biofeedback, stretching exercises, transcutaneous electrical nerve stimulation, stress management techniques, friction massage, or posture training.

A patient who is suffering emotional or psychological problems that contribute to his or her TMD must address those problems before expecting relief of TMD symptoms.

Phase II treatment

By definition of the American Dental Association, Phase II treatment is non-reversible, invasive therapy. Its purpose is to definitively correct any discrepancies in the TMJ. Modalities include adjustment of the occlusion, orthodontics, reconstruction of the teeth, surgery, or a combination of these treatments.

In the 1980s, synthetic implants were used to replace the TMJ disc, but the implants proved to be too fragile to withstand jaw pressure. By 1999, all implants were taken off the market by the FDA. A new implant design was approved by the FDA in 2000.

Any patient considering Phase II treatment should be advised to get a second and possibly third opinion, and to proceed cautiously.

Prognosis

The prognosis for recovery from TMD is excellent for almost all patients. Most do not need any form of long-term treatment. In the case of patients with TMD associated with arthritis or fibromyalgia, the progression of the condition determines whether TMD can be eliminated.

Health care team roles

Every member of the dental team should be alert for TMD symptoms in patients, though only the dentist can prescribe treatment. A dental hygienist or assistant can use a skull or charts to help the patient understand the function and action of the TMJ. Additionally, dental auxiliaries can educate the patient about correct posture and modifying behavior such as gum chewing and fingernail biting.

If the dentist determines a splint is necessary, the hygienist or assistant can take impressions of the teeth and prepare plaster casts from the impressions. A **dental laboratory technician** then constructs the splint, and the dentist places it, checking to ensure an exact fit.

KEY TERMS

Arthrography—A testing technique in which a special dye is injected into the joint, which is then x rayed.

Bruxism—Habitual clenching and grinding of the teeth, especially during sleep.

Condyle—An articular prominence of a bone.

Electromyographic biofeedback—A method for relieving jaw tightness by monitoring the patient's attempts to relax the muscle while the patient watches a gauge. The patient gradually learns to control the degree of muscle relaxation.

Fibromyalgia—A complex, chronic condition which causes widespread pain and fatigue, as well as a variety of other symptoms.

Malocclusion—The misalignment of opposing teeth in the upper and lower jaws.

Mandible—The lower jaw.

Orofacial—Pertaining to the mouth and face.

Osteoarthritis—A type of arthritis marked by chronic degeneration of the cartilage of the joints, leading to pain and sometimes loss of function.

Rheumatoid arthritis—A chronic autoimmune disorder marked by inflammation and deformity of the affected joints.

Temporal bones—The compound bones that form the right and left sides of the skull above the ears.

Tinnitus—A sensation of ringing or roaring in the ears that can only be heard by the individual affected.

Transcutaneous electrical nerve stimulation—A method for relieving the muscle pain of TMD by stimulating nerve endings that do not transmit pain. It is thought that this stimulation blocks impulses from nerve endings that do transmit pain.

Prevention

To prevent TMD from developing, suggestions to patients can include:

- Avoid overuse of the jaw. Gum chewing is the major culprit, along with fingernail biting.

- Try not to grind the teeth. Follow the "lips together, teeth apart" rule. Upper and lower teeth should meet only for chewing. Make a conscious effort to keep the masseter (cheek) muscles relaxed.

- Sleep on the back. Sleeping on either side can put pressure on the TMJ.

- Manage stress. **Relaxation** exercises and biofeedback can help.

- Use correct posture. Carrying the head in a forward position has been shown to affect TMD. Also, correct bad ergonomic habits such as holding a telephone receiver between the ear and shoulder.

Resources

BOOKS

"Disorders of the Temporomandibular Joint." In *Merck Manual of Medical Information: Home Edition*, edited by Robert Berkow, et al. Whitehouse Station, NJ: Merck Research Laboratories, 1997.

PERIODICALS

Guthrie, Catherine. "Peace for Troubled Jaws?" *Health* (March 2001): 90-94.

"Temporomandibular Joint (TMJ) Syndrome." *Clinical Reference Systems* (Annual 2000): 1565.

Walling, Anne D. "Review of Diagnosis and Treatment of TMJ Disorders." *American Family Physician* (November 1998): 1841-2.

Wright, Edward F., Manuel A. Domenech, and Joseph R. Fischer, Jr. "Usefulness of Posture Training for Patients with Temporomandibular Disorders." *Journal of the American Dental Association* (February 2000): 202-11.

ORGANIZATIONS

American Academy of Head, Neck and Facial Pain. 520 West Pipeline Road, Hurst, TX 76053.

American Dental Association. 211 E. Chicago Ave., Chicago, IL 60611. (312) 440-2500. <http://www.ada.org>.

OTHER

"An Overview of the Fundamental Features of Fibromyalgia Syndrome." *The National Fibromyalgia Partnership Inc. website* <http://www.fmpartnership.org/FMPartnership.htm> (1999 edition).

"Treatment of TMJ." *The American Academy of Head, Neck and Facial Pain Website.* <http://www.drshankland.com/treatment.html> (April 3, 2001).

Cathy Hester Seckman, R.D.H.

TENS (Transcutaneous electrical nerve stimulation) *see* **Electrotherapy**

TENS unit *see* **Transcutaneous electrical nerve stimulation unit**

Tension headache

Definition

This most common type of headache is caused by severe muscle contractions triggered by **stress** or exertion. It affects as many as 90% of adult Americans.

Description

While most American adults get a tension headache from time to time, women and people with more education are slightly more likely to suffer from them. People who are so anxious that they grind their teeth or hunch their shoulders may find that the physical strain in their body can be experienced as **pain** and tension in the muscles of the neck and scalp, producing almost constant pain.

Causes and symptoms

Tension headaches are caused by tightening in the muscles of the face, neck, and scalp because of stress or poor posture. They can last for days or weeks and can cause pain of varying intensity. The tightening muscles cause more expansion and constriction of **blood vessels**, which can make head pain worse. Eyestrain caused by dealing with a large amount of paperwork or reading can cause a tension headache as well.

Many people report the pain of a tension headache as a kind of steady ache (as opposed to a throb) that forms a tight band around the forehead, affecting both sides of the head. Tension headaches usually occur in the front of the head, although they also may appear at the top or the back of the **skull**.

Tension headaches often begin in late afternoon and can last for several hours; they can occur every day and last throughout most of the day. When this happens, the headache is called a chronic tension headache. Unlike migraines, tension headaches do not cause nausea and vomiting, and sufferers do not exhibit sensitivity to light or signs of any kind of aura before the headache begins.

Diagnosis

Diagnosis of tension headaches is made from a medical history, discussion of symptoms, and elimination of other types of headaches or underlying disorders.

Very few headaches are the sign of a serious underlying medical problem. However, sufferers should call a physician at once if they:

- Have more than three headaches a week.
- Take medication for pain almost every day.
- Need more than the recommended dose of pain medication.
- Have a stiff neck and/or **fever** in addition to a headache.
- Are dizzy, unsteady, or have slurred speech, weakness, or numbness.
- Have confusion or drowsiness with the headache.
- Have headaches that began with a head injury.
- Have headaches triggered by bending, coughing, or exertion.
- Have headaches that keep getting worse.
- Have severe vomiting with a headache.
- Have the first headache after age 50.
- Awaken with headache that gets better as the day goes on.

Treatment

There are many different treatments for tension headaches, which respond well to both medication and massage. If these headaches become chronic, however, they are best treated by identifying the source of tension and stress and reducing or eliminating it.

Medication

Tension headaches usually respond very well to over-the-counter medicines such as aspirin, ibuprofen, or acetaminophen. However, some of these drugs (especially those that contain **caffeine**) may trigger rebound headaches if their use is discontinued after they are taken for more than a few days.

More severe tension headaches may require combination medications, including a mild sedative such as butalbital. These should be used sparingly, though. Chronic tension headaches may respond to low-dose amitriptyline taken at night.

Massage

Massaging the tense muscle groups may help ease pain. Instead of directly massaging the temple, persons will get more relief from rubbing the neck and shoulders, because tension headaches often arise from tension in this area. In fact, relaxing the muscles of the neck can cut the intensity and duration of tension headaches at least in half.

KEY TERMS

Acupressure—An ancient Chinese method of relieving pain or treating illness by applying pressure to specific areas of the body.

Acupuncture—An ancient Chinese method of relieving pain or treating illness by piercing specific areas of the body with fine needles.

To relax these muscles, the neck should be rotated from side to side as the shoulders shrug. Some people find that imagining a sense of warmth or heaviness in the neck muscles can help. Taking three very deep breaths at the first hint of tension can help prevent a headache.

Other therapy

If tension headaches are a symptom of either depression or **anxiety**, the underlying problem should be treated with counseling, medication, or a combination of both.

Alternative treatment

Eliminating the sources of the tension as much as possible will help prevent tension headaches. Acupuncture or **acupressure** may be helpful in treating some chronic tension headaches. Homeopathic remedies and botanical medicine can also help relieve tension headaches. Valerian (*Valeriana officinalis*), skullcap (*Scutellaria lateriflora*), and passionflower (*Passiflora incarnata*) are three herbal remedies that may be helpful. A tension headache can also be relieved by soaking the feet in hot water while an ice cold towel is wrapped around the neck.

Prognosis

Reducing stress and relying less on caffeine-containing medications can reduce the number of tension headaches for most people. Also, reducing the intake of products such as coffee, tea, and soft drinks that contain caffeine often reduces headaches.

Health care team roles

Many headaches are identified and treated at home using over-the-counter products. Physicians become involved in diagnosing and treating the underlying causes of tension headaches. Therapists and psychiatrists are involved in processing underlying stress.

Prevention

Tension headaches can often be prevented by managing everyday stress and making some important lifestyle changes. Those who are prone to tension headaches should:

- Take frequent "stress breaks."
- Get regular **exercise**. Even a brisk 15-minute walk can help prevent tension headaches.
- Get enough sleep.
- Release angry feelings.

Resources

BOOKS

Adams, Raymond D, Maurice Victor, and Allen H. Ropper. *Adams & Victor's Principles of Neurology*, 6th ed. New York: McGraw Hill, 1997.

Aminoff, Michael J. *Neurology and General Medicine*, 3rd ed. London: Churchill Livingstone, 2001.

Cutrer, F. Michael, and Michael A. Moskowitz. "Headaches and Other Head Pain." In *Cecil Textbook of Medicine*, 21st ed. Ed. by Lee Goldman and J. Claude Bennett. Philadelphia: W.B. Saunders, 2000, 2072-2074.

Lance, James W., and Peter J. Goadsby. *Mechanism and Management of Headache*, 6th ed. Woburn, MA: Butterworth-Heinemann Medical, 1998.

Raskin, Ned H. "Headache." In *Harrison's Principles of Internal Medicine*, 14th ed. Ed. by Anthony S. Fauci, et al. New York: McGraw-Hill, 1998, 68-73.

PERIODICALS

Bansevicius, D., R. H. Westgaard, and O. M. Sjaastad. "Tension-type headache: Pain, fatigue, tension, and EMG responses to mental activation." *Headache* 39, no. 6 (1999): 417-425.

Carruthers, A., J. A. Langtry, J. Carruthers, and G. Robinson. "Improvement of tension-type headache when treating wrinkles with botulinum toxin A injections." *Headache* 39, no. 9 (1999): 662-665.

Diamond, S., T. K. Balm, and F. G. Freitag. "Ibuprofen plus caffeine in the treatment of tension-type headache." *Clinical Pharmacological Therapy* 68. no. 3 (2000): 312-319.

McCrory, P. "Headaches and exercise." *Sports Medicine* 30, no. 3 (2000): 221-229.

Rokicki, L. A., E. M. Semenchuk, S. Bruehl, K. R. Lofland, and T. T. Houle. "An examination of the validity of the IHS classification system for migraine and tension-type headache in the college student population." *Headache* 39, no. 10 (1999): 720-727.

Smetana, G. W. "The diagnostic value of historical features in primary headache syndromes: A comprehensive review." *Archives of Internal Medicine* 160, no. 18 (2000): 2729-2737.

Sparano, N. "Is the combination of ibuprofen and caffeine effective for the treatment of a tension-type headache?" *Journal of Family Practice* 50, no. 1 (2001): 10-17.

Torelli, P., D. Cologno, and G. C. Manzoni. "Weekend headache: A possible role of work and life-style." *Headache* 39, no. 6 (1999): 398-408.

ORGANIZATIONS

American Council for Headache Education, 19 Mantua Road, Mt. Royal, NJ 08061. (856) 423-0258. Fax: (856) 423-0082. <http://www.achenet.org/>. achehg@talley.com.

National Headache Foundation, 428 West St. James Place, 2nd Floor, Chicago, IL 60614-2750. (888) 643-5552 or (800) 843-2256. Fax: (312) 525-7357. <http://www.headaches.org/index.html>. info@headaches.org.

OTHER

American Academy of Family Physicians. <http://family-doctor.org/handouts/172.html>.

Mental Health Help Net. <http://mentalhelp.net/articles/mood2.htm>.

Merck Manual. <http://www.merck.com/pubs/mmanual/section14/chapter168/168d.htm>.

National Library of Medicine. <http://www.nlm.nih.gov/medlineplus/ency/article/000797.htm>.

University of Illinois. <http://www.mckinley.uiuc.edu/health-info/dis-cond/headache/ten-head.html>.

University of Iowa School of Nursing. <http://www.nursing.uiowa.edu/sites/AdultPain/GenePain/tenHAnt.htm > and <http://pedspain.nursing.uiowa.edu/GenePain/tenHAnt.htm>.

University of Maryland. <http://umm.drkoop.com/conditions/ency/article/000797.htm>.

University of Michigan School of Medicine. <http://cme.med.umich.edu/headache/office/disorders/tension.html>.

US Food and Drug Administration. <http://www.fda.gov/bbs/topics/CONSUMER/CON00168.html>.

L. Fleming Fallon, Jr., MD, DrPH

Testicular scan *see* **Scrotal nuclear medicine scan**

Testicular ultrasound *see* **Scrotal ultrasound**

Testosterone test *see* **Sex hormones tests**

Thallium heart scan

Definition

A thallium **heart** scan is a diagnostic test that uses a special perfusion-scanning camera and a small amount of thallium-201, a radioactive substance, injected into the bloodstream to produce an image of the **blood** flow to the heart.

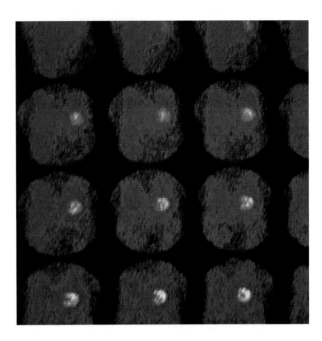

A thallium scan of the human heart. This set of pictures was taken over time. The dark areas receive an inadequate supply of blood. *(Custom Medical Stock Photo. Reproduced by permission.)*

Purpose

A thallium heart scan is used to evaluate the blood supply to the heart muscle. It can identify areas of the heart that may have a reduced blood supply as a result of damage from a previous **myocardial infarction** (heart attack) or blocked coronary arteries. While **exercise** testing has long been a standard examination in the diagnosis of **coronary artery disease**, in some instances, the thallium scan may provide more sensitive and more specific information. In other words, the test may be better able to detect a problem and to differentiate one condition from another. For example, a thallium heart scan may more accurately detect ischemic heart disease. A thallium scan is most likely to aid diagnosis in cases where the exercise test is inconclusive, the patient cannot exercise adequately, or a quantitative evaluation of blood flow is required. In addition to evaluating coronary artery disease, thallium scanning can help to evaluate coronary blood flow following coronary artery bypass graft surgery or **angioplasty**.

Precautions

Radioisotopes such as thallium 201 should not be administered during **pregnancy** because they may be harmful to the fetus.

Description

The thallium scan is performed in conjunction with an exercise **stress test**. At the end of the stress test (once the patient has reached the highest level of exercise he or she can comfortably achieve), a small amount of the radioisotope thallium 201 is injected into the patient's bloodstream through an IV (intravenous) line. The patient then lies down under a gamma scintillation camera, which generates photographs from the gamma rays emitted by the thallium.

Thallium attaches to the red blood cells and is carried throughout the body in the bloodstream. It enters the heart muscle by way of the coronary arteries and accumulates in the cells of the heart muscle. Since the thallium can only reach those areas of the heart with an adequate blood supply, it can help to detect perfusion defects. In patients with perfusion defects, no thallium will show up in poorly perfused areas of the heart. Instead, these areas show up as "cold spots" on the thallium scan. The patient is then given a second injection of thallium. Several hours later, the gamma scintillation camera takes more pictures in order to obtain an image of the heart when the patient is at rest.

Cold spots that appear at rest as well as during exercise often indicate an area of previously damaged heart tissue or scars that have resulted from a prior myocardial infarction. Sometimes perfusion is adequate during rest but cold spots appear during exercise, when the heart has to work harder and has a greater demand for blood. This cold spot indicates ischemia resulting from a blockage in the coronary arteries. In ischemia, the heart temporarily does not get enough blood flow. Patients with perfusion defects, especially perfusion defects that appear only during exercise, have the greatest risk of future cardiac events such as myocardial infarctions.

In recent years, there have been improvements in heart scanning. Many centers now use a single photon emission computed tomographic (SPECT) camera, which provides a clearer image. Some centers also use, in place of thallium, a chemical called sestamibi. Sestamibi is used along with a radioactive compound called technetium. While thallium may still be better for some uses, such as providing a better image of the heart muscle itself, sestamibi may produce clearer images in overweight patients and is more useful in assessing how well the heart pumps blood.

When patients are unable to exercise because of another medical condition, such as arthritis or lung disease, they may be given a pharmacological thallium test instead of an exercise thallium stress test. In the pharmacological test, a drug is administered to mimic the effects of exercise on the heart such as dipyridamole (Persantine), which dilates the coronary arteries, or dobutamine, which increases blood flow through the heart muscle.

Preparation

Patients should be instructed not to drink alcoholic or caffeinated beverages, smoke tobacco, or ingest other nicotine products for 24 hours before the test. These substances can affect test results. Patients should also be advised not eat anything for at least three hours before the test. They may also be instructed to stop taking certain medications during the test that may interfere with test results. **Patient education** preceding a thallium scan may be performed by a nurse or cardiovascular laboratory technician.

Aftercare

In most cases, another set of scans may be needed (one in conjunction with exercise, one at rest), and the patient may be given special instructions regarding eating and test preparation. In most cases, patients are free to return to their normal daily activities.

Complications

Radioisotopes such as thallium 201 should not be administered during pregnancy because they may be harmful to the fetus.

Results

A normal thallium scan shows healthy blood flow through the coronary arteries and normal perfusion of the heart muscle, without cold spots, both at rest and during exercise.

Cold spots on the scan, where no thallium shows up, indicate areas of the heart that are not getting an adequate supply of blood. Cold spots appearing both at rest and during exercise may indicate areas where the heart tissue has been damaged. However, "reversible" cold spots, appearing only during exercise, usually indicate some blockage of the coronary arteries.

Health care team roles

A thallium scan is generally ordered by a primary care physician or cardiologist and is performed

KEY TERMS

Angioplasty—The reconstruction of damaged blood vessels.

Coronary bypass surgery—Surgery in which a section of blood vessel is used to bypass a blocked coronary artery and restore an adequate blood supply to the heart muscle.

Perfusion—The passage of fluid (such as blood) through a specific organ or area of the body (such as the heart).

Radioisotope—A radioactive form of a chemical element, which is used in medicine for therapeutic or diagnostic purposes.

by a trained technician. All healthcare providers performing or monitoring cardiac tests should be prepared to provide emergency medical intervention, such as defibrillation. The exam is interpreted by a radiologist, cardiologist, or nuclear medicine physician.

Patient education

Patients must be well prepared for a thallium scan. They should not only know the purpose of the test, but also signs and symptoms that indicate the test should be stopped. Physicians, nurses, and ECG technicians can ensure patient safety by encouraging them to immediately communicate discomfort at any time during the scan.

Resources

BOOKS

The Faculty Members at the Yale University School of Medicine. "Myocardial Perfusion Scan." In *The Patient's Guide to Medical Tests*. Ed. by Barry L. Zaret, et al. Boston: Houghton Mifflin Company, 1997, 99-101.

Thelan, Lynne A., et al. *Critical Care Nursing Diagnosis and Management*. St. Louis, MO: Mosby, 1998, pp. 438.

ORGANIZATIONS

American Heart Association. 7272 Greenville Ave., Dallas, TX 75231. (214) 373-6300. <http://www.amhrt.org>.

National Heart, Lung, and Blood Institute Information Center. PO Box 30105, Bethesda, MD 20824-0105. (301) 951-3260. <http://www.nhlbi.nih.gov>.

Barbara Wexler

Therapeutic drug monitoring

Definition

Therapeutic drug monitoring (TDM), or simply drug monitoring, is the measurement of drug levels in the **blood**.

Purpose

TDM is employed to measure blood drug levels so that the most effective dosage can be determined and toxicity can be prevented. Drug monitoring is not needed for most drugs. Many drugs have a wide therapeutic window, meaning that the difference between the therapeutic and toxic level is large. Often, the physician can measure an expected outcome to see if a drug is working. For example, body temperature can be measured to evaluate an antipyretic drug. Monitoring is mainly used for drugs that can be toxic or cause severe side effects. Examples are antiepileptic drugs, antiarrhythmic agents, oral anticoagulants, theophylline, tricyclic antidepressants, lithium, antineoplastics, aminoglycoside **antibiotics**, cardiac glycosides, and drugs to prevent transplant rejection. TDM is also utilized to identify noncompliant patients (i.e., those patients who, for whatever reason, either cannot or will not comply with **drug dosages** as prescribed by the physician).

Precautions

Many different factors influence blood drug levels, and the following points should be taken into consideration during TDM: the age, sex, and weight of the patient; the route of administration of the drug; the drug's absorption rate, excretion rate, delivery rate, and dosage; other medications the patient is taking; other diseases the patient has; the patient's compliance regarding the drug treatment regimen; and the laboratory methods used to measure the drug.

Drugs taken orally should not be measured until the processes of absorption and elimination have nearly reached a steady state. The steady state is reached when the drug in the next dose is sufficient to replace the drug that is eliminated. This requires approximately five drug elimination half-lives. Some drugs such as tricyclic antidepressants may be decreased by the gel in serum separator tubes. Since drug levels rise and then fall in between oral, bolus intravenous, and intramuscular doses, the interpretation of blood drug levels requires strict adherence to the appropriate time of collection. Blood collected at an improper time will provide misleading information. Blood should not be taken from an intravenous line immediately following infusion of medication. Before collecting a sample from an intravenous line, at least 3 mL of blood should be collected from the line and discarded to clear the line of heparin, IV contents, and medication.

Description

TDM is a practical tool that can help the physician provide effective and safe drug therapy in patients who need medication. Monitoring can be used to confirm that a blood drug concentration is within the therapeutic range. If the desired therapeutic effect of the drug is not as expected, two blood levels can be used to determine the drug's half-life in the body. This data along with dose information can be used to calculate the change in dose or dosing interval needed to bring the concentration into the therapeutic range.

Blood drug levels are influenced by five processes: liberation, absorption, distribution, **metabolism**, and excretion. Liberation is the release of the drug in the body (usually the gastrointestinal tract) and absorption is the transport of the drug to the blood. These variables determine the fraction of the dose that is bioavailable. Many drugs are absorbed by the portal circulation and transported directly to the **liver**, where they are partly metabolized to inactive forms. This process reduces the amount of drug available to the target tissues. Distribution refers to the volume of body fluids in which the drug becomes diluted. Metabolism refers to the chemical transformation of the drug performed by the liver. Most drug metabolites are water soluble and removed by the **kidneys**. Individual differences in any of these processes alters the relationship between dose and drug blood levels, called drug pharmacokinetics. For example, persons with decreased renal function will have a longer drug half-life (decreased clearance) causing the blood level (and tissue level) of drug to be higher than expected. Drugs in the blood are mainly protein-bound, and therefore, inactive. Decreased albumin, abnormal blood pH, or displacement of one drug by another may alter protein binding increasing the blood level of free (active) drug. Persons may metabolize a drug more slowly than expected due to genetic factors or liver disease. Smoking, **stress**, and drug formulation (generic versus trade name) can alter pharmacokinetic properties, making some drugs ineffective or toxic at usual doses. In such cases TDM can explain the discordance between dose and outcome and provide data needed to safely make changes in drug administration.

Blood specimens for drug monitoring can be taken at two different times, called peak and trough levels. Blood for peak level is collected at the drug's highest therapeutic concentration within the dosing period. For drugs given intravenously, the peak level is drawn 30 minutes after completion of the dose. For drugs given orally, this time varies with the drug because it is dependent upon the rates of absorption, distribution and elimination. For intravenous drugs, peak levels can be measured immediately following complete infusion. Trough levels (occasionally called residual levels) are measured just prior to administration of the next dose, and are the lowest concentration in the dosing interval. Too low a dose or too great a dose interval will produce a trough level that is below the therapeutic range, and too great a dose or too close a dose interval will show a peak level greater than the therapeutic range. Most therapeutic drugs have a narrow trough to peak difference, and therefore, only trough levels are needed to detect blood levels that are too low or too high. Peak levels are needed for some drugs, especially aminoglycoside antibiotics. A concentration below the therapeutic range will not resolve the bacterial **infection**. However, too high a level can cause damage to the kidneys, bone marrow and acoustic nerves.

Many methods are available to measure the concentration of specific drugs. The most widely used methods are immunoassay and chromatography.

Preparation

In preparing for this test, the following guidelines should be observed:

- For patients suspected of symptoms of drug toxicity, the best time to draw the blood specimen is when the symptoms are occurring.

- If there is a question as to whether an adequate dose of the drug is being achieved, it is best to obtain trough levels.

- Peak (highest concentration) levels are usually obtained 30 minutes after an intravenous dose, one hour after intramuscular (IM) administration, and approximately one to two hours after oral dosing. However, slow-release formulas for many drugs will not produce peak levels for several hours after ingestion.

Complications

Risks for this test are minimal, but may include slight bleeding from the blood-drawing site, fainting or feeling lightheaded after blood is drawn, or accumulation of blood under the puncture site (hematoma).

KEY TERMS

Absorption—Uptake of drug into the circulation.

Bioavailability—The amount of drug in a dosage that can be absorbed by the patient.

Distribution—The division of the drug into different parts of the body such as the liver, blood, spinal fluid and urine.

Elimination—The final excretion of a drug and its metabolites.

Half-life—The amount of time that is needed to reduce a drug level to one half of what was absorbed in the blood.

Maintenance dose—The amount of drug that is needed to keep the patient's blood levels at a steady state.

Metabolism—The breakdown of a drug into its metabolites.

Metabolites—Compounds that the drug is broken down into, usually done by the liver.

Peak concentration—The highest level of drug reached in the blood.

Slow release—A preparation of the drug that allows for slow absorption, over hours or days.

Therapeutic range—Levels of a drug that will yield the desired effect without toxicity.

Toxic—Poisonous; a drug is toxic when levels in the body are too high.

Trough concentration—The lowest level of a drug in the plasma, usually seen right before the next dose is given.

Aftercare

Bruising may occur at the puncture site or the person may feel dizzy or faint. Pressure should be applied to the puncture site until the bleeding stops to reduce bruising. Warm packs can also be placed over the puncture site to relieve discomfort. Drug dose, dosing schedule, or medication changes may be required if the blood drug level is outside the therapeutic range.

Health care team roles

Physicians will determine the initial dose of drug. A nurse or phlebotomist collects the specimen by venipuncture documenting the time of draw. Pharmacists may assist by providing information about drug half-life, recommended peak collection time, therapeutic ranges, side-effects, and **drug interactions**. Clinical laboratory scientists, CLS(NCA)/medical technologists, MT(ASCP) or clinical laboratory technicians, CLT(NCA) or medical laboratory technicians, MLT(ASCP) perform drug assays. They are responsible for notifying the physician when critical values are exceeded.

Patient education

Patients should be educated on the importance of complying with their physician's orders for medications, and should be told to report any complications or side effects they may experience. Patients should also be told about the frequency of their drug monitoring tests, and why keeping their appointment is important.

Resources

BOOKS

Burtis, Carl A., and Edward R. Ashwood. *Tietz Fundamentals of Clinical Chemistry,* 4th edition. Philadelphia: W.B. Saunders, 1999.

Kaplan, Lawrence A., and Amadeo J. Pesce. *Clinical Chemistry, Theory, Analysis and Correlation,* 3rd edition. St. Louis: Mosby Publishing, 1996.

Lane, Keryn A.G. *The Merck Manual of Medical Information.* Merck Research Laboratories, 1997.

Pagana, Kathleen D. *Mosby's Manual of Diagnostic and Laboratory Tests.* St. Louis: Mosby, Inc., 1998.

Jane E. Phillips

Therapeutic exercise

Definition

Therapeutic **exercise** is a **physical therapy** intervention encompassing a broad range of activities designed to restore or improve musculoskeletal, cardiopulmonary and/or neurologic function.

Purpose

Some form of therapeutic exercise is indicated in almost every physical therapy case. Physical therapists may assist clients in designing therapeutic exercise programs to prevent injury or secondary impairments. In addition, physical therapists use therapeutic exercise as one component of patient care to improve functional ability and general well-being in those who are experiencing limitations or disability due to a disease, disorder, trauma, or surgery.

Precautions

Therapeutic exercise includes a broad spectrum of activities, from passive range of motion and breathing exercises to high-speed agility drills. Precautions, therefore, are specific to each individual depending upon his or her condition. The physical therapist must use his or her specialized knowledge to determine exercises that are appropriate for a patient or client's level of ability, age, endurance, severity of injury and/or stage of recovery. Outlined below, however, are a few examples of situations in which general precautions should be observed.

Post-operative

A progression of therapeutic exercise is usually more gradual in a patient recovering from surgery than in one who did not require surgery, especially in order to allow inflamed tissues to heal. In general, specific joint motions and weightbearing are often restricted. High-intensity stretching and resistance exercise is usually limited for at least six weeks to allow adequate healing time for muscles or tendons that have been repaired.

Osteoporosis

In **osteoporosis**, bone resorption has taken place at a much higher rate than bone formation, resulting in weakened osseous structures. The risk for pathologic fracture resulting from very minor **stress** is high. In patients with osteoporosis, low-impact weight-bearing and endurance exercises should be introduced. Caution should be taken when adding resistive exercises, and explosive or twisting movements should be avoided altogether.

Pregnancy

There are several high-risk conditions that are contraindications to exercise. These include: incompetent cervix, vaginal bleeding, **placenta previa**, preterm rupture of membranes, premature labor, and maternal **heart** disease, diabetes, or **hypertension**. Precautions need to be taken when women present with the following: multiple gestation, anemia, systemic **infection**, extreme fatigue, musculoskeletal **pain**, overheating, phlebitis, diastisis recti, or uterine contractions which last several hours after exercise. In these cases, women who participate in exercise should be monitored closely by both physician and therapist.

Resistance exercise

Resistance exercise is often a key part of a therapeutic exercise program; however, considerations must be made regarding risk factors. Resistive exercise should not be performed when there is muscle or joint inflammation, or when severe pain is present during or after exercise. Precautions should be taken with high-risk cardiovascular patients. All patients should be taught to avoid the Valsalva maneuver, excessive fatigue, and overwork.

Joint mobilization

Joint mobilization techniques are often used to increase range of motion by passively distracting or gliding the joint surfaces. Gentle, small-grade oscillatory movements may be used to inhibit pain and relax the patient; however, larger movements are contraindicated in the cases of hypermobility, joint effusion and inflammation. In addition, precautions should be taken when any of the following exist: malignancy, unhealed fracture, connective tissue or bone disease, total joint replacements, or weakened connective tissue (due to recent trauma, surgery, disuse, or medication).

Description

Therapeutic exercise can be an intervention used in a physical therapy plan of care or as part of a recommendation in client consultation. The physical therapist uses a thorough examination including subjective and objective data to assess each patient's specific needs. It is clear that an 80-year-old woman with osteoporosis with a history of **fractures** is going to require a much different program from a 20-year-old athlete who wants to return to sports following a knee injury.

The main goal of therapeutic exercise is to improve or maintain functional ability, including daily living skills, through the application of careful and gradual forces to the body. Often, this overall goal is achieved through the objectives of developing, improving, restoring or maintaining one or more of the following: strength, endurance, flexibility, stability, coordination and/or balance.

Strength

Strength in muscular tissue is improved through graded and deliberate overloading of the targeted muscle(s). When the main focus is strength, exercise is usually performed against heavy loads with relatively few repetitions. Physiologically, this training leads first to an increase in the number of motor units being fired, which increases force output.

Gradually, the cross-sectional size of individual skeletal muscle fibers increases as well, which produces bulk and improves strength capacity.

Endurance

Endurance affords individuals the ability to perform activities over a relatively prolonged period. When muscular endurance is developed, a muscle can generate and sustain a larger number of contractions over a period of time. With total body endurance, an individual develops the ability to participate in a period of low-intensity conditioning such as walking, jogging, and other aerobic activity. Cardiovascular and pulmonary fitness are increased through this means. In a program directed at improving endurance, large muscle groups are recruited for prolonged periods of time (at least 15 minutes).

Flexibility

Contractile and noncontractile tissues both are susceptible to tightening when injured or exposed to a neurological disease process that causes weakening and/or spasticity. Prevention, through careful and regular movement and stretching, is key to maintaining flexibility. Consideration, however, must be taken regarding restrictions to mobility in post-operative or post-traumatic healing. Muscular flexibility may be increased or maintained through active or passive stretching, while connective tissue mobility requires passive procedures.

Stability

Stability is required in order to provide a stable base for functioning. Usually, stability concerns are focused on proximal musculature in the trunk, shoulders, and hips to allow for movement of the extremities.

Coordination and balance

The ability to execute complex patterns of movement with the right timing and sequencing is essential to motor function, as is the ability to maintain one's center of gravity over the available base of support. Coordination and balance are usually trained using motor learning principles, and are important components of a therapeutic exercise program designed to increase function.

Along with training in the above areas, therapeutic exercise may include education about body mechanics, gait and locomotion training, neuromuscular re-education, developmental activities and **relaxation** strategies. It is important to note also that, although trunk and

KEY TERMS

Motor learning—A set of processes related to practice or experience that results in relatively permanent changes in the ability to produce a skilled action.

Neuromuscular re-education—The training of an individual to recover or develop effective sensory and motor strategies for task demands.

extremity musculature may be the first to come to mind when discussing strength and endurance, physical therapists may also address ventilatory and pelvic-floor issues with therapeutic exercise.

Because the ultimate goal is function, any discussion about therapeutic exercise has to include the topic of closed-chain exercise, which is the movement of the body over a fixed distal segment such as the hand or foot. Open-chain exercise, in which the distal segment moves freely in space, is the traditional form seen in weight rooms; however, it does not train the patient to perform functional weight-bearing activities such as walking, stair climbing, or jumping. If there is a restriction on weight bearing, closed-chain exercises should be delayed or modified to comply with restrictions. Modifications may include performing the exercise in a pool or while sitting instead of standing.

Results

Depending on the individual, the anticipated outcomes may include:

- increase in physical function following a trauma or surgery
- maintenance of, or minimizing loss of, function with respect to a disease process
- prevention of complications post-operatively or after an injury
- prevention of future or further limitations or disability

These outcomes may be reached through increases in strength, endurance, flexibility, mobility, stability, coordination, and/or balance. Numerous tests and measures are available to assist in assessing desired outcomes. Strength may be measured using **electromyography**, dynamometry, and/or manual **muscle testing**. Muscular endurance may be assessed with physical capacity tests, timed activity tests, and/or functional muscle tests. Aerobic endurance is often measured using cardiovascular and pulmonary signs and symptoms, ergometry, step tests, and timed walk/run, treadmill, or wheelchair tests. Flexibility can be measured by observation of functional range of motion, goniometry, inclinometry, and joint play movements. In addition, many motor control and function tests assess stability, coordination, and balance.

Health care team roles

The physical therapist is responsible for evaluating the patient or client and developing a plan of care that includes appropriate therapeutic exercise intervention. The physical therapist also must teach, assist, and monitor the patient with the exercise program. Modifications must be made as the patient shows signs of distress, inappropriate fatigue, or progress. The physical therapist assistant, under the supervision of a physical therapist, may participate in all aspects of care except for initial evaluation, modifications outside of the plan of care, or interventions requiring the specific expertise of the physical therapist.

Resources

BOOKS

American Physical Therapy Association. *Guide to Physical Therapist Practice,* 2nd ed. Fairfax, VA: American Physical Therapy Association, 2001.

Hall, Carrie M., and Lori Thein Brody. *Therapeutic Exercise: Moving Toward Function.* Philadelphia: Lippincott Williams & Wilkins, 1999.

Kisner, Carolyn, and Lynn Allen Colby. *Therapeutic Exercise: Foundations and Techniques.* 3rd ed. Philadelphia: F. A. Davis Company, 1996.

PERIODICALS

Drake, Nicholas. "Breakthrough for People with Osteoporosis." *IDA Personal Trainer* 11, no. 10 (October 2000): 9.

Huffman, Grace Brooke. "Guidelines: Prescribing Exercise for the Older Patient." *American Family Physician* 62 (1 September 2000): 1166.

Sadovsky, Richard. "Physical Therapy and Exercise for Osteoarthritis of the Knee." *American Family Physician* 61 (15 June 2000): 3727.

ORGANIZATIONS

American Physical Therapy Association, 1111 North Fairfax St., Alexandria, VA 22314-1488. (703) 684-2782. <http://www.apta.org>.

Peggy Campbell Torpey, MPT

Therapeutic nutrition *see* **Medical nutrition therapy**

Therapeutic touch

Definition

Therapeutic touch, or TT, is a noninvasive method of healing that was derived from an ancient laying on of hands technique. In TT, the practitioner alters the patient's energy field through an energy transfer from the hands of the practitioner to the patient.

Origins

Therapeutic touch was developed in 1972 by Dora Kunz, a psychic healer, and Dolores Krieger, Ph.D., R.N, a nurse and professor of nursing at New York University. The year before in 1971, when Krieger was working as a **registered nurse** in a hospital, she became very frustrated when one of her patients, a 30-year-old female, lay dying from a **gallbladder** condition. In desperation, she tried what she was learning from Kunz. Within one treatment, the patient's condition began to shift, and she lived, surprising the other hospital staff. Krieger and Kunz met during the study of Oskar Estebany, a world-renowned healer. They had invited Estebany to form a study for three years, observing his work with patients. In this study, Estebany practiced laying on of hands healing on various patients. Using her psychic and intuitive abilities, Kunz would observe and assist in the healing, while Krieger recorded the activities of the healing session and created profiles of the patients.

As the study progressed, Kunz began teaching Krieger how to heal, based on her perceptions of Estebany's healing techniques. During her research of ancient healing methods, Krieger concluded that the energy transfer between the healer and the healed that takes place in a TT session is prana, an Eastern Indian concept representing energy, vitality, and vigor. Krieger then combined her research with Kunz's techniques to create TT.

TT was initially developed for persons in the health professions, but is currently taught worldwide to anyone who is interested in learning the technique. As of 1998, an estimated 100,000 people around the world have been trained in TT; 43,000 of those persons are health care professionals, many of whom use TT in conjunction with traditional medicine, as well as osteopathic, chiropractic, naturopathic, and homeopathic therapies. TT is taught in over 100 colleges, universities, and medical schools.

Benefits

The major effects of TT are **relaxation**, **pain** reduction, accelerated healing, and alleviation of psychosomatic symptoms. Studies have shown that TT has a beneficial effect on the **blood** as it has the ability to raise hemoglobin values. It also affects **brain** waves to induce a relaxed state. TT can induce the relaxation response often within five minutes.

Krieger has said that it is not individual illnesses that validate the effectiveness of TT, but rather, it is questioned which systems are most sensitive to TT. She and others have found that the most sensitive is the **autonomic nervous system** (ANS), which, for example, controls urination, and is followed by dysfunctions of lymphatic and circulatory systems, and then finally musculoskeletal systems. In addition, the female **endocrine system** is more sensitive to TT than the corresponding male system. Thus, TT helps with dysmenorrhea, amenorrhea, problems with **contraception**, and the course of **pregnancy**.

TT is reported to have a positive effect on the **immune system** and thus accelerates the healing of **wounds**. Nurses use therapeutic touch in operating rooms to relax patients before surgery and in recovery rooms on postoperative patients to help speed the healing process. TT is used in the treatment of terminally ill patients, such as those with **cancer** and acquired immune deficiency syndrome (**AIDS**), to relieve **anxiety** and **stress**, create peace of mind, and reduce pain.

Many nurses use TT in the nursery. The conditions of many premature babies who received TT reportedly improved rapidly. TT has been used to calm colicky infants, assist women in **childbirth**, and increase milk let-down in breast-feeding mothers.

Other claims of TT include relief of acute pain, nausea, **diarrhea**, tension and migraine headaches, **fever**, and joint and tissue swelling. TT has been used to treat thyroid imbalances, ulcers, psychosomatic illnesses, premenstrual syndrome, **Alzheimer's disease**, stroke and **coma** patients, **multiple sclerosis**, measles, infections, **asthma**, and bone and muscle injuries.

Therapeutic touch is performed in many different locations, including healing centers, delivery rooms, hospitals, hospice settings, accident scenes, homes, and schools.

Description

Therapeutic touch treats the whole person: relaxes the mind, heals the body, and soothes the spirit. The principle behind it is that it does not stop at the skin: the human body extends an energy field, or aura, several inches to several feet from the body. When illness occurs, it creates a disturbance or blockage in the vital energy field. The TT practitioner uses her/his hands to sense the blockage or disturbance. In a series of gentle strokes, the healer removes the disturbance and rebalances the energy to restore health.

The TT session generally lasts about 20–30 minutes. Although the name is therapeutic touch, there is generally no touching of the physical body, only the energetic body or field. It is usually performed on fully clothed patients who are either lying down on a flat surface or sitting up in a chair.

Each session consists of five steps. Before the session begins, the practitioner enters a state of quiet **meditation** where he/she becomes centered and grounded in order to establish intent for the healing session and to garner the compassion necessary to heal.

The second step involves the assessment of the person's vital energy field. During this step, the practitioner places the palms of his/her hands 2–3 in (5–8 cm) from the patient's body and sweeps them over the energy field in slow, gentle strokes beginning at the head and moving toward the feet. The practitioner might feel heat, coolness, heaviness, pressure, or a prickly or tingling sensation. These cues, as they are called, each signal a blockage or disturbance in the field.

To remove these blockages and restore balance to the body, the practitioner then performs a series of downward, sweeping movements to clear away any energy congestion and smooth the energy field. This is known as the unruffling process and is generally performed from head to feet. To prevent any energy from clinging to him/her, the practitioner shakes his/her hands after each stroke.

During the next phase, the practitioner acts as a conduit to transfer energy to the patient. The energy used is not solely the energy of the practitioner. The practitioner relies on a universal source of energy so as not to deplete his/her own supply. In short, the healer acts as an energy support system until the patient's immune system is able to take over.

The practitioner then smoothes the field to balance the energy and create a symmetrical flow. When the session is over, it is recommended that the patient relax for 10–15 minutes in order for the energies to stabilize.

Side effects

The side effects reported occur when an excess of energy enters the body for an extended period of time creating restlessness, irritability, and hostility, or increasing anxiety and pain. **Burns** are sensitive to therapeutic touch, and it is recommended that TT be performed on burned tissue for short periods, generally two to three minutes at a time.

Research and general acceptance

Therapeutic touch is not generally accepted by Western medical professionals. Basic and anecdotal research has been performed on TT since its development in 1972, although little quantitative research has been carried out. It is based on a theory derived from formal research. It began as the basis of Dolores Krieger's postdoctoral research.

Dolores Krieger has performed extensive research on TT, including with pregnant women, and has noted that the following changes occur in a patient after short, consistent treatment: relaxation within the first five minutes of a session, a reduction of pain, and the acceleration of the healing process.

One study was created to determine the effect TT would have on wounds that resulted from a biopsy of the upper arm. Forty-four patients placed their injured arms through a hole in a door. Twenty-two of them received TT on their arms. The other half received no treatment. The wounds treated with TT healed more quickly than the wounds that received no treatment.

In 1998, a study was performed on 27 patients with **osteoarthritis** in at least one knee. For six weeks, the patients were treated with therapeutic touch, mock therapeutic touch, or standard care. According to *The Journal of Family Practice*, the journal who published the study, the results showed that the group who had received TT had "significantly decreased pain and improved function as compared with both the placebo and control groups."

Therapeutic touch can be combined with a number of different therapies, including **acupressure**, massage, mental imagery, **physical therapy**, and **yoga**. When combined with massage and physiotherapy, TT may reduce tension headaches, back pain, stress-related problems, circulatory problems, and constipation. **Shiatsu** and TT may help sinusitis, digestive disorders, muscle cramps, menstrual difficulties, and insomnia. Yoga and TT may be beneficial in the treatment of bronchitis, asthma, **blood pressure**, fatigue, and anxiety.

TT is practiced in over 70 countries worldwide: by Egyptians and Israelis during fighting in the Gaza Strip; in South Africa to reduce racial strife; and in Poland, Thailand, and the former Soviet Union.

Training and certification

Therapeutic touch is taught at over 100 universities and nursing and medical schools around the United States and Canada. Although it was developed primarily for nurses, anyone can learn TT.

State laws vary regarding the practice of TT. In general, laypersons are allowed to practice TT within their families. Therapeutic touch is considered an extension of health care skills, so most health care professionals are covered under the state medical practice act.

Many hospitals have established policies allowing nurses and staff to perform TT on patients at no extra charge. The American Nurse's Association often holds workshops on TT at national conventions. Therapeutic touch classes are often held for the general public through community education, healing clinics, and holistic schools.

Resources

BOOKS

Krieger, Dolores, Ph.D., R.N. *Accepting Your Power to Heal. The Personal Practice of Therapeutic Touch.* Bear & Company, 1993.

Krieger, Dolores, Ph.D., R.N. *The Therapeutic Touch. How to Use Your Hands to Help or to Heal.* Prentice Hall Press, 1979.

Macrae, Janet, Ph.D., R.N. *Therapeutic Touch: A Practical Guide.* Knopf, 1998.

PERIODICALS

Rosa, Linda, Emily Rosa, Larry Sarner, and Stephen Barrett. "A Close Look At Therapeutic Touch." *JAMA, The Journal of the American Medical Association* (April 1, 1998): 1005–11.

OTHER

The Nurse Healers Professional Associates International (NH-PAI), the Official Organization of Therapeutic Touch. 3760 S. Highland Dr. Salt Lake City, UT 84106. (801) 273–3399. nhpai@therapeutic-touch.org. <http://www.therapeutic-touch.org>.

Jennifer Wurges

Therapeutic ultrasound

Definition

Ultrasound refers to sound waves with a frequency greater than 20,000 Hertz, which is above the range of human hearing. Therapeutic ultrasound is the application of sound waves to the human body to treat various medical conditions.

Purpose

Ultrasound can be used for a variety of therapeutic applications, including healing soft-tissue injuries and skin wounds, destroying tumors and calculi, and delivering medications. Ultrasound is the most commonly used therapeutic heat modality in sports medicine, and an emerging modality in minimally invasive surgery. Specific applications of therapeutic ultrasound include:

- healing musculoskeletal and soft-tissue injuries
- relieving joint pain associated with arthritis
- relieving chronic low back pain, and pain associated with plantar fascitis and bursitis
- stimulating bone fracture healing
- treating kidney stones, gallstones, and other calculi via extracorporeal shock wave lithotripsy (ESWL)
- enhancing the action of "clot-busting" drugs (thrombolysis) during treatment of stroke and heart attack
- halting internal bleeding associated with trauma (acoustic hemostasis)
- ablating cardiac tissue to treat arrhythmia
- destroying tissue to treat cancerous tumors, uterine fibroids, and benign prostatic hyperplasia (BPH).

Precautions

Therapeutic ultrasound should be delivered by a clinician trained and experienced in its use. Improper selection of treatment parameters may result in tissue damage. Its use may be contraindicated in pregnant patients, or for over the spine or brain.

Description

Therapeutic ultrasound typically uses sound waves in the range of 1 to 3 MegaHertz (MHz), or 1,000,000 to 3,000,000 vibrations per second. This mechanical energy is approximately 1,000 times that of the ultrasound energy commonly used for diagnostic imaging purposes. Lower frequencies are used for healing applications, while higher frequencies are used for deep heating and tissue destruction.

Low-frequency ultrasound stimulates healing by breaking up scar tissue and adhesions, improving blood flow, and reducing inflammation. High-frequency ultrasound, often referred to as high-intensity focused ultrasound (HIFU), causes the formation of tiny bubbles within tissue (cavitation) that vibrate and collapse, or induces coagulation of tissue and blood.

A therapeutic ultrasound system is generally portable or mobile, and consists of a control unit and a handheld probe with a crystal transducer through which sound waves are delivered through the patient's skin. In some ESWL systems, the patient is submerged in a water bath, and sound waves are delivered through the water. The clinician delivering the therapy selects the treatment parameters (e.g., intensity and duration). The patient usually experiences a comfortable feeling of heating or no sensation at all. The treatment time is 5–10 minutes, but may be longer depending on the condition being treated.

Recently, a focused ultrasound ablation system for use with magnetic resonance imaging (MRI) was introduced to non-invasively treat benign and cancerous tumors. This system is in development as a possible alternative to conventional surgery or radiation therapy.

Preparation

Therapeutic ultrasound for healing purposes, involves little patient preparation. A coupling gel is usually applied to the patient's skin to facilitate transmission of sound waves from the probe into the body. ESWL and HIFU procedures may require epidural or general anesthesia.

Aftercare

No aftercare is necessary for healing applications. HIFU and ESWL procedures involving anesthesia require that the patient recover in a post-anesthesia care unit.

Complications

Tissue damage may result from improper administration of therapeutic ultrasound. Complications related to anesthesia may occur following HIFU and ESWL procedures.

Results

The application of therapeutic ultrasound should result in relief of pain, faster healing, and/or resolution of the medical condition being treated.

Health care team roles

Therapeutic ultrasound for healing injuries or other rehabilitative/sports medicine applications is administered by a trained physical therapist or credentialed athletic trainer. Therapeutic ultrasound for healing chronic wounds is administered by a healthcare professional specializing in wound management and therapeutic wound healing modalities. For chronic pain applications, chiropractors, physical therapists, or pain management specialists may administer therapeutic ultrasound.

Specialists are usually involved in HIFU procedures. ESWL for kidney stones is generally performed by a urologist, and ESWL for gallstones by a gastroenterologist. A urologist also performs HIFU for prostate cancer and benign prostatic hyperplasia. HIFU for other cancer applications may be performed by an oncologist or surgeon with ultrasound training. HIFU for arrhythmia ablation is performed by an interventional cardiologist. Nursing staff are generally required for HIFU and ESWL procedures.

Resources

PERIODICALS

Cummings, Jennifer E., Antonio Pacifico, John L. Drago, et al. "Alternative Energy Sources for Ablation of Arrhythmias." *Pacing and Clinical Electrophysiology.* 28 (May 2005): 434–443.

Jolesz, FA, K. Hynynen, N. McDannold, and C. Tempany. "MR Imaging-Controlled Focused Ultrasound Ablation: A Noninvasive Image-Guided Surgery."
Magnetic Resonance Imaging Clinics of North America. 13(August 2005) 545–560.

Ouellette, Jennifer. "New Ultrasound Therapies Emerge." *The Industrial Physicist.* American Institute of Physics. (September 1998): 30–33.

Uhlemann, C., B. Heinig, and U. Wollina. "Therapeutic Ultrasound in Lower Extremity Wound Management." *International Journal of Lower Extremity Wounds.* 2 (September 2003): 152–157.

ORGANIZATIONS

International Society for Therapeutic Ultrasound. http://www.istus.org/istu/index.asp.

American Physical Therapy Association. 1111 North Fairfax Street, Alexandria, VA 22314-1488. (800) 999-2782. Fax: (703) 684-7343. http://www.apta.org.

National Athletic Trainers' Association. 2952 Stemmons Freeway, Dallas, TX 75247. (214) 637-6282. Fax: (214) 637-2206. http://www.nata.org.

OTHER

Abella, H.A. "Focused Ultrasound Fries Pancreatic Cancer." *Diagnostic Imaging Online.* November 1, 2005. www.dimag.com/showNews.jhtml?articleID=172901932.

Klein, Milton J. "Deep Heat." *eMedicine.* December 12, 2001. http://www.emedicine.com/pmr/topic203.htm.

Jennifer Sisk, M. A.

Thermometer

Definition

A thermometer is a device used to monitor temperature.

Purpose

A thermometer is used to establish a baseline on the admission of a patient to a health care facility, to detect any abnormalities from the normal state, and to establish if current medication is having the desired effect.

Temperature is recorded to check for pyrexia or monitor the degree of hypothermia present in the body. The body's normal temperature is 98.6 °F (37 °C). A **fever** is a temperature of 101 °F (38.3 °C) or higher in an infant younger than three months or above 102 °F (38.9 °C) for older children and adults. Hypothermia is recognized as a temperature below 96 °F (35.5 °C).

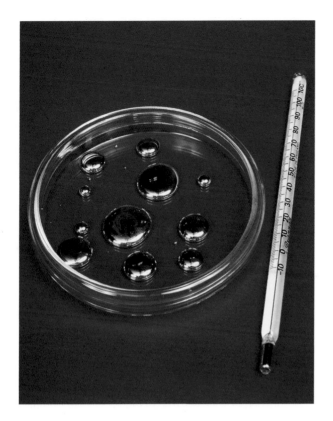

Mercury drops in a petri dish with a thermometer. Mercury is a dense metal that is liquid at room temperature. It has a high surface tension, so small droplets form almost perfect spheres, which accounts for its quick-flowing motion when spilled. Despite its toxicity, mercury's sensitivity to temperature changes and uniform expansion explain its use in bulb thermometers. *(Andrew Lambert Photography / Photo Researchers, Inc. Reproduced by permission.)*

Description

A thermometer can be mercury, liquid-in-glass, electronic with digital display, infrared or tympanic, or disposable dot-matrix. It can be used in a clinical or emergency setting or at home.

A mercury thermometer consists of a narrow glass stem approximately 5 in (12.7 cm) in length with markings along one or both sides indicating the temperature scale in Fahrenheit, Centigrade or both. Mercury is held in a reservoir bulb at one end that rises when the glass chamber is placed in contact with the body. Mercury thermometers are not used in modern clinical settings.

Electronic thermometers can record a wide range of temperatures between 94–105 °F (35–42 °C) and can be used orally, axillary (under the arm), or rectally. They have temperature sensors inside round-tipped probes and can be covered with disposable guards to prevent **infection** passing from one patient to another. The sensor is connected to the container housing the central processing unit, and the information gathered by the sensor is then shown on the display screen. Some models have other features such as **memory** recall of the last recording and a large display screen for easy reading. The thermometer probe is placed under the arm, tongue, or placed in the rectum and held in place for a few seconds, depending on the model used. The device will beep when the peak temperature is reached. The time required for obtaining the reading is between a few seconds to thirty seconds.

A tympanic thermometer has a round-tipped probe containing the sensor that can be covered with disposable guards to prevent infection from one patient to another. It is placed in the ear canal for one second while an infrared sensor records the body heat radiated by the eardrum. The reading then appears on the unit's screen.

Digital and tympanic thermometers should be used in accordance with the manufacturer's guidelines.

Disposable thermometers are plastic strips that have chemicals impregnated in dots on the surface. They are sticky on one side to adhere to the skin and prevent slippage and are worn under the armpit. The dots change color at different times as the chemicals respond to the body heat. The temperature is readable after two to three minutes, depending on the manufacturer's guidelines. Some products are disposable, reusable, or can be used continuously for up to 48 hours. These devices are useful for children, and the temperature can be recorded even while the child is asleep.

Operation

The patient should be sitting or lying comfortably to ensure that the readings are taken in similar positions each time and that there is little excitement to affect the results.

The manufacturer's guidelines should be followed when taking a temperature with a digital, tympanic, or disposable thermometer. Dot-matrix thermometers are placed next to the skin and usually held in place by a sticky strip. With the tympanic thermometer, caregivers should ensure that the probe is properly inserted into the ear in order to allow an optimal reading. The reading will be less accurate if the sensor cannot accurately see the tympanic membrane or if the view is obscured by wax and debris in the ear canal.

A mercury thermometer can be used to monitor a temperature by three methods:

- Axillary.

- Orally or sub-lingually. This method is never used with infants.

- Rectally. This method is used with infants. The tip of the thermometer is usually blue-tipped to distinguish it from the silver tip of an oral/axillary thermometer.

Before recording a temperature using a mercury thermometer, the mercury is shaken down by holding the thermometer firmly at the clear end and flicking it quickly a few times in a downward motion toward the silver end. The mercury level should be below 96 °F (35.5 °C) before taking a temperature.

The silver tip is placed under the patient's right armpit, with the arm clamping it in place against the chest. The thermometer should stay in place for six to seven minutes. During this waiting period, the remaining **vital signs** may be recorded.

When the time has elapsed, the thermometer is removed and held at eye level. The mercury will have risen to a mark that indicates the temperature of the patient.

To record oral temperature, the procedure is the same as the axillary method, except that the silver tip of the thermometer is placed beneath the tongue for four to five minutes before reading.

In both cases, the thermometer is wiped clean and stored in an appropriate container to prevent breakage.

To record rectal temperature, a rectal thermometer is used and shaken down as described above. A small portion of a water-based lubricant is placed on the colored tip of the thermometer. With the infant lying on his back, the nurse holds him securely in place. The tip of the thermometer is inserted into the child's rectum no more than 0.5 in (1.3 cm) and held there for two to three minutes. The thermometer is removed, read as before, and wiped with an antibacterial wipe. It is then stored in an appropriate container to prevent breakage, as ingestion of mercury can be fatal.

Liquid-in-glass thermometers contain alternatives to mercury (such as alcohol) and are used in the same manner.

Maintenance

Many digital and infrared thermometers are self-calibrating. To ensure accuracy, mercury thermometers should be shaken down prior to every use and left in place for at least three minutes. They require

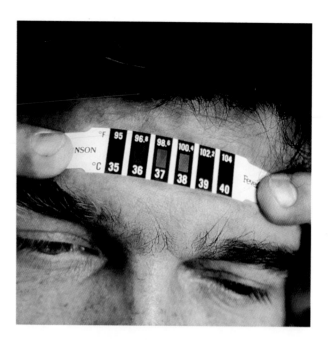

A man using a thermochromic strip thermometer. This kind of thermometer consists of patches that change color at different temperatures. *(Francoise Sauze / Photo Researchers, Inc. Reproduced by permission.)*

careful storage to prevent breakage and require cleaning after each use to prevent cross-infection.

Currently, there is a nationwide initiative to ban the sale of mercury thermometers and **blood pressure** monitors. Health activists are concerned about mercury contaminating the environment after it has been disposed of. A mercury thermometer contains 0.7g (0.025 oz) of mercury; one gram of the substance can contaminate a 20-acre lake. Several states have banned the use of products containing mercury, and stores such as Wal-Mart, CVS, and Kmart have already stopped selling mercury thermometers. According to a study by the Mayo Clinic in March 2001, mercury-free devices can monitor information without compromising accuracy. In October 1999, the Environmental Protection Agency (EPA) advised using alternative mercury products to avoid the need for increased regulations in years to come and to protect human health and wildlife by reducing unnecessary exposure to mercury.

Health care team roles

Patients may ask questions about specific concerns they have regarding aspects of vital signs or a particular disease. The nurse can provide counseling on the prevention of illness or direct the person to their doctor.

The nurse should make the patient comfortable and reassure them that recording temperature is part

KEY TERMS

Axillary—Under the armpit.

Hypothermia—A body temperature below 96 °F (35.5 °C).

Orally—By mouth.

Pyrexia—A temperature of 101 °F (38.3 °C) or higher in an infant younger than three months or above 102 °F (38.9 °C) for older children and adults.

Rectally—By the rectum.

of normal health checks and that it is necessary that their health be correctly monitored. Any abnormalities in the temperature must be reported to the medical staff.

Training

Staff should be given appropriate training in the device used in the clinical setting.

Resources

OTHER

"Eleven of the Nation's Leading Retailers and Manufacturers Give Mercury Fever Thermometers the Heave-Ho." 8 August 2001. <http://www.nurses.com/content/news/article.asp?DocID = {1CDF3C1E-9521-11D4-8C66-009027DE0829}>.

"Getting the Right Reading with Thermometers." 8 August 2001. <http://www.nurses.com/content/news/article.asp?DocID = {BE5A4CA0-00ED-11D4-8C2D-009027DE0829}>.

"Rectal Thermometer Use." 8 August 2001. <http://www.healthsquare.com/mc/fgmc0922.htm>.

"Reducing Mercury Use in Health Care." EPA document. 8 August 2001. <http://www.epa.gov/glnpo/bnsdocs/merchealth/index.html>.

Margaret A. Stockley

Thermoregulation

Definition

Thermoregulation refers to the mechanisms and control systems used by the body to balance thermal inputs and thermal losses so as to maintain its core temperature nearly constant.

Description

In a healthy individual, the temperature of the core of the body is regulated by feedback control mechanisms that maintain it nearly constant around 98.6 °F (37 °C) throughout the day, week, month, or year. This thermoregulation is efficiently coordinated by the **central nervous system** (CNS) as long as the temperature of the surroundings ranges between 68 °F (20 °C) and 130 °F (54 °C).

The body increases and lowers its core temperature using a temperature control system that works like a thermostat. Increased body temperature activates mechanisms promoting heat loss, and lowered body temperature activates mechanisms enabling the accumulation or production of heat. Such a system is called a feedback control system, because it uses as input the total or partial output of the system, meaning that the consequences of the process dictate how it will go on further. A feedback system has three components: sensors that register the change, a control center that receives the signals of the sensors, and an effector mechanism, meaning a pathway for the commands of the control center when it responds to the information received from the sensors. In thermoregulation, the control center is located in the hypothalamus, a tiny cluster of **brain** cells located in the brain just above the **pituitary gland**. It also contains the key temperature sensors. Other sensors, located all over the body, record whether the body temperature is too high or too low. There are three main effector mechanisms involved in thermoregulation. The first is the vasomotor system, which consists of the nerves that act on vascular smooth muscle to control **blood** vessel diameter; the second is provided by metabolic effectors, which are substances produced by the body to increase its activity. The third main effector mechanism is provided by the sweat glands. The vasomotor system is responsible for two physiological responses called vasodilation and vasoconstriction. The first increases blood flow in the tissues and the second decreases it.

Heat production, also called thermogenesis, is the result of several different body functions. One of them is the action of the thyroid gland, located in the neck. Hormones released by this gland increase the body's metabolism, meaning the activity of the body. Increased production of heat is thus achieved by increasing the metabolic processes in which energy is released in the form of heat. Other producers of heat are the **skeletal muscles**, the **liver**, the internal organs, and the brain. Muscles play a major role in thermogenesis. Because of their weight, they are able to produce very large amounts of heat very rapidly during increased physical activity. Digestion also results in an increased production of heat.

Heat is lost from the body in four different ways: by conduction, convection, evaporation, and radiation. Heat loss by conduction occurs because there is a gradient between the body temperature and the temperature of the surrounding environment. When the external temperature is lower, heat flows from the body to the colder external environment. The body also loses heat by evaporation, mainly through sweating. This mechanism occurs especially during phases of increased heat production, for example during physical **exercise**. The sweat glands are controlled by cholinergic impulses through the sympathetic nerve fibers. During intensive sweating, up to one liter of sweat may be formed. When the humidity of the environment is higher, heat loss through sweating is easier. When the body needs to accumulate heat, adrenergic impulses restrict the blood flow through the skin, with the result that the skin becomes an insulator, thus decreasing heat loss to a minimum. The body can also lose heat by convection, through the circulatory system. With this mechanism, heat flows from each cell to the surrounding extracellular fluid (ECF) and afterwards to the circulating blood. Heat loss is modulated by the amount of blood that circulates through the body surface. The high flow occurring through the subcutaneous area and the skin transfers the heat carried by the blood to the environment through the body surface. Finally, the body can lose heat by simply radiating it away.

Several conditions can influence body temperature, such as exercise, the time of day, the environmental temperature, digestion and the level of water consumption. For example, body temperature varies in the narrow range between 97.7° and 99.5°F (36.5° and 37.5°C). It slightly increases during the day, reaching a peak between 6:00 to 10:00 p.m. and a low between 2:00 and 4:00 a.m. This diurnal variation depends on the body activity throughout the day. Diurnal variations do not change in persons that work at night and sleep during the day and they also occur when **fever** is present. Fever reaches a peak in the evening, and decreases during the night so that, in the morning, even a very sick person may have an almost normal temperature. Body temperature changes are also more intensive in young people than in older people. Physical activity also increases body temperature, in some cases very significantly. For example, the average body temperature of marathon runners may increase to 102.2–105.8°F (39–41°C). The feedback control system responsible for thermoregulation is very complex, but overall, it can be summarized as follows:

When the surroundings are hot or when the body is vigorously exercising:

- The body core temperature starts to rise.
- This increase in temperature is detected by heat sensors in the body.
- These sensors send signals to the CNS.
- The CNS stimulates the sweat glands.
- This increases the production of sweat.
- This activates the evaporation of sweat.
- Evaporation promotes heat loss by evaporation.
- The CNS also signals the vasomotor system to dilate the capillaries underlying the skin.
- Vasodilation occurs and the capillaries become larger.
- More blood flows underneath the skin surface.
- Blood flow promotes heat loss by conduction, radiation, and convection.
- The body core temperature returns to normal.

When the surroundings are cold or when the body is resting:

- The body core temperature starts to drop.
- This is detected by cold sensors in the body.
- These sensors send signals to the CNS.
- The CNS slows down the activity of the sweat glands.
- This lowers the production of sweat.
- Lowered production of sweat decreases the evaporation of sweat.
- Lowered rates of evaporation reduces heat loss.
- The CNS also signals the vasomotor system to constrict the capillaries underlying the skin.
- Vasoconstriction occurs and the capillaries become narrower.
- Less blood flows underneath the skin surface.
- This reduces heat loss by conduction, radiation, and convection.
- The body core temperature returns to normal.

Function

The major function of thermoregulation is to help maintain homeostasis, meaning the stability of the body's internal environment. A wide variety of body systems and organs interact to maintain the body's

KEY TERMS

Acetylcholine—Neurotransmitter produced by an enzyme in the body that stimulates muscle tissue.

Adrenaline—A hormone produced by the adrenal medulla that causes vasodilation of the small arteries in muscle and increases cardiac output.

Adrenergic—Substance that has an effect similar to that of adrenaline.

Antagonist—A substance that cancels or counteracts the action of another.

Capillaries—The smallest blood vessels of the body.

Central nervous system (CNS)—One of two major divisions of the nervous system. The CNS consists of the brain, the cranial nerves and the spinal cord.

Cholinergic—Substance that has an effect similar to that of acetylcholine.

Conduction—Heat transfer by means of molecular agitation within a material without any motion of the material as a whole. If one end of a metal piece is at a higher temperature, then heat will be transferred down the piece toward the colder end.

Convection—Heat transfer by motion of a fluid when the heated fluid is caused to move away from the source of heat, carrying energy with it.

Dermis—Layer of connective tissue underlying the skin. Contains smooth muscle tissue, nervous tissue and blood vessels.

Endocrine glands—Glands secreting substances that are released directly into the bloodstream and that regulate metabolism and other body functions.

Endocrine system—The system of glands in the body that secretes hormones directly into the circulatory system.

Enzyme—A type of protein produced by the body that speeds up chemical reactions. Some enzymes regulate certain functions due to their ability to change their activity by modifying their structure.

Extracellular fluid (ECF)—The fluid found outside of the cells and between the cells in body tissues.

Feedback system—A feedback system uses as input the total or partial output of the system. Feedback systems are used to control and regulate processes. They use the consequences of the process (for example, too much or too little produced) to regulate the rate at which the process occurs (decrease or increase the rate of the process).

Homeostasis—Stability of the body's internal environment, achieved by a system of integrated control systems activated by feedback systems. Homeostasis is thus the maintenance of a constant internal environment (the immediate surroundings of cells) in response to changes occurring in the conditions of the external environment and the internal body environment.

Hormone—A naturally occurring substance secreted by specialized cells that affects the metabolism or behavior of other cells possessing receptors for the hormone.

Hypothalamus—The hypothalamus is a tiny cluster of brain cells just above the pituitary gland that is involved in the regulation of body temperature.

Metabolic effectors—Substances, such as hormones, that can increase the metabolism of the body or of a target organ.

Metabolism—The sum of all the physical and biochemical processes occurring in the body to produce what is required to maintain life. This includes the transformation of nutrients into energy and the use of energy by the body.

Nervous system—The entire system of nerve tissue in the body. It includes the brain, the brainstem, the spinal cord, the nerves and the ganglia and is divided into the peripheral nervous system (PNS) and the central nervous system (CNS).

Peripheral nervous system (PNS)—One of the two major divisions of the nervous system. The PNS consists of the somatic nervous system (SNS), which controls voluntary activities, and of the autonomic nervous system (ANS), which controls regulatory activities. The ANS is further divided into sympathetic and parasympathetic systems.

Radiation—Heat transfer that occurs by the emission of electromagnetic waves which carry energy away from the emitting object.

Thermogenesis—Production of heat.

Thermoregulation—Regulation of body temperature so as to maintain it nearly constant at 98.6 °F (37 °C).

Thyroid gland—A butterfly-shaped endocrine gland located in the neck on both sides of the windpipe. It controls the rate at which the body produces energy from nutrients. It secretes the hormones triiodothyronine (T3) and thyroxine (T4) which increase the rate of metabolism and cardiac output.

Vasoconstriction—The decrease in the internal diameter of a blood vessel resulting from tightening the smooth muscle located in the walls of the vessel. Vasoconstriction decreases the blood flow.

Vasodilation—The increase in the internal diameter of a blood vessel resulting from relaxation of the smooth muscle located in the walls of the vessel. Vasodilation increases the blood flow.

Vasomotor system—The neural systems which act on vascular smooth muscle to control blood vessel diameter.

internal environment (the immediate surroundings of cells) constant in response to changes that occur either in the conditions of the external environment or in the conditions of the internal body environment. Thermoregulation is one of these essential homeostatic mechanisms.

Role in human health

Thermoregulation is of the utmost importance in maintaining health, because human life is only compatible with a narrow range of temperatures. Core temperature changes of the order of 6 °F (3 °C) will not interfere with physiological functions, but any variation outside that range has very serious effects. For example, at 82.4 °F (28 °C), the muscles can no longer respond; at 86 °F (30 °C), confusion occurs and the body can no longer control its temperature; at 91.4 °F (33 °C), loss of consciousness occurs; at 107.6 °F (42 °C), the CNS breaks down with irreversible brain damage; and at 111.2 °F (44 °C), death occurs, the result of the body **proteins** starting to denature.

Common diseases and disorders

- Fever—Increase in body core temperature. Fever is not an illness but a natural reaction to a number of illnesses.

- Hyperthermia—Overheating of the body caused only by an external factor, as for example a hot environment, or a hot bath.

- Hypothermia—A low body temperature, as caused by exposure to cold weather or a state of low temperature of the body induced by decreased **metabolism**.

- Hypothyroidism—Hypothyroidism refers to a condition in which the amount of thyroid hormones in the body is below normal. Since the thyroid hormones are important in thermoregulation, hypothyroidism affects the body's capacity to control temperature.

Resources

BOOKS

Imber, G. *Body Temperature.* Scranton, PA: William Morrow & Co, 2001.

Jessen, K. *Temperature Regulation in Humans and Other Mammals.* New York: Springer Verlag, 2001.

PERIODICALS

Boulant, J. A. "Role of the preoptic-anterior hypothalamus in thermoregulation and fever." *Clinical Infectious Diseases* 31: Suppl. 5 (October 2000): S157–S161.

Febbraio, M. A.; R. Wallis; D. A. Schoeller; J. Nedergaard; V. Golozoubova; A. Matthias; A. Asadi; A. Jacobsson; B. Cannon; T. B. VanItallie. "Alterations in energy metabolism during exercise and heat stress." *Sports Medicine* 31 (2001): 47–59.

Sawka, M. N.; E. F. Coyle. "Influence of body water and blood volume on thermoregulation and exercise performance in the heat." *Exercise & Sport Science Review* 27 (1999): 167–218.

Schoeller, D. A.; J. Nedergaard; V. Golozoubova; A. Matthias; A. Asadi; A. Jacobsson; B. Cannon; T. B. VanItallie. "The importance of clinical research: the role of thermogenesis in human obesity." *American Journal of Clinical Nutrition* 73 (March 2001): 511–516.

OTHER

Temperature Regulation of the Human Body. *Hyperphysics Website.* <http://hyperphysics.phy-astr.gsu.edu/hbase/thermo/heatreg.html>.

Monique Laberge, Ph.D.

▌ Thiamine

Description

Thiamine, also known as vitamin B_1, was the first of the water-soluble B-vitamin family to be discovered. It is an essential component of an enzyme, thiamine pyrophosphate, that is involved in metabolizing **carbohydrates**. Thiamine works closely with other B **vitamins** to assist in the utilization of **proteins** and **fats** as well, and helps mucous membranes and the **heart** to stay healthy. The **brain** relies on thiamine's role in the conversion of **blood** sugar (glucose) into biological energy to function properly. Thiamine is also involved in certain key metabolic reactions occurring in nervous tissue, the heart, in the formation of red blood cells, and in the maintenance of smooth and skeletal muscle.

General use

The recommended daily allowance (RDA) of thiamine is 0.3 mg for infants less than six months old, 0.4 mg for those from six months to one year old, 0.7 mg for children ages one to three years, 0.9 mg for those four to six years, and 1.0 mg for those seven to 10 years. Requirements vary slightly by gender after age ten. Males need 1.3 mg from 11-14 years, 1.5 mg from 15-50 years, and 1.2 mg when over age 50 years. Females require 1.1 mg from 11-50 years of age, and 1.0 mg if older than 50 years. The RDA is slightly higher for women who are pregnant (1.5 mg) or lactating (1.6 mg). Adults need a minimum of 1.0 mg of thiamine a day, but the requirement is increased by approximately 0.5 mg for each 1,000 calories of daily dietary intake over a 2,000-calorie base.

Thiamine has limited therapeutic use apart from supplements for people who are deficient or have significant risk factors for deficiency, such as **alcoholism**. High doses are used to treat some metabolic disorders, including certain enzyme deficiencies, Leigh's disease, and maple syrup urine disease. People suffering from diabetic neuropathy may sometimes benefit from additional thiamine. This should be undertaken with the advice of a healthcare provider. Claims have been made that it can also help people with **Alzheimer's disease**, epilepsy, canker sores, depression, fatigue, **fibromyalgia**, and motion sickness. Improvement of these conditions based on supplementation with thiamine is unsubstantiated. Although a deficiency of thiamine may cause canker sores, taking extra of the vitamin after they appear does not appear to help them resolve.

Preparations

Natural sources

While all plant and animal foods have thiamine, higher levels of thiamine are found in many nuts, seeds, brown rice, seafood, and whole-grain products. Sunflower seeds are a particularly good source. Grains are stripped of the B vitamin content during processing, but it is often added back to breads, cereals, and baked goods. Legumes, milk, beef liver, and pork are other foods with high vitamin B_1 content. Thiamine is destroyed by prolonged high temperatures, but not by freezing. Food should be cooked in small amounts of water so that thiamine and other water-soluble vitamins do not leach out. Do not add baking soda to vegetables, and do eat fresh foods to avoid sulfite preservatives. Both of these chemicals will break down the thiamine content found in foods. Drinking tea or alcohol with a meal will also drastically decrease the amount of thiamine that is absorbed by the body.

Supplemental sources

Thiamine is available in oral, **intramuscular injection**, and intravenous formulations. Injectable types are usually preserved for the severely deficient. Supplements should always be stored in a cool dry place, away from direct light, and out of the reach of children.

Deficiency

A deficiency of thiamine leads to a condition known as beriberi. Once common in sailors, it has become rare in the industrialized parts of the world except in the cases of alcoholism and certain disease conditions. The syndrome typically causes poor appetite, abdominal **pain**, heart enlargement, constipation, weakness, swelling of limbs, muscle spasms, insomnia, and **memory** loss. Under treatment, the condition can resolve very quickly. Untreated beriberi will lead to Wernicke-Korsakoff syndrome. These patients experience confusion, disorientation, inability to speak, gait difficulties, numbness or tingling of extremities, **edema**, nausea, vomiting, visual difficulties, and may progress to psychosis, **coma**, and death. Even in advanced states, this condition can be reversible if thiamine is given, nutritional status is improved, and use of alcohol is stopped.

Risk factors for deficiency

The leading risk factor for developing a deficiency of thiamine is alcoholism. Generally, alcoholics eat poorly, and therefore have low dietary intake of thiamine and other vitamins to begin with. Alcohol also acts directly to destroy thiamine, and increases the excretion of it. People with cirrhosis of the liver, malabsorption syndromes, diabetes, kidney disease, chronic infections, or hypermetabolic conditions also have increased susceptibility to deficiency. The elderly are more prone to poor nutritional status, as well as difficulties with absorption, and may need a supplement. Others with nutritionally inadequate diets, or increased need as a result of **stress**, illness, or surgery may benefit from additional vitamin B₁ intake since utilization is higher under these conditions. Those who diet or fast frequently may also be at risk for low levels of thiamine. Use of tobacco products or carbonate and citrate food additives can impair thiamine absorption. A shortage of vitamin B₁ is likely to be accompanied by a shortage of other B vitamins, and possibly other nutrients as well. A supplement containing a balance of B complex and other vitamins is usually the best approach unless there is a specific indication for a higher dose of thiamine, or other individual vitamins.

Precautions

Thiamine should not be taken by anyone with a known allergy to B vitamins, which occurs rarely.

Side effects

In very unusual circumstances, large doses of thiamine may cause rashes, itching, or swelling. This is more likely from intravenous injection than oral supplements. Most people do not experience any side effects from oral thiamine.

Interactions

Oral contraceptives, **antibiotics**, sulfa drugs, and certain types of diuretics may deplete thiamine. Consult a health care professional about the advisability of supplementation. Taking this vitamin may also intensify the effects of neuromuscular blocking agents that are used during some surgical procedures. B vitamins are best absorbed as a complex, and magnesium also promotes the absorption of thiamine.

Resources

BOOKS

Bratman, Steven, and David Kroll. *Natural Health Bible.* Rocklin, CA: Prima Publishing, 1999.

Feinstein, Alice. *Prevention's Healing with Vitamins.* Emmaus, PA: Rodale Press, 1998.

Griffith, H. Winter. *Vitamins, Herbs, Minerals & Supplements: The Complete Guide.* Tucson, AZ: Fisher Books, 1998.

Jellin, Jeff, Forrest Batz, and Kathy Hitchens. *Pharmacist's Letter/Prescriber's Letter Natural Medicines Comprehensive Database.* Stockton, CA: Therapeutic Research Faculty, 1999.

Pressman, Alan H., and Sheila Buff. *The Complete Idiot's Guide to Vitamins and Minerals.* New York: Alpha Books, 1997.

Judith Turner

Thoracentesis

Definition

Thoracentesis is a procedure by which pleural fluid is removed from the space between the lung and the chest wall. The space in which this fluid collects is called the pleural space. It is formed in between the serous membrane covering each lung, called the visceral pleura, and the serous membrane covering the chest wall, called the parietal pleura. Normally very little fluid is present in the pleural space, and it serves to lubricate the two pleural surfaces, so they can easily slip across each other during respiration.

Purpose

Abnormal quantities of pleural fluid may accumulate in various conditions. Removal of pleural fluid for analysis is commonly performed in order to determine the cause of fluid accumulation. Sometimes the effusion is so large that it interferes with normal lung function. In such cases, thoracentesis may be performed to relieve the respiratory distress caused by lung compression.

An excess of pleural fluid is called an effusion. Laboratory analysis is directed at distinguishing between two types of effusion, transudates and exudates. Transudates are caused by hemodynamic changes outside the **lungs** that increase the movement of fluid from the capillaries in the parietal pleura into the pleural space. These include increased hydrostatic pressure (i.e., high **blood pressure**); decreased oncotic pressure (i.e., low plasma protein due to **liver** or renal disease); increased pleural capillary permeability; and lymphatic obstruction. Exudates are caused by injury, **infection**, inflammation, or malignancy. Exudates usually involve the lungs, but in some cases such as esophageal rupture or **pancreatitis**, they do not.

A recent report suggests that thoracentesis is preferred to pericardiocentesis for pericardial and pleural effusion caused by central venous catheterization in neonates. Thoracentesis is as effective and less invasive.

Precautions

Practitioners should be aware that many pleural fluids display some characteristics of both transudates and exudates. These conditions have many causes which may be present concurrently, making the distinction complicated. The physician performing thoracentesis must take great care to avoid puncturing the lung, which can cause air to enter the pleural space (pneumothorax) and result in lung collapse. A **blood** sample should be collected at the time of thoracentesis to provide a basis for comparison to certain pleural fluid results. When collecting pleural fluid or blood, the physician and other members of the health care team should observe **universal precautions** for the prevention of transmission of bloodborne pathogens. If pH is to be measured, the syringe containing the fluid must be capped, placed in an ice bath, and sent immediately to the laboratory.

Preparation

Written consent should be obtained before the procedure is begun. X ray of the chest is performed prior to the procedure. A special view of a pleural effusion, called a lateral decubitus film, may be ordered. In this view, the patient lies down on the side on which the effusion is known to exist. If the effusion is "free-flowing," gravity will cause it to spread up the lateral chest wall. If an effusion is not free-flowing, it may be more difficult to access for thoracentesis, and ultrasound or CT guidance may be helpful. A thorough history is performed to determine if any conditions such as a bleeding disorder are present that may complicate the procedure. The history should also document the medications that the patient is currently taking, and **allergies** to drugs or anesthetics. Prior to the procedure, a blood sample should be collected and a platelet count and prothrombin time should be performed. These tests determine whether there is an abnormally high risk of uncontrolled bleeding from the site that may contraindicate the procedure.

Description

Generally the effusion has been identified already on **chest x ray**, and may be noticeable by percussion of the chest wall. Traditionally, if there has been any question about the location of the excess fluid, ultrasound or computed tomography (CT) may be used as a guide for the procedure. In recent years, studies have shown that ultrasound-guided thoracentesis results in fewer complications than thoracenteses performed with no image guidance during the procedure.

The patient should be seated upright, generally on the edge of a bed or chair, with arms propped up on a stable surface. The lateral chest wall is scrubbed with an antiseptic preparation, **local anesthesia** is administered, and a needle inserted between two ribs known to overlie the effusion. Generally the needle enters the chest below the armpit. Using a syringe, the appropriate amount of fluid is removed. The fluid should be collected in a heparinized syringe or transferred to a tube containing heparin or EDTA, and delivered to the lab for analysis. If the effusion is large, recurrent, or particularly concerning (e.g., very low pH and signs of infection), a chest tube may be placed and attached to a one-way system to promote continued drainage and prevent air from entering the pleural space. A **pulse oximeter** can be used to monitor the patient's oxygenation, and oxygen can be administered via a nasal cannula if needed. Generally **oxygen therapy** is not required, but if a pneumothorax occurs as a complication, or a large volume of pleural fluid is removed in a short period of time, lung function can be compromised.

Transudates form from diseases that occur outside the lungs. They are most frequently caused by congestive **heart failure** which accounts for up to 90% of all pleural effusions, pulmonary embolism (which sometimes causes exudates), cirrhosis of the liver, myxedema (hypothyroidism) or kidney disease. Exudates are generally due to infection, malignancy, trauma, pulmonary infarction, ruptured esophagus, pancreatitis systemic lupus erythematosus, and rheumatoid arthritis.

Sometimes bloody fluid is found in the pleural space. This may be due to major trauma that has severed **blood vessels** in the chest. This is termed a hemothorax, and will produce a **hematocrit** that approximates that of blood. Malignancies involving the pleural fluid cause an increased red blood cell count but usually do not cause massive bleeding into the pleural space. Occasionally a thoracentesis sample may appear milky (chylothorax). This can be caused by a perforated or torn thoracic duct that carries lymph from the intestines to the **heart**. Chylothorax can also be caused by an aggressive **cancer** that blocks the flow of lymph. A similar appearance to the fluid can result from necrosis, which causes formation of a pseudochylous effusion. Such fluids are characterized by foul odor, cholesterol, and high cellularity. Chylous effusions are odorless and have high triglycerides.

Malignancy is a common cause of pleural effusions and exudative fluids should always be examined for malignant cells. Approximately 35% of lung cancers, 25% of breast cancers, and 10% of lymphatic cancers shed cells into the pleural fluid.

Laboratory evaluation

Pleural fluid is generally evaluated for gross appearance and volume, protein, specific gravity, glucose, lactate dehydrogenase, blood cell counts, pH, cytology, culture and **Gram stain**. Other tests may be requested such as lactate, amylase, flow cytometry, triglycerides, complement, other enzymes, bilirubin, and tumor markers.

Normal pleural fluid has a volume of 3-5 mL, but effusions of several hundred milliliters are not uncommon. The fluid should be clear and light yellow (straw-colored). Turbidity can be caused by a traumatic tap or by an abnormal condition. Bloody taps are associated with streaking of the fluid as it is collected, and a clear supernatant after centrifugation. Turbidity can result from infection, mucin, or fat in the fluid. It takes very little blood to turn the pleural fluid red. In addition to a traumatic tap, red tinged fluids are caused by trauma, malignancy, and pulmonary infarction. Turbid, yellow fluids are associated with infection. Turbid, green fluids are associated with rheumatoid arthritis, and milky-white fluids with lymph containing chyle. The specific gravity of the fluid should be equal to or less than plasma. Exudates are associated with a specific gravity of 1.015 or higher, but transudates sometimes overlap this cutoff.

Chemistry tests are performed on pleural fluid by the same methods used for plasma. The pleural fluid glucose should be the same as the plasma glucose. Low levels are significant. Pleural fluid glucose below 40 mg/dL are associated with infection, malignancy, and rheumatic disease (i.e., rheumatoid arthritis) and systemic lupus erythematosus. LD is the single best test to differentiate transudates from exudates. Pleural fluid LD in excess of 200 U/L or a fluid to serum LD ratio of 0.6 or higher indicates an exudate. Lactate levels are increased in exudative fluids as well but cannot differentiate between the causes. Total protein in pleural fluid is increased when the fluid is exudative, but the interpretation is difficult whenever there is bleeding or a traumatic tap. A total protein of less than 3.0 g/dL is consistent with a transudate. Pleural fluid amylase is increased in both chronic and acute pancreatitis, in amylase producing cancers

that infiltrate the pleura, and in rupture of the esophagus. pH is below 7.45 in exudative fluids and is extremely low (7.0-7.3) in malignancy, bacterial infection, rupture of the esophagus, **tuberculosis**, and rheumatoid arthritis. A pH below 7.0 is seen only in empyema (bacterial infection with a white count greater than 10,000 per microliter), esophageal rupture, and rheumatoid arthritis. Triglycerides are increased (greater than 110 mg/dL) in chylous effusions.

The white blood cell (WBC) count of pleural fluid is performed manually. Transudates have a WBC count of less than 1,000 per microliter. Exudates have a WBC count of 10,000 per microliter or higher. WBC counts in excess of 50,000 per microliter signal infection of the pleura. A WBC differential is always performed on pleural fluid using a method to concentrate the cells. No single cell type should predominate. A predominance of lymphocytes (greater than 50%) occurs in lymphoid cancers (lymphoma), lymphocytic leukemias, and tuberculosis. Greater than 50% neutrophils occurs in acute infections, acute injuries (such as pulmonary infarction and rupture of the esophagus), malignancies, and granulocytic leukemia. Increased eosinophils are seen in pneumothorax, pulmonary infarction, congestive heart failure, parasitic infestation, and some infections. Red blood cell counts are also performed manually. Red counts in excess of 100,000 per microliter are associated with trauma, malignancy, and pulmonary infarctions.

A Gram stain and culture should be performed on the sediment of all pleural fluids. The Gram stain of sediment is positive in about 50% of persons with pleural infections. Cultures for tuberculosis are frequently requested because this disease is associated with approximately 8% of pleural fluid effusions. Cultures should be performed using blood agar plates, chocolate (heated blood) agar plates, and thioglycolate broth. Transudative fluids are usually negative for growth. The most common bacterial isolates are *Staphylococcus aureus* and gram negative bacilli.

Cytological analysis of pleural fluid is usually requested and should be performed on a concentrate of any fluid that is exudative. As with microbiological culture, the sensitivity of cytology is proportional to the volume of fluid concentrated. Metastatic carcinoma, **sarcomas**, mesothelioma, and Hodgkin's and non-Hodgkin's lymphomas and leukemias can cause cellular infiltration of the pleura and produce exudative effusions. Activated and phagocytic mesothelial cells are often seen in inflammatory pleural fluids, and are difficult to distinguish from malignant mesothelial cells. Cytology is performed on both Wright and Papanicolaou stains. Special cytochemical stains and flow cytometry are often used to differentiate reactive from malignant mesothelial cells and identify the type of other malignant cells present.

Aftercare

Vital signs are assessed every fifteen minutes until stable. A chest x ray is ordered to document changes in the appearance of the lung fields, and to look for possible pneumothorax. Examination of the chest with a **stethoscope** is also useful for documenting bilateral breath sounds that make pneumothorax unlikely. The site of the needle puncture is covered with a simple dressing and monitored for bleeding or drainage.

Complications

With any procedure which breaks the skin, bleeding and infection are possibilities, although unlikely if careful and sterile technique are followed. Pneumothorax is a very real complication, and may need to be treated with a chest tube. If very large effusions are drained quickly, pulmonary **edema** and low oxygen levels can occur, requiring oxygen and possibly other support measures for the patient. A chest x ray should be ordered right after the procedure. If the pH and glucose are very low (e.g., pH below 7.2), white blood cells are found to be greater than 25,000 per microliter, or there are other signs of frank infection, a chest tube may need to be placed.

Results

Representative normal values for pleural fluid are shown below:

- Volume: less than 10 mL.
- Appearance: clear, light yellow.
- Specific gravity: less than 1.015.
- Protein: less than 3.0 g/dL.

- Lactate dehydrogenase: less than or equal to 200 U/L.
- Pleural fluid:serum LD ratio: less than 0.6.
- pH: 7.65 (transudates 7.4-7.5).
- Glucose: greater than 60 mg/dL (pleural fluid:serum ratio greater than 0.5).
- Triglycerides: 13-107 mg/dL.
- WBC count: less than 1,000 per microliter.
- Neutrophils: less than 50%.
- Lymphocytes: less than 50%.
- Eosinophils: less than 10%.

Health care team roles

A physician performs the thoracentesis, and orders and interprets the results of the laboratory tests. Nursing staff will be involved in documenting a patient's response to the procedure, and providing support and instruction for the patient during thoracentesis. Careful observation of respiratory status and pulse oximetry is important to aid in speedy intervention if necessary. Clinical laboratory scientists/medical technologists perform all of the laboratory tests done on the pleural fluid with the exception of cytological evaluation, which is performed by a pathologist. Radiologic technologists will perform x rays and other imaging studies before and after thoracentesis.

Resources

BOOKS

Light, Richard W. "Disorders of the Pleura, Mediastinum, and Diaphragm." In *Harrison's Principles of Internal Medicine.* Edited by Kurt Isselbacher, et al. New York: McGraw-Hill, 1998.

Malarkey, Louise M., and Mary Ellen McMorrow. *Nurse's Manual of Laboratory Tests and Diagnostic Procedures,* 2nd ed. Philadelphia: W.B. Saunders Company, 2000: 301–303.

Tierney, Lawrence M., Stephen J. McPhee, and Maxine A. Papadakis. *Current Medical Diagnosis and Treatment 2001.* Lange Medical Books/McGraw-Hill, 2001: 339–343.

PERIODICALS

Miller, Karle. "Is Ultrasound-guided Thoracentesis Safer?" *American Family Physician* (Sept. 1, 2003): 947.

"Thoracentesis Is a Less-invasive Neonatal Approach." *Heart Disease Weekly* (Sept. 26, 2004): 19.

Erika J. Norris
Teresa G. Odle

Thoracoscopy

Definition

Thoracoscopy is an endoscopic examination of the chest cavity. In the procedure, a specialized endoscope is inserted by a surgeon through a tiny incision in the patient's chest wall. Thoracoscopy is used to visually examine regions and organs of the chest cavity including the lungs, mediastinum, and pleura. When thoracoscopy is performed on a specific organ, it is often given another, more specific name. For example, when performed on the lungs it is called pleuroscopy.

Purpose

Thoracoscopy allows a physician to examine the interior of the chest cavity without making a large incision. Thus, it eliminates many possible complications that sometimes result from invasive procedures such as open chest surgery and surgical lung biopsy. The procedure also reduces pain, length of hospital stay, and recovery time at home. Thoracoscopy is performed to assess lung cancer; analyze possibly abnormal lung tissues; determine the cause of fluid in the cavity; treat accumulated air bubbles, blood, fluids, or pus; insert medications or other therapeutic treatments directly into the cavity; and remove adhesions (scar tissue). Thoracoscopy is often used to examine lungs and other organs that contain tumors or a metastatic growth of cancer.

Precautions

The surgical team must be aware of any potential patient who should not be considered for thoracoscopy. The procedure cannot be performed on anyone who cannot receive sufficient oxygen from only one lung (because one lung is deflated during the procedure). In addition, patients who had previous thoracic surgery or have blood-clotting problems are generally not suitable for thoracoscopy.

Thoracoscopy provides only a limited views of organs and regions of the chest cavity; primarily, it is only able to evaluate abnormalities near the surface of organs.

Description

Thoracoscopy is traditionally performed in hospitals and under general anesthesia but recently has been performed more frequently as an outpatient procedure and under local anesthesia. The procedure generally takes from two to four hours to perform.

The patient is positioned on his or her side on the operating table. The surgeon makes several (usually two to four) small incisions on the patient's side in the chest wall, usually spaced between the ribs to minimize damage to muscles, nerves, and ribs. A suction tube is inserted into one of the incisions to remove blood. A bronchoscope is inserted into the airway to check for structural abnormalities. A Y-shaped endotracheal tube (with two inner tubes) is inserted into the trachea, and one inner tube is inserted into each bronchus. The other end is connected to a ventilator. The lung is then partially deflated to create an empty volume between the lungs and chest wall. The patient breathes with a single inflated lung along with help from the ventilator.

An endoscope is inserted through one incision and surgical instruments inserted through other incisions. The doctor examines the surfaces of the areas and structures within the chest cavity, makes a cut through the pleura, and removes (as needed) biopsies, cultures, and tissue samples of the pleura, lung, and other areas. The remaining open incision is used to insert a drainage tube. When all examinations are completed, the deflated lung is re-inflated. All incisions are closed except for one to drain fluids and residual air. The incisions are closed with sutures or staples. Bandages are placed over the incisions to keep the area clean and to prevent infection.

The biopsies, samples, and cultures removed during the procedure are examined under a microscope. Samples are sent to a laboratory for analysis and evaluation. If a cancerous tumor is suspected, biopsies are delivered to a pathology laboratory.

Preparation

Patients who undergo thoracoscopy usually have all or some of the following preliminary procedures performed: chest x ray, electrocardiogram (anyone over 35 years of age), various blood and urine tests, pulmonary function analysis, and arterial blood gas analysis.

No foods or liquids should be consumed for twelve hours before the thoracoscopy because the anesthesia can cause vomiting. The physician should be informed of any medications taken by the patient, especially aspirin, blood pressure medicine and heart pills, diabetes pills and insulin, and ibuprofen.

KEY TERMS

Biopsy—Removal of sample of living tissue for examination.

Bronchoscope—Flexible tube less than 0.5 inches (1.3 centimeters) wide and about 2 feet (0.6 meters) long that is inserted into the trachea during a diagnostic procedure called bronchoscopy.

Bronchus—Tube leading from trachea to a lung.

Endoscope—Illuminated optic instrument with long, narrow-diameter tube (which may be rigid or flexible) that is attached to camera, which allows a surgical team to view inside chest cavity on video screen.

Endoscopy—Process to view interior of body.

Endotracheal—Within or passed through windpipe (trachea).

Mediastinum—Region in chest containing heart, trachea, and other organs that separate the two lungs.

Metastatic—Malignant.

Pleura—Membrane surrounding the lungs.

Thoracic—Of or about chest cavity.

Ventilator—Mechanical device that assists patient with breathing.

Aftercare

The patient remains in the recovery room for about one to two hours after the surgery. When drainage of fluid stops, the tube is removed. The patient will remain in the hospital several days (two to five days, on average) to recuperate. Medications will be given on an as-needed basis. Patients should rest when returning home and should lift only light objects for at least one month.

Complications

The main complication comes from the use of the general anesthesia. Another complication that sometimes occurs is excessive internal bleeding. Blood clots can form and travel to the lungs. A lung may also deflate (pneumothorax) when the drainage tube is removed. There is usually some chest discomfort after the procedure because of the surgical incisions.

Results

A partial diagnosis can be made by observing the internal structures of the chest cavity. A normal chest cavity contains a small amount of lubricating fluid. Normal functioning lungs will appear free of abnormalities. An abnormal chest cavity will show excess fluid. Abnormal looking tissue will be biopsied to determine if it is malignant. Results of the biopsy will be returned from the laboratory for the physician to determine any future course of action. If cancer is found in any biopsies, open chest surgery may be performed to remove the malignancy.

Health care team roles

The health care team performs preliminary tests on the patient in preparation for surgery. The surgeon (usually a chest surgeon or pulmonary specialist) and the surgical team perform the procedure usually in a hospital. The health care team will follow up with post-surgical care. A member of the health care team will inform the patient about the results of the procedure.

Resources

BOOKS

Shannon, Joyce Brennfleck, editor. *Medical Tests Sourcebook: Basic Consumer Health Information about Medical Tests.* Detroit, MI: Omnigraphics. 1999.

Shtasel, Philip. *Medical Tests and Diagnostic Procedures: A Patient's Guide to Just What the Doctor Ordered.* New York: HarperPerennial, 1991.

Zaret, Barry, editor. *The Patient's Guide to Medical Tests.* New York: Houghton Mifflin Company, 1997.

OTHER

Health A to Z, Medical Network, Inc. "Thoracoscopy," 2002. http://www.healthatoz.com/healthatoz/Atoz/ency/thoracoscopy.jsp (December 15, 2005).

HealthSquare, Physicians' Desk Reference. "Thoracoscopy: What You Should Know." http://www.healthsquare.com/mc/fgmc1001.htm (December 15, 2005).

William Arthur Atkins

Thorax, bones of

Definition

The skeleton of the thorax or chest is a cage that encloses and protects the main organs of respiration and circulation. It has a conical shape, being narrower at the top and broader at the bottom, and longer behind than in front. It consists of the sternum and the ribs.

Description

The bones of the thorax include the sternum, commonly called the breastbone, and the ribs.

The sternum is a narrow, elongated, flattened bone that forms the center of the front of the chest. It consists of three parts: an upper section called the manubrium, a middle section called the body, and a lower section called the xiphoid process that projects down. The junction of the manubrium and body is called the sternal angle. In early life, the xiphoid process is not a bone, but a piece of cartilage. Cartilage is a type of connective tissue containing collagen, a protein substance that forms tough and elastic fibers. It is a softer and more flexible material than bone. As the child grows, the xiphoid process slowly hardens into bone and by adulthood, it has become fused to the body of the sternum. The sides of both manubrium and body are notched so as to attach to seven costal cartilages. These are strips of strong cartilage that prolong into ribs and provide elasticity to the thorax. The upper section of the sternum supports the clavicles (shoulder blades). It contains a notch called the clavicular notch that allows it to articulate with the clavicle. The average length of the adult sternum is about 6.7 in (17 cm), and it is usually somewhat longer in the male than in the female.

The ribs are flexible, long bones that look like arches, and they form a large part of the thoracic skeleton. There are 12 ribs on each side and they are located one below the other in such a way that spaces called intercostal spaces occur between them. The first seven (1-7) are called the true ribs or the vertebro-sternal ribs. They connect in the back to the **vertebral column**, and in front to the sternum, through the costal cartilages. The following three ribs (8-10) are called the false ribs or the vertebro-chondral ribs. These ribs have their costal cartilages attached to the cartilage of the true rib above. The last two ribs (11-12) are only attached to the vertebral column and are thus called the floating or vertebral ribs.

All ribs have many structural features in common:

- Head. The head of the rib is the flat surface that connects with the vertebrae in the vertebral column.

- Neck. The neck of the rib is a flattened section that has a length of about 1 in (2.5 cm). It is located between the head and the tubercle. Its inferior surface is flat and smooth and its superior surface is rough for the attachment of ligaments.

- Tubercle. The tubercle is a bony eminence, or growth, that comes right after the neck of the rib. It has two sections, one that serves as a point of attachment to the vertebrae and another that attaches to ligaments.

- Body. The body—or shaft—is the longest part of a typical rib.

- Angle. The angle is the point at which the body of the rib starts to curve, just after the tubercle.

- Costal groove. The costal groove is located on the inner surface of the body of a rib. It provides a seat and protection for the intercostal nerve bundle.

Ribs present some degree of variability. For example, they vary in their angle, the upper ribs being less oblique than the lower. Characteristic features of some special ribs include:

- Rib 1. The first rib is the most curved of all ribs; it is also the broadest, shortest and widest rib. The head is small, rounded, and only has a single bony projection for articulation with the first thoracic vertebra.

- Rib 2. The second rib is much longer than the first, and its body is not flat like that of the other ribs. It has a rough section near its angle for attachment of a large back muscle and also attaches to the sternal angle of the sternum.

- Rib 10. This rib only has one point of attachment to the vertebrae.

The upper opening of the thorax is broader from side to side than from front to back. It is formed by the first thoracic vertebra in the back, the upper section of the sternum in front, and the first rib on either side. It slopes downward and forward, so that the front part of the opening is on a lower level than the back part. The lower opening of the thorax is formed by the twelfth thoracic vertebra in the back, by the eleventh and twelfth ribs on the sides, and by the costal cartilages of the tenth, ninth, eighth, and seventh ribs in the front. The lower opening is closed by the diaphragm, the thin muscle located below the **lungs** and **heart**, that forms the floor of the thorax.

Function

The major function of the thorax bones is to form the thoracic cavity that encloses and protects the most important organs of the circulatory and respiratory systems, the heart and lungs. The rib cage has a very special function—it allows breathing to take place, which occurs as a result of the rib cage moving up and down as air is inhaled and exhaled.

Role in human health

Besides its role in protecting major organs and in breathing, the thorax also provides a structural frame for the attachment of the trunk muscles, which are

KEY TERMS

Cartilage—Connective tissue containing collagen, the protein substance that forms tough and flexible fibers. Cartilage is more flexible and compressible than bone and often serves as a bone precursor, becoming mineralized as the body ages.

Costal cartilages—Cartilage that prolongs the ribs forward and connects each rib to the sternum.

Diaphragm—The thin muscle located below the lungs and heart that separates the chest from the abdomen.

False ribs—The three ribs, 8-10, that attach to the costal cartilage of the seventh true rib.

Floating ribs—The two last ribs, 11-12, that are not attached to the sternum. Also called the vertebral ribs.

Manubrium—The upper section of the sternum, it articulates with the shoulder blades and connects to the first seven ribs.

Ribs—The long, elastic bones resembling arches that are part of the thoracic skeleton. There are 12 ribs on either side of the thorax.

Sternum—One of the bones of the thorax, located in front of the chest. It has three sections: the manubrium, the body, and the xiphoid process.

Thorax—The bones that surround and form the chest cavity. The thorax includes the sternum and the ribs.

True ribs—The first seven ribs, 1-7, directly attached to the sternum.

Vertebra—Flat bones that make up the vertebral column. The spine has 33 vertebrae.

needed for movement. Thus, it also plays a role in body locomotion.

Common diseases and disorders

Injuries to the bony structures of the thorax are very serious because of the relationship of the thorax to the spine as a whole and because of the importance of the major respiratory and circulatory organs that the thoracic cavity contains. For example, broken ribs can cause disease by mechanical interference with internal organs, irritation of surrounding soft tissues, straining ligaments, impinging nerves, or blocking **blood vessels**. Likewise, the sternum is a very strong bone and requires great force to fracture. But the main

danger in this type of injury is not so much the fracture itself, but the risk that the broken bone may be driven into the heart, which lies just behind it. Some thoracic diseases and disorders include:

- Asphyxiating thoracic dystrophy. Also known as Jeune's syndrome, this is a form of dwarfism characterized by an abnormally long and narrow thorax with a reduced thoracic cage capacity that results in the lungs not having enough room for respiration to occur.

- Chondrosarcoma. Chondrosarcoma is a **cancer** that can arise in the costal cartilage of the ribs.

- Costochondritis. Also called Tietze's syndrome, it is an inflammation of the costochondral or costosternal joints that causes localized **pain** and tenderness. Any of the seven rib junctions may be affected, and more than one site is affected in 90% of cases.

- Luxation of ribs. A luxation is a sprain of a rib. It is the result of twisting a rib about its head in such a way that the rib departs from its normal conformation.

- Pleurisy. Pleurisy is an inflammation of the membrane that covers the inside of the thorax.

- Thorax hematoma. This is bruising due to the breaking of **blood** vessels that results in a localized accumulation of blood.

Resources

BOOKS

Putz, R., et al, eds. *Sobotta Atlas of Human Anatomy: Thorax, Abdomen, Pelvis, Lower Limb.* 12th English ed. Philadelphia: Lippincott, Williams & Wilkins, 1997.

Roussos, C. *The Thorax.* New York: Marcel Dekker Inc., 1995.

Simon, Seymour. *Bones: Our Skeletal System.* New York: Morrow (Harper-Collins), 1998.

OTHER

"The Thorax." Bartleby.com edition of *Gray's Anatomy of the Human Body.* <http://www.bartleby.com/107/26.html>.

Monique Laberge, PhD

Throat culture

Definition

A throat culture is a technique for identifying disease-causing microorganisms in material taken from the throat. Most throat cultures are performed

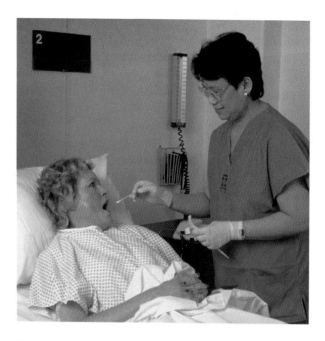

This nurse is taking a throat culture from a patient for laboratory analysis. *(Photograph by David Weinstein & Associates, Custom Medical Stock Photo. Reproduced by permission.)*

to identify infections caused by group A beta-hemolytic streptococci, which cause **strep throat**.

Purpose

The primary purpose of a throat culture is to isolate and identify organisms from the throat that cause **infection** of the posterior pharynx and tonsillar areas. Since most sore throats are caused by viral infections rather than by **bacteria**, a correct diagnosis is important to prevent unnecessary use of **antibiotics**. The bacterium that most often causes a **sore throat** is *Streptococcus pyrogenes* or group A beta-hemolytic streptococcus. In many circumstances, the throat culture is performed for the purpose of identifying this organism only. Throat cultures are also performed to identify people who are carriers of the organisms that may cause **meningitis** (*Neisseria meningitidis, Streptococcus pneumoniae*) and whooping cough (*Bordetella pertussis*).

Precautions

Throat cultures should be taken before the patient is given any antibiotic medications. In addition, the patient's immunization history should be checked to evaluate the possibility that diseases other than strep are causing the sore throat. The health care provider should use a mask and gloves for **infection control**, as the patient may cough or gag when the throat is swabbed. Swabs for rapid strep tests should be made of dacron or rayon.

Description

Throat cultures are performed for isolation of bacteria that cause throat infections. Throat washings or swabs are also required for culture of **viruses** that cause throat infections, but these viral cultures are not commonly performed. Most bacterial throat infections are caused by group A streptococci. Strep throat is more common in children (ages five to 15) than in adults, and is spread by droplets of mucus and other respiratory secretions. The tonsils and the back of the throat often appear red, swollen, and streaked with pus. The symptoms usually appear within three days after being exposed to group A strep and include an abrupt sore throat, headache, **fever**, loss of appetite, and malaise. Group A strep infections may be associated with complications called sequelae if not treated promptly with antibiotic therapy. In addition to causing sore throat (pharyngitis), this group of strep can also cause scarlet fever, rheumatic fever, glomerulonephritis, or abscesses around the tonsils

Other bacteria may cause pharyngitis, but do so less frequently. These include groups B, C and G streptococci, *Neisseria gonorrhoeae, Corynebacterium diptheriae, Haemophilis influenzae, Mycoplasma pneumonia*, and *Clamydia trachomatis*. In addition, anaerobic bacteria are often implicated as the cause of Vincent's angina, a form of tonsillitis. Many other pathogenic bacteria can be isolated from sites in the upper respiratory tract other than the pharynx such as the sinuses, nasopharynx, and epiglottis.

The specimen for culture is obtained by swabbing the throat with a sterile swab. The patient is asked to tilt the head back and open the mouth wide. A tongue depressor is used to hold down the tongue and the swab tip is rubbed against the area behind the uvula (posterior pharynx) and tonsillar areas on both sides of the throat. Any red or whitish patches on the throat should also be swabbed. The swab is removed gently without touching the teeth, gums, or tongue. It is then placed in a sterile tube for immediate delivery to a laboratory. For optimal recovery, especially if the laboratory is located off-site, the tube should contain Stuart's or Cary-Blair transport medium in order to maintain the viability of the organisms. The swab tip is used to break the ampoule and is immersed in the fluid. If a rapid strep test (streptococcal antigen test) is being performed, two swabs should be taken of the throat. One is used for the rapid test, and the other is used for culture should the rapid test result be negative. Obtaining the specimen takes less than 30 seconds. The swabbing procedure may cause gagging but is not painful. The physician or nurse should indicate if any disease organisms other than strep are suspected, because some bacteria require special culture media and growth conditions.

S. pyogenes, group A beta hemolytic streptococcus, is cultured on a growth medium called blood agar. Agar is a gel that is made from the cell walls of red algae. Blood plates are made from agar that contains a low carbohydrate nutrient such as trypticase soy and 5% sheep red blood cells. When the throat swab reaches the laboratory, it is wiped across a blood agar plate. An inoculating loop is used to streak the plate and stab the agar. This process separates the bacteria so that individual colonies can be isolated. An antibiotic disk containing bacitracin (A disk) is placed on the agar in an area containing the initial inoculum. Blood agar allows differentiation of streptococci based upon the characteristic hemolysis that they produce. Beta hemolytic strep releases products into the medium called beta hemolysins, which lyse the red blood cells and cause a clear zone to form around the colonies. Alpha strep releases alpha hemolysins, which causes a green discoloration to the blood around the colonies. Gamma hemolysis (no hemolysins produced) refers to no zone of discoloration around the colonies. Blood agar is nonselective and permits the growth of normal throat flora as well as other potential pathogens. For identification of group A strep, a selective medium such as strep selective agar (SSA) is used. This medium contains colistin, crystal violet, and trimethoprin-sulfamethoxazole (SXT). These antibiotics inhibit the growth of most normal flora and all streptococci except groups A and B. Plates are allowed to incubate for 18 hours at 95°F (35°C) in 10% carbon dioxide or under anaerobic conditions.

Plates should be examined after 18 hours of incubation, and if negative, again after an additional 24 hours incubation. Group A streptococci produce small oval-shaped transparent colonies that produce beta hemolysis and will not grow around the bacitricin disk. The colonies are catalase and coagulase negative and pyroglutamyl aminopeptidase (PYR) positive which differentiates them from the genera *Staphylococcus* and *Micrococcus*, which may appear similar on blood agar. Colonies of beta hemolytic strep isolated from the medium should be tested with group specific antibodies to confirm that they are group A. Antibiotic susceptibility testing is not usually necessary because group A strep are susceptible to penicillin and related antibiotics such as ampicillin. Persons who are allergic to penicillin may be given erythromycin.

Rapid strep tests are enzyme immunoassays that detect group A streptococcal antigens. The specificity of these tests is very high (approximately 98%), but the sensitivities have been reported to be from 60-96%. Consequently, negative tests can occur in the presence of group A streptococcal infections, and culture should be performed on samples that test negative. These tests can be performed in a medical office or clinic and results can be available within 10 minutes, allowing for quicker diagnosis and treatment. Usually, the physician will order a throat culture if the rapid strep test is negative, but the patient has clinical symptoms that are suggestive of strep infection. If the rapid strep test is positive, then treatment is ordered immediately.

Rapid strep tests are based upon the principle of double antibody sandwich immunoassay. The first step of a rapid strep test is the extraction of specific group A streptococcal antigen from the swab. The swab is placed in a test tube containing the extracting reagents (usually dilute acid). The swab is rotated vigorously in the solution while pressing the tip against the sides of the test tube. After all fluid is pressed from the swab, it is discarded and the extract is applied to a nitrocellulose membrane containing both immobilized antibodies and non-immobilized antibodies to different regions of the group A strep antigen. The non-immobilized antibodies are conjugated to colored particles or colloidal gold. If Group A streptococcal carbohydrate antigen is present in the extract, the conjugated antibodies bind to it, forming antigen-antibody complexes. These migrate along the pad until they reach the reaction zone containing immobilized antibodies to the same group A strep antigen. These antibodies capture the antigen-antibody complexes, forming a colored bar or line in the reaction zone area.

Preparation

Recent gargling or treatment with antibiotics will adversely affect the culture results. The laboratory should be notified if the patient has recently taken antibiotic medications.

Aftercare

No specific aftercare is needed.

KEY TERMS

Antibiotic—A drug given to stop the growth of bacteria. Antibiotics are ineffective against viruses.

Antigen—A substance that interacts with an antibody and causes an immune reaction.

Carrier—A person harboring an infectious disease who may be immune to it but who can transmit the disease to others.

Diphtheria—A serious disease of the throat, nose, and lungs caused by a bacterium, *Corynebacterium diphtheriae*.

Streptococcus—A category (genus) of sphere-shaped bacteria that occur in pairs or chains.

Thrush—A disease occurring in the mouth or throat that is caused by a yeast, *Candida albicans*, and is characterized by a whitish growth and ulcers.

Whooping cough—An infectious disease of the respiratory tract caused by a bacterium, *Bordetella pertussis*.

Complications

There is a minor risk to the health care provider collecting the specimen of contracting a viral or bacterial infection from the patient.

Results

The results from throat cultures identify the presence of any pathogenic bacteria growing on the media. Non-disease-producing organisms that grow in healthy throat tissues include non-hemolytic and alpha-hemolytic streptococci, some *Neisseria* species, *Moraxella catarrhalis*, coagulase negative staphylococci, and diphtheroids. These organisms are described on the culture report as normal flora. Group A streptococci are identified as described previously. Unless the culture is done solely for the identification of group A strep, any other potential pathogen (e.g., *Haemophilus influenzae, Neisseria gonorrhoeae*) is isolated on appropriate growth media, and the colonies that grow are identified by a selection of biochemical tests. Antimicrobial susceptibility testing is performed on a standardized growth of the isolated organism to determine which antibiotics will be effective in treating the infection.

Health care team roles

A physician, nurse, or physician assistant collects the throat swab. A health care provider such as a nurse will usually perform the rapid strep test in the outpatient setting. Cultures are performed by a clinical laboratory scientist CLS(NCA)/medical technologist MT(ASCP). Culture results are reported directly to the ordering physician who will select the appropriate antibiotic therapy if required.

Patient education

Because strep is highly contagious, the health care provider should stress that other family members and close contacts of patients diagnosed with strep throat also seek medical attention if they have similar symptoms. The health care provider should stress that the patient should wash hands frequently (especially after coughing or sneezing), stay home, and follow the treatment regimen prescribed by the physician.

Resources

BOOKS

Fischbach, Frances. "Throat Cultures (Swab or Washings)." In *A Manual of Laboratory & Diagnostic Tests*, 6th ed. Philadelphia: Lippincott Williams & Wilkins, 2000, pp. 551-553.

Forbes, Betty A., Daniel F. Sahm, and Alice S. Weissfeld. "Streptococcus, Enterococcus, and Similar Organisms." In *Bailey & Scott's Diagnostic Microbiology*, 10th ed. St. Louis: Mosby, 1998, pp. 620-635.

PERIODICALS

Hayes, Cynthia S., and Harold Williamson, Jr. "Management of Group A Beta-Hemolytic Streptococcal Pharyngitis." *American Family Physician* 63 (April 15, 2001): pp.1557-1565.

ORGANIZATIONS

The American Society for Clinical Laboratory Science. 7910 Woodmont Ave., Suite 523, Bethesda, MD 20814. (301) 657-2768. <http://www.ascls.org>.

Division of Bacterial and Mycotic Diseases, National Center for Infectious Disease, Centers for Disease Control and Prevention. 1600 Clifton Road NE, Atlanta, GA 30333. (800) 311-3435. <http://www.cdc.gov>.

National Institute of Allergy and Infectious Diseases, National Institutes of Health. Building 31, Room 7A-50, 31 Center Drive MSC 2520, Bethesda, MD, 20892. <http://www.niaid.nih.gov>.

Linda D. Jones, B.A., PBT (ASCP)

Throat swab *see* **Throat culture**

Thrombocyte count *see* **Complete blood count**

Thrombosis risk tests

Definition

Thrombosis risk tests check for defects in the anticoagulant system (hypercoagulability) that can cause a predisposition to thrombosis. The D-dimer test is used to screen for the presence of fibrin associated with deep vein and other forms of thrombosis.

Purpose

The purpose of thrombosis risk tests is to establish whether someone has a predisposition for developing thrombosis or has suffered a thrombotic episode, so that appropriate interventions can be instituted. The most common thrombosis risk tests are the D-dimer test, protein C test, protein S test, factor V Leiden test, prothrombin 1 + 2 (prothrombin 1.2) test, and the antithrombin test. These tests can be ordered individually but are usually ordered as a part of a panel.

Common indications for testing include:

- venous thrombosis
- pulmonary embolism
- cerebral **brain** thrombosis
- transient ischemic attack or premature stroke
- peripheral vascular disease
- prior to **pregnancy**, oral contraceptive prescription, estrogen therapy or major surgery if there is a family history of thrombosis
- relative with known genetic predisposition to thrombosis
- history of thrombosis and presence of a known genetic predisposition to thrombosis
- previous laboratory finding of activated protein C resistance (indication for factor V Leiden DNA test)
- premature **myocardial infarction** in a female patient (indication for prothrombin DNA test)
- history of multiple unexplained miscarriages

Precautions

Treatment with Coumadin, an anticoagulant, can interfere with the protein C and protein S tests. Ideally, the patient should discontinue treatment with Coumadin two weeks prior to undergoing these tests. If this is not possible then, an alternate panel of risk tests should be used. Alternatively heparin therapy can replace Coumadin therapy for two weeks prior to the tests, although heparin anticoagulant therapy can sometimes result in false positive antithrombin III test results. Protein S assays are not reliable during pregnancy. Heterophilic antibodies and rheumatoid factor are known to cause false positive reactions for D-dimer.

Description

The D-dimer test is the only laboratory test that is used to screen for the presence of deep vein thrombosis. The test is positive only when fibrin has formed. The D fragment of fibrinogen is produced by the action of plasmin on fibrinogen. Thrombin activates factor XIII, which stabilizes the fibrin clot by dimerizing the D fragments. In disseminated intravascular coagulation, pulmonary embolism, deep vein thrombosis, sickle cells disease and other conditions such as post surgical thrombus formation, the D-dimer level will be elevated in serum or plasma. D-dimer is measured by immunoassay, either latex agglutination or enzyme immunoassay (EIA). Latex agglutination is a qualitative assay that is not sufficiently sensitive to screen for deep vein thrombosis. Levels measured by EIA below 200 ng/ml indicate that thrombosis is unlikely in patients with no apparent signs of deep vein thrombosis.

Prothrombin fragment 1 + 2 (1.2), like D-dimer, is a marker for thrombotic disease. Prothrombin fragment 1 + 2 (1.2) can be measured by enzyme immunoassay. This fragment is produced when factor Xa activates prothrombin. The prothrombin fragment is increased in persons at risk for thrombotic episodes.

Other thrombosis risk tests check for mutations in the genes or **proteins** that are involved in the anticoagulant system. The anticoagulant system is designed to regulate coagulation and prevent excess **blood** clotting. Each anticoagulant protein is produced by a different gene. Each person possesses two copies of each anticoagulant gene. Mutation in an anticoagulant gene can cause it to produce abnormal protein, an increased or decreased amount of normal protein or can cause it to stop producing protein altogether. The common anticoagulant abnormalities (protein S, protein C, antithrombin III, prothrombin and factor V Leiden) are autosomal dominant, since only one gene of a pair needs to be altered to cause an increased risk of thrombosis. Someone with one normal copy of an anticoagulant gene and one changed copy of an anticoagulant gene (heterozygote) will have a moderately increased risk of thrombosis. Someone with both copies of an anticoagulant gene changed (homozygous) will have a significantly increased risk of thrombosis. People who have changes in multiple anticoagulant genes also have a significantly increased risk of thrombosis. There are other genetic and environmental factors that affect the risk of thrombosis, making it difficult to predict the exact risk in an individual with an anticoagulant gene mutation.

In some cases a thrombosis risk test checks for a change in the anticoagulant gene. In other cases, it is not feasible to check for a gene change and the activity of the protein is assayed.

Proteins C and S

Mutation in the genes that produce protein C and protein S can cause an increased risk of thrombosis. The frequency of protein C deficiency in the general population is 0.5% or less and the frequency of protein S deficiency is approximately 0.7%. Activated protein C (APC) is involved in inactivating **blood coagulation** factors V and VIII. Inactivation of these factors decreases blood coagulation. Activated protein S is a cofactor that enhances the activity of protein C. A deficiency in activated factors C or S can result in increased levels of factor Va and VIIIa, which increases the risk of thrombosis.

As of 2001, DNA testing for proteins C and S deficiencies is not available on a clinical basis. Proteins C and S can be measured by immunoassay which determines the mass of protein present, or by one of two functional tests. Protein C is a serine protease that inactivates factors Va and VIIIa. In the chromogenic substrate assay, plasma is mixed with *Agkistrodon* snake venom, an activator of protein C. The activated protein C splits a synthetic anilide substrate, producing a yellow product called p-nitroaniline. The amount of color is proportional to the concentration of functional protein C. However, this test does not detect all abnormal forms of protein C and will be normal in those cases where the defect occurs in the binding of protein C to protein S. All forms of protein C deficiency can be detected using a coagulation test in which protein C-deficient plasma is mixed with *Agkistrodon* snake venom and the patient's plasma. **Calcium** chloride and activated thromboplastin are added and the time required for clot formation is measured. The clotting time is proportional to the concentration of functional protein C in the sample.

Protein S is a cofactor required for enzymatic activity of protein C. Protein S can be measured by immunoassay or by a coagulation test using protein S deficient plasma, activated protein C, activated factor V, and calcium. The time required for a clot to form is proportional to protein S activity.

Factor V Leiden

A mutation in the gene that produces factor V protein, called a factor V Leiden mutation, causes this factor to become resistant to inactivation by protein C (APC resistance). APC resistance increases the risk of thrombosis. If another type of factor V mutation, called an R2 mutation, is found in one copy of the factor V gene, and a Leiden mutation is found in the other copy, the risk of thrombosis is further increased. An R2 mutation alone does not cause an increased risk of thrombosis. R2 mutation testing is, therefore, only performed if a Leiden mutation is found in one copy of the factor V gene. Factor V Leiden has normal coagulation activity when activated, and therefore, does not affect clotting tests such as the prothrombin time. It is detected by the polymerase chain reaction (PRC) using a probe that recognizes the point mutation in the factor V gene. Factor V Leiden is the most common inherited risk factor for hypercoagulability. Its prevalence is 2–7% in the general population.

Prothrombin (factor II)

A mutation in the gene that produces prothrombin can also result in an increased risk of thrombosis. Prothrombin is the precurser to thrombin. Thrombin, when activated, converts fibrinogen to fibrin, which forms the clot. A mutation called G20210A in the gene that produces prothrombin results in increased prothrombin plasma levels and an increased risk of thrombosis. Prothrombin mutation is the second most common inherited risk factor for hypercoagulability; the point mutation occurs in approximately 2% of the general population. The changed gene is detected by PCR analysis of DNA.

Antithrombin III

Mutation in the gene that produces Antithrombin III can result in increased thrombosis. Antithrombin III (AT), when activated by heparin, neutralizes thrombin and other activated coagulation factors. A deficiency in this protein results in increased levels of coagulation factors which is associated with an increased risk of thrombosis. The frequency of antithrombin deficiency in the general population is approximately 17%. As of 2001, DNA testing for antithrombin III deficiency was not available on a clinical basis. Testing typically involves measuring antithrombin activity. Antithrombin is measured by a chromogenic substrate assay. Antithrombin is a serine protease inhibitor that blocks the enzymatic activity of factor Xa and thrombin. The plasma is mixed with heparin causing formation of the antithrombin-heparin complex. Factor Xa is added and incubated with the antithrombin-heparin complex. After incubation, an anilide-conjugated substrate is added. This reacts with factor Xa that has not been inhibited by the antithrombin-heparin complex producing a yellow product. Therefore, the amount of color is inversely proportional to the antithrombin activity of the sample.

Specimen requirements

DNA tests require 5 mL of whole blood in an EDTA (lavender top) tube and protein activity tests require 3 mL of fresh or frozen citrated plasma. Thrombosis risk panels require 5 mL of whole blood in an EDTA (lavender top) tube and 3 mL of fresh or frozen citrated plasma in 1 mL aliquots. The turn around times for thrombosis risk tests range from one to five days.

Thrombosis risk panels

Two thrombosis risk panels are used, one for patients not receiving Coumadin therapy and one for those who are.

Panel for patients not on Coumadin therapy:

- factor V Leiden DNA test
- prothrombin (Factor II) DNA test
- antithrombin activity
- protein C activity
- protein S activity

(This panel is less accurate and should only be used if discontinuation of therapy is not possible.) Panel for patients on Coumadin therapy:

- factor V Leiden DNA test
- prothrombin (Factor II) DNA test
- antithrombin activity
- protein C/factor IX antigen ratio
- protein S/factor IX antigen ratio

Preparation

If possible, Coumadin anticoagulant therapy should be discontinued at least two weeks prior to undergoing the thrombosis risk tests.

Aftercare

There are no post-test procedures required.

Complications

Excessive bleeding, bruising, soreness around the puncture site, fainting, and lightheadedness are possible complications of the blood draw. **Infection** is also an occasional complication.

Results

The type of results, interpretation, and management recommendations vary by type of thrombosis risk. Factor V and prothrombin DNA testing is fairly definitive. Test results for protein S, C, and antithrombin deficiencies are more difficult to interpret since environmental factors can influence the results. The clinical history and family history should be used to aid in the interpretation. It is important to rule out acquired protein S, C, and antithrombin deficiency prior to establishing a diagnosis. Acquired protein S deficiency is quite common and can be caused by factors such as: the lupus anticoagulant, pregnancy, **liver** disease, inflammatory conditions, nephritic syndrome, and thromboembolism. Liver disease can decrease protein C levels and oral contraceptives can increase protein C levels. Acquired antithrombin deficiency can result from mild liver disease, acute thrombosis, and heparin anticoagulant therapy. When the results are borderline, repeat testing and comparative studies of other family members may be appropriate. Protein activity testing cannot definitively differentiate those with one abnormal copy from those with two abnormal copies of an anticoagulant gene.

Normal values

These may be defined in mass units for immunoassay methods or as the percentage of normal for functional assays. Values presented below are representative of immunoassay and functional assays but will vary depending upon the method employed.

- antithrombin III: 20-30 mg/dL or 80-120% of normal
- D-dimer: less than 200 ng/mL
- protein C: 3-4 µg/mL or greater than 65% of normal
- protein S: 0.7-1.4 µg/mL or greater than 65% of normal

Health care team roles

The main role for the nurse is **patient education**. Patients with positive results need to be informed of the increased risk of thrombosis. Patients need to be reassured, however, that many people with a genetic predisposition to thrombosis remain free of symptoms for their entire life. Women should be informed that they have an increased risk of second- or third-term pregnancy loss and obstetrical complications such as preeclampsia, fetal growth retardation, and placental infarction. Patients also need to be counseled about the common environmental risk factors for thrombosis. Thrombosis risk tests are performed by a clinical laboratory scientist CLS(NCA)/ medical technologist MT(ASCP) or clinical laboratory technician CLT(NCA) or medical laboratory technician MLT(ASCP). Results of a thrombosis risk panel or test is interpreted by a physician. The physician also determines if further tests (e.g., Doppler ultrasound) are needed and directs any anticoagulant therapy.

Common environmental risk factors for thrombosis include:

- pregnancy
- oral contraceptive use
- estrogen therapy
- medications that are estrogen receptor modulators such as Tamoxifan and Raloxifene
- obesity
- **diabetes mellitus**
- presence of lupus anticoagulant
- smoking
- cancer
- surgery
- prolonged bed rest

Smoking should be discouraged in all patients with positive test results. Oral contraceptive use should be strongly discouraged in patients who are homozygous for the prothrombin or factor V Leiden mutations or who have a severe C, S, or antithrombin deficiency. Patients who are heterozygous for factor V Leiden or prothrombin G20210A or who have a mild deficiency in protein C, S, or antithrombin should be informed of the risks associated with oral contraceptive use.

It is important that the patient be informed of the hereditary nature of the disorder. Heterozygotes have a 50% chance of passing on the changed gene to their offspring and homozygotes have a 100% chance of passing on a changed gene. Homozygotes have inherited a changed gene from each parent. Heterozygotes have usually inherited the changed gene from either their father or mother. In some cases the gene change will occur spontaneously in the embryo at the time of conception. In these cases siblings and parents are not at increased risk.

KEY TERMS

Anticoagulant—A medication that prevents blood clotting.

Blood clot—The solid clump of accumulated blood factors that results when blood coagulates.

Cerebral brain thrombosis—Thrombus that forms within a blood vessel in the brain.

DNA testing—Testing for a change or changes in a gene or genes.

Embolism—A blood clot that has traveled from a different location.

Gene—A building block of inheritance, made up of a compound called DNA (deoxyribonucleic acid) and containing the instructions for the production of a particular protein.

Heterozygous—Changes in one copy of a gene.

Homozygous—Changes in both copies of a gene.

Mutation—Change in a gene.

Peripheral vascular disease—Narrowing of the blood vessels that carry blood to the extremities such as the arms and legs.

Neonatal purpura fulminans—A life-threatening condition in the neonate that results in small hemorrhages in the skin.

Placental infarction—An area of dead tissue in the placenta that is due to an obstruction of circulation in the area.

Preeclampsia—Pregnancy-induced high blood pressure that is associated with edema and protein in the urine.

Protein— A substance produced by a gene that is involved in creating the traits of the human body or is involved in controlling the basic functions of the human body such as blood coagulation.

Thrombosis—The development of a thrombus.

Thrombus—An accumulation of blood factors that often causes a vascular obstruction. Often used synonymously with the term blood clot.

Transient ischemic attack—A temporary blockage of an artery which supplies blood to the brain and lasts less than 24 hours. Often called a "mini-stroke."

Patients with positive test results should be encouraged to inform first degree relatives of their risks. It can sometimes be helpful to provide the patient with an informational letter about their test results that they can give to other family members.

Resources

BOOKS

Goodnight, Scott, and John Griffin. "Hereditary Thrombophilia." In *Williams Hematology,* 6th ed. Ed. by Ernest Beutler, Barry Coller, Marshall Lichtman, and Thomas Kipps. New York: McGraw-Hill, 2001, pp. 1697-1714.

Rodgers, George. "Thrombosis and Antithrombotic Therapy." In *Wintrobe's Clinical Hematology,* 10th ed. Edited by Richard Lee, John Foerster, John Lukens, Frixos Paraskevas, John Greer, and George Rodgers. Baltimore, MD: Williams and Wilkins, 1999, pp. 1781-1818.

PERIODICALS

Baglin, Trevor. "Thrombophilia testing: What do we think the tests mean and what should we do with the results?" *Journal of Clinical Pathology* 53, no. 3 (March 2000): 167-170.

Barger, A.P., and R. Hurley. "Evaluation of the hypercoagulable state. Whom to screen, how to test and treat." *Postgrad Medicine* 108, no. 4 (September 15, 2000): 59-66.

OTHER

Kimball Genetics. *Inherited Hypercoagulability Testing.* <http://www.kimballgenetics.com/tests-hypercoagul.html>.

Taylor, Annette. "Venous Thrombosis and the Factor V (Leiden) Mutation." *Genetic Drift* 14. <http://www.mostgene.org/gd/gdvol114b.htm> (Spring 1997).

Yeon, Christina. *Hereditary Thrombotic Disorders.* <http://www.medsch.ucla,edu/residencies/medres/ChiefFil/Heredita.htm> (October 3, 2000).

Lisa Maria Andres, M.S., GCG

Thyroid-stimulating hormone test *see* **Thyroid function tests**

Thyroid function tests

Definition

Thyroid function tests are **blood** tests used to evaluate how effectively the **thyroid gland** is working. These tests include the thyroid-stimulating hormone test (TSH), free and total thyroxine tests (FT_4, T_4), the free and total triiodothyronine tests (FT_3, T_3), the thyroxine-binding globulin test (TBG), and the T-uptake test.

Purpose

Thyroid function tests are used to:

- Help diagnose an underactive thyroid (hypothyroidism) and an overactive thyroid (hyperthyroidism).

- Evaluate thyroid gland activity.

- Monitor response to thyroid therapy.

Thyroid hormones regulate the rate of cellular activity and affect body temperature, appetite, sleep, and mental health. A low level of thyroid hormone results in myxedema. Although the severity of disease may range from very mild to severe, symptoms associated with hypothyroidism are anemia, malaise, intolerance to cold, hyperlipidemia, fluid retention, and depression. A high level of thyroid hormone causes hyperthyroidism. Classical symptoms include insomnia, intolerance to heat, weight loss, and rapid **heart** rate.

Both hypo- and hyperthyroidism can be caused by several mechanisms. Primary hypo- and hyperthyroidism are caused by conditions intrinsic to the thyroid, while secondary hypo- and hyperthyroidism are caused by pituitary-hypothalmic failure. T_4 is present in much higher concentrations than T_3, but T_3 is physiologically more potent. Thyroid hormones are active only when not protein bound (i.e., as free hormone). Circulating free hormone levels are regulated by pituitary release of thyroid stimulating hormone (TSH). The release of TSH is controlled by negative feedback. Increased blood levels of free hormone inhibit pituitary release of TSH.

Precautions

Many drugs affect the results of thyroid function tests without causing thyroid disease. Some common drugs known to depress thyroid hormone levels are dopamine, **corticosteroids**, lithium, salicylates, anticonvulsants, and androgens. Thyroid hormone levels may be increased by estrogens, clofibrate, and opiates. TSH, TBG, and T-uptake levels are also affected by many of the drugs cited above. In addition, acute and chronic illnesses and **pregnancy** also affect thyroid function tests. Such conditions may be confused with clinical hypo- or hyperthyroidism. When possible, patients may be asked to discontinue medications that are known to interfere with the tests several days or more prior to testing.

While most drugs that interfere with thyroid function tests do so by altering thyroxine-binding protein concentrations, peripheral conversion of T_4 to T_3, and other *in vivo* mechanisms, a few substances (mainly heterophile and autoantibodies) may interfere directly with the analysis. Such interference should be suspected by a physician who sees a test result that is inconsistent with the patient's symptoms or other thyroid function test results.

Description

Currently, thyroid testing is performed on plasma or serum specimens using immunoassay methods including enzyme-multiplied immunoassay technique (EMIT), cloned enzyme donor immunoassay (CEDIA), radioimmunoassay (RIA), fluorescence polarization immunoassay (FPIA), and chemiluminescence.

The high-sensitivity thyroid-stimulating hormone (TSH) test is the most sensitive and specific screening test for thyroid disease. TSH levels change exponentially with changes in T_4 and T_3 and are less likely to be elevated or depressed by nonthyroid illnesses or drugs.

This strategy is more cost-effective than a panel approach (e.g., TSH + FT_4 or FT_4 + FT_3) but necessitates the use of a TSH assay with a functional sensitivity below 0.02 mU/L. This level of sensitivity is required to differentiate primary hyperthyroidism, which causes levels to be near undetectable from the low end of the reference range, which is only 0.4 mU/L. A normal TSH level rules out clinical thyroid disease. Low TSH levels may result from primary hyperthyroidism or secondary hypothyroidism caused by pituitary TSH deficiency. High TSH levels are caused by primary hypothyroidism or secondary hyperthyroidism resulting from pituitary adenoma. Abnormal TSH levels are followed by measurements of T_3 and T_4 (preferably free T_4) to confirm the diagnosis. For example, a person with a low TSH who has primary hyperthyroidism will have an elevated T_3 and usually an elevated free T_4; a person with a low TSH caused by pituitary disease will have low levels of these hormones. Measurement of T_4 (and FT_4) is considered a more specific indicator of hypothyroidism than T_3, while T_3 (and FT_3) are more sensitive in detecting cases of hyperthyroidism than is T_4.

TSH levels are sometimes abnormal in persons with subclinical thyroid disease and in patients with severe acute or chronic illness (called euthyroid sick syndrome). These cases may require the thyrotropin-releasing hormone stimulation test (TRH stimulation test) and reverse T_3 test to determine if underlying thyroid disease is present. TRH stimulation is performed by measurement of the TSH level followed by IV administration of thyrotropin releasing factor. The TSH is measured 30 and 60 minutes after the injection. Persons with primary hypothyroidism show an excessive TSH response. The TRH stimulation test is usually normal in persons with euthyroid sick syndrome. Reverse T_3 forms from peripheral conversion of T_4 to T_3. Levels of rT_3 are low in persons with hypothyroidism and usually increased in persons with euthyroid sick syndrome.

Pregnancy, certain diseases (e.g., viral hepatitis), and several drugs (e.g., steroids) affect the level of thyroxine-binding **proteins**. In such cases, the level of total hormone will be abnormal, but the level of free hormone will be unaffected. FT_4 and FT_3 improve diagnostic accuracy for detecting hypo- and hyperthyroidism in patients with thyroid hormone-binding abnormalities that compromise the diagnostic utility of total hormone tests.

In cases where abnormal levels of thyroxine-binding proteins is suspected, two tests are helpful, the T-uptake test and measurement of thyroxine binding globulin (TBG). The T-uptake test [historically called the triiodothyronine resin uptake (T3RU) test] measures the available binding sites on TBG. The test is reported as the thyroid hormone-binding ratio (THBR). The THBR is determined by dividing the percent T-uptake of the patient by that for a normal sample. The ratio is high in hyperthyroidism and low in hypothyroidism. When thyroxine-binding proteins are reduced, the THBR is high; and when binding proteins are elevated, the THBR is low.

The thyroxine-binding globulin (TBG) test measures blood levels of this substance, which is manufactured in the **liver**. TBG binds to T_3 and T_4, and prevents the **kidneys** from filtering the hormones from the blood. Bound hormone is not physiologically active. The hormone-protein complex is reversible, and in equilibrium with free hormone levels. Therefore, when binding proteins such as TBG are increased, there will be an increase in the amount of total hormone.

Additional tests:

- Ultrasound exams of the thyroid gland are used to detect signs of growth and other irregularities.

- Thyroid scans using radioactive iodine or technetium (a radioactive metallic element) reveal the size and activity of the gland. Growths or nodules are seen and can be classified as inactive (cold) or active (hot) depending upon the amount of radioactivity present.

- Thyroid-specific autoantibodies. Autoimmune disease is the most frequent cause of both hypo- and hyperthyroidism. Commonly performed tests for thyroid autoantibodies are thyroid peroxidase antibody (TPOAb), thyroglobulin antibody (TgAb), and TSH receptor antibodies (TRAb). Although low levels of these antibodies may be found in healthy persons, elevated levels point to the presence of autoimmune disease that involves the thyroid.

- Thyroglobulin (Tg) methods are critical for the postoperative management of patients with differentiated thyroid carcinoma (DTC).

KEY TERMS

Cirrhosis—Progressive disease of the liver, associated with failure in liver cell functioning and blood flow in the liver. Tissue and cells are damaged, the liver becomes fibrous, and jaundice can result.

Clofibrate (Altromed-S)—Medication used to lower levels of blood cholesterol and triglycerides.

Graves' disease—The most common form of hyperthyroidism, characterized by bulging eyes, rapid heart rate, and other symptoms.

Hepatitis—Inflammation of the liver.

Hyperthyroidism—Overactive thyroid gland; symptoms include irritability/nervousness, muscle weakness, tremors, irregular menstrual periods, weight loss, sleep problems, thyroid enlargement, heat sensitivity, and vision/eye problems. The most common type of this disorder is called Graves' disease.

Hypothyroidism—Underactive thyroid gland; symptoms include fatigue, difficulty swallowing, mood swings, hoarse voice, sensitivity to cold, forgetfulness, and dry/coarse skin and hair.

Myxedema—Hypothyroidism, characterized by thick, puffy features, an enlarged tongue, and lack of emotion.

Nephrosis—Any degenerative disease of the kidney (not to be confused with nephritis, an inflammation of the kidney due to bacteria).

Reverse T_3 (rT_3)—An isomer of T_3 that is formed from deiodination of T_4 in the blood. It is not physiologically active.

Salicylates—Aspirin and certain other nonsteroidal anti-inflammatory drugs (NSAIDs).

T_3—Also called triiodothyronine. The more active of the two thyroid hormones.

T_4—The principal thyroid hormone, called tetraiodothyronine.

T-uptake test—Also known as the T_3 resin uptake test, this test measures the number of available binding sites on TBG.

Thyroid gland—A butterfly-shaped gland in front and to the sides of the upper part of the windpipe; influences body processes like growth, development, reproduction, and metabolism.

Thyroid-stimulating hormone (TSH)—A pituitary polypeptide that regulates the activity of the thyroid gland.

Thyrotropin-releasing hormone (TRH)—A neuropeptide produced by the hypothalamus that stimulates pituitary synthesis of TSH.

Thyroxine-binding globulin (TBG)—The primary thyroxine binding protein in blood.

Preparation

There is no need to make changes in diet or activities. The patient may be asked to stop taking certain medications until after the test is performed. Venipuncture is performed in the usual manner following standard precautions for prevention of exposure to bloodborne pathogens.

Aftercare

Aftercare consists of routine care of the area around the puncture mark. Pressure is applied for a few seconds, and the wound is covered with a bandage.

Complications

Generally, thyroid function tests are easily interpreted by a physician. However, under certain circumstances interpretation of results is less straightforward. According to an article published in the February 2001

issue of *Lancet*, one or more of the following features should prompt further investigation:

- abnormal thyroid function in childhood
- familial disease
- thyroid function results inconsistent with the clinical picture
- an unusual pattern of thyroid function tests results
- transient changes in thyroid function

Results

Not all laboratories measure all of the thyroid function tests that are available. Different methods may result in different normal ranges. Each laboratory will provide a range of values that are considered normal for each test. Some acceptable ranges are listed below.

TSH

Normal TSH levels for adults are 0.4-5.0 mU/L.

T_4

Normal T_4 levels are:

- 10.1-2.0 microg/dl at birth
- 7.5-16.5 microg/dl at 1-4 months
- 5.5-14.5 microg/dl at 4-12 months
- 5.6-12.6 microg/dl at 1-6 years
- 4.9-11.7 microg/dl at 6-10 years
- 4-11 ug/dl at 10 years and older

Levels of free T_4 (thyroxine not attached to TBG) are higher in teenagers than in adults.

Normal T_4 levels do not necessarily indicate normal thyroid function. T_4 levels can register within normal ranges in a patient who:

- is pregnant
- has recently had contrast x rays
- has nephrosis or cirrhosis

T_3

Normal T_3 levels are:

- 90-170 ng/dl at birth
- 115-190 ng/dl at 6-12 years
- 110-230 ng/dl in adulthood

TBG

Normal TBG levels are:

- 1.5-3.4 mg/dl or 15-34 mg/L in adults
- 2.9-5.4 mg/dl or 29-54 mg/L in children

T-Uptake (THBR)

Normal THBR levels are:

- 0.75 - 1.05 at birth
- 0.83 - 1.15 at 1-15 years
- 0.85 - 1.11 for adult males
- 0.80 - 1.04 for adult females
- 0.68 - 0.87 for second half of pregnancy

LATS

Long-acting thyroid stimulator is found in the blood of only 5% of healthy people.

Health care team roles

Thyroid function tests are ordered and interpreted by a physician. In difficult cases, an endocrine specialist may be needed. A phlebotomist, or sometimes a nurse, collects the blood, and a clinical laboratory scientist CLS(NCA)/medical technologist MT(ASCP) or clinical laboratory technician CLT(NCA)/medical laboratory technician MLT(ASCP) performs the testing.

Resources

BOOKS

Burtis, C.A., and E.R. Ashwood, eds. *Tietz Textbook of Clinical Chemistry,* 3rd ed. Philadelphia, PA: Saunders, 1999.

Fischbach, Frances Talaska. *A Manual of Laboratory and Diagnostic Tests,* 5th ed. Philadelphia, PA: J.B. Lippincott Co., 1996.

Pagana, Kathleen Deska, and Timothy James Pagana. *Mosby's Diagnostic and Laboratory Test Reference,* 3rd ed. St. Louis, MO: Mosby-Year Book, Inc., 1997.

Shaw, Michael, ed. *Everything You Need to Know About Medical Tests.* Springhouse, PA: Springhouse Corp., 1996.

PERIODICALS

Boschert, S. "Drugs can alter thyroid function test results." *Family Practice News* 29, no. 11 (June 1, 1999): 34.

Dayan, C.M. "Interpretation of thyroid function tests." *The Lancet* 357, no. 9256 (Feb 24, 2001): 619.

Kendall-Taylor, P., et. al. "Thyroid function tests. (Letter to the Editor)." *British Medical Journal* 321, no. 7268 (Oct 28, 2000): 1080.

O'Reilly, D. "Thyroid function tests time for a reassessment." *BMJ* 320 (May 13, 2000):1332-1334.

Tate, J., and F. Tasota. "Assessing thyroid function with serum tests." *Nursing* 31, no. 1 (Jan 2001): 22.

ORGANIZATIONS

The American Thyroid Association, Inc. Montefiore Medical Center, 111 E. 210th St., Bronx, NY 10467. <http://www.thyroid.org>.

The Thyroid Foundation of America, Inc. Ruth Sleeper Hall, RSL350, 40 Parkman St., Boston, MA 02114-2698. (800) 832-8321. <http://www.tfaeweb.org/pub/tfa>.

OTHER

Spencer, C. "Assay of Thyroid Hormones and Related Substances." <http://www.thyroidmanager.org/FunctionTests/assay-frame.htm>. Revised Aug. 1, 1999.

Victoria E. DeMoranville

Thyroid gland

Definition

The thyroid gland is a bilobed organ of the **endocrine system** located in the front of the neck. It secretes hormones that are involved in human development, growth, and **metabolism**.

Description

The thyroid gland is a small, butterfly-shaped gland made up of two lobes separated by tissue called the isthmus, which lies across the trachea. The lobes of the thyroid are each approximately 2 inches (5 cm) in length, and the isthmus is approximately 2 inches (5 cm) in width and length. The thyroid gland weighs approximately 1 ounce (28 g). Each lobe of the thyroid gland wraps around and is affixed by fibrous tissue to one side of the trachea. A narrow projection of thyroid tissue, called the pyramidal lobe, is often present and originates at the isthmus and extends up to and lays on the surface of the thyroid cartilage (Adam's apple). The upper projections of the right and left lobes are called the upper poles of the gland while the lower projections of the lobes are called the lower poles. The lobes of the thyroid lie between the larynx and trachea medially and the sternomastoid muscles and carotid sheath laterally. The thyroid gland can be felt through palpitation of the neck, unless the neck is very thick and short or the sternomastoid muscles are very well developed.

A thin capsule of connective tissue surrounds the thyroid and divides it into a cluster of globular sacks called follicles. The gland does not, however, have any true subdivisions, and the follicles are packed together like a bag of berries. The follicles are lined with follicular cells that secrete hormones called thyroxine (T4) and triiodothyronine (T3) and enclose a glutinous material called colloid. Colloid is primarily made of a protein called thyroglobulin that is involved in the formation of T4 and T3. Cells called parafollicular cells or C-cells, which secrete the hormone calcitonin, are found between the follicles.

Function

T3 and T4 hormones

The primary function of the thyroid gland is to produce and secrete T4 and T3, which are hormones involved in many aspects of growth, development, and metabolism. T4 and T3 are produced from thyroglobulin attached to iodide. Iodine obtained from the diet is absorbed through the **small intestine**, converted into iodide, and transported through the **blood** stream to the thyroid. The iodide absorbed by the thyroid attaches to thyroglobulin and forms monoiodotyrosine (MIT) and diiodotyrosine (DIT). T4 is formed when two DITs join together, and T3 is formed when

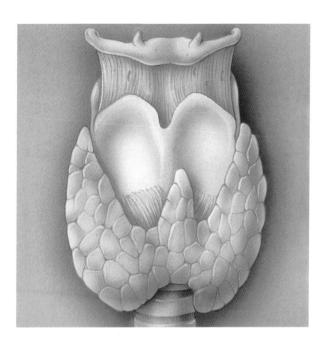

The thyroid gland releases hormones that are involved in growth, development, and metabolism. It lies on top of the trachea in the throat. (*K. Sommerville/Custom Medical Stock Photo. Reproduced by permission.*)

one MIT joins to one DIT. At this point the T3/T4 are still attached to the thyroglobulin. The thyroglobulin containing T4 and T3 is then transported to the center of the follicle where it forms colloid. When there are low levels of T4 and T3 in the blood, the follicular cells are stimulated to ingest colloid, and digest the thyroglobulin. This ultimately results in the release of T4 and T3 into the bloodstream.

REGULATION OF T3 AND T4 SYNTHESIS AND RELEASE. Thyroid stimulating hormone (TSH), which is also called thyrotropin, is the main regulator of thyroid hormone synthesis and release. TSH is produced by the **pituitary gland**. Binding of TSH to receptors on the thyroid gland stimulates the synthesis and release of T4 and T3. High concentrations of TSH result in increased thyroid hormone synthesis and release into the bloodstream, and low levels of TSH result in decreased synthesis and decreased release into the blood stream. The amount of TSH secreted is controlled by the thyroid-releasing hormone, which is produced by an organ called the hypothalamus. When the amount of thyroid hormones in the blood exceeds a certain level, the hypothalamus stops secreting thyroid-releasing hormone. This stops the secretion of TSH, which stops the secretion of T3 and T4. This process is called a negative feedback loop. When the levels of thyroid hormones in the blood stream decrease to below a predetermined level then the negative feedback is stopped and the secretion of thyroid-releasing hormone resumes. This ultimately results in resumed secretion of T4 and T3. The amount of T4 and T3 produced can also be influenced by dietary factors, such as the amount of iodine consumed and the total caloric intake, and can also be affected by inhibitory drugs such as the thionamides.

Calcitonin

The thyroid gland also secretes calcitonin. The thyroid's C-cells are stimulated to secrete calcitonin when there is a high concentration of **calcium** in the blood stream. The function of calcitonin is to inhibit the amount of resorption of calcium from the bone and to regulate the amount of calcium in the blood stream.

Role in human health

The hormones T4 and T3 produced by the thyroid gland are involved in growth, development, and metabolism, and it is likely that most cells are targets for these hormones. Some researchers feel that T4 is only an inactive prohormone, while T3 is the biochemically active form of the thyroid hormone. Some T3 is produced in the thyroid, but most of it is produced from the conversion of T4 outside of the **liver**. Receptors on cells bind some T4 but preferentially bind T3. The thyroid hormones stimulate the metabolic activities of most tissues and cause an increase in basal metabolic rate. Normal levels of T4 and T3 are necessary for normal development of the **brain** and normal growth in childhood. The thyroid hormones are also involved in regulating **heart** rate and increasing cardiac contractility and output. These hormones also have effects on the **central nervous system**, since decreased thyroid hormone levels are associated with decreased ability to concentrate and think, and increased levels are associated with **anxiety**. The reproductive system also requires normal thyroid hormone levels, and decreased levels of these hormones can result in **infertility**.

Common diseases and disorders

Iodine deficiency or excess

Dietary intake of iodine is necessary for the normal synthesis of T3 and T4. A deficiency or excess consumption of iodine can result in a deficiency in these hormones (hypothyroidism) or an excess of these hormones (hyperthyroidism). Iodine deficiency is less common in developed countries where table salt contains iodine. Disorders which lead to a deficiency

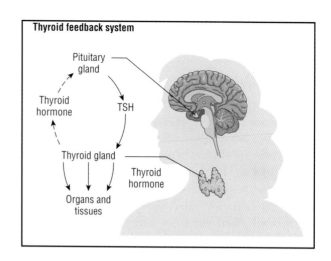

Thyroid feedback system

The thyroid gland produces T4 and T3 in response to a production of thyroid stimulating hormone (TSH) from the pituitary gland. (Delmar Publishers, Inc. Reproduced by permission.)

of iodide in the thyroid can also cause hypothyroidism.

Hypothyroidism

Hypothyroidism is the most common disease of the thyroid and results in deficient production of T4/T3 by the thyroid, or defects, which result in the inability of the body to respond to T4/T3. The clinical manifestations of hypothyroidism include:

- goiter
- fatigue
- constipation
- weight gain
- memory and mental impairment and decreased concentration
- depression
- loss of libido
- coarseness or loss of hair
- dry skin and cold intolerance
- irregular or heavy menses
- infertility
- hoarseness
- myalgias
- hyperlipidemia
- reflex delay
- bradycardia
- hypothermia
- ataxia

Hypothyroidism is usually confirmed when serum levels of T4 are decreased and serum levels of TSH are increased. In some cases, patients with hypothyroidism can have normal T4 or TSH levels or even low TSH levels. Hypothyroidism is typically treated by oral administration of a synthetic form of T4 called levothyroxine. Hypothyroidism can be classified into primary hypothyroidism, central hypothyroidism and peripheral hypothyroidism.

PRIMARY HYPOTHYROIDISM. Primary hypothyroidism is the most common form of hypothyroidism. Primary hypothyroidism is caused by factors affecting the thyroid gland itself, such as thyroid dysgenesis, environmental damage to the thyroid, inherited metabolic defects, and environmental factors such as medications that affect thyroxin synthesis. Primary hypothyroidism generally results in low serum levels of T4 and high serum levels of TSH.

The most common cause of primary hypothyroidism in adults in developed countries is autoimmune thyroiditis (Hashimoto's thyroiditis). Hashimoto's thyroiditis results when the body forms antibodies against the TSH receptors in the thyroid gland. This results in a decreased stimulation of T4/T3 production by the thyroid gland.

CENTRAL HYPOTHYROIDISM. Central hypothyroidism results from insufficient stimulation of the thyroid gland by the thyroid-stimulating hormone (TSH). Central hypothyroidism can result from abnormalities that interfere with the pituitary release of TSH or factors that affect the regulation of TSH by thyropin releasing hormone (TRH). Central hypothyroidism generally results in low serum levels of T4 and normal to low serum levels of TSH.

PERIPHERAL HYPOTHYROIDISM. Peripheral hypothyroidism is extremely rare and results when the body is unable to respond to thyroxin. The most common cause is thyroid hormone resistance, a rare, autosomal dominant disorder that results from mutations in the thyroid hormone receptor (Trbeta). Increased secretions of T4 and increased T4 in sera and increased levels of TSH characterize this disorder. Patients with this disorder have a 50% chance of passing it on to their offspring. Peripheral hypothyroidism can also be caused by massive infantile hemangiomas that excrete high levels of type 3 deiodinase, which inactivates T4.

Congenital hypothyroidism

Infants born with hypothyroidism are said to be affected with congenital hypothyroidism. In addition to the typical manifestations of hypothyroidism, congenital hypothyroidism, if untreated, can cause stunted growth, apathy, distended abdomen, swollen tongue, and mental retardation.

Eighty to 90% of cases of congenital hypothyroidism are caused by thyroid dysgenesis. Ten to 15% are due to inherited inborn errors of thyroid hormonogenesis, which are usually autosomal recessive and have a 25% recurrence risk. Congenital hypothyroidism can sometimes be caused by maternal radiation treatment during **pregnancy** or uncontrolled maternal hypothyroidism or hyperthyroidism during pregnancy.

Hyperthyroidism

Hyperthyroidism results from an excess amount of T4 and T3 in the bloodstream. The major symptoms of hyperthyroidism include nervousness, tremors, sweating, heat intolerance, palpitations, weight loss with normal caloric intake, amenorrhea, and muscle weakness. In the presence of clinical symptoms, the diagnosis of hyperthyroidism can be confirmed when serum measurements indicate increased T4 and/or decreased TSH levels. Hyperthyroidism can be treated through medications such as thionamides, which inhibit the synthesis of T4 and T3; and beta blockers, which block the action of thyroid hormones on peripheral cells. Patients who cannot be treated with medications are treated through radioiodine destruction of the thyroid or surgical removal of the thyroid. Surgical removal of the thyroid and sometimes radioiodine treatment can leave the patient permanently hypothyroid.

GRAVES' DISEASE. Graves' disease, the most common cause of hyperthyroidism, is an autoimmune disease resulting from the formation of antibodies against the TSH receptors in the thyroid gland. The only difference between Hashimoto's thyroiditis and Graves' disease is that Graves' disease results when these antibodies stimulate thyroid hormone synthesis rather than inhibiting it. Graves' disease results in increased synthesis of T4 and T3, and can result in exophthalmos, thyroid enlargement and goiter, and vitiligo. People with Graves' disease may pass on a genetic predisposition and a slightly increased chance of developing Graves' disease to their offspring.

OTHER CAUSES OF HYPERTHYROIDISM. Toxic adenoma of the thyroid results from a thyroid nodule that produces additional T4 and T3. This excess production of thyroid hormones results in increased concentrations of T3 and/or T4 in the bloodstream and suppression of TSH. Toxic adenoma can be treated through surgical removal of the thyroid, treatment

KEY TERMS

Adenoma—A benign glandular epithelial tumor.

Autosomal dominant—Mutation of only one gene of a pair is required to cause abnormal functioning.

Autosomal recessive—Mutations in both genes of a pair are required to cause abnormal functioning.

Basal metabolic rate—The number of calories that the body consumes when at rest.

Bradycardia—Slowing of the pulse.

Colloid—The gelatinous material made up primarily of thyroglobulin which is found in the follicles of the thyroid.

Cardiac contractility—The ability of the muscles of the heart to contract in the presence of a stimulus.

Endocrine system—A group of organs that secrete hormones directly into the circulatory system and affect metabolism and other body functions.

Exophthalmos—Protrusion of the eyeball.

Goiter—An enlarged thyroid gland resulting in a swelling on the front of the neck.

Hemangioma—Benign tumor made of newly formed blood vessels.

Hormone—A chemical produced by the body which is involved in regulating specific bodily functions such as growth, development, and reproduction.

Hormonogenesis—The production of hormones.

Lobe—Well defined segment of an organ.

Metabolism—Activity by which cells obtain energy from nutrients or use energy to perform basic body functions.

Thyroglobulin—Protein found in the follicles of the thyroid which is involved in the formation of the T4 and T3 hormones produced by the thyroid.

Trachea—Windpipe.

Vitiligo—A skin disorder characterized by depigmented white patches that can have a hyperpigmented border.

---

with radioactive iodine, and injection of ethanol into the nodule.

Hyperthyroidism can also be caused by a toxic multinodular goiter. Toxic multinodular goiter is common in areas of iodine deficiency. The multinodular goiter usually results from a goiter caused by hypothyroidism that eventually develops multiple nodules. These nodules produce excess T4 and T3

hormone independent of the TSH levels. Treatment usually involves radioactive iodine or surgery. Hyperthyroidism can also occasionally be caused from abnormalities such as adenomas of the pituitary gland, which result in an increased production of TSH. Infections of the thyroid gland can also result in hyperthyroidism. Uncontrolled maternal hyperthyroidism in pregnancy can cause hyperthyroidism in the fetus. In the past hyperthyroidism was occasionally induced when individuals ingested hamburgers containing ground up bovine thyroid gland.

Resources

BOOKS

Braverman, L. E., and R. D. Utiger, eds. *The Thyroid: A Fundamental and Clinical Text.* Philadelphia, PA: Lippincott Williams and Wilkins, 2000.

Falk, S.A., ed. *Thyroid Disease: Endocrinology, Surgery, Nuclear Medicine and Radiotherapy,* 2nd edition. Philadelphia, PA: Lippincott-Raven, 1997.

Fisher, D. A. "Thyroid Disorders." In *Principles and Practice of Medical Genetics.* Edited by D. L. Rimoin, J. M. Connor, and R. E. Dyeritz. New York: Churchill Livingstone, 1997, pp.1365–1377.

ORGANIZATIONS

The American Thyroid Association, Inc. Townhouse Office Park, 55 Old Nyack Turnpike, Suite 611, Nanuet, NY 10954. Fax: 914–623–3736. <http://www.thyroid.org/>.

OTHER

American Association of Clinical Endocrinology (AACE). *Clinical Practice Guidelines for Evaluation and Treatment of Hyperthyroidism and Hypothyroidism.* <http://www.aace.com/clin/guides/thyroid_guide.html> (1996).

De Groot, Leslie J., and Georg Hennemann, eds. *The Thyroid Manager.* <http://www.thyroidmanager.org/> (February 1, 2001).

Lisa Maria Andres, M.S., CGC

Thyroid radionuclide scan

Definition

A thyroid nuclear medicine scan is a diagnostic imaging procedure to evaluate the **thyroid gland**, which is an endocrine gland consisting of two lobes located in the front of the neck anterior to the trachea. The two lobes are connected by a thin band of tissue called the isthmus. The thyroid gland is stimulated by hormones and secretes other hormones that govern the body's **metabolism**. In a radionuclide scan, a radioactive tracer that is selectively absorbed by the thyroid is administered either orally or intravenously. Special equipment that can detect radioactive emissions from the thyroid is used to image the gland, or to measure the concentration of the radioactive tracer in the thyroid gland. The data collected are interpreted to evaluate thyroid function and to diagnose the presence of thyroid disease.

The radionuclides that are used in thyroid scans are two isotopes of iodine, I-131 and I-123, and an isotope of technetium known as 99 m Tc. Technetium scanning is preferred for some diagnostic workups because it is relatively fast and does not require the patient to fast beforehand. Some professionals prefer to reserve I-131 for follow-up evaluations of **cancer** patients, and use I-123 for thyroid uptake tests and routine thyroid scans. The reason for the distinction is the higher radiation burden of I-131.

Purpose

Thyroid scans are performed to determine the size, shape, location, and relative function of the thyroid gland. More specifically, a thyroid scan may be ordered by a physician to assess thyroid nodules; to diagnose the cause of thyrotoxicosis (excessive thyroid secretion); to evaluate patients with a history of radiation therapy of the head or neck; or to assess a goiter. A thyroid scan is also used to detect the presence of ectopic thyroid tissue. If the patient had abnormal results from a **blood** test that measures circulating thyroid hormone levels, a scan may be required to aid in diagnosis of the presence of thyroid disease. In some instances, an additional study performed in conjunction with a thyroid scan, called a radioactive iodine uptake, or RAIU, is required to determine the level of glandular functioning.

Precautions

Although thyroid scans use only low doses of radioactive substances, women who are pregnant are cautioned not to have these tests unless the physician indicates that the benefit outweighs the risk. If the patient is breastfeeding, she may be advised to interrupt nursing, depending upon the radionuclide used and the dose administered for the test.

Description

Thyroid scans are most often performed in a nuclear medicine or radiology facility, either in an outpatient x-ray center or a hospital department. If radioactive iodine is given, it is administered either in the form of a tasteless liquid or a capsule. If radioactive technetium is used, the patient is given an intravenous injection. Images of the thyroid gland are obtained at a specified amount of time afterward, depending on the radionuclide administered.

Typically, if radioactive iodine is used, an RAIU is also performed. Uptakes are usually obtained at two and 24 hours after administration of the radioactive iodine. The patient is positioned in front of a piece of equipment that measures the concentration of radioactive substance in the thyroid gland. The uptake procedure takes only a few minutes and the scan is most often performed at 24 hours after administration. If technetium is administered, the scan is performed approximately 20–30 minutes after the injection.

For the thyroid scan, the patient is positioned lying down on his or her back, with the head tilted slightly backward. The radionuclide scanner, also called a gamma camera, is positioned above the thyroid area. This procedure takes 30–60 minutes. There is no discomfort involved with either the uptake test or the scan.

Preparation

Some medications may interfere with thyroid studies. If a patient is taking thyroid replacement hormone or anti-thyroid medication, the medication must be discontinued for a specified period of time, usually several weeks. Other recent nuclear medicine scans can affect thyroid studies if there is any residual radiation in the patient's body. In these cases the thyroid scan is postponed for a specified period of time, depending upon the other radioactive material that was used.

X-ray studies using contrast material containing iodine that were performed within the previous 60–90 days will affect thyroid studies using radioactive iodine. Patients should tell their doctors if they have had either of these types of studies before a thyroid scan.

Some over-the-counter medications, herbal supplements, and **vitamins** contain large amounts of iodine or such iodine-rich substances as kelp (a type of seaweed), and therefore should be discontinued for a specified time prior to a thyroid scan.

Some institutions prefer that the patient have nothing to eat or drink after midnight on the day before the scan. Most departments provide detailed written instructions regarding preparation for the scan, including dietary restrictions. A normal diet can usually be resumed two hours after the radioisotope is taken. Jewelry and other metallic objects worn around the neck must be removed before the scanning. No other physical preparation is necessary. Patients should understand that there is no danger of radiation exposure to themselves or others. Only very small amounts of the radioactive tracer are used. The total amount of radiation absorbed is often less than the dose received from ordinary x rays. The scanner or camera does not emit any radiation, but detects and records it from the patient.

Aftercare

No isolation or special precautions are needed after a thyroid scan. The patient should check with his or her physician about restarting any medications that were stopped before the scan. Nursing mothers should inquire about resumption of breastfeeding.

Complications

There are no complications with this type of diagnostic study.

Results

Normal findings will show a thyroid gland of normal size, shape, and position. The amount of radionuclide concentrated by the thyroid will be within established laboratory guidelines. There should be no areas where the concentration of radionuclide is increased or decreased. An area of increased radionuclide uptake may be called a hot nodule or "hot spot," and may represent a hyperfunctioning nodule. An area of decreased radionuclide uptake may be called a cold nodule or "cold spot." This finding indicates that a particular area of the thyroid gland is underactive or low-functioning. A variety of conditions, including cysts, localized inflammation, or cancer may produce a cold spot.

Abnormal findings for an RAIU would include abnormally high and abnormally low uptake of the radioactive iodine. A low RAIU suggests hypothyroidism; a high RAIU points to a hyperthyroid condition.

A thyroid scan is rarely sufficient to establish a clear diagnosis by itself. The data collected from a thyroid scan are usually combined with data from blood tests that measure circulating thyroid hormone levels to establish the diagnosis. If nodules are present, a **thyroid ultrasound** may be performed.

The data collected are typically stored in a computer, and the images of the thyroid gland are made on

---

KEY TERMS

Ectopic thyroid—Congenital thyroid tissue found outside the normal location of the thyroid gland, usually under the breastbone or the tongue.

Endocrine—A type of gland that secretes internally into the blood or lymph.

Goiter—Enlargement of the thyroid gland along the front and sides of the neck.

Isotope—One of two or more forms of a chemical element having the same atomic number but having different atomic weights.

Nodule—A small, rounded lump or mass of tissue.

Radionuclide—A substance that emits radiation as it disintegrates.

Technetium—A synthetic element obtained from the fission of uranium. Technetium is used for some types of radionuclide thyroid scans.

Thyrotoxicosis—A disorder characterized by an enlarged thyroid, rapid pulse, and increased basal metabolism due to excessive thyroid secretion. Thyrotoxicosis is sometimes called Graves' disease.

---

film or paper. The results for an RAIU are expressed as a mathematical equation and are reported as a percentage.

Health care team roles

A nuclear medicine technologist administers the radioactive substance to the patient and operates the equipment that produces the scan. The nuclear medicine technologist obtains pertinent medical history from the patient and will explain the nature of the test. All data collected by the technologist are interpreted by a physician who is a specialist in nuclear medicine or a radiologist. Patients usually obtain the test results from their physician or the physician who requested the thyroid tests.

Resources

BOOKS

Goldsmith, Stanley J. "Endocrine System." In *Nuclear Medicine*, ed. D. R. Bernier et al. St. Louis, MO: Mosby, 1997.

Klingensmith, William C. III, Dennis Eshima, and John Goddard. *Nuclear Medicine Procedure Manual 2000-2001*. Englewood, CO: Oxford Medical Inc., 2000.

OTHER

Feld, Stanley. *AACE Clinical Practice Guidelines for the Diagnosis and Management of Thyroid Nodules*. New York: American Association of Clinical Endocrinologists, 1996.

Christine Miner Minderovic, B.S., R.T., R.D.M.S.

Thyroid sonogram *see* **Thyroid ultrasound**

Thryoid ultrasound

Definition

A thyroid ultrasound, or sonogram, is a diagnostic imaging technique used to evaluate the structure of the **thyroid gland**. The thyroid is an endocrine gland, which means that it releases its secretions directly into the bloodstream or lymph. It consists of two lobes located in the front of the neck that are connected by a thin band of tissue called the isthmus, which lies in front of the trachea (windpipe). Ultrasound procedures utilize high frequency sound waves to obtain images of various anatomical structures. Ultrasonography is the most common imaging technique used to evaluate the thyroid because it is not invasive, does not expose patients to radioactive materials, is less expensive than **CT scans** or MRI, and is more effective in detecting small lesions on the thyroid.

Purpose

An ultrasound of the thyroid is performed to evaluate thyroid nodules discovered during a **physical examination** or revealed by a radionuclide study (thyroid scan). A sonogram is most useful when the physician must distinguish between cystic lesions and solid ones, or evaluate any mass in the neck. In many cases the ultrasound examination identifies additional nodules in the thyroid that are too small for the doctor to feel during the external physical examination.

Most thyroid cysts are benign; however, ultrasound imaging cannot be used to differentiate between benign cysts or nodules and **cancer**. Specialized thyroid sonograms, such as color Doppler flow studies, can add valuable information. By showing an image of the **blood** circulation in the gland, this study can assess some ambiguous masses in greater detail. The shade and intensity of the color indicate the direction and the velocity of the flow. The physician may insert a needle in order to remove some tissue for laboratory evaluation (needle biopsy or fine needle aspiration).

Ultrasound is used during this procedure to help the physician guide the needle into the mass under evaluation. The use of color Doppler flow helps the physician to avoid puncturing a blood vessel while collecting the tissue sample.

Thyroid ultrasound can measure the size of the gland with great precision, and may be done periodically to assess the results of treatment. An enlarged thyroid gland or a benign nodule should decrease in size with appropriate medication. In addition, patients who have had **radiotherapy** of the head or neck may be monitored at regular intervals using thyroid ultrasound. Patients who had radiation treatment in these areas in childhood or adolescence have a 30% risk of developing thyroid cancer or other glandular abnormalities in adult life. In the early stages, these conditions may not cause symptoms or be discovered during a physical examination. They may, however, be detected by ultrasound.

Precautions

Thyroid ultrasound is safe for people of all ages. It is the preferred procedure to evaluate suspected disease in pregnant women because no radioactive materials are involved.

Description

Thyroid ultrasonograms may be performed in an outpatient facility or in a hospital department. The patient usually lies on his or her back, although the procedure can also be done with the patient in a sitting position. A pillow or rolled towel is placed under the shoulders and upper back, allowing the head to tilt back (hyperextend). A gel that enhances sound transmission is spread over the thyroid area. The technologist then gently places a transducer, an instrument that both emits and receives sound waves, against the skin. The transducer is about the size of an electric shaver and is moved over the thyroid area. The most common frequencies used for thyroid ultrasound are between 7.5 and 10 megahertz (mHz). The patient should not experience any discomfort from the procedure. The examination takes 15–30 minutes.

The high-frequency sound waves emitted by the transducer are transmitted or reflected differently by different body tissues and structures. Bone and cartilage block the passage of the sound waves, producing a very bright signal. The windpipe, which is filled with air, does not transmit ultrasound waves. Most tissues do, however, transmit the sound waves to a greater or lesser extent. Fluid-filled structures, such as cysts,

KEY TERMS

Endocrine—A type of gland that secretes internally into the blood or lymph.

Fine needle aspiration (FNA)—A technique for diagnosing thyroid nodules by withdrawing, or aspirating, a sample of thyroid tissue cells through a 22–29-gauge needle.

Goiter—Enlargement of the thyroid gland along the front and sides of the neck.

Nodule—A small, rounded lump or mass of tissue.

Sonogram—Another word that is sometimes used for an ultrasound examination.

Thyroiditis—Inflammation of the thyroid gland. Chronic thyroiditis is sometimes called Hashimoto's disease.

Transducer—A device that converts a signal from one form of energy to another. In an ultrasound examination, the transducer converts an electrical current to sound waves and echoes from the sound waves back into electrical current.

have a uniform appearance. Muscles, organs, and other fleshy structures have a ground-glass appearance; that is, they appear to diffuse light.

Preparation

Some facilities recommend limiting food and drink for one hour before the study to prevent discomfort. No other preparation is needed.

Aftercare

No special restrictions or procedures are needed after a thyroid ultrasound.

Complications

There are no risks or complications with this procedure.

Results

A normal study will demonstrate a thyroid gland of normal size, shape, position, and uniform echotexture. A thyroid gland that measures outside of the normal limits suggests a goiter. If the overall echotexture or pattern of reflected sound waves is mottled and uneven, the pattern may indicate the presence of thyroiditis or other inflammatory disease. Lesions, both solid and cystic, are easily visualized on ultrasound examination.

Health care team roles

The ultrasound examination is performed by an ultrasound technologist, or diagnostic medical sonographer. The sonographer will review any medical history provided and may need to obtain additional information from the patient. All information obtained from the ultrasound is interpreted by a physician who is a radiologist or, in some cases, an endocrinologist. Patients typically receive the results of the examination from the doctor who ordered the test. This physician will correlate the results of the sonogram with the patient's history as well as findings from the physical examination, **thyroid function tests**, and nuclear medicine tests.

Resources

BOOKS

Kawanamura, Diane M., PhD, ed. *Abdomen and Superficial Structures*, 2nd ed. Philadelphia: Lippincott, 1997.

PERIODICALS

Rifat, Sami F., and Mack T. Ruffin. "Management of Thyroid Nodules." *American Family Physician* 50 (September 15, 1994): 785-791.

OTHER

Blum, Manfred, MD. *Ultrasonography of the Thyroid*, revised March 2001. <http://www.thyroidmanager.org>.

Feld, Stanley, MD. *AACE Clinical Practice Guidelines for the Diagnosis and Management of Thyroid Nodules*. New York: American Association of Clinical Endocrinologists, 1996.

Christine Miner Minderovic, B.S., R.T. R.D.M.S.

Thyroid x ray *see* **Thyroid radionuclide scan**

Thyroxine test *see* **Thyroid function tests**

Tics *see* **Movement disorders**

Tilt table test

Definition

Tilt table testing is a medical test designed to study how the human **heart** adapts to changes in position.

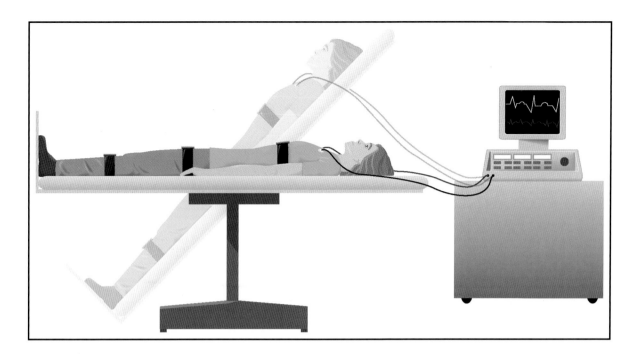

(Illustration by GGS Information Services, Inc. The Gale Group.)

Purpose

The American College of Cardiology considers the use of head-up tilt table testing to be the best means of evaluating symptoms and potential treatment for vasovagal **syncope**. More than 7 million Americans suffer from common fainting spells, but only recently has this standardized method been used to determine the root cause of these episodes. Syncope accounts for about 3% of all emergency room visits and nearly 6% of hospital admissions. Overall, it is believed that 6 million Americans are affected, and that vasovagal fainting (common fainting) is the most common type of syncope.

Syncope can be described as a pathological brief loss of consciousness caused by a temporary deficiency of oxygen in the **brain**. It is called by many other names, including:

- neurally-mediated hypotension
- fainting reflex
- neurocardiogenic syncope
- vasodepressor syncope
- vasovagal reflex
- autonomic dysfunction

The **autonomic nervous system** normally compensates for the fact that **blood** pools in the legs when a person suddenly stands up, decreasing the volume of blood available to the heart and eventually the brain.

Communication between the brain and the rest of the body causes a rush of adrenaline to be sent into the bloodstream. This speeds up the heart rate and causes the blood to be pumped rapidly and efficiently to necessary areas, especially the heart and brain. When the necessary communication from the brain does not occur or is not received, the person feels light-headed or faint and may actually faint. This is basically what happens when someone gets out of bed or a hot tub too fast. When this occurs, it can often lead to difficulty in functioning and to injuries.

Tilt table testing is designed to study the human body's heart rate and **blood pressure** adaptations to changes in position. To perform the test, patients lie on their back on a table, which is then tilted to a 60° angle, and then an 80° angle. This positioning is an attempt to bring on an episode of fainting to determine whether the fainting spells are common or malignant. Malignant syncope, possibly caused by a heart arrhythmia or flutter, cannot be reproduced by a tilt table test.

The application of the tilt test as a diagnostic tool in the United States has doubled in the past decade. However, it is often not paid for by insurers, including **Medicare**.

Precautions

Precautions are few with the tilt table test, as the person is constantly monitored. However, when any drug is used with this test, the appropriate precautions for that particular drug should be observed. The physician should also be informed of any **allergies** to any sympathomimetic drugs, including several of the diet pills on the market, or of any serious heart-rhythm disorders, or that the person is not feeling well during the test.

Description

The tilt table test takes approximately one hour. Patients lie on their backs and are secured to the table by three straps, under the arm and across the abdomen, across the pelvis, and across the knees. While the person is in a prone position, blood pressure and pulse are taken and electrodes are put in place to monitor the heart. An intravenous line is started in order to provide fluids as necessary during the test. Special electrodes that measure the amount of oxygen going to the brain are placed on the forehead. The head of the table is then tipped upward to a maximum of 75° angle while heart rhythm, pulse, blood pressure, and oxygen saturation at the brain are continuously monitored. Isoproterenol, or Isuprel, a medication with similar properties to adrenaline, is often injected intravenously during the test to duplicate the normal reaction of the body.

Preparation

In order for a patient to make informed decisions about any diagnostic test or procedure, detailed information and description of the test to be performed need to be provided. The patient should understand the purpose of the tilt table test and the diagnosis that the physician is trying to confirm or rule out.

Aftercare

After the procedure, the patient is asked to move from the supine position to a sitting position, and is observed for a short period of time. When ready, the individual transfers from the sitting position to standing. After additional observation and taking of **vital signs**, the individual is allowed to go home.

Complications

Complications as a result of a tilt table test are very infrequent, but could potentially include significant changes in blood pressure while in the supine position, and any adverse reactions to any drugs administered during the tilt table test.

KEY TERMS

Sympathomimetic—A drug that mimics the effects of stimulation of organs and structures by the sympathetic nervous system.

Syncope—A loss of consciousness over a short period of time, caused by a temporary lack of oxygen in the brain.

Results

Normal results of the tilt table test should help the physician in assessing what may or may not be the cause of the syncope. Abnormal results include any pathologic reactions to the position changes or sensitivity enhancing techniques such as the administration of isoproterenol or other related drugs.

Health care team roles

In most cases, a licensed physician will be in charge of conducting a tilt table test; the physician may be a cardiologist or neurologist. Both registered nurses (RNs) and licensed practical nurses (LPNs) may assist the patient in understanding and preparing for the test, and monitor vital signs during the test. An RN may start the intravenous infusion, or attach and monitor electrocardiogram leads and oxygenation-measuring equipment.

Resources

PERIODICALS

Benditt, D. G., D. W. Ferguson, and B. P. Grubb. "Tilt Table Assesses Common Fainting Spells." *Journal of American Cardiology* 28 (1996): 263-75.

ORGANIZATIONS

National Dysautonomia Research Foundation. P. O. Box 211153, Eagan, MN 55121-2553.

OTHER

"Neurally-Mediated Hypotension Working Group." *Johns Hopkins Hospital.*

Joan M. Schonbeck

Tissue typing *see* **Human leukocyte antigen test**

TMJ *see* **Temporomandibular joint disorders**

Tocopherol *see* **Vitamin E**

Tongue *see* **Dental anatomy**

Tonsillitis *see* **Sore throat**

Tooth bleaching *see* **Cosmetic dentistry**

Tooth decay *see* **Dental caries**

Tooth development, permanent

Definition

Permanent teeth, which are also known as adult teeth, are the second and final set of teeth in the human mouth. There are generally 32 permanent teeth in an adult mouth—16 in the upper jaw and 16 in the lower jaw. The permanent teeth replace the 20 primary teeth, which are also known as baby teeth, milk teeth, or deciduous teeth.

Description

In the mouth, a combination of hard and soft tissue areas form the occlusion (bite). The teeth, along with upper and lower jaw bones, are among the hard tissues. The soft tissue includes the gums, tongue, and salivary glands.

Teeth, both primary and permanent, are used to chew and swallow food. Each tooth is divided into a crown and root. The crown is visible. The root grows below the gum and is attached to the jawbone. A pulp chamber located in the center of the crown houses pulp tissue.

The crown is covered with enamel, the hardest substance in the body. It is 95% calcified (mineralized). Cementum, a thinner material, surrounds a portion of the root.

Types of teeth

The shape of the crown determines the purpose of the tooth:

- Incisors have a straight edge to incise or cut food. The two central incisors in each jaw are also known as the front teeth, indicating their location in the mouth. A lateral incisor is located on each side of the front teeth. There is one root in each incisor.

- The canine teeth are located in the corners of the mouth, with two in each jaw. The canine teeth have pointed crowns and are longer than the other teeth. These teeth are used to grip and tear food. They are

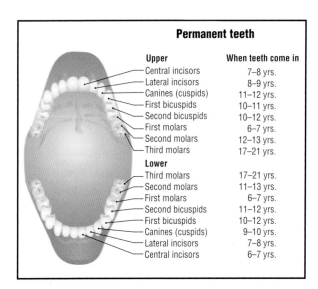

Permanent teeth

Upper	When teeth come in
Central incisors	7–8 yrs.
Lateral incisors	8–9 yrs.
Canines (cuspids)	11–12 yrs.
First bicuspids	10–11 yrs.
Second bicuspids	10–12 yrs.
First molars	6–7 yrs.
Second molars	12–13 yrs.
Third molars	17–21 yrs.
Lower	
Third molars	17–21 yrs.
Second molars	11–13 yrs.
First molars	6–7 yrs.
Second bicuspids	11–12 yrs.
First bicuspids	10–12 yrs.
Canines (cuspids)	9–10 yrs.
Lateral incisors	7–8 yrs.
Central incisors	6–7 yrs.

(Illustration by GGS Information Services, Inc. The Gale Group.)

also known as cuspids or eye teeth. Each canine tooth has a single heavy root.

- On each side of the six front teeth (incisors and canines) are five molars known as the back teeth. The crowns have wider surfaces that are used to chew food. On the surface of the molar are two or more cusps, slight elevations in the crown that are used to grind and pulverize food before it is swallowed.

- The premolars, which are also known as bicuspids, are located behind the cuspids (canine teeth). They help the canine teeth to grip and tear food. There are eight premolars in the adult mouth, with half in the upper jaw and half in the lower jaw. A premolar has one or two roots.

- The remaining molars in each jaw are used to grind food. The first molar, also known as the six-year molar, is adjacent to the second bicuspid. On the other side of the first molar is the second molar, the twelve-year molar. At the back of the mouth are the third molars, which are also known as wisdom teeth. The upper molars generally have three roots, and there are usually two or three roots in the lower molars. These roots help bolster the teeth for the heaviest pressure of chewing and grinding food.

Permanent tooth development

The development of both primary and permanent teeth starts long before these teeth are visible. When a child is born, the primary teeth are partially formed, and development of permanent teeth has started in the jaw bone.

At about the age of six, a child begins losing primary teeth and permanent teeth erupt (appear). The primary teeth fall out (exfoliate) to make room for the permanent teeth to erupt. Generally, girls' teeth develop before boys, and lower teeth grow through the gums before upper teeth. Development of this second set of teeth can sometimes continue into adulthood. A delay in the development process of two years or more could be a symptom of hormonal deficiencies.

TOOTH DEVELOPMENT IN THE UPPER JAW. According to the American Dental Association (ADA), permanent teeth in the upper jaw generally erupt in this order:

• Between the ages of 6 and 7, the permanent first molars erupt. These teeth erupt behind the child's primary second molars.

• Between the ages of 7 and 8, central incisors appear.

• Lateral incisors erupt between the ages of 8 and 9.

• Between the ages of 10 and 11, the first premolars (first bicuspids) appear.

• The second premolars appear between ages of 10 and 12.

• Between the ages of 11 and 12, the canine teeth (cuspids) erupt.

• Between the ages of 12 and 13, second molars erupt.

• Between the ages of 17 and 21, the molars known as wisdom teeth appear.

TOOTH DEVELOPMENT IN THE LOWER JAW. According to the ADA, permanent teeth in the lower jaw generally erupt in this order:

• Between the ages of 6 and 7, the permanent first molars and central incisors erupt.

• Between the ages of 7 and 8, lateral incisors appear.

• Between the ages of 9 and 10, the canine teeth (cuspids) erupt.

• Between the ages of 10 and 12, the first premolars (bicuspids) appear.

• Between the ages of 11 and 12, second premolars (bicuspids) erupt.

• Between the ages of 11 and 13, second molars erupt.

• Between the ages of 17 and 21, third molars (wisdom teeth) erupt.

CHARACTERISTICS OF PERMANENT TOOTH DEVELOPMENT. Permanent teeth tend to have a yellowish color and are generally larger than primary teeth. Since permanent teeth are larger, their development could crowd other teeth. For example, permanent incisors may be more closely spaced together than primary teeth, particularly in the lower jaw.

There could be space between the upper incisors. The eruption of the upper canine teeth will generally push those incisors together.

The premolars are smaller than the primary premolars. After the adult teeth erupt, the permanent first molars move and fill the space left by the exfoliated premolar.

The third molars are the last teeth to erupt, and there may not be room in the mouth for some or all four of the wisdom teeth. These molars have a tendency to be impacted (out of alignment) and may be unable to erupt. Extraction (removal) of unerupted wisdom teeth may be required.

MISSING PERMANENT TEETH. Some people may not develop all permanent teeth. This lack of teeth is believed to be genetic. The teeth most often missing include the lateral incisors, second premolars, and third molars. The absence of wisdom teeth is generally not a problem unless the third molars in the opposite jaw over-erupt.

EXTRA PERMANENT TEETH. Supernumerary teeth are those teeth in excess of the usual 32 permanent teeth. Most frequently, a supernumerary tooth erupts between the two central incisors in the upper jaw. This extra incisor is called a mesiodens (middle tooth). The presence of these extra teeth has been linked to two hereditary conditions, Gardners's syndrome and cleidocranial dysostosis. Because extra teeth can cause orthodontic problems, dentists generally remove them.

Function

Humans are omnivores, which means they eat meat and vegetables. Permanent and primary teeth make this possible. The location and shape of the tooth indicates its role in separating food into smaller pieces that can be swallowed and digested. The incisors incise or cut food; the canine teeth tear the food; premolars crush the food; and permanent molars grind it into pieces that can be swallowed.

Role in human health

Teeth allow a person to bite and chew food. Without them, a person could eat only soft foods. Teeth also contribute to understandable speech. For example, when a person speaks, the sound of a letter such a "t" is conveyed by the tongue striking the back teeth.

Permanent teeth: development and eruption

		Hard tissue formation begins	Eruption (years)	Root completed (years)
Maxillary	Central incisor	3–4 mos.	7–8	10
	Later incisor	10 mos.	8–9	11
	Canine	4–5 mos.	11–12	13–15
	First premolar	1.5–1.75 yrs.	10–11	12–13
	Second premolar	2–2.25 yrs.	10–12	12–14
	First molar	at birth	6–7	9–10
	Second molar	2.5–3 yrs.	12–13	14–16
	Third molar	7–9 yrs.	17–21	18–25
Mandibular	Central incisor	3–4 mos.	6–7	9
	Lateral incisor	3–4 mos.	7–8	10
	Canine	4–5 mos.	9–10	12–14
	First premolar	1.75–2 yrs.	10–12	12–13
	Second premolar	2.25–2.5 yrs.	11–12	13–14
	First molar	at birth	6–7	9–10
	Second molar	2.5–3 yrs.	11–13	14–15
	Third molar	8–10 yrs.	17–21	18–25

SOURCE: Ash, M.M. *Wheeler's Dental Anatomy, Physiology, and Occlusion.* 6th ed. Philadelphia: W.B. Saunders Co., 1984.

Common diseases and disorders

Tooth decay and injury can result in the loss of or damage to permanent teeth. Dentists should advise patients about how to prevent decay and injury, advice that includes cautions about sugar and the use of protective athletic gear.

Dental health

As permanent teeth develop, it is advisable for the dentist to see the patient every six months. The dental appointment includes the application of fluoride because newly erupted teeth are prone to tooth decay. The areas most susceptible to tooth decay are the chewing surface of the back teeth, the area where adjacent teeth meet, and the surface closest to the gumline.

The dentist may use a sealant (plastic coating) on the permanent back teeth (molars and premolars). The sealant protects against plaque, which produces tooth decay. If the dentist finds tooth decay, the patient's cavities should be treated with fillings. Small tooth-colored composites are recommended.

An adolescent patient also may experience gum inflammation known as **gingivitis**. Most cases are mild. However, the dental staff needs to remind the patient about the importance of a nutritional diet and **oral hygiene**. In addition, some teenagers may smoke

and should be cautioned that tobacco can harm the teeth and gums.

Accidents and injuries

Accidents and injuries can result in the loss of permanent teeth. As with oral hygiene, prevention is the best method of combating injury. Children and teenagers should be advised to wear sports equipment such as a baseball catcher's mask and a football helmet with a mouth guard.

If a tooth is broken or knocked out, the patient and tooth should be taken to the dentist as soon as possible. In some cases, the tooth can be repaired or reinserted.

Irregular development

Teeth may not develop according to the traditional pattern. A difference in the shape or size of teeth can affect the spacing of teeth. In addition to problems with the alignment of adjacent teeth, there may be a misalignment in the meshing of teeth in the upper and lower jaws. Common problems include large central incisors, or the "peg" lateral incisor that is thinner and has a sharper point than the normal incisor.

Missing teeth may also affect the alignment of teeth. Adjacent teeth can drift towards the empty area. This situation can also cause over-eruption of the opposing teeth in the other jaw. If several side teeth are missing, the person may have a collapsed bite.

Health care team roles

In the case of irregular tooth development or missing teeth, orthodontic treatment could provide adjustments. Regular dental appointments and daily oral hygiene that includes brushing the teeth and flossing can help fight tooth decay. Patients should also be advised to play safely.

Resources

BOOKS

Guerini, Vincenzo. *A History of Dentistry From the Most Ancient Times Until the End of the Eighteenth Century*. Boston, MA: Longwood Press, 1977.

Leonardi Darby, Michele, ed. *Mosby's Comprehensive Review of Dental Hygiene*. St. Louis, MO: Mosby, Harcourt Health Sciences, 1998.

Taintor, Jerry, and Mary Jane Taintor. *The Complete Guide to Better Dental Care*. New York: Facts on File, Inc., 1997.

Teabord, Mark, et al, eds. *Development, Function, and Evolution of Teeth*. New York: Cambridge University Press, 2000.

ORGANIZATIONS

Academy of General Dentistry. 211 E. Chicago Ave., Chicago, IL 60611. (312) 440-4300. <http://www.agd.org>.

American Dental Association. 211 E. Chicago Ave., Chicago, IL 60611. (312) 440-2500. <http://www.ada.org>.

American Dental Hygienists' Association. 444 N. Michigan Ave., Suite 3400, Chicago, IL 60622. (312) 440-8900. <http://www.adha.org>.

Centers for Disease Control and Prevention. National Center for Chronic Disease Prevention and Health Prevention. Division of Oral Health, MS F-10. 4770 Buford Highway, NE. Atlanta, GA 30341. (888) CDC-2306. <http://www.cdc.gov>.

National Institute of Dental & Craniofacial Research. National Institutes of Health. Building 45, Room 4AS-18. 45 Center Drive MSC 6400, Bethesda, MD 2089-6400. <http://www.nidr.nih.gov>.

Liz Swain

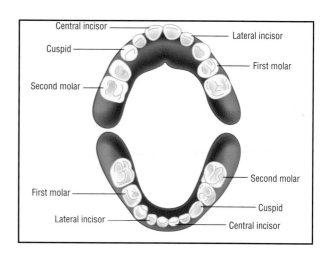

Primary, or "baby," teeth. *Illustration courtesy of Gale Group.*

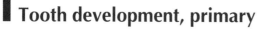

Tooth development, primary

Definition

Primary dental development involves the development of the primary, first, or baby teeth.

Description

The primary teeth usually begin to appear about six months after birth. Most children have all 20 primary teeth by age two. The eruption of teeth is associated with teething, a process often causing symptoms such as drooling, disturbed sleep, irritability, swollen gums, and, sometimes, a low-grade **fever**. While there are typical patterns of tooth eruption, these patterns can vary greatly from child to child.

Tooth development in the upper jaw

The primary teeth in the upper jaw are:

- Central incisors, which erupt between ages seven and 12 months and fall out around 6 to 8 years of age.

- Lateral incisors, erupting between nine and 13 months of age and falling out by the time a child reaches seven or eight years of age.

- Canines or cuspids, which appear around 16 to 22 months of age and fall out at 10 to 12 years old.

- First molars, emerging between 18 and 19 months and falling out at 9 to 11 years of age.

- Second molars, which come in at 25 to 33 months old and fall out at 10 to 12 years of age.

Tooth development in the lower jaw

The primary teeth in the lower jaw are:

- Central incisors, which erupt at six to 10 months and fall out at five to six years.

- Lateral incisors, erupting at seven to 16 months and falling out between seven to eight years of age.

- Canines, which come in at 16 to 23 months of age and fall out between nine and 12 years of age.

- First molars, emerging at 12 to 18 months and falling out at nine to 11 years of age.

- Second molars, which erupt between 20 and 31 months and fall out at 10 to 12 years of age.

Function

Teeth are for chewing and crunching food. They are attached to the tooth root, which anchors them to

Primary teeth: development and eruption

		Hard tissue formation begins (weeks in utero)	Eruption (months)	Root completed (years)
Maxillary	Central incisor	14	8–12	1.5
	Later incisor	16	9–13	2
	Canine	17	16–22	3.25
	First molar	15.5	13–19 boys 14–18 girls	1.5
	Second molar	19	25–33	3
Mandibular	Central incisor	14	6–10	1.5
	Lateral incisor	16	10–16	1.5
	Canine	17	17–23	3.25
	First molar	15.5	14–18	2.25
	Second molar	18	23–31 boys 24–30 girls	3

SOURCE: Lunt, R.C. and D.B. Law. "A review of the chronology of eruption of deciduous teeth." *J. Am. Dent . Assoc.* 89 (Oct. 1974): 872.

the jaw bone. The visible part of the tooth is the crown and its hard covering is enamel, which is the hardest substance in the body. The enamel covers a material, called dentin, which makes up the majority of each tooth. Deeper inside the tooth is the pulp, which includes nerve sensations and provides nutrients to the tooth. Baby teeth, like permanent teeth, include pointier incisor and cuspid teeth capable of tearing meats and rounder, flatter molars for grinding foods such as vegetables.

Role in human health

Primary teeth have many roles. They allow children to chew properly, helping them to maintain sound **nutrition**. Primary teeth are important for good pronunciation and speech and are a key aesthetic facial feature. Another function of primary teeth is that they guide permanent teeth and contribute to healthy jaw development.

Common diseases and disorders

Premature primary tooth loss

At times, primary teeth fall out or are knocked out too early. The resulting space might become too small for the erupting tooth, so dentists often fill the space with a space maintainer to ensure adequate room for permanent tooth eruption.

Dental decay or caries

Dental decay often begins in childhood. Caries, also known as cavities, start as an interaction between **bacteria**, which normally occurs on teeth, and sugars in the diet. The bacteria and sugars produce an acid, which causes teeth that are exposed to it to lose mineral. Cavities that form in the primary teeth can spread into the developing permanent teeth below. To treat the decay, the dentist has to remove it and fill the tooth with silver- or tooth-colored materials. The fluoride found in drinking water helps prevent cavities and has resulted in far fewer children developing **dental caries**. Dentists also use sealants to prevent decay. Sealants are clear or shaded plastic materials, which dentists apply to the chewing surfaces of the back teeth. The sealants coat the teeth and form a barrier to protect against bacteria.

Early childhood dental caries

Early childhood dental caries is a dental problem that frequently develops in infants that are put to bed with a bottle containing a sweet liquid. Bottles containing liquids such as milk, formula, fruit juices, sweetened drink mixes, and sugar water continuously bathe an infant's mouth with sugar during naps or at night. The bacteria in the mouth use this sugar to produce acid that destroys the child's teeth. The upper front teeth are typically the ones most severely damaged; the lower front teeth receive some protection from the tongue. Pacifiers dipped in sugar, honey, corn syrup, or other sweetened liquids also contribute to early childhood dental caries. The first signs of damage are chalky white spots or lines across the teeth. As decay progresses, the damage to the child's teeth becomes obvious.

Injuries, such as falls

Falls and athletic injuries can result in damage to the primary teeth and gums. Dentists should examine these injuries as soon as possible after they occur because they can often save teeth even if they have been knocked out of the socket.

Amelogenesis imperfecta

Amelogenesis imperfecta is a genetic defect in tooth enamel formation. It can appear as a localized row or pits of linear depressions or as generalized tooth discoloration, varying from white to translucent brown. Some children have no enamel at all, or their teeth might look hard or rough on the surface. Sometimes, the enamel of children with amelogenesis imperfecta looks soft and mottled. It can also appear

KEY TERMS

Amelogenesis imperfecta—An enamel formation defect.

Canines or cuspids—Second to last primary teeth on each side of the back of the upper and lower jaw.

Caries—Another word for dental cavity or decay.

Dentition—Development and eruption of teeth.

Fluoride—A chemical compound containing fluorine that is used to treat water or applied directly to teeth to prevent decay.

Malocclusions—Bite problems caused by malpositioned teeth.

Sealant—A thin plastic substance that is painted over teeth as an anti-cavity measure to seal out food particles and acids produced by bacteria.

honey-colored, yellow, orange, or brown. Dentists often treat amelogenesis imperfecta by placing crowns or fillings to restore the primary teeth. Fluoride supplements can help. Regular dental care to monitor amelogenesis imperfecta is important. It is not known how this condition affects the permanent teeth.

Bite problems and growth and development disturbances

Bite problems, or malocclusions, can be hereditary or caused by missing or extra teeth from birth, thumb sucking, or early loss of baby teeth. Bite problems can affect a child's appearance, as well as his or her ability to talk, eat, and digest foods properly. Dentists or orthodontists can help correct malocclusions.

Developmental abnormalities

Discoloration or deformation of teeth can occur in the primary dentition. The problem might affect a few of the teeth or the entire dentition. These defects can affect normal chewing, disrupt normal tooth development, and adversely affect appearance. Illness, high fevers, or some medications can cause unerupted teeth to erupt discolored.

Resources

ORGANIZATIONS

American Academy of Pediatric Dentistry. 211 East Chicago Ave., Suite 700, Chicago, IL 60611-2663. (312) 337-2169. <http://www.aapd.org>.

American Dental Association. 211 E. Chicago Ave., Chicago, IL 60611. (312) 440-2806. <http://www.ada.org>.

Dental Health Foundation. 26 Harcourt Street. Dublin 2. Ireland. 01-473-0466. <http://www.dentalhealth.ie>.

OTHER

"Dental Development." Dr. Sean McSorley's Web site. <http://www.gatewest.net/~mcsorley/tooth.html>

Lisette Hilton

Tooth extraction

Definition

Tooth extraction is the removal of a tooth from its socket in the bone. It is performed to control disease, improve function, or treat **malocclusion**.

Purpose

Tooth extraction is performed for many reasons. Teeth are often removed because they are impacted, that is, they cannot erupt normally on their own. Teeth become impacted when they are prevented from growing into their normal position in the mouth by gum tissue, bone, or other teeth. Wisdom teeth sometimes are impacted and require extraction. Teeth might also require extraction if they cause **pain** or cause crowding of other teeth.

Teeth may also be extracted to make more room in the mouth prior to straightening the remaining teeth (orthodontic treatment), or to make room for the placement of dental implants or dentures. Sometimes, teeth are extracted because they are so badly positioned that straightening is impossible. Extraction may be necessary because of severe gum disease or because the teeth are so badly decayed or broken that they cannot be restored. Patients also sometimes choose extraction as a less expensive alternative to filling or placing a crown on a severely decayed tooth.

Precautions

Tooth extractions may sometimes need to be postponed temporarily. Such situations include:

• When an **infection** has progressed from the tooth into the bone. Infections may make anesthesia difficult and can be treated with **antibiotics** before the tooth is extracted.

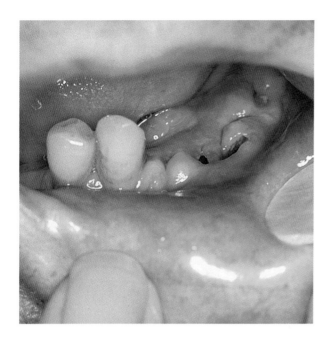

A close-up view inside a person's mouth following the extraction of the lower right molar. *(Custom Medical Stock Photo. Reproduced by permission.)*

- When a patient takes blood-thinning medications (anticoagulants), such as warfarin (Coumadin) or aspirin. The patient may need to stop using these medications for three days prior to extraction if medically advisable.

- When patients have had any of the following procedures in the previous six months: **heart** valve replacement, open-heart surgery, prosthetic joint replacement, or placement of a medical shunt. Such patients may be given antibiotics to reduce the risk of bacterial infection.

Description

Once the area has been numbed with a local anesthetic, an instrument called an elevator is used to loosen (luxate) the tooth, widen the space in the bone, and break the tiny elastic fibers that attach the tooth to the bone. When the tooth is dislocated from the bone, it can be lifted and removed with forceps.

If the extraction is likely to be difficult, the dentist may refer the patient to an oral and maxillofacial surgeon, a specialist trained to give intravenous sedatives or **general anesthesia** to relieve pain. Examples of difficult procedures are extracting an **impacted tooth** or a tooth with curved roots. This typically requires cutting through gum tissue to expose the tooth and

may also require removing portions of bone to free the tooth. Some teeth must be cut and removed in sections. The extraction site may require one or more stitches to close the incision.

Preparation

Before an extraction, the dentist takes the patient's medical history, noting **allergies** and prescription medications. A dental history is also taken, with particular attention to previous extractions and reactions to anesthetics. The dentist may then prescribe antibiotics, or consult with the physician and recommend stopping certain medications prior to the extraction. The tooth is x-rayed to determine its full shape and position, especially if it is impacted.

If the patient is going to have deep anesthesia, loose clothing should be worn that allows access for an intravenous line. The patient should not eat or drink anything for at least six hours before the procedure. Arrangements should be made for a friend or relative to drive the patient home afterwards.

Women who take oral contraceptives are twice as likely to develop dry socket, a common complication in which a **blood** clot does not properly fill the empty socket after extraction. Women taking birth control pills should try to schedule their extractions during the last week of their cycle to coincide with low estrogen levels.

Aftercare

An important goal of aftercare is achieving clot formation at the extraction site. The patient should put pressure on the area by biting gently on a roll or wad of gauze for several hours after surgery. Once the clot is formed, it should not be disturbed. The patient should not rinse, spit, drink with a straw, or smoke for at least 24 hours after the extraction and preferably longer. Vigorous **exercise** should be avoided for the first three to five days.

For the first two days after the procedure, the patient should drink liquids without using a straw and eat only soft foods. Any chewing should be done on the side away from the extraction site. The mouth may be gently cleaned with a toothbrush, but the extraction area should not be scrubbed.

Facial swelling is a normal part of the healing process and is most pronounced in the first 48 to 72 hours. Wrapped ice packs can be applied to help it. As swelling subsides, the patient may experience muscle stiffness. Moist heat and gentle exercise usually

KEY TERMS

Dental implants—Anchors placed on bone, which are used to secure bridges, partials or dentures.

Dry socket—A painful condition following tooth extraction in which a blood clot does not properly fill the empty socket. Dry socket leaves the underlying bone exposed to air and food.

Extraction site—The empty tooth socket following removal of the tooth.

Impacted tooth—A tooth that is in an abnormal position or is growing against another tooth or a bone so that it cannot erupt normally.

Luxate—To loosen or dislocate the tooth from the socket.

Oral and maxillofacial surgeon—A dentist who specializes in surgical procedures of the mouth, including extractions.

Orthodontic treatment—The process of straightening teeth to correct orofacial appearance and function.

Wisdom teeth—The third molars.

restores normal jaw movement. The dentist may prescribe medications to relieve postoperative pain.

Complications

Potential complications of tooth extraction include temporary numbness from nerve irritation and jaw joint pain, which usually resolve with time but can be treated with over-the-counter pain-killing medications. Antibiotics are given if postoperative infection develops. If dry socket occurs, the dentist must wash out the area and pack the socket with an antiseptic paste and cover it with a dressing. These dressings must typically be changed a few times by the dentist before the problem resolves. Jaw fracture or bone fragments left behind in the gum are unusual complications that may require further surgical intervention.

Results

After an extraction, the wound usually closes in about two weeks. It takes three to six months for the bone and soft tissue to restructure. Complications such as infection or dry socket may prolong the healing time.

Health care team roles

Dental assistants and dental hygienists can assist with taking pre-extraction x rays. Dental assistants usually prepare the room for the procedure and assist the dentist during the extraction, as well as educate patients about postoperative **home care**.

Resources

ORGANIZATIONS

Academy of General Dentistry, 211 East Chicago Ave., Chicago, IL 600611. (312) 440-4800. <http://www.agd.org>.

American Association of Oral and Maxillofacial Surgeons. 9700 West Bryn Mawr Avenue, Rosemont, IL 60018-5701. (847) 678-6200. <http://www.aaoms.org>.

Lisette Hilton

Tooth grinding *see* **Bruxism**

Tooth numbering *see* **Dental and periodontal charting**

Tooth polishing

Definition

Tooth polishing is the smoothing of all exposed tooth surfaces with a rubber cup, a brush, or by an air polisher driven by a slow-speed hand piece or water unit.

Purpose

According to the *Journal of Periodontology* an oral prophylaxis is the removal of plaque, calculus, and stains from the exposed and unexposed surfaces of the teeth by scaling and polishing as a means to prevent periodontal disease. A cleaning involves removing debris and extraneous matter from the teeth. Polishing makes the surfaces of teeth smooth. As a result of these procedures, the teeth are smooth and clean at the end of treatment.

Precautions

Historically polishing has been part of the oral prophylaxis appointment. Dental polishing was considered important for the removal of plaque and stain prior to a fluoride treatment to insure adequate uptake of fluoride in the enamel. Recent research by the American Dental Association has shown that

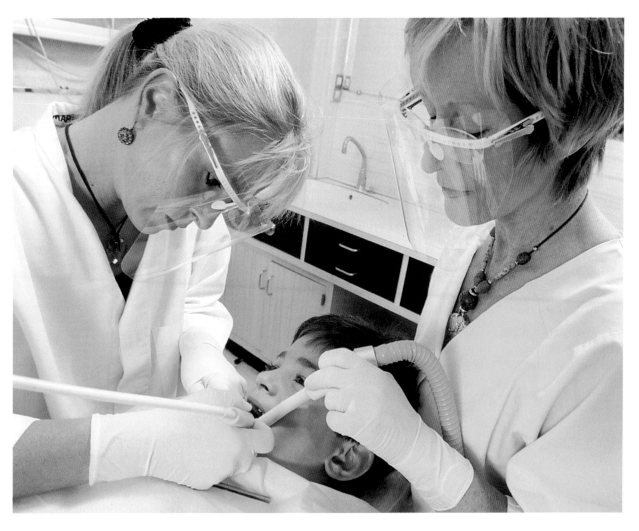

A dentist and her assistant clean a child's teeth. *(Mendil / Photo Researchers, Inc. Reproduced by permission.)*

polishing does not improve the uptake prior to a professionally applied fluoride treatment. Polishing prior to a sealant application has also been considered important, but recent research by the ADA again has shown that other methods of plaque removal are equally efficient.

The American Dental Hygienist Association (ADHA) considers that polishing of the teeth is a cosmetic procedure with little therapeutic benefit. Some have argued that continuous polishing over time can cause morphological changes in the teeth by abrading tooth structure and removing fluoride in the outer layers of the enamel. In some cases, polishing is required where there is heavy staining that cleaning with hand instruments will not take care of, but polishing should not be considered a routine part of the oral prophylaxis and the dentist and dental hygienist must assess each patient for the amount, type, and location of stain present to determine the need for polishing.

Air polishing was introduced in the mid-1980s. It is a technique for cleaning tooth surfaces efficiently removing stain and soft tissue deposits. The technique consists of directing a stream of air, water, and sodium bicarbonate particles at the tooth surface to be cleaned. Compared with conventional polishing methods using a rotating rubber cup or brush, together with a polishing paste, air polishing is less abrasive on the teeth, more efficient, faster, and allows better access to difficult-to-reach areas. Concerns over airborne pathogens associated with the air polisher have arisen, causing the ADA to study data on the matter. Data suggest that an aerosol reduction device attached to the air polishing unit is effective in reducing the number of aerosol microorganisms generated during air polishing, and that the air polisher is a safe unit to use.

Description

Dental polishing, or more commonly called coronal polishing, is performed when scaling has removed the hardened tartar buildup. The patient is assessed by the dentist and hygienist to determine whether coronal polishing is necessary. If it is deemed necessary, a coronal polishing will remove any stain buildup not removed by the scaling procedure. The duration of a polishing appointment can vary, depending on the amount of plaque and tartar buildup. Commonly, prophylaxis is scheduled for 45 minutes of the hygienist's time and 10 minutes of the dentist's time. The coronal polishing is billed as part of the oral prophylaxis and is considered a preventive measure, most commonly covered by major insurance companies at 100%.

Preparation

Premedication with **antibiotics** prior to the polishing treatment is required for those patients with **heart** disease or a history of rheumatic **fever**. This is a preventive measure, since toxins released during the cleaning and polishing may enter the **blood** stream and travel to the heart. Premedication prescriptions can be written by the dentist or obtained from the patient's medical doctor.

Aftercare

The patient is advised not to eat or drink for 30 minutes following a cleaning/polishing appointment, to allow sufficient time for fluoride uptake.

Complications

There are usually no complications associated with coronal polishing.

Results

The results of coronal polishing are smooth teeth free of tartar and plaque buildup. The results with the air polisher are smooth teeth, above and below the gum tissue.

Health care team roles

Licensed dental hygienists and dentists are best qualified to perform polishing procedures. Currently, 23 states in the United States allow dental assistants to perform coronal polishing. This raises concerns by the ADA and the ADHA because only half of these states require education or an examination in

---

KEY TERMS

Abrade—To rub off or wear away by friction.

Enamel—Outer most layer or coat of a tooth.

Pathogen—An agent such as bacteria that causes disease.

Registered dental assistant (RDA)—An individual trained for the specific purpose of assisting the dentist in dental procedures.

Registered dental hygienist (RDH)—An individual trained for the specific purpose of oral hygiene who performs teeth cleanings and gives home care instructions.

Scaling—The removal of food and debris from the portion of the tooth above the gum line.

Sealant—A clear coating placed over permanent premolars and molars to guard against tooth decay.

---

polishing for dental assistants. There is also a lack of standardization for education, examination, or certification for dental assistants among states. The ability to judge appropriately which patients should or should not be polished, is compromised if the practitioner is not knowledgeable about the procedure.

Air polishing should only be performed by a dental hygienist or dentist, as the direct flow and the exact amount of water used is crucial, depending on how much staining and tartar buildup is present.

Patients need to be made aware that coronal polishing research has changed today's procedures. Patients expecting to have their teeth polished after scaling might feel neglected and unsatisfied with the treatment. **Patient education** with literature and pamphlets relating to the research and the effects of coronal polishing, will help alleviate any concerns and greatly improve patient relationships.

Resources

PERIODICALS

Chava, Vijay K. "An Evaluation of the Efficacy of a Curved Bristle and Conventional Toothbrush. A Comparative Clinical Study." *Journal of Periodontology* 71 (May 2000). <http://www.electronicipc.com/JournalEZ/ detail.cfm?code=02250010710514>.

Muzzin, Kathleen B. "Assessing the Clinical Effectiveness of an Aerosol Reduction Device for the Air Polisher." *JADA: Journal Of The American Dental Association*

(September 1999): 1354. <http://www.ada.org/prof/pubs/jada/9909/ab-8.html>.

ORGANIZATIONS

American Dental Association. 211 East Chicago Avenue, Chicago, IL 60611. (312) 440-2500. <http://www.ada.org>.

American Dental Hygienist Association. 444 North Michigan Avenue, Suite 3400, Chicago, IL 60611. <http://www.adha.org>.

OTHER

ADHA Professional Issues. Position Paper on Polishing (2001). <http://www.adha.org/profissues/polishingpaper.htm>.

Deldent Ltd. (2000). *Air Polishers.* <http://www.deldent.com/air%20polisher.htm?tm>.

Cindy F. Ovard, RDA

Toothbrush *see* **Oral hygiene aids**

Toothpicks *see* **Oral hygiene aids**

Topical anesthetic *see* **Anesthesia, local**

Topical antifungal drugs *see* **Antifungal drugs, topical**

Topical medicine application

Definition

A topical medicine is a form of medication meant to be administered externally onto the body rather than ingested or injected into the body. Medicines administered to the eye, ear, and nose are considered topical medicines, will be discussed in separate articles. Topical medicine in this article refers to medicines applied externally onto the skin. Topical medicines available for external application include lotions, creams, ointments, powders (talc), and solutions (liquids). A specific dose of medication is prepared and suspended into a transport media such as a lotion. Topical lotions are water based and thin. They are absorbed quickly into the skin and are often invisible after application. Topical creams are thicker and are visible on the skin after application. They require more time for the medication to be absorbed into the skin. Ointments or unguents are the thickest form of topical medication. The medicine is suspended in a greasy substance that adheres to the skin until the medicine is absorbed.

Purpose

The purpose of using topical medicine is to deliver medication directly onto areas of the skin that are irritated, inflamed, itching, or infected. Topical medicines are often applied directly onto a rash or a irritated area on the skin for rapid relief of symptoms.

Precautions

Topical skin medicines should not be applied near the eyes or the mouth. They can cause stinging and irritation in the eyes and are not meant to be taken orally.

Description

To apply topical medicine, the health care provider places a small amount on gloved finger tips or a sterile gauze pad and spreads a thin layer of lotion, cream, or ointment across the affected area. Cover the affected area and overlap slightly onto the unaffected skin. A thin layer is usually sufficient. A thick coating may prevent air that is necessary for healing from reaching the wound.

Preparation

The health care provider should wash his or her hands and put on a glove before applying topical medicine. The medication label should be checked each time to avoid medication errors. Be sure it is the right medicine, the right dose (strength), the right time, the right person and the right method. Look at the expiration on the label. Do not use outdated medicine. Cleanse the affected area on the skin with warm water or a gentle soap and water. This will remove drainage and the residue of old medication. Rinse and allow the skin to air dry.

Aftercare

After applying topical medicine, the health care provider should place the glove and/or gauze used to apply the medicine in a trash bag that can be closed and discarded. The hands should be washed. If topical medicines are applied to skin on the hands, the hands may need to be wrapped in gauze to prevent the patient from accidentally rubbing the medicine into their eyes or mouth. **Wounds** or rashes with a lot of drainage may require special dressings after the topical medicine is applied. Wrapping the area with a sealed dressing such as saran wrap will increase the absorption of the medicine. Follow the physician's or advanced practice nurse's directions in these matters.

Complications

Applying excessive amounts of topical medicine can cause adverse skin reactions such as redness, itching, and inflammation.

Results

Most topical medicines, when applied properly, will produce the desired results within a few days. Contact the leader of the health care team if the skin condition deteriorates or the original condition does not improve.

Health care team roles

Administering any medicine is generally the responsibility of a licensed nurse (R.N. or L.P.N.). Unlicensed staff can be trained to administer topical medicine under the direction of a **registered nurse** in some health care settings. A licensed nurse, however, must observe the affected area routinely to evaluate the outcome of medication application. The patient or a patient family member can be instructed on how to apply topical medicine in the home setting.

Resources

OTHER

"Betamethasone/Clotrimazole. *Drug Information Corner: Johns Hopkins Health Online*. 2000. <http://www.healthandage.com/john_hopkins/drugs/betamethasonecl>.

"Corticosteroids-Medium to Very High Potency (Topical)." *Drug Information: Mayo Clinic Online*. August 2000. <http://www.mayohealth.org/>.

"Getting the Most Out of Your Medicines." *Drug Information: Mayo Clinic Online*. November 2000. <http://www.mayohealth.org/>.

Lesar, Timothy, PharmD. "Following Medication Instructions." *Albany Medical Center Health Update Online*. 2000. <http://www.amc.edu/gethealthupdates.cfm?healthupdatesid = 72>.

"Skin, Hair and Nails. First Aid and Self-Help." *Mayo Clinic Online*. April 2000. <http://www.mayohealth.org/>.

"Topical Skin Medications." *The Merck Manual Home Edition Online*. 2001. <http://www.merck.no/pubs/mmanual_home/>.

Mary Elizabeth Martelli, R.N., B.S.

TORCH test

Definition

The TORCH test, which is sometimes called the TORCH panel, consists of tests for antibodies to four organisms that cause congenital infections transmitted from mother to fetus. The name of the test is an acronym for the organisms detected by this panel: *Toxoplasma gondii* (toxoplasmosis), rubella (German measles), cytomegalovirus (CMV), and herpes simplex virus (HSV).

Purpose

Although the four diseases are not particularly serious for adults who are exposed and treated, women who are become affected with any of these diseases during **pregnancy** are at risk for **miscarriage**, still birth, or for a child with serious birth defects and/or illness. Thus, this test is performed before or as soon as pregnancy is diagnosed to determine the mother's history of exposure to these organisms. The test is also performed on neonatal serum when the newborn presents with symptoms consistent with a congenitally acquired **infection** by one of the organisms above.

Precautions

TORCH screening can be associated with both false negative and false positive results. False negative IgM tests can result from IgG antibodies to the organism binding to the antigen used in the test or from **immunodeficiency** syndromes that reduce the antibody response to these organisms. False positive test results can result from rheumatoid, autoimmune, or heterophile antibodies in the mother's serum. When testing neonates, the IgG antibody levels may be detected as a result of prior infection or current maternal infection, and therefore does not mean the neonate is infected. Maternal antibodies to HSV and CMV may not adequately protect the fetus. TORCH screening requires **blood** from the mother and if needed, the neonate. The nurse or phlebotomist performing the venipuncture should observe **universal precautions** for the prevention of transmission of bloodborne pathogens.

Description

The TORCH panel is performed on women before or during pregnancy and on newborns if warranted by risk of infection during pregnancy. Samples from infants are usually obtained by the heelstick procedure when only a small quantity of blood is

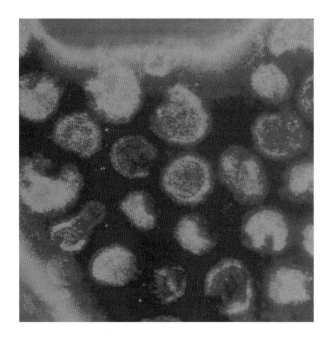

A colored electron micrograph of the rubella virus. (Custom Medical Stock Photo. Reproduced by permission.)

needed. The baby's foot is wrapped in a warm cloth for five minutes, to make the blood flow more easily. The foot is then wiped with an alcohol swab and a lancet is used to stick the baby's heel on one side. Blood is collected from adults by venipuncture. The blood is collected by a nurse or phlebotomist from a vein located in the crease of the arm. Serum, the liquid portion of the blood after it clots, is used for the test.

When a person is infected with a pathogen, the normal **immune response** results in the production of immunoglobulin M (IgM) antibodies followed by immunoglobulin G (IgG) antibodies. IgM antibodies against TORCH organisms usually persist for about three months, while IgG antibodies remain detectable for a lifetime, providing immunity and preventing or reducing the severity of reinfection. Thus, if IgM antibodies are present in a pregnant woman, a current or recent infection with the organism has occurred. If IgM antibodies are absent and IgG antibodies are present and do not demonstrate an increase on serial testing several weeks later, it can be assumed that the person has had a previous infection by the corresponding organism, or has been vaccinated to prevent an infection. If the serum of a person has no evidence of either IgM or IgG antibodies specific for the organism, then the person is at risk of infection if exposed because they do not have any demonstrable immunity.

TORCH testing is most often performed by enzyme linked immunsorbent assay (ELISA). These are double antibody sandwich enzyme immunoassays in which the antigens or organisms are bound to a solid phase such as the bottom of a plastic well. Dilutions of the patient's serum are prepared and incubated with the antigens. Any specific antibodies to the antigen will bind forming antibody-antigen complexes. The wells are washed to remove unbound serum **proteins**, and enzyme-conjugated antihuman immunoglobulin is added. The wells are washed again to remove any unbound reagent antibody and a substrate is added. If antibodies to the organism are present, the enzyme converts the substrate to a colored product that can be measured. Assays for IgM or IgG antibodies are available. Alternative procedures include latex agglutination, indirect immunofluorescence assay for toxoplasma antibodies, chemiluminescence immunoassay, DNA amplification, and viral culture.

The TORCH panel is used to determine the immune status of a pregnant female for *Toxoplasma gondii,* rubella, cytomegalovirus, and herpes simplex virus. If IgG antibodies are present at a concentration that indicates immunity against each of these organisms, the female is in no danger of contracting a toxoplasma or rubella infection during pregnancy and transmitting it to the fetus. In addition, there is a low probability of transmitting a herpes simplex or CMV infection, although the antibodies detected by the test may not be fully protective. If antibodies are absent, the patient will be observed closely during the pregnancy for any sign of suspected infection. Should an infection occur, it will need to be treated aggressively to prevent transmission to the fetus.

The organisms which comprise the TORCH panel are commonly encountered. Most people are exposed the them during childhood. In most healthy persons exposed to *Toxoplasma gondii*, the organism causes an asymptomatic infection or mild self-limiting illness resembling infectious mononucleosis. The same pattern occurs for CMV infection. Rubella causes an acute infection with **fever** and rash, but is self-limiting with symptoms subsiding in two to three days. Children and young adults are typically infected. Herpes simplex 1 typically causes fever blisters. The infections caused by TORCH organisms are grouped together because they may all result in stillbirth or serious birth defects when transmitted from an infected mother to her fetus during pregnancy.

The symptoms of the TORCH infections in neonates include:

• small size for gestational age (SGA)

• enlarged **liver** and spleen

- low level of platelets in the blood

- skin rash

- **central nervous system** involvement, including encephalitis, **calcium** deposits in the **brain** tissue, and seizures

- jaundice

This group of defects is called the TORCH syndrome. As such, other organisms causing serious congenital infections such as **syphilis**, human immunodeficiency virus, parvovirus, and enterovirus are sometimes considered part of this group. A newborn baby with these symptoms will be given a TORCH test and may be tested for some of these other infections as well.

In addition to these symptoms, each of the TORCH infections has its own characteristic symptoms in newborns.

Toxoplasmosis

Toxoplasmosis is caused by *Toxoplasma gondii*, a parasite that can acquired from ingesting cysts from the feces of infected cats, drinking unpasteurized milk, or eating contaminated meat containing the cyst or trophozoites. The infection is transmitted to the infant through the placenta, and can cause eye deformity, eye infections and mental retardation by invading brain tissue. The later in pregnancy the mother is infected, the higher the probability that the fetus will be affected. On the other hand, toxoplasmosis exposure early in pregnancy is more likely to cause a miscarriage or serious birth defects. The incidence of toxoplasmosis in newborns is between one to eight per 1,000 live births in the United States.

Rubella

Prior to the 1970s the incidence of congenital rubella infection was approximately 6.3 per 10,000 births. Ten years following the introduction of the vaccine the rate dropped six-fold to approximately one in 10,000 births. The rate of fetal infection varies depending on when in gestation the exposure occurred. Approximately 85% of neonates who develop birth defects as a result of infection during pregnancy contract the virus during the first eight weeks of gestation. Infants born with rubella may show signs of **heart** disease, retarded growth, ocular defects, or **pneumonia** at birth. They may also develop problems later in childhood, including autism, **hearing loss**, brain involvement, **immune system** disorders, or thyroid disease.

Cytomegalovirus

Cytomegalovirus belongs to the herpes virus group of infections. It can be transmitted through body secretions, as well as by sexual contact; some newborns acquire CMV through breast milk. Of newborns in the United States infected with CMV, 10% will have measurable symptoms. The mortality rate for these symptomatic newborns is 20-30%. Surviving infants with CMV may suffer from **hearing** loss (15%) or mental retardation (30%). Newborns that acquire CMV during the birth process or shortly after birth may develop pneumonia, hepatitis, or various blood disorders.

Herpes simplex virus

Herpes virus infections are among the most common viral infections in humans. They are spread by oral, as well as genital, contact. It is estimated that between one in 1,000 and one in 5,000 infants are born with HSV infections. About 80% of these infections are acquired during the birth process itself; the virus enters the infant through its eyes, skin, mouth, and upper respiratory tract. Of infants born with HSV infection, about 20% will have localized infections of the eyes, mouth, or skin. About 50% of infected infants will develop disease spread throughout the body (disseminated) within nine to 11 days after birth. Disseminated herpes infections attack the liver and **adrenal glands**, as well as other body organs. Without treatment, the mortality rate is 80%. Even with antiviral medication, the mortality rate is still 15-20%, with 40-55% of the survivors having long-term damage to the central nervous system. It is critical for the doctor to diagnose HSV infection in the newborn as soon as possible, for effective treatment.

TORCH testing is most effectively utilized to determine the mother's immune status and monitor those pregnant females who do not demonstrate immunity. TORCH testing of neonates is difficult to evaluate, since maternal IgG from either present or past exposure crosses the placenta and will often produce higher levels in the neonate than in maternal serum. The infant's IgM response may or may not be developed sufficiently at birth to be definitive, and false positive and negative results are known to occur. When neonates are tested, the TORCH screen should include testing for specific IgM antibodies, and should be repeated within two to three weeks to demonstrate a rise in concentration indicative of active infection. Viral cultures or DNA probe tests are required to make a definitive diagnosis of the specific infection. CMV can be cultured from urine and white blood cells; herpes simplex can be cultured from vesicles on the skin or conjunctiva (mucus membranes inside the eyelids); both CMV and rubella may be cultured from cerebrospinal fluid, but culture time for rubella can take several weeks. Cultures are performed by inoculating living cells such as primary monkey kidney.

Preparation

No special preparation, other than sterile technique, is required.

Aftercare

There is no special aftercare specific to the test itself. Discomfort or bruising may occur at the puncture site, or the person may feel dizzy or faint. Pressure to the puncture site until the bleeding stops reduces bruising. Applying warm packs to the puncture site relieves discomfort.

Complications

For the mother, minor temporary discomfort may occur with any blood test, but there are no complications specific to TORCH testing. For the infant, complications associated with the TORCH test are those resulting from the heelstick technique/venipuncture. These risks include scarring, infection, cellulitis (inflammation of cellular tissue), and small lumpy calcium deposits. Results of serological tests (antibody tests) on the neonate may be inconclusive. Follow-up testing may be needed to demonstrate a rise in antibody titre (concentration). Additional diagnostic testing and/or treatment is determined on a case-by-case basis, depending on results.

Results

A normal result is undetectable IgM antibody in the blood of either mother or neonate. The presence of IgM indicates recent or current infection. When specific IgM antibodies to TORCH antigens are found in the neonate, this indicates a very high probability of infection with the respective organism, and should be followed up by subsequent testing to demonstrate either a rise in titre or by viral culture or DNA tests.

For rubella and *Toxiplasma gondii*, the presence of a significant IgG titer in maternal serum indicates immunity for both mother and fetus. The presence of IgG antibody to CMV and herpes simplex in maternal serum may or may not be fully protective. When neonatal infection is suspected, TORCH testing of the

---

KEY TERMS

Antibody—A protein molecule produced by the immune system that is specific to a disease agent, such as CMV. The antibody combines with the antigen on the organism and facilitates its destruction or removal from the host.

Perinatal—Referring to the period of time surrounding an infant's birth, from the last two months of pregnancy to the first 28 days of life. The TORCH panel tests for perinatal infections.

Small-for-gestational-age (SGA)—A term used to describe newborns who are below the 10th percentile in height or weight for their estimated gestational age. The gestational age is based upon the date of the mother's last menstrual period. SGA is one of the symptoms of TORCH syndrome.

Titre (titer)—The concentration of a substance in a given sample of blood or other tissue fluid.

---

neonate may not be definitive. IgG antibodies in fetal serum may result from either current or prior maternal infection or **vaccination**. In such cases, an IgM level should be measured in both maternal and neonatal serum, and viral cultures or DNA testing should be performed.

Results for TORCH antibodies may be interpreted as negative, equivocal, or positive. Equivocal results occur when antibody levels fall within an index value below the low positive standard but above the negative standard. Testing by another method is recommended. In addition, serum from the patient should be collected and retested after waiting an additional 10-14 days.

Health care team member roles

The test is typically ordered and interpreted by a physician. Blood samples for the TORCH screen are collected by a nurse or phlebotomist. Pregnant women found to be exposed should receive treatment and a thorough explanation of potential consequences by their obstetrician. Counseling may be helpful. TORCH testing is performed by a clinical laboratory scientist/medical technologist.

Resources

BOOKS

Cruse, Julius M., and Robert E. Lewis. *Illustrated Dictionary of Immunology*. New York: CRC Press, 1995.

"Pediatrics and Genetics: Disturbances in Newborns and Infants." In vol. II, edited by Robert Berkow, et al. Rahway, NJ: Merck Research Laboratories, 1992.

"Procedures: Heelstick (Capillary Blood Sampling)." In *Neonatology: Management, Procedures, On-Call Problems, Diseases, and Drugs*. 4th edition. Edited by Tricia Lacy Gomella, et al. Norwalk, CT: Appleton & Lange, 1999.

OTHER

Pittsburgh.com. *Illustrated Health Encyclopedia*. <http://www.pittsburgh.com/shared/health/adam/ency/article>.

Rachael T. Brandt

Total body hydraulic lift usage

Definition

Total body hydraulic lifts are devices used to transfer patients from a bed to a wheelchair, bedside commode, bathtub, etc. They are also known as Hoyer lifts. (Hoyer was one of the first companies to manufacture the lifts.)

Purpose

Total body hydraulic lifts are typically used with patients who cannot bear weight, have physical limitations such as amputations or quadriplegia, or who are extremely heavy and cannot be safely transferred by members of the health care team or the patient's caregivers. These portable lifts support all of the patient's weight using a sling that is attached to a stand on wheels.

Precautions

Several precautions should be taken prior to using a total body lift. The weight capacity of the lift should be taken into consideration before using it with any patient. Proper positioning of the sling must be insured, as well as proper positioning of the patient, maintaining good body alignment.

Description

Total body lifts are used in many maximal assistance patient transfers. Most lifts work through hydraulic devices that involve pumping or cranking the lift by hand. Many of the newer lifts, however, have an electric motor that is controlled by a hand control, eliminating the need for hand pumping. Consisting of a metal frame with a heavy canvas swing capable of suspending the patient, total body lifts are often a safer patient transferring option for both the patient and the caregiver.

When a patient is manually lifted, the health care professional or other caregiver must rely on their own strength to carry out the transfer. This frequently means that the caregiver is working beyond their physical capabilities. This increases the risk for mishandling or even dropping the patient during a manual lift. The majority of Hoyer lifts used are quite stable, require little force to move the lift with the patient in it, and are designed with slings that decrease the potential for skin tears or abrasions. In addition, most lifts can be operated by one person, which can free up other staff members to care for other patients.

The health care professional or other patient caregiver can safely transfer a patient utilizing a total body, or Hoyer, lift by following these steps:

- Assess the patient's weight, making sure it falls within the weight limits of the particular lift being used.

- Obtain assistance from another caregiver if needed. Move the lift to the bedside and the object the patient is being transferred into to a convenient location.

- Raise the bed. Turn the patient on the side and place the canvas sling under the body, from head to knees.

- Instruct the patient to keep the arms crossed over the body. Position the lift with the legs spread and under the bed. Attach the lift chains to the sling, and adjust the sling, evenly distributing the patient's weight.

- Raise the lift, elevating the sling just off of the bed.

- Maneuver the patient's legs over the side of the bed. Insure that the patient's head and extremities are protected from injury.

- Guide the lift over the object so the patient is positioned appropriately. Release the lift valve slowly, and lower the patient. Release the lift chains.

Preparation

Prior to transferring a patient using a total body lift, instruct the patient on the procedure, and how he or she can assist by keeping the arms folded.

Aftercare

Assess the patient after the transfer is completed, noting how the patient tolerated the procedure.

Health care team roles

Many members of the health care team may use a total body lift to transfer a patient, including nurses and nursing assistants, and physical therapists. Health care professionals are responsible for knowing how to correctly and safely use the lift device to transfer patients.

Resources

PERIODICALS

Goldsmith, Connie. "Watch Your Back." *Nurseweek* (January 8, 2001).

Owen, Bernice Dr. "Preventing Injuries Using an Ergonomic Approach." *AORN Journal* (December 2000).

OTHER

Simonton, Kevin, and Dana Wilcox. "Frequently Asked Questions About Portable Total Body Patient/Resident Lifts." *Department of Labor and Industries: Nursing Home Initiative.* <http://www.wa.gov/lni/hip/liftfaq.html>.

Deanna M. Swartout-Corbeil, R.N.

Total protein test *see* **Plasma protein tests**

Toxemia *see* **Preeclampsia and eclampsia**

Toxicology

Definition

Toxicology is the scientific study of poisons or toxins. The National Library of Medicine describes toxicology as "the study of the adverse effects of chemicals or physical agents on living organisms." How these toxins affect humans is based in understanding these basic relationships.

Description

The Swiss physician and alchemist Philippus Aureolus, also known as Paracelsus (1493–1541) and said to be the father of the modern science of toxicology, wrote, "All things are poison, and nothing is without poison, the dose alone makes a thing not a poison." In other words, if **poisoning** is to be caused, an exposure to a potentially toxic chemical must result in a dose that exceeds a physiologically determined threshold of tolerance. Smaller exposures do not cause poisoning.

The dose of toxin is a crucial factor to consider when evaluating effects of a toxin. Small quantities of a substance like strychnine taken daily over an extended period of time might have little to no effect, while one large dose in one day could be fatal. In addition, some toxins may only affect a particular species of organism, such as pesticides and **antibiotics** killing insects and microorganisms with significantly less harmful effects to humans.

Organisms vary greatly in their tolerance of exposure to chemicals. Even within populations of the same species great variations in sensitivity can exist. In rare cases, some individuals may be extremely sensitive to particular chemicals or groups of similar chemicals, a phenomenon known as hypersensitivity. Organisms are often exposed to a wide variety of potentially toxic chemicals through medicine, food, water, and the atmosphere.

The study of the disruption of biochemical pathways by poisons is a key aspect of toxicology. Poisons affect normal physiology in many ways; but some of the more common mechanisms involve the disabling of enzyme systems, induction of cancers, interference with the regulation of **blood** chemistry, and disruption of genetic processes.

Toxic agents may be physical (for example, radiation), biological (for example, poisonous snake bite), or chemical (for example, arsenic) in nature. In addition, biological organisms may cause disease by invading the body and releasing toxins. An example of this is tetanus, in which the bacterium *Clostridium tetanus* releases a powerful toxin that travels to the nervous system.

Toxic agents may also cause systemic or organ-specific reactions in the body. Cyanide affects the entire body by interfering with the body's capacity for utilizing oxygen. Lead has three specific target organs: the **central nervous system**, the **kidneys**, and the hemopoietic (blood-cell generating) system. The target organ is affected by the dose and route of the toxin. For example, the initial effects of a chemical may affect the nervous system; repeated exposure over time might cause chronic damage to the **liver**.

Function

The toxicologist employs the tools and methods of science to understand more completely the consequences of exposure to toxic chemicals. Toxicologists typically assess the relationship between toxic chemicals and environmental health by evaluating such factors as:

• Risk—To assess the risk associated with exposure to a toxic substance, toxicologists first measure the exposure characteristics and then compute the doses that enter the human body. Then they compare these numbers to derive an estimate of risk, sometimes based on animal studies. In cases where human data exist for a toxic substance, such as benzene, more straightforward correlations with human risk of illness or death are possible.

• Precautionary strategies—Given recommendations from toxicologists, government agencies sometimes decide to regulate a chemical based on limited evidence from animal and human epidemiological studies that the chemical is toxic.

• Clinical data—Some toxicologists devise new techniques and develop new applications of existing methods to monitor changes in the health of individuals exposed to toxic substances. For example, one academic research group in the United States has spent many years developing new methods for monitoring the effects of exposure to oxidants (for example, free radicals) in healthy and diseased humans.

• Epidemiological evidence—Another way to understand the environmental factors contributing to human illness is to study large populations that have been exposed to substances suspected of being toxic. Scientists then attempt to tie these observations to clinical data. Ecological studies seek to correlate exposure patterns with a specific outcome. Case-control studies compare groups of persons with a particular illness with similar healthy groups, and seek to identify the degree of exposure required to bring about the illness. Other studies may refine the scope of environmental factor studies; or, examine a small group of individuals in which there is a high incidence of a rare disease and a history of exposure to a particular chemical.

• Evidence of bioaccumulation—When a chemical is nonbiodegradable, it may accumulate in biosystems, resulting in very high concentrations accumulating in animals at the top of food chains. Chlorinated pesticides such as dieldrin and DDT, for example, have been found in fish in much greater concentrations than in the seawater where they swim.

Role in human health

Humans are exposed to complex mixtures of chemicals, many of which are synthetic and have been either deliberately or accidentally released into the environment. In some cases, people actively expose themselves to chemicals that are known to be toxic, such as smoking cigarettes, drinking alcohol, or taking recreational drugs. Voluntary exposure to chemicals also occurs when people take medicines to deal with illness, or when they choose to work in an occupation that involves routinely dealing with dangerous chemicals. Most exposures to potentially toxic chemicals are inadvertent, and involve living in an environment that is contaminated with small concentrations of pollutants, such as those associated with pesticide residues in food, lead from gasoline combustion, or sulfur dioxide and ozone in the urban atmosphere.

Drugs given to improve health can lead to toxicity even when given in appropriate doses. Conditions such as **dehydration** and other forms of physiological compromise can make the patient more vulnerable to toxicity. Drugs like digoxin, lidocaine, and lithium are common examples of drugs with potentially toxic effects. Interactions of substances in the body may also produce toxic effects. For example, if two central nervous system depressants are taken at once, as in the case of combining alcohol and a tranquilizer, the effects are additive and could lead to extreme depression of the central nervous system functions.

The health care system's role related to toxicology includes education and prevention as well as treatment of both acute and chronic effects of toxins. Agencies such as the Food and Drug Administration (FDA) and the Occupational Safety and Health Administration (OSHA) work with health care and industry to offer guidelines and restrictions on the manufacture and use of pharmaceuticals, foods, and other substances.

Health care workers are involved by being aware of these regulations, and staying informed. They also provide education, such as, teaching new parents about the dangers of lead paint consumption by children, and help prevent exposure to toxins, such as, tetanus **vaccination**, or monitoring for signs of lithium toxicity. The Poison Control Center uses nurses and other allied health workers to inform the public of immediate actions to take in the event of a poisoning emergency. Emergency interventions at the hospital include blood and urine tests, gastric lavage with administration of absorbent activated charcoal, and administration of antidotes when available.

Common diseases and disorders

Toxicologists have ranked the most commonly encountered toxic chemicals in the United States. In descending order of frequency of encounter, they are as follows:

- Arsenic—Toxic exposure occurs mainly in the workplace, near hazardous waste sites, or in areas with high natural levels. A powerful poison, arsenic can, at high levels of exposure, cause death or illness.

- Lead—Toxic exposure usually results from breathing workplace air or dust, or from eating contaminated foods. Children may be exposed to lead from eating lead-based paint chips or playing in contaminated soil. Lead damages the nervous system, kidneys, and the immune systems.

- Mercury—Toxic exposure results from breathing contaminated air, ingesting contaminated water and food, and possibly having dental and medical treatments. At high levels, mercury damages the **brain**, kidneys, and developing fetuses.

- Vinyl chloride—Toxic exposure occurs mainly in the workplace. Breathing high levels of vinyl chloride for short periods can produce dizziness, sleepiness, unconsciousness, and, at very high levels, death. Breathing vinyl chloride for long periods of time can give rise to permanent liver damage, immune reactions, nerve damage, and liver **cancer**.

- Benzene—Benzene is formed in both natural processes and human activities. Breathing benzene can produce drowsiness, dizziness, and unconsciousness. Long-term exposure affects the bone marrow and can produce anemia and leukemia.

- Polychlorinated biphenyls (PCBs)—PCBs are mixtures of chemicals. They are no longer produced in the United States, but remain in the environment. They can irritate the nose and throat, and cause acne and rashes. They have been shown to cause cancer in animal studies.

- Cadmium—Toxic exposure to cadmium occurs mainly in workplaces where cadmium products are made. Other sources of exposure include cigarette smoke and cadmium-contaminated foods. Cadmium can damage the **lungs**, cause kidney disease, and irritate the digestive tract.

Resources

BOOKS

Klaassen, Curtis D. *Casarett & Doull's Toxicology: The Basic Science of Poisons.* New York: McGraw Hill, 2001.

ORGANIZATIONS

American Association of Poison Control Centers (AAPCC). <http://www.aapcc.org>.

OTHER

National Library of Medicine Toxicology Tutor Web site. <http://sis.nlm.nih.gov/ToxTutor;> and, TOXNET, <http://www.nlm.nih.gov/toxnet>.

Katherine Hauswirth, A.P.R.N.

Toxoplasmosis test *see* **TORCH test**

Trace metal tests

Definition

Trace metals are a group of metals that include both heavy and transitional elements present in submilligram quantities in the **blood**. There are two groups, the micronutrients that are essential for health and those that have no known biological function. The essential micronutrients that may be measured include arsenic, chromium, cobalt, **copper**, **iron**, manganese, nickel, selenium, and **zinc**. Rarely, molybdenum, tin, and vanadium may also be measured. The nonessential metals that may be measured are lead, mercury, aluminum, thallium, and cadmium.

Purpose

All trace metals have the potential to be toxic when present in excessive concentrations. Trace metal tests are required when the patient has symptoms of toxicity or when the patient is in a high risk category for environmental exposure to a toxic metal. Excessive amounts of a trace metal can cause specific diseases or abnormalities that will require medical intervention and removal of the metal by chelation therapy. Deficiencies of micronutrients including iron, zinc, copper, and selenium are common and can lead to significant medical problems. Tests for these metals are sometimes needed in order to diagnose essential trace metal deficiency and its cause.

Precautions

A blood sample or urine sample is required for trace metal testing. When performing venipuncture, the nurse or phletobomist collecting the sample should observe **universal precautions** for prevention of transmission of bloodborne pathogens. Trace metal contamination is a potentially serious problem with samples for trace metal analysis. Metals are present in the materials used to manufacture rubber stoppers and lubricants used in blood collection tubes. Therefore, special tubes with lubricant-free stoppers are required. Samples for lead analysis require whole blood because the lead is primarily within the red blood cells. Special tubes containing heparin or EDTA (ethylenediaminetetraacetic acid) are used for this purpose. These have a tan colored stopper and are certified to be lead free. Other trace metals are usually measured in serum or urine. If serum is used, the blood must be collected in a tube having a navy blue stopper. The only exception is iron, which is present in sufficient concentration in serum or plasma to allow use of regular blood collection tubes. In addition, when performing analysis of any trace metal, the water used must by Type I purity, and the reagents must meet or exceed American Chemical Society (ACS) purity standards.

Description

Measurement techniques

With the exception of iron, the method of choice for routine trace metal measurement is atomic absorption spectrophotometry with a graphite furnace atomizer. The instrument should be capable of background absorbance correction. Iron is the trace metal in highest concentration in plasma and can be measured by colorimetric methods. Other suitable methods for trace metal analysis include inductively coupled plasma mass spectroscopy and emission spectroscopy.

The following list represents both essential and nonessential trace metals that are measured in the medical laboratory. The most commonly measured metal and the only one routinely measured as part of a comprehensive metabolic profile is iron. The principal reason for measuring iron is to detect iron deficiency states that lead to anemia, or excessive iron ingestion that leads to tissue damage caused by excessive deposition of iron in tissues such as the **liver**. The most commonly measured nonessential metal is lead. There are many environmental sources of lead, but it is especially prevalent in paint chips, lead pipes, car exhaust, and cigarette smoke. Young children are at greatly increased risk because they absorb up to five times more lead from the intestinal tract than adults. Since lead exposure during childhood can result in diminished intellectual ability, many medical centers have established lead screening programs in high prevalence areas.

A brief description of the major effects of the trace metals listed above follows:

- Aluminum (Al): Toxic levels are found in patients with **chronic kidney failure** who have received hemodialysis over long periods of time; the dialysis solutions contain aluminum. Also at risk are diabetic patients (aluminum is present in medications) and those who ingest large quantities of **antacids** containing aluminum. Excess aluminum is deposited in the **brain** and in bone. Aluminum is a potent inhibitor of parathyroid hormone and induces osteomalacia. **Central nervous system** toxicities include convulsions, behavior, and speech disturbances.

- Arsenic (As): The organic form of arsenic is nontoxic but the ionic form is toxic. Arsenic is found in some herbicides, pesticides, insecticides, and seafood. Excessive amounts usually result from ingestion of poisons containing arsenic. Symptoms vary depending upon whether exposure is acute or chronic. Acute toxicity causes nausea, vomiting, abdominal **pain**, **diarrhea**, cardiac arrhythmia, and kidney damage; and very high doses can induce **coma**. Chronic exposure causes dermatitis, abnormal nail growth pattern, headache, drowsiness, confusion, and bone marrow failure.

- Cadmium (Cd): Cadmium is used to manufacture batteries and is used extensively in automotive spray painting. It is also prevalent in industrial pollution and in cigarette smoke. Breathing excessive amounts can cause lung damage (**emphysema**). Ingestion or inhalation causes dizziness, headache, and intestinal irritation. Chronic exposure causes damage to the renal tubules known as heavy metal nephrosis.

- Chromium (Cr): Chromium is used to manufacture stainless steel, tan leather, and dye fabrics. Breathing excessive amounts can cause **lung cancer**. Chromium is also a skin irritant and excessive exposure to skin leads to ulceration.

- Cobalt (Co): Cobalt is used in various industrial processes, and inhalation of cobalt in dust can cause **asthma**. Symptoms include goiter, nerve damage, excessive blood cell production, and cardiomyopathy.

- Copper (Cu): Copper is the third most abundant trace metal and deficiency is more common than toxicity. The most common cause of copper deficiency is total **parenteral nutrition**. This leads to anemia, bone loss, hyperlipidemia, impaired immune function, and glucose intolerance. Copper toxicity is associated with a genetic deficiency of ceruloplasmin, Wilson's disease. This results in copper accumulation in the liver, eyes, kidney, and brain which is fatal without chelation therapy.

- Iron (Fe): Iron is the most abundant trace metal and is needed to make hemoglobin. Iron deficiency results in anemia and is most commonly seen in children with inadequate dietary intake; adults who exhibit chronic blood loss; and multiparous females who have not received iron supplementation. Iron excess is most often caused by increased ingestion and absorption of iron supplements or exposure from iron pots used for cookware. Some persons absorb excessive iron for unknown reasons. Accumulation of iron in the tissues leads to hemochromatosis which results in renal damage, cirrhosis, and an enlarged spleen and liver. The **pancreas** may become damaged leading to **diabetes mellitus** and deposition in other tissues causes inflammatory damage (e.g., deposits in joints cause arthritis).

- Lead (Pb): Lead is found in old paint, some ceramic products, lead-soldered water pipes, industrial waste, car exhaust, and cigarette smoke. Excessive amounts cause anemia, renal tubular nephrosis, diminished intellectual capacity and developmental delays in children, headache, drowsiness, and gastrointestinal upset.

- Manganese (Mn): Manganese is found in paint, cleaners for laboratory glass, and red brick. Excessive exposure to manganese dust in miners can cause pneumonitis. Chronic **poisoning** usually results from industrial exposure. Manganese accumulates in the brain causing symptoms similar to Parkinson's disease.

- Mercury (Hg): Mercury is used in the manufacture of paper, plastics, paint, and dental amalgams. The two most common sources of exposure are industrial pollution and ingestion of seafood containing methyl mercury, which is toxic. Excessive exposure can cause pulmonary, brain, kidney, liver, and gastrointestinal damage.

- Nickel (Ni): Nickel is used in industrial processes as a catalyst and as an alloy for steel and other metals. Skin contact causes eczema in sensitive individuals.

Ingestion of toxic levels can result in headache, vomiting, vertigo, and nausea. Inhalation of toxic levels can cause asthma and a pneumonia-like condition.

- Selenium (Se): Selenium is a micronutrient needed for normal **heart** function, and deficiency leads to cardiomyopathy. Selenium deficiency is seen in regions where soil and water are depleted of **minerals**. It occurs in persons with gastrointestinal malabsorption, patients with kidney disease receiving dialysis, and patients receiving total parenteral **nutrition**. Excess toxicity is most commonly caused by excessive dietary supplementation and causes cirrhosis, enlarged spleen, hair loss, and gastrointestinal bleeding.

- Thallium (Tl): Thallium is used during the lead smelting process and as a rodent killer. Excessive amounts can cause hair loss, confusion, seizures, **paralysis**, and kidney failure.

- Zinc (Zn): Zinc is the second most abundant trace metal. Zinc deficiency is usually associated with total parenteral nutrition and drugs that prevent absorption, but a genetic deficiency causing reduced gastrointestinal absorption is also a rare cause. Deficiency causes dermatitis, diarrhea, impaired growth, hypogonadism, anemia, enlarged liver, hair loss, and decreased immune function. Zinc is used in metal plating and excessive exposure can cause **fever**; and skin, throat, and gastrointestinal irritation.

Lead poisoning

Children are often screened for lead poisoning since even very low levels of lead in their body can impact growth, learning, and intelligence. Before 1970, high levels of lead were routinely found in paints. A child has an increased risk of lead exposure if he or she lives in an older, dilapidated house that contains lead paint. As the paint chips and peels, young children, especially those six months to six years old, are at particular risk since they are young enough to put chips, dust, or their contaminated fingers in their mouths. The daily diet normally contains a small amount of lead, approximately 300 micrograms per day. Adults absorb 1-10% of ingested lead, but children absorb lead more efficiently putting them at greater risk for toxicity.

Suspected cases of lead poisoning can be presumptively diagnosed with two surrogate tests. Lead blocks the incorporation of iron into protoporphyrin, resulting in the inability to form heme, the iron-containing component of hemoglobin. This results in increased levels of erythrocyte zinc protoporphyrin

(ZPP) in which protoporphyrin is bound to zinc instead of iron and free erythrocyte protoporphyrin (FEP). Both ZPP and FEP can be measured by fluorometric analysis. However, both are also increased in iron deficiency, aluminum poisoning, and erythropoietic porphyria as well as lead poisoning.

Preparation

Usually, there is no special preparation for the patient before testing.

Aftercare

Since only a small sample of blood (or urine) is collected, no complex aftercare is required. The patient should be comforted (especially young children), and direct pressure should be applied to the venipuncture or finger stick site for several minutes or until the bleeding has stopped.

Complications

In normal circumstances, a blood draw for a heavy metal test takes only a few minutes, and the patient experiences minor discomfort and a minute puncture wound at the site of the needle stick.

Results

Reference ranges for specific metals are provided based on the type of testing performed by the laboratory, the specimen provided, and the type of metal tested. Representative ranges are shown below:

- Aluminum: less than 6 micrograms per liter.
- Arsenic: in urine less than 100 micrograms per liter (in whole blood less than 70 micrograms per liter).
- Cadmium: less than 5 micrograms per liter.
- Chromium: 0.5-2.1 micrograms per liter (urine 0.5-5.0 mcg/L).
- Copper: 75-150 micrograms per liter.
- Iron: 500-1500 micrograms per liter.
- Lead: Normal in children: less than 100 micrograms/L; Normal in adults: less than 300 micrograms/L.
- Lead (in ZPP testing for lead poisoning): Normal in children and adults: 15–77 micrograms/dL; Average: less than 35 micrograms/dL.
- Manganese: less than 7.9 micrograms per liter.
- Mercury: less than 5 micrograms per liter.
- Nickel: less than 5.2 micrograms per liter urine.

KEY TERMS

Edematous—The state of swelling (edema) caused by the collection of excess fluid within tissues.

Hematoma—Swelling and subsequent bruising when blood leaks from a vein into local tissues; can be caused by improper venipuncture when the needle has gone through a vein or when the needle has been inserted incorrectly.

Hemodialysis—Procedure used to filter toxins and waste products from the blood while the blood circulates outside the body; dialysis is used for patients with kidney failure.

Venipuncture—Puncture of a vein with a needle for the purpose of withdrawing a blood sample for analysis.

- Selenium: 95-160 micrograms per liter.
- Thallium: less than 10.1 micrograms per liter.
- Zinc: 50-150 micrograms per liter.

Health care team roles

A physician orders trace metal tests and interprets the results. The nurse, physician assistant, or nurse practitioner may participate in the medical examination of the patient, and should perform a careful history in order to document any environmental source of metal exposure (such as working in a battery manufacturing plant, automobile paint shop, etc.) that could be linked to the symptoms. A nurse or phlebotomist collects the specimen for trace metal tests. Trace metal analysis is performed by clinical laboratory scientists/medical technologists with special training in the use of atomic absorption spectrophotometry.

Additionally, health care providers should contact community health officials if the poisoning is acquired by an industrial or environmental exposure that may affect other people.

Patient education

The health care provider's role in educating patients about trace metal poisoning is crucial, especially in cases of suspected lead poisoning in children. The health care provider should explain how lead poisoning is acquired, and work with the parents to determine the lead source. Since the health complications for children are serious, it is vital that the parents understand that treatment may be needed immediately and further testing will be required to monitor the lead level and its effects. The health care provider can work with adult patients to determine the source of metal in their homes or work environments and inform them about treatment and follow-up testing requirements.

Resources

BOOKS

Fischbach, Frances. "Lead." In *A Manual of Laboratory & Diagnostic Tests*. 6th ed. Philadelphia: Lippincott Williams & Wilkins, 2000, pp.398- 400.

Kee, Joyce LeFever. "Lead (Blood)" and "Zinc Protoporphyrin (ZPP) (Blood)." In *Laboratory & Diagnostic Tests with Nursing Implications*. 5th ed. Stamford, CT: Appleton & Lange, 1999, pp.281-282, 460-461.

Mofenson, Howard C., et al. "Acute Poisonings: Lead." In *Conn's Current Therapy 2001*. edited by Robert E. Rakel and Edward T. Bope. Philadelphia: W.B. Saunders Company, 2001, pp.1230-1235.

Moyer, Thomas P. "Toxic Metals." In *Tietz Textbook of Clinical Chemistry*. 3rd ed., edited by Carl A. Burtis and Edward R. Ashwood. Philadelphia: W. B. Saunders Company, 1999, pp.982-998.

Sacher, Ronald A., Richard A. McPherson, with Joseph M. Campos. "Heavy Metals." In *Widmann's Clinical Interpretation of Laboratory Tests*. 11th ed. Philadelphia: F. A. Davis Company, 2000, pp.919-921.

ORGANIZATIONS

Alliance to End Childhood Lead Poisoning. 227 Massachusetts Ave., N.E., Suite 200, Washington, D.C. (202) 543-1147. <http://www.aeclp.org>.

Lead Poisoning Prevention Branch, Division of Environmental Hazards and Health Effects, National Center for Environmental Health, Centers for Disease Control and Prevention. 1600 Clifton Rd., Mailstop E25, Atlanta, GA. (404) 498-1420. <http://www.cdc.gov/nceh/lead>.

Linda D. Jones, B.A., PBT (ASCP)

Tracheostomy *see* **Tracheotomy**

Tracheostomy care

Definition

A tracheostomy is a surgically created opening in the trachea. A tracheostomy tube is placed in the incision to secure an airway and to prevent it from closing. Tracheostomy care is generally done every eight hours and involves cleaning around the incision, as well as replacing the inner cannula of the tracheostomy tube. After the site heals, the entire tracheostomy tube is replaced once or twice per week, depending on the physician's order.

Purpose

The goals of tracheostomy care are to maintain the patency of the airway, prevent breakdown of the skin surrounding the site, and prevent **infection**. Sterile technique should be used during the procedure.

Precautions

Extra precautions should be taken when performing site care during the first few days after the tracheostomy is surgically created. The site is prone to bleeding and is sensitive to movement of the tracheostomy tube. It is recommended that another health care professional securely hold the tube while site care is performed. Tracheostomy care should not be done while the patient is restless or agitated, since this increases the chance that the tube may be pulled out and the airway lost.

Description

Tracheostomy care starts with suctioning the patient's airway, both via the tracheostomy and orally. Sterile technique must be used when suctioning the tracheostomy. The gauze dressing is removed from the tracheostomy site, and the amount and color of drainage should be noted. Using sterile technique, the skin and external portion of the tube are cleaned with hydrogen peroxide. Cotton-tipped applicators should be used to clean closely around the stoma. The condition of the skin and stoma should be noted. The area is then wiped with gauze dampened in 0.9% sodium chloride and a new tracheostomy dressing is applied.

If the patient has a disposable inner cannula, the old cannula can simply be removed and discarded. A new cannula is inserted using sterile technique. If the inner cannula is not disposable, it must be cleaned with hydrogen peroxide, rinsed with 0.9% sodium chloride, and reinserted. Sterile technique must be used, and the cannula should be tapped against the side of the sterile container to remove excess fluid. It should not be completely dried, as the film of saline facilitates reinsertion.

Preparation

All supplies needed for tracheostomy care should be at the bedside prior to beginning the procedure.

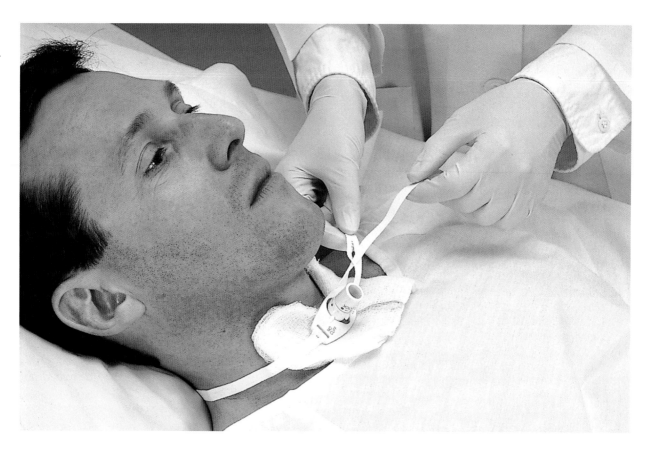

A health care professional changes tracheostomy dressings as a part of patient care. *(Delmar Publishers, Inc. Reproduced by permission.)*

There are prepackaged tracheostomy care kits available that contain gauze pads, cotton-tipped applicators, a tracheostomy dressing, and hydrogen peroxide. In addition, a container of 0.9% sodium chloride solution, a suction kit, and sterile gloves are needed. The velcro strap that holds the tracheostomy tube in place may be soiled and need to be replaced as well.

The patient should be preoxygenated with 100% oxygen prior to suctioning. If the patient is agitated, a sedative should be given or the procedure should be rescheduled for a later time when the patient is calm. **Pain** medication may be offered, especially during the first few days after surgery when manipulating the incision can cause discomfort.

Aftercare

After tracheostomy care is finished, the soiled dressing and supplies should be discarded, either in the garbage or in a biohazard container if there is a large amount of **blood**. The patient may need to be suctioned again, and his or her respiratory status

> ## KEY TERMS
>
> **Inner cannula**—Smaller tube that fits inside the tracheostomy tube, which can be removed quickly if it becomes obstructed. This is often used for patients who have copious secretions.
>
> **Tracheostomy tube**—An indwelling tube used to maintain patency of the tracheostomy. It can be made of metal (for long term use) or disposable plastic. The tube can be cuffed (a balloon is inflated to keep the tube in place) or uncuffed (air is allowed to flow freely around the tube). It can also be fenestrated, which allows the patient to speak.

should be reassessed. Again, pain medication should be offered as appropriate.

Complications

Tracheostomy care is a relatively benign procedure. The greatest risk is that the tube may be inadvertently removed and the airway lost.

Results

The anticipated outcomes of tracheostomy care include continual patency of the airway, prevention of skin breakdown around the stoma, and prevention of infection.

Health care team roles

The nurse has the primary role in tracheostomy care, as her or she is responsible for the care in the acute care setting. The respiratory therapist may assist the nurse during the procedure and during respiratory assessment. Some patients may be sent home with a tracheostomy. In this case, the nurse and respiratory therapist are both responsible for teaching patients and their families how to perform site care at home.

Resources

BOOKS

McGovern, Kate & Marguerite Ambrose. "Providing Tracheostomy Tube Care." In *Critical Care Skills: A Nurse's PhotoGuide*, edited by June Norris. Springhouse: Springhouse Corporation, 1996, pp. 298-311.

Thelan, Lynne, et al. *Critical Care Nursing: Diagnosis and Management.* St. Louis, MO: Mosby, 1998.

Abby Wojahn, RN, BSN, CCRN

Tracheotomy

Definition

A tracheotomy is surgery in which a cut is made into the skin of the throat and then into the windpipe (trachea). The surgeon inserts a breathing tube into the opening. The purpose may be to bypass an obstruction (such as a chunk of meat stuck in the throat) and thus allow air to get into the **lungs**, or it may be to remove secretions.

Since about 1950, the term "tracheostomy" has been preferred to "tracheotomy," but many surgeons still use the older term. The suffix "-tomy" is derived from the Greek for "cutting," and thus "tracheotomy" means simply "cutting the trachea." The Latin for "mouth," is *os, oris,* and so "tracheostomy" comes to mean "cutting an (artificial) mouth into the trachea." "Tracheostomy" thus has the advantage of being more specific than "tracheotomy."

Purpose

A tracheotomy is performed if there is a blockage in the pharynx or in the upper trachea, or if the patient is having problems with mucus and other secretions getting into the windpipe (trachea). There are many reasons why the pharynx or the upper trachea may be blocked. The patient's windpipe may be blocked by a swelling; by a severe injury to the neck, nose, or mouth; by a large foreign object; by **paralysis** of the throat muscles; or by a tumor. Patients who need help to breathe may be in a **coma**, or, because of spinal injury affecting the cervical nerves that control breathing, the patients may need a ventilator to pump air into the lungs for a long time.

Precautions

Doctors perform emergency tracheotomies as last-resort procedures. They are only done if the patient's windpipe is obstructed and the situation is life-threatening.

Description

Emergency tracheotomy

There are two different procedures that are called tracheotomies: emergency tracheotomies and non-emergency (elective) tracheotomies. The first is done only in extreme emergency situations and must be performed quite rapidly. It may be done anywhere, even in a restaurant, if the person would likely die while being transported to a proper operating room. The surgeon (sometimes, a non-surgeon must perform the tracheotomy) makes a cut into a thin part of the voice box (larynx) called the cricothyroid membrane. A tube is inserted and connected to an oxygen bag. This emergency procedure is sometimes called a cricothyrotomy. Cricothyrotomy is associated with a few immediate complications, such as hemorrhage and collapsed lung (pneumothorax).

Non-emergency (elective) tracheotomy

The second type of tracheotomy takes more time and is usually done in an operating room. The most common reason for performing a non-emergency (elective) tracheotomy is the need for the patient to undergo long-term mechanical ventilation. In this situation, the tracheotomy replaces a tube which had been inserted into the trachea through the patient's nose or mouth (an endotracheal tube). Other valid reasons for non-emergency (elective) tracheotomy include life-threatening aspiration **pneumonia**, poor clearance of bronchial secretions, and sleep apnea.

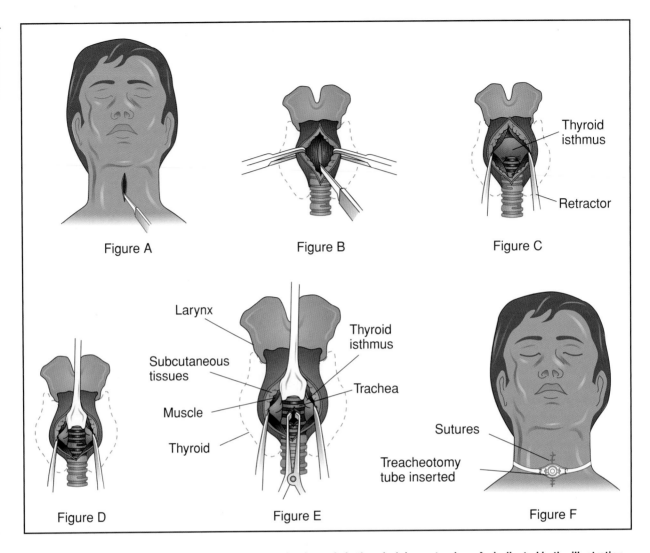

Figure A

Figure B

Figure C
Thyroid
isthmus

Retractor

Figure D

Figure E
Larynx

Subcutaneous
tissues

Muscle

Thyroid

Thyroid
isthmus

Trachea

Figure F
Sutures

Treacheotomy
tube inserted

Tracheotomy is a surgical procedure in which an opening is made in the windpipe or trachea. As indicated in the illustration above, the physician or surgeon will follow these steps in performing this procedure: Figure A: A vertical incision is made through the skin. Figure B: Another incision is made through the subcutaneous tissues and muscles of the neck. Figure C: The neck muscles are separated using retractors. Figure D: The thyroid isthumus is either cut or retracted. Figure E: The surgeon identifies the rings of cartilage that make up the trachea and cuts into the walls. Figure F: A metal or plastic tube is inserted into the opening and sutures are used to hold the tube in place. *(Illustration by Electronic Illustrators Group. The Gale Group.)*

The surgical procedure itself is basically the same in the emergency and non-emergency (elective) tracheotomy. The surgeon first makes a cut (incision) into the skin of the neck that lies over the trachea. This incision is made in the lower part of the neck, between the Adam's apple and the top of the breastbone. The neck muscles are separated, and the **thyroid gland**, which overlies the trachea, is usually cut down the middle. The surgeon identifies the rings of cartilage that make up the trachea and cuts into the tough walls. A metal or plastic tube, called a breathing tube (tracheotomy tube), is inserted through the opening. This tube acts as an artificial windpipe and thus allows the patient to breathe. Oxygen or a mechanical ventilator may be hooked up to the tube to bring oxygen more effectively to the lungs. A dressing is placed around the opening. Tape or stitches (sutures) are used to hold the tube in place.

After a non-emergency tracheotomy, the patient usually stays in the hospital for one or two days, unless there is a complicating condition.

Preparation

Emergency tracheotomy

In the emergency tracheotomy, there is no time to explain the procedure or the need for it to the patient. The patient is placed on his or her back with face upward (supine), with a rolled-up towel (if available) between the shoulders. This positioning of the patient makes it easier for the doctor to feel and see the structures in the throat. A local anesthetic (if available, for example in the emergency room of a hospital, but not in a proper operating room) is injected across the cricothyroid membrane. In a setting such as a restaurant, a rescue worker would cut without anesthesia. If the person would otherwise die within five minutes from lack of oxygen, the **pain** and risks are justified.

Non-emergency (elective) tracheotomy

In a non-emergency tracheotomy, there is time for the doctor to discuss the surgery with the patient, to explain what will happen and why it is needed, and to get the patient's **informed consent**. The patient is then given anesthesia (sometimes general, sometimes local or topical). The neck area and chest are then disinfected as preparation for the operation, and surgical drapes are placed over the area, setting up a sterile field.

Aftercare

Postoperative care

A **chest x ray** is often taken, especially in children, to check whether the tube has become displaced, or, of course, in any patient when complications are known to have occurred. The doctor may prescribe **antibiotics** to reduce the risk of **infection**. If the patient can breathe on his or her own, the whole room is humidified; otherwise, if the tracheotomy tube is to remain in place, the air entering the tube from a ventilator is humidified. During the hospital stay, the patient and his or her family members will learn how to handle the problems that the tracheotomy tube causes, including mechanically sucking mucus out of the throat and keeping the tube itself clear. Tracheotomy initially prevents easy swallowing because the larynx is no longer elevated. Secretions are removed by passing a smaller, sterile tube (catheter) into the tracheotomy tube and extending it down into one of the two main bronchi. The tracheotomy tube itself generally requires several cleanings every day. An aseptic, or preferably a sterile, technique must be used. It is important that the skin around the opening (stoma) be carefully maintained to prevent secondary infection and disintegration caused by moisture (such softening and disintegration is called "maceration").

It takes most patients several days to adjust to breathing through the tracheotomy tube. At first, it will be hard even to make non-speech sounds. If the tube allows some air to escape and pass over the vocal cords, then the patient may be able to speak by holding a finger briefly over the tube. A patient on a ventilator will not be able to talk at all.

The tube will be removed if the tracheotomy is temporary. Then the wound will heal quickly, and only a small scar may remain. If the tracheotomy is intended to be permanent, the hole stays open. If eventually it is no longer needed, it will be surgically closed.

Home care

After the patient is discharged, he or she will need help at home to manage the tracheotomy tube. Warm compresses can be used briefly to relieve pain at the incision site. However, in general, the patient is advised to keep the area dry, lest prolonged moisture cause disintegration of the skin (maceration).

It is recommended that the patient wear a loose scarf over the opening when going outside. He or she must drink fluids to avoid **dehydration** and must eat to maintain proper **nutrition**. At the same time, he or she must keep water, other fluids, small food particles, and powdery substances from entering the tube and thus causing serious breathing problems. The doctor may prescribe pain medication and antibiotics to minimize the risk of infections.

If the tube is to be kept in place permanently, the patient can be referred to a speech therapist in order to learn to speak with the tube in place. The tracheotomy tube may be changed four to ten days after surgery.

Patients are encouraged to resume most of their normal activities once they leave the hospital. Vigorous activity is restricted for about six weeks. However, swimming and rough contact sports would be life-threatening. Even when taking a shower, the patient must keep the tracheotomy covered. If the tracheotomy is permanent, further surgery may be needed to widen the opening, which narrows with time.

Risks

Immediate risks

There are several short-term risks associated with tracheotomies. Severe bleeding is one possible complication. The voice box or the esophagus may be damaged during surgery. Air may become trapped in the tissues surrounding a lung, causing it to collapse. The tracheotomy tube can be blocked by **blood** clots, mucus, or the pressure of the airway walls. Blockages can be prevented by suctioning, humidifying the air, and selecting the appropriate tracheotomy tube. Serious infections are rare unless suction tubes are inserted without aseptic (or preferably sterile) technique. In cases of such carelessness, one is introducing **bacteria** into the suction catheter.

Long-term risks

Over time, other complications may develop following a tracheotomy. The windpipe itself may become damaged for a number of reasons, including pressure from the tube, bacteria that cause infections and form scar tissue, or friction from a tube that moves too much. Sometimes the opening does not close on its own after the tube is removed. This risk is higher in tracheotomies with tubes remaining in place for 16 weeks or longer. In these cases, if the breathing tube is to be removed because it is no longer necessary, the wound is surgically closed.

High-risk groups

The risks associated with tracheotomies are higher in the following groups of patients:

- children, especially newborns and infants
- smokers
- alcoholics and other substance-abusers
- obese adults
- persons over 60
- persons with chronic respiratory diseases or respiratory infections
- persons taking **muscle relaxants**, sleeping medications, tranquilizers, or cortisone

The overall risk of death from a tracheotomy is less than 5%.

Results

Normal results include uncomplicated healing of the incision (even in an emergency tracheotomy) and successful maintenance of long-term tube placement in a non-emergency (elective) tracheotomy.

Health care team roles

A variety of allied health personnel is likely to be involved in the care of patients requiring a tracheotomy. In the case of an emergency tracheotomy, an emergency-room nurse or **nurse anesthetist** will assist the surgeon. A respiratory nurse or therapist will provide information to the patient and family about how

---

KEY TERMS

Cartilage—A tough, fibrous connective tissue that forms various parts of the body, including the trachea and the larynx.

Cricothyrotomy—An emergency tracheotomy that consists of a cut through the cricothyroid membrane to open the patient's airway as quickly as possible.

Larynx—A structure in the throat made basically of cartilage, ligaments, and muscle, that connects the pharynx with the trachea. The larynx contains the vocal cords.

Maceration—Softening and eventual disintegration of tissue because of constant exposure to moisture.

Stoma—Artificially created opening between a body cavity and the surface of the body. ("Stoma" is Greek for the mouth.)

Trachea—The tube made of cartilage and other connective tissue that leads from the voice box (larynx) to two major air passages (the main bronchi) that bring oxygen to the lungs. The trachea is sometimes called the windpipe.

Ventilator—A machine that helps patients to breathe. It is sometimes called a respirator.

---

to properly clean and maintain the tracheotomy tube if the tube is to be used long-term. This specialist will also provide information about administration of food and water and other issues. A nurse will likely provide information to the patient about how to prevent infection at the site of tube placement. A nurse specializing in the healing of **wounds** may work with the patient whether the tube is intended to be short-term or long-term. In many cases, a speech therapist is used to help the patient resume verbal communication following the trauma of the tracheotomy. This is more likely to occur in patients who will need long-term mechanical ventilation.

Resources

BOOKS

Fagan, Johannes J., et al. *Tracheotomy*. Alexandria, VA: American Academy of Otolaryngology—Head and Neck Surgery Foundation, 1997.

"Foreign Bodies of the Larynx and Tracheobronchial Tree." In *Current Surgical Diagnosis and Treatment*. Norwalk, CT: Appleton & Lange, 1994.

"Tracheotomy and Cricothyrotomy." In *Current Medical Diagnosis and Treatment 2001*, edited by Lawrence M. Tierney, et al. New York: Lange, 2001.

OTHER

"Answers to Common Otolaryngology Health-Care Questions." University of Washington School of Medicine, Department of Otolaryngology—Head and Neck Surgery. <http:weber.u.washington.edu/~ otoweb/trach.html>.

Sorce, James J. "Acute Airway Management and Tracheotomy." <http:hsinfo.ghsl.nwu.edu/otolink/ trach.html>.

Mark Mitchell

Traction *see* **Spinal traction**

Tranquilizers, major *see* **Antipsychotic drugs**

Tranquilizers, minor *see* **Antianxiety drugs**

Transcranial Doppler ultrasonography

Definition

Transcranial **Doppler ultrasonography** (TCD) is a noninvasive method of evaluating cerebrovascular **blood** flow (CBF), the flow of blood in the vessels of the **brain**. The TCD technology allows changes in the rate of blood flow (velocity) over time to be easily followed, documented, and analyzed. Ultrasonography (ultrasound) is a diagnostic imaging technology that directs high-frequency sound waves into the body, where they either bounce off or pass through body tissues and fluids. Echoes from the tissues and fluids return to the ultrasound machine, where changes in pitch and direction are instantly measured and displayed on a monitor as a picture (image) of the tissue or body organ being scanned. Doppler ultrasonography measures what is called the Doppler effect, the frequency change that occurs when ultrasound is directed toward **blood vessels** and reflected back to the source. Unlike reflected ultrasound signals that are received as an image, reflected Doppler waves make an audible sound that corresponds to the **heart** beat.

The Doppler principle is a wave theory first described by an Austrian physicist, Christian Doppler, in 1842. It relates to the velocity of objects and wave frequencies either transmitted or received by these objects. In Doppler ultrasound, the rate and direction of blood flow in the vessels can be determined by the frequency of the reflected sound, which indicates the rate of blood flow in the reflecting vessel (blood vessel sending back the sound waves). While Doppler ultrasound has been in use since 1965 to monitor fetal heart rates and blood flow in the carotid artery in the neck, it has only been in use since 1981 to measure blood flow velocity in the arteries of the head.

Purpose

TCD has proven to be a safe, fast, and reliable procedure for measuring the rate of CBF, especially as an assessment of risk for stroke. Individuals at risk for stroke usually have high blood velocities in the vessels of the brain. The rates of flow can be up to three or four times normal. Restrictions in blood flow may occur with the narrowing of blood vessels (stenosis), clot formation (thrombosis), blockage of blood vessels (embolism), or blood vessel rupture (hemorrhage). Lack of sufficient blood flow (ischemia) threatens brain tissue and may cause a stroke or other types of brain damage.

While ultrasonography typically receives inaudible echoes from tissues or organs and displays them as images, TCD measures changes in the frequency of transmitted waves, which are received as audible sounds. Just as a siren's pitch sounds higher when its source is moving toward the listener and lower as it moves away, so will ultrasound waves change pitch, or frequency, as they bounce off the blood flow in veins and arteries. Faster blood flow causes a greater change in frequency. These frequency shifts can be used to measure both the direction and the speed of blood flow in even the smallest of blood vessels.

Combined with other tests, this information can be used to locate restrictions in the blood vessels in the brain, and to track changes in blood flow over time. Ultrasound images can also be produced by the TCD equipment (as in ultrasound exams that view other body tissues or organs) from the reflected sound so that a vascular lesion (site of damage, blockage, or blood clot) can be found and examined. In this way, TCD can offer valuable information about the location of blockage or a clot that has caused a stroke and can help monitor the patient's response to therapy after a stroke. TCD is also used to evaluate the contraction of blood vessels that may occur if a blood vessel ruptures. Besides helping to diagnose stroke, TCD is used to evaluate brain death, **head injury**, abnormalities in veins and arteries, detection of blockage or rupture of vessels, and in surgical procedures such as heart bypass surgery or procedures requiring anesthesia.

Precautions

Ultrasonography procedures, including TCD, are noninvasive and painless. They are considered to be safe procedures with no known side effects. There are no special precautions.

Description

A TCD machine is an ultrasound scanner with Doppler capability. It is usually portable and is easy to set up in an examining room or at the patient's bedside. The first step in a TCD exam is to find an ideal location on the head (called an accoustic window) where the ultrasound beam can pass through the **skull** and allow the best transmission of sound waves. Because bone absorbs sound waves, areas where the bone is thinner are best for TCD exams. Children have thinner bones, and it is possible to obtain good signals from a large area of the head. The elderly have thicker bones, making it more difficult to obtain a good evaluation of blood flow velocity.

TCD is done with probes called transducers, which transmit and receive the ultrasound signals. These probes are placed against the skin of the head at the selected windows. The sonographer spreads a clear gel on the areas where a probe will be placed. Typical sites are the temple, the base of the skull at the back of the neck, and over the closed eyelid. These sites have the least amount of thick protective bone and will allow the best sound wave transmission. The sonographer adjusts the probe position and orientation to direct the sound waves toward the blood vessels of interest. Finding the best approach may take some time. A compression test may be performed during the exam. In this test, the main artery in the neck (carotid artery) is briefly compressed, and changes in blood flow patterns are observed. A full TCD exam may last 30 to 45 minutes, although a longer examination may be necessary in patients with known cerebrovascular disease.

Preparation

No special preparation is needed. The patient should remove **contact lenses**, and may wish to avoid the use of eye makeup, since the gel is likely to smear it. For convenience and comfort during the procedure, the patient should wear loose, comfortable clothing and no earrings or hair ornaments.

Aftercare

The gel is washed off with soap and water. No other aftercare is needed.

Complications

TCD is noninvasive and has no notable complications. A compression test is occasionally, though very rarely, hazardous for a patient with narrowed arteries (atherosclerosis), since the increased pressure may dislodge a piece of the substance that causes the narrowing (plaque).

Results

Normal results

TCD ultrasonography calculates blood flow velocity, which, in turn, helps determine direction of flow and restrictions in flow. The sound being measured will vary depending on the direction and rate of flow through the vessel being examined. Each of the vessels in the brain has a characteristic direction of flow, which can be altered in various conditions. Flow rates are variable from person to person depending upon the condition of the vessels in the brain and the rate of blood flow from the heart. A normal result will correspond to typical flow rates and direction of flow for each of the brain's blood vessels. Blood flow velocity may be measured in several sites, after which a peak flow velocity and an average velocity will be calculated.

Abnormal results

Diminished blood flow indicates that a vessel has been blocked to some extent. Lack of a signal may mean no blood flow due to complete blockage, although absence of a signal may also mean that sound waves have been absorbed by bone. If blood in a certain vessel flows in the wrong direction or alternates between normal and reverse flow, it may indicate a blockage elsewhere in the brain. This happens because blood is rerouted when a blockage causes differences in intracranial pressure.

An increased rate of flow may mean that blood is flowing through a restricted area just "upstream" from the probe. Although it seems that a restricted blood vessel would cause the speed of blood flow to slow down, the opposite is true. This is because the same amount of blood going through a narrower opening must go faster. Increased speed is also seen if a vessel is carrying rerouted blood.

KEY TERMS

Cerebrovascular—The blood vessels that make up the vascular system of the brain, including all veins and arteries that carry blood.

Doppler ultrasonography—Measures frequency changes that occurs when ultrasound signals are directed toward blood vessels and reflected back to their source. Transcranial Doppler ultrasonography (TCD) pertains to frequency changes measured in the blood vessels of the brain.

Frequency—The number of cycles of a wave over time, such the frequency of a sound wave.

Transcranial—Scanning through the skull.

Transducer—Also called a probe, a hand-held instrument that transmits and receives sound waves, which can then be measured by electronic equipment. In an ultrasound examination, a transducer is used to scan the body.

Ultrasonography—Also called ultrasound scanning or sonography; a safe, non-radiologic, non-invasive diagnostic imaging technology in which high frequency sound waves are bounced off or passed through body tissues to obtain a visual image of the tissue or body organs being evaluated.

Ultrasound image—Also called a scan or a sonogram; created on a computer monitor when high frequency sound waves are transmitted into the body and the resulting echoes are recaptured and displayed by the ultrasound system.

Health care team roles

Ultrasound procedures, including TCD, are usually performed by a sonographer in an ultrasound or radiology department in a hospital or in a separate diagnostic imaging facility. When these procedures are performed during surgery, they may be performed by an anesthesiologist or other physician. The sonographer will explain the procedure to the patient, describing each step in a reassuring manner. A radiologist, who is a physician experienced in diagnostic imaging examinations, such as radiology (x ray) and ultrasound exams, will usually analyze the Doppler results and simultaneous images of the vessels examined. The testing physician will use the information to aid in diagnosis and treatment of the patient.

Training

Sonographers are specifically trained to understand and use ultrasound equipment, including Doppler equipment, and to perform a broad range of ultrasound exams. They will have a good understanding of ultrasound electronics, of computer functions in the ultrasound scanning equipment, and they will be able to observe ultrasound images and interpret results, although they will neither diagnose nor advise patients.

Resources

BOOKS

Samuels, M.A. and Feske, S. eds. *Office Practice of Neurology*. New York: Churchill Livingstone, 1996.

ORGANIZATIONS

American Society of Neuroimaging. 5841 Cedar Lake Road, Ste. 204 Minneapolis, MN 55416. (952) 545-6291.
Society for Diagnostic Medical Sonographers (SDMS). 12770 Coit Road, Ste. 708, Dallas, TX 75251. (800) 229-9506.

L. Lee Culvert

Transcutaneous electrical nerve stimulation *see* **Electrotherapy**

Transcutaneous electrical nerve stimulation unit

Definition

A transcutaneous electrical nerve stimulation (TENS) unit is used to apply electrical currents through the skin to the nerves via electrodes in order to reduce chronic and acute **pain** from various causes.

Purpose

TENS is a noninvasive therapeutic **pain management** modality that is used alone or in conjunction with pain medications or other pain-management techniques. A TENS unit is used to transmit low-voltage electrical currents through the skin to the underlying nerves at the area where pain occurs. TENS is used to treat both chronic and acute pain associated with musculoskeletal problems (e.g., arthritis, low back pain), dental problems and procedures, **bursitis**, menstruation, urinary incontinence, surgical procedures, labor and delivery, fracture pain, and traumatic injuries. TENS is also used as an adjunct

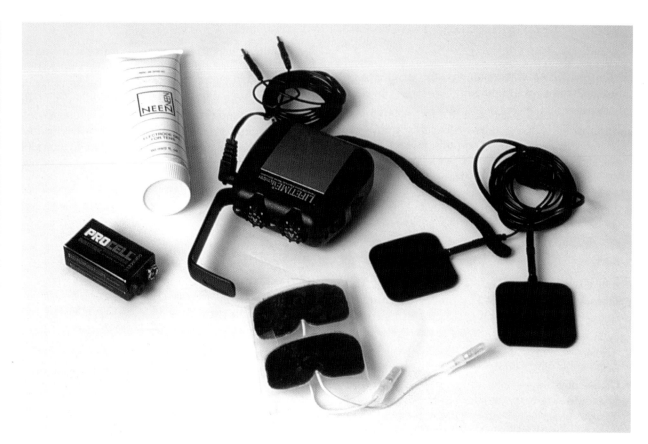

Transcutaneous Electrical Nerve Stimulation (TENS) equipment, used for painkilling if analgesic drugs (painkillers) are not working well enough. The main TENS unit (at center) is powered by a battery (at center left). The electrodes (at lower right and lower center) are placed on skin once it has been covered in a gel (at upper right), which aids conductivity. The TENS unit delivers minute electrical impulses through the electrodes. These pulses are thought to stop pain messages from reaching the brain. *(Faye Norman / Phopto Researchers, Inc. Reproduced by permission.)*

treatment for chemotherapy-induced nausea and vomiting.

Description

A TENS unit consists of an electronic stimulus generator, which transmits electrical current to electrodes placed directly on the patient's skin. Most TENS units use two or four electrodes to transmit electrical impulses. The number of impulses (frequency), the pulse duration, and intensity can be adjusted. Some TENS units offer modulation, which allows the frequency, duration, and intensity to be intermittently changed, and a burst mode, which allows groups of rapid pulses to be applied at regular intervals. The treatment parameters (i.e., rate of stimulation, pulse intensity and duration, other settings) are based on the type of TENS unit used, the patient's medical condition, and response to stimulation.

The physiological mechanism of TENS pain relief is not fully understood, but two theories are have been proposed to explain it: gate control and endorphin release.

According to the gate-control theory, pain is experienced when certain small unmyelinated fibers are stimulated (the "gate" is opened). Pain is not felt when larger myelinated fibers that inhibit the feeling of pain are stimulated (the gate is closed). The electrical currents produced by a TENS unit stimulate these large myelinated fibers, blocking pain stimuli transmitted by the smaller unmyelinated fibers.

According to the endorphin release theory, TENS is believed to stimulate the release of endorphins, peptides in the body that help inhibit the transmission of painful stimuli.

TENS units are available in desktop, handheld, portable, and wearable configurations, depending on the manufacturer and clinical applications for which the unit is designed. For example, some TENS units dedicated to treating premenstrual pain and dysmenorrhea are smaller and configured with a belt clip and battery operation so the patient can wear the unit for the duration of pain treatment.

TENS is used in **physical therapy**, rehabilitation, primary care, hospital, chiropractic care, long-term care, and home-care settings, and is initially administered with close supervision of the patient to evaluate their response to treatment. Depending on their pain and associated medical condition, the patient may then given instructions on how to use the TENS unit at home according to a prescribed schedule.

Operation

To use a TENS unit, electrodes are placed on the patient's skin in the painful area, on either side of the spine, in peripheral nerve areas, or at trigger points, depending on the nature of the patient's pain. Electrodes should be kept at least 3 centimeters (1.18 inches) apart. The most common type of electrode supplied with the TENS unit is made of soft rubber that may require conducting gel before application. Other types of electrodes include those made of disposable foam or sponge that must be moistened with water, conductive self-adhesive polymer, or reusable pregelled material. Leads are then plugged into one end of each electrode and into output sockets on the electronic generator unit. Pulse rate, intensity, and duration are then adjusted according to the patient's condition; a vibration or tingling sensation may be felt and the muscles may twitch as the electrical pulses are delivered.

TENS should not be used in patients with **tuberculosis**, malignant tumors, high or low **blood pressure**, high **fever**, carotid sinus hypersensitivity, or acute inflammatory disease. Electrodes should not be applied over the eyes, the front of the throat, directly over a wound, on skin wet from bathing or sweating, over broken skin, or over psoriasis and similar skin conditions. Because TENS may interfere with pacemaker operation, electrodes should not be applied in the vicinity of a pacemaker, and TENS use in patients with **pacemakers** should be carefully supervised.

There are very few side effects associated with the use of a TENS unit. Minor skin irritation may occur from the electrodes; proper cleaning of the patient's skin and changing the electrodes daily can alleviate irritation. Some sensitive patients may have an allergic reaction to gel or the electrode material. If TENS is applied in areas with poor sensation, skin **burns** may occur.

KEY TERMS

Dysmenorrhea—Painful menstruation.

Electrode—A conductor used to complete the electrical circuit between the TENS unit and the patient.

Endorphins—A group of naturally occurring peptides that, when released, act like a painkiller by inhibiting the transmission of pain impulses.

Lead—Insulated wires that connect the TENS unit to the electrode.

Trigger points—Areas on the skin that, when stimulated electrically, produce sensations at that point or elsewhere on the body.

Maintenance

TENS units are, in general, low-maintenance systems that need only periodic battery checks to ensure effective delivery of the electrical pulses. Many TENS units have self-testing features that detect defective leads and electrodes; if the unit does not have self-testing features, leads and electrodes should be checked frequently to avoid potential shocks. Rubber electrodes can last years with proper cleaning and use; the leads should not be detached between uses, as this increases wear on the rubber and the connection. Pregelled reusable electrodes can be used for approximately one month or 100 hours.

Health care team roles

Depending on where the patient is being treated for pain and how TENS treatment is prescribed, a number of healthcare professionals could be involved. In physical therapy and rehabilitation settings, the therapist, nurse, or clinical assistant could administer TENS. In the hospital and primary care settings, physicians and/or nurses could administer TENS. Chiropractors, naturopathic physicians, and pain-management professionals (e.g., anesthesiologists) may also prescribe and administer TENS. The nurse or other clinician trained in the use of TENS can instruct patients using TENS at home, ensuring that they understand how to apply TENS and are compliant with their pain-management protocol.

Training

Training in the use of the TENS unit is provided by the manufacturer for administration by clinical staff. Detailed manuals on maintenance and use are provided with the unit.

Resources

BOOKS

Walsh, Deirdre M., and Eric T. McAdams. *TENS: Clinical Applications and Related Theory*. New York: Churchill Livingstone, 1997.

PERIODICALS

Bertoti, Dolores B. "Electrical Stimulation: A Reflection on Current Clinical Practices." *Assistive Technology* 12, no. 1 (2000): 21–32.

ORGANIZATIONS

American Academy of Pain Management. 13947 Mono Way #A, Sonora, CA 95370. (209) 533-9744. <http://www.aapainmanage.org>.

American Society of Anesthesiologists. 520 North Northwest Highway, Park Ridge, IL 60068-2573. <http://www.asahq.org>.

Society for Pain Practice Management. 4801 College Boulevard, Leawood, KS 66211. (913) 491-6451. <http://www.sppm.org>.

OTHER

American Society of Anesthesiologists. "Practice Guidelines for Chronic Pain Management." *Anesthesiology* 86 (1997): 995-1004. <http://www.asahq.org/practice/chronic_pain/chronic_pain.html>.

Reeve, Janis, and Paula Corabian. "Transcutaneous Electrical Nerve Stimulation (TENS) and Pain Management." Canadian Coordinating Office for Health Technology Assessment. April 1995.

Jennifer E. Sisk, M.A.

Transesophageal echocardiography

Definition

Transesophageal **echocardiography** (TEE) is a diagnostic test in which an **endoscope** with an ultrasound transducer at its tip is inserted into the patient's esophagus by means of a catheter (thin tube). Sound waves are transmitted and received by the transducer to produce a clear image of the **heart** muscle and other parts of the heart.

Purpose

Since the esophagus is located directly behind the heart, transesophageal echocardiography provides a very clear image of the heart. It can provide information on the size of the heart, its pumping strength, and the location and extent of any damage to its tissues. TEE can also detect the presence of abnormal tissue growth around the heart valves. It is useful for identifying abnormalities in the pattern of **blood** flow, such as the backward flow of blood through partly closed heart valves (regurgitation). TEE is especially useful in cases in which conventional echocardiography (a test in which the transducer is moved across the patient's chest) cannot offer a good image, as when the patient is obese or has a thick chest wall. TEE is also used to monitor heart function during cardiac surgery; to detect blood clots in the left atrium of the heart; and to diagnose infections in pacemaker lead infections.

TEE is performed with portable devices and equipment, and it is safer and less expensive than aortography, an invasive procedure performed in a **cardiac catheterization** laboratory. TEE is less expensive than computed tomography and **magnetic resonance imaging**, two diagnostic imaging modalities commonly used for cardiac studies; in addition, it allows a more direct evaluation of the heart. Finally, results from a TEE examination are available within 15 minutes, which offers the physician another advantage over **CT scans**.

The convenience, safety, and promptness of TEE make it the diagnostic procedure of choice in patients suspected of aortic dissection, especially those who are in unstable condition. TEE can also be used for long-term follow-up of these patients.

Precautions

Transesophageal echocardiography should be performed only by physicians who have received the necessary postgraduate training. It is a highly specialized technique requiring advanced skills in interpreting results as well as performing the procedure.

TEE should not be performed in patients with **dysphagia** (difficulty swallowing), indications of gastroesophageal disease, or injuries to the esophagus. Before the procedure, the patient should be asked about any drug **allergies** and current medications, since some medications may entail risks during the procedure. For example, patients on anticoagulant therapy are at risk for bleeding complications.

Patients should avoid consuming alcohol for a day or so before and after TEE, since alcohol may amplify the effects of the sedative used with the procedure.

Description

TEE uses the same principles as conventional echocardiography to produce images of the heart, namely high-frequency sound waves. TEE produces sharper images, however, because the transducer is positioned directly behind the heart, not on the chest wall as in conventional echocardiography.

A TEE examination generally lasts 15–30 minutes. The patient is given a mild sedative intravenously, and the back of the throat is sprayed with a local anesthetic in order to suppress the gag reflex. The patient is positioned on the left side. A special viewing tube called an endoscope, which contains a transducer at the tip, is inserted through the mouth and into the esophagus. The instrument is carefully moved until it is positioned directly next to the heart. Essentially a modified microphone, the transducer directs ultrasound waves into the heart, some of which are reflected (or echoed) back to the transducer. Tissues of different densities and blood all reflect ultrasound waves differently. These sound waves can be translated into an image of the heart, displayed on a monitor, or recorded on paper or tape. The transducer may be moved several times during the test to help the doctors get a better view of the heart.

TEE can be performed as an outpatient procedure in an echocardiography laboratory; as an inpatient procedure in an operating room; or as an emergency procedure in an intensive care unit or emergency department.

Preparation

The patient is asked not to eat or drink for six hours before the TEE examination. Patients who wear dentures must remove them before the test. The patient may be given a mild sedative intravenously before the procedure, and an anesthetic is sprayed into the back of the throat in order to suppress the gag reflex.

Aftercare

After the test, the patient must refrain from eating or drinking until the gag reflex has returned—otherwise, he or she may accidentally inhale some of the food or beverage. In addition, patients should not drive or operate heavy machinery for at least 10–12 hours if they have been given a sedative. They should avoid consuming alcohol for a day or so, since alcohol may amplify the effect of the sedative.

KEY TERMS

Aneurysm—A dilatation of the aorta or other artery, caused by a weakening of the vessel wall.

Aorta—The main artery of the circulatory system, conveying blood from the left ventricle of the heart.

Dissection—Separation of the layers of arterial tissue in the aorta, resulting from blood being forced out into the wall of the aorta through a tear in the innermost layer of tissue.

Dysphagia—Difficulty in swallowing.

Endoscope—An instrument used to visualize and examine the inside of a body cavity or organ.

Gag reflex—A normal reflex consisting of elevation of the palate, retraction of the tongue, and contraction of the throat muscles.

Regurgitation—The backward flow of blood through a partly closed valve.

Transducer—A device that converts electrical signals into ultrasound waves and the echoes back into electrical impulses.

Ultrasound—Sound waves at a frequency of 2–10 megahertz (mHz), often used for diagnostic imaging.

Complications

Transesophageal echocardiography may cause gagging and discomfort when the endoscope is inserted down into the throat. Patients may also experience a **sore throat** for a few days after the test. In rare cases, the procedure may cause bleeding or perforation of the esophagus, or an inflammatory condition known as infective **endocarditis**. The patient may also have an adverse reaction to the sedative or local anesthetic.

Results

A normal transesophageal echocardiogram shows a normal heart structure and normal patterns of blood flow through the valves and chambers of the heart.

In terms of abnormal findings, a transesophageal echocardiogram may show a number of abnormalities in the structure and function of the heart, such as thickening of the wall of the heart muscle (especially the left ventricle). Other abnormal findings may include aneurysms or dissections of the aorta, regurgitation, or blood clots in the left atrium of the heart.

Health care team roles

TEE is performed by a cardiologist trained and experienced in the applications of cardiac sonography. A cardiac ultrasonographer may assist during the procedure. Nurses are present during TEE to monitor the patient's **vital signs**. During cardiac surgery, TEE may be performed by the cardiac surgeon or by a cardiovascular anesthesiologist.

Resources

BOOKS

Faculty Members of the Yale University School of Medicine. *The Patient's Book of Medical Tests*. Boston and New York: Houghton Mifflin Company, 1997.

PERIODICALS

Lopez-Candales, Angel. "Assessing the Aorta with Transesophageal Echocardiography: Update on Imaging Capabilities with Today's Technology." *Postgraduate Medicine* 106, no. 4 (October 1, 1999): 157-172. <http://www.postgradmed.com/issues/1999/10_01_99/lopez.htm>.

Report by the American Society of Anesthesiologists and the Society of Cardiovascular Anesthesiologists Task Force on Transesophageal Echocardiography. "Practice Guidelines for Perioperative Transesophageal Echocardiography." *Anesthesiology* 84 (1996): 986-1006.

Rose, Verna L. "American College of Cardiology and American Heart Association address the use of echocardiography." *American Family Physician* 56 (October 7, 1997): 1489-90.

ORGANIZATIONS

American College of Cardiology. Heart House, 9111 Old Georgetown Road, Bethesda, MD 20814-1699. (800) 253-4636. <http://www.acc.org>.

American Heart Association National Center. 7272 Greenville Avenue, Dallas, TX 75231. (800) AHA-USA1. <http://www.americanheart.org>.

American Society of Echocardiography. 1500 Sunday Drive, Suite 102, Raleigh, NC 27607. (919) 787-5181. <http://asecho.org>.

Jennifer E. Sisk, M.A.

Transferrin test *see* **Iron tests; Plasma protein tests**

Transfusion therapy

Definition

Transfusion therapy refers to the process of administering whole **blood** or blood components to a patient through an intravenous (IV) needle or catheter placed in a patient's vein. Blood and blood products may be autologous (comprised of the patient's own blood), homologous (blood donated from another person), or synthetic (blood products developed in a laboratory). Some of the types of blood products available for transfusion include: whole blood, plasma, platelets, packed red blood cells (RBCs), leukocyte-poor RBCs, white blood cells (WBCs), clotting factors (II, VII, VIII, IX and X complex), anti-inhibitor coagulant complex, human antithrombin III, and human Rh (D) immune globulin.

Purpose

The most common purpose for administering a transfusion is to replace lost blood volume. Transfusions are also given to increase the blood's ability to carry oxygen to the tissue, to improve immunity, or to correct blood-clotting problems. Some specific purposes of transfusions include:

- Replacement of blood volume lost due to trauma or surgery.
- Correction of anemia caused by chronic conditions.
- Treatment of immune suppression.
- Treatment of thrombocytopenia.
- Replacement of missing clotting factors.
- Correction of coagulation deficiencies.
- Treatment of **hemophilia** or other congenital clotting deficiencies.
- Treatment of chronic hypoproteinemia.
- Suppression of active antibody response in Rh negative patients exposed to Rh positive blood.

Precautions

Donor blood must be compatible to the recipient of the transfusion. Compatibility blood testing (type and cross match) must be performed before administering homologous blood to avoid serious transfusion reactions. This blood test assures that the donor blood matches and is compatible with the recipient blood (including the blood type and the **Rh factor**). In an emergency when there is no time for matching blood, type O, Rh-negative blood (universal donor) is used until compatibility testing can be performed.

To minimize the chance of giving a patient the wrong product and causing a severe transfusion reaction, blood and blood products are labeled with patient name, number, type, and Rh factor by the blood bank. The clinician should check and record the blood bag name, number, type, and Rh factor against the patient's identification armband and the lab slip numbers twice with another nurse before administering blood products. The nurse should recheck the physician's order and the expiration date on the blood product before giving the blood product.

Patients must understand and sign an **informed consent** form before receiving a blood transfusion. Blood is never given without the patient's consent. When a patient is unable to give consent, the closest family member should sign the form. The consent assures that the patient or family member is aware of the risks involved in blood transfusions, including the potential for an allergic reaction, transfusion reaction, and/or the possibility of contracting an **infection** from the transfusion.

Special equipment is used for blood transfusions to assure proper flow of the blood product and to filter out impurities or small clots. Use appropriate blood tubing, filter tubing, and/or needle filters as directed by the policy of the medical setting. The tubing may vary according to the blood product being administered. Blood and blood products require a separate IV line, separate IV lumen in a multi-lumen central line, or an IV line that has been thoroughly flushed with normal saline. Blood and blood products are not compatible with IV solutions other than normal saline. Drugs should not be administered through the IV line while blood or blood products are running. Drugs may be given in some medical settings through a separate lumen of a multi-lumen central IV line if the lumen is flushed with normal saline before and after drug administration.

Blood should be given to the patient within 30 minutes of receiving it from the blood bank. If there is a delay because of IV line issues or other patient needs, the blood should be returned to the blood bank until the staff is ready to administer the blood. This decreases the chance of **bacteria** growing in the blood bag and helps prevent confusion and errors. Never transfuse blood for longer than four hours to minimize risks of infection.

Nurses monitor patients receiving blood or blood products closely by checking their **vital signs** every 15 minutes during the first hour of the transfusion and hourly thereafter or as dictated by the policy of the medical setting. Transfusion reactions most often occur within the first 15 minutes of the blood administration. If signs such as high **fever**, rapid pulse, wheezing, shortness of breath, flushed face, chest **pain**, flank pain, hematuria or restlessness occur, the nurse should stop the transfusion, change the IV tubing, and run in normal saline slowly. The nurse should keep the line open in the event that drug therapy is needed to reverse the reaction. He or she should elevate the head of the bed, administer oxygen if needed, monitor the patient's vital signs, and contact the physician immediately. The reaction should be documented and the blood bag and tubing returned to the blood bank for testing. There is usually a transfusion reaction protocol in the medical setting for collecting post-reaction blood or urine specimens. If the patient develops itching and a rash during a transfusion, the nurse should slow the flow rate and contact the physician before stopping the blood. The physician may elect to administer **antihistamines** and continue the blood transfusion. If the patient develops a low-grade fever during transfusion, the nurse should slow the flow rate down and contact the physician before stopping the blood. The physician may elect to administer an antipyretic and continue the transfusion.

Fluid overload can occur (especially in children or the elderly) as a result of a transfusion running too rapidly. The nurse should run blood in slowly (generally over two hours) and monitor the patient closely for restlessness, rapid pulse, or respiratory distress. The flow rate should be adjusted according to the physician's order or the policy of the medical setting. Flow rates may vary according to the product. For instance, the rate for whole blood may be different than the rate for packed cells.

Description

The blood or blood product is checked by two nurses, two times to be sure the label on the bag matches the patient and the lab slip. The patient should state his name, and the armband should be checked to avoid errors. The nurse should check the expiration date on the unit, to make sure to not give blood products past their expiration dates. He or she should gently rotate the bag in the hands to mix the blood or blood components and then connect the blood or blood product to the IV line in place of the normal saline. If a Y-tubing is in use, the saline line is shut off and the blood product line is opened. Blood products are usually started slowly at 5-10 ml per minute for the first 15 minutes. The line and the patient should be checked frequently during the first 15 minutes of the transfusion to assure that the line is intact, the rate is correct, and the patient is not displaying signs of a reaction. After 15 minutes, vital signs should be obtained and compared to pre-transfusion vital signs to detect any changes. The blood flow rate can then be increased to the correct flow

KEY TERMS

Antipyretic—A medication used to reduce fever.

Autologous transfusion—The collection, filtration and re-administration of a person's own blood. The blood for an autologous transfusion is collected, filtered, and stored for a patient prior to surgery or may sometimes be salvaged after a traumatic injury or during major surgery.

Clotting factors—Plasma proteins normally found in the blood that work with platelets to help blood clot.

Coagulation—The process of thickening or clotting of the blood.

Hematuria—The appearance of blood or blood cells in the urine.

Hemolytic reaction—A serious transfusion reaction that occurs when donor blood type or Rh factors are not compatible with the recipient's blood. Red blood cell destruction within the body causes symptoms such as shaking, chills, fever, chest pain, difficulty breathing, flank pain, and abnormal bleeding. Hemolytic reactions can lead to major organ failure, shock, and death.

Homologous transfusion—The intravenous delivery of blood or blood products donated by one person (donor) to another person (recipient).

Hyperkalemia—An excess of potassium in the blood which can cause heart muscle irritability and arrhythmias.

Hypocalcemia—A deficiency of calcium in the blood which can cause symptoms of muscle tingling or cramps, nausea, vomiting, lowered blood pressure, and seizures.

Hypoproteinemia—A deficiency of protein in the blood.

Hypothermia—An abnormally low body temperature, usually below 92 °F (33.3 °C).

Non-hemolytic febrile reaction—An antigen antibody reaction that occurs in 1% of all transfusions. Symptoms include a temperature elevation, chills, palpitations, back pain, chest pain, or headache.

Plasma—The liquid portion of the blood.

Platelets—Small disc-shaped substances in the blood that assist in blood clotting.

Red blood cells—Cells found in the blood that contain hemoglobin, transport oxygen to body tissue, and are responsible for the red coloring of the blood.

Rh factor—An antigen found on the membrane of red blood cells that will mount an immune response to transfused blood or blood products if not matched correctly before transfusion.

Thrombocytopenia—A persistent deficiency of blood platelets that leads to problems with blood clotting.

White blood cells—White or colorless cells found in the blood that do not contain hemoglobin, but contain a nucleus and help protect the body from infections and disease.

rate for the product being delivered. The patient's vital signs, affect, IV site, and transfusion flow rate should be checked and recorded every 15 minutes for the first hour of the transfusion and then hourly until the completion of the transfusion or according to the medical setting policy.

Preparation

A blood specimen is drawn from the patient, so that the blood bank can type, match, and prepare the appropriate blood product. In most settings an arm-band is placed on the patient's wrist at the time of the blood draw with a number and name that will later match the blood product label. A physician or nurse will explain the procedure to the patient and obtain a signed informed consent for the transfusion. A physician or nurse will insert either a peripheral or central IV line and connect it to a normal saline drip with appropriate blood tubing and filters in place. If the patient has a peripherally inserted central catheter (PICC), it is better to start another peripheral IV to deliver blood because a PICC line has such a long narrow tubing that blood flows slowly through it and has a tendency to clog the line. Blood will flow most easily through a large bore (#18 or #19) needle or catheter. A blood pump, pressure bag, or blood warmer should be obtained if necessary. Blood warmers are most often used in the surgical or neonatal setting. Most IV pumps will pump blood without damaging the cells, but the medical center's policy should be checked for using blood pumps. The nurse should take and record a set of base-line vital signs, including the patient's **blood pressure**, temperature, pulse, and respirations prior to transfusion. The patient should be placed in a comfortable position in bed during a transfusion to enhance **relaxation** and decrease resistance to the blood flow.

Aftercare

When the transfusion is complete, the IV line is flushed with normal saline and discontinued or changed to other IV solutions with new IV tubing for ongoing IV therapy. The patient should be observed for 30 minutes after a transfusion for delayed reactions. A final set of vital signs is taken and recorded 30 minutes after the transfusion is finished. Blood slips are returned to the lab. Fresh IV tubing should be used for subsequent units of blood or blood products. Gloves should be worn when handling used blood supplies. Blood bags, tubing, and catheters are placed in a contaminated trash bag that can be sealed and discarded. Needles are placed (without recapping) in a puncture-proof contaminated needle box.

Complications

Complications of transfusion therapy are not frequent but can include:

- allergic reactions
- hemolytic reactions
- non-hemolytic febrile reactions
- circulatory overload
- hypothermia
- hypocalcemia
- hyperkalemia
- microbial contamination
- disease transmission (**AIDS**, hepatitis C, or bacterial infection)

Results

The results of transfusion therapy are usually rapid and positive. Blood volume is expanded, missing factors are replaced, clotting problems are corrected, or immunity is improved. In some cases, a patient may need multiple transfusions to reach desired effect. Most transfusions are safe; however, mild febrile and allergic reactions occur in about 1-2% of all transfusions. Severe or fatal transfusion reactions are rare. Autologous transfusions are the safest type of transfusion and pose the least risk for infection or reaction. Autologous blood, however, is not always available when needed.

Health care team roles

Transfusion therapy is usually performed by a **registered nurse** in a controlled medical setting because of the need for ongoing assessment and the potential for transfusion reaction. Transfusions are occasionally administered in the home by a registered nurse who has access to appropriate equipment, emergency medical back-up, and immediate contact with a physician.

Resources

BOOKS

"Blood and Blood Products." In *Medication Administration. Nurse's Clinical Guide.* Pennsylvania: Springhouse Corporation, 2000.

OTHER

"Blood Transfusion." *The Merck Manual of Medical Information—Home Edition Online,* 2001. <http://www.merck.com/pubs/mmanual_home/sec14/153.htm>.

Fitzpatrick, Linda, R.N. "Blood Transfusion: Keeping Your Patient Safe." Nursing Interventions. *Nursing 97.* Springnet Online. August 1997. <http://www.springnet. com/ce/p708b.htm>.

"Transfusion of Blood and Blood Products." *Your Surgery Online,* 2001. <http://www.yoursurgery.com/data/Procedures/blood_transfusion/p_blood_transfusion.cfm>.

"Transfusion Procedures." *University of Michigan Hospitals and Health Centers Online,* December 2000. <http://141.214.6.15/bloodbank/bb_book/bbch_6/default.htm>.

"Transfusion Therapy." Chapter 27. *Lippincott Manual of Nursing Practice.* Books at Ovid Online. 2001. <http://pco.ovid.com/lrppco/>.

Mary Elizabeth Martelli, R.N., B.S.

Transplant reaction screening test *see*
Cytomegalovirus antibody screening test

Traumatic amputations

Definition

Traumatic amputation is the accidental severing of some or all of a body part. A complete amputation totally detaches a limb or appendage from the rest of the body. In a partial amputation, some soft tissue remains attached to the site.

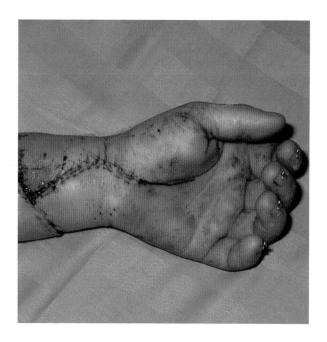

This man's hand was surgically reattached following a traumatic amputation. *(Photograph by Michael English, M.D., Custom Medical Stock Photo. Reproduced by permission.)*

Description

Trauma is the second leading cause of amputation in the United States. About 30,000 traumatic amputations occur in this country every year. Four of every five traumatic amputation victims are male, and most of them are between the ages of 15 and 30.

Traumatic amputation most often affects limbs and appendages such as the arms, ears, feet, fingers, hands, legs, and nose.

Causes and symptoms

Farm and factory workers have greater-than-average risks of suffering injuries that result in traumatic amputation. Automobile and motorcycle accidents and the use of lawnmowers, saws, and power tools are also common causes of traumatic amputation.

Blood loss may be massive or minimal, depending on the nature of the injury and the site of the amputation. Persons who lose little blood and have less severe injuries sometimes feel more **pain** than those who bleed heavily and whose injuries are life-threatening.

Diagnosis

When an injured person and the amputated part(s) reach the hospital, an emergency department physician will assess the probability that the severed tissue can be successfully reattached.

The mangled extremity severity score (MESS) assigns numerical values to such factors as body temperature, circulation, numbness, **paralysis**, tissue health, and the person's age and general health. This is one of the diagnostic tools used to determine the probability of success for reattachment surgery. The total score is doubled if blood supply to the amputated part has been absent or diminished for more than six hours.

A general, emergency, or orthopedic surgeon makes the final determination about whether surgery should be performed. The surgeon also considers an injured person's wishes and lifestyle. Additional concerns are how and to what extent the amputation will affect an individual's quality of life and ability to perform everyday activities.

Treatment

First aid or emergency care given immediately after the amputation has a critical impact on both a physician's ability to salvage and reattach the severed part(s) and a person's ability to regain feeling and function.

Muscle tissue dies quickly, but a well-preserved body part can be successfully reattached as much as 24 hours after the amputation occurs. Tissue that has not been preserved will not survive for more than six hours.

Initial response

The most important steps to take when a traumatic amputation occurs are:

- Contact the nearest emergency services provider, clearly describe what has happened, and follow any instructions given.

- Make sure the injured person can breathe. If not, clear an airway and administer **CPR** as necessary.

- Use direct pressure to control bleeding, but minimize or avoid contact with blood and other body fluids.

- Persons should not be moved if back, head, leg, or neck injuries are suspected or if motion causes pain. If none are found by an emergency medical technician (EMT), put the injured person in a supine (back down) position flat with the feet raised 1 ft (0.3 m) above the surface.

- Cover the person with a coat or blanket to prevent shock.

The injured site should be cleansed with a sterile solution and wrapped in a clean towel or other thick material that will protect the wound from further injury. Tissue that is still attached to the body should not be forced back into place. If it cannot be gently replaced, it should be held in its normal position and supported until additional care is available.

Saving a person's life is always more important than recovering the amputated part(s). Transporting the injured person to a hospital or emergency center should never be delayed until missing pieces are located.

Preserving tissue

No amputated body part is too small to be salvaged. Debris or other contaminating material should be removed, but the tissue should not be allowed to get wet.

An amputated body part should be wrapped in bandages, towels, or other clean, protective material and sealed in a plastic bag. Placing the sealed bag in a cooler or in a container that is inside a second container filled with cold water or ice will help prevent tissue deterioration.

Prognosis

Possible complications of traumatic amputation include:

- excessive bleeding
- infection
- muscle shortening
- pulmonary embolism

Improved medical and surgical care and rehabilitation have improved the long-term outlook for persons experiencing a traumatic amputation.

Phantom pain

About 80% of all amputees over the age of four experience tingling, itching, numbness, or pain in the place where the amputated part used to be. Phantom sensations may begin immediately after the amputation, or they may develop months or years later. They often occur after an injury to the site of the amputation.

These intermittent feelings may:

- occur frequently or infrequently
- be mild or intense
- last for a few minutes or several hours
- help injured persons adjust more readily to an artificial limb (prosthesis)

Health care team roles

Emergency medical technicians often provide initial assistance to persons experiencing traumatic amputation. These people are evaluated by emergency room physicians and surgeons (trauma, plastic and neurosurgeons) to establish a plan for treatment. During surgery, they are supported by anesthesiologists, nurses, and surgical assistants. Plastic surgeons may perform many other operations to restore injured body parts to a more normal condition and appearance. Infectious disease specialists may be called upon to treat infections that may accompany an accident and subsequent traumatic amputation.

After surgery, rehabilitation professionals begin to assist. Doctors trained in physical medicine and rehabilitation (physiatrists) design a general course of therapy. Physical therapists work to regain lost physical functions. Occupational therapists may assist with redeveloping fine motor coordination and control.

If a prosthetic limb (arm or leg) is needed, an orthotist may be called upon to fit such a device to an injured person. Physical and occupational therapists will assist recovering amputees to learn how to use their new artificial limbs.

Most persons who experience a traumatic amputation require some form of counseling to help them adjust to their loss and altered appearance. Psychiatrists, counselors and other therapists may conduct therapy sessions. These may continue for many months.

Physiatrists monitor and evaluate the status of reattached limbs over time. They may also be called upon to treat phantom pain.

Prevention

The best way to prevent traumatic amputation is to observe common-sense precautions such as using seat belts and obeying speed limits and other traffic regulations. It is important to take special precautions when using potentially dangerous equipment. Guards should be securely fastened over blades, belts, gears, and other moving parts. Machinery should be turned off and disconnected before attempting to service or repair it. Appropriate protective clothing should be worn at all times. Personal clothing such as scarves, ties, and other loose items of jewelry that might become entangled in machinery should not be worn.

Resources

BOOKS

Ferrera, Peter C., Steven A. Colucciello, John Marx, and Cince Verdile. *Trauma Management: An Emergency Medicine Approach.* St. Louis: Mosby, 2000.

Leung, K.S., and P.Y. Ko. *Practical Manual for Musculoskeletal Trauma.* New York: Springer–Verlag, 2001.

Mattox, Kenneth L., David V. Feliciano, and Ernest E. Moore. *Trauma,* 4th Ed. New York: Appleton & Lange, 1999.

Scaletta, Thomas A., and Jeffery J. Schaider. *Emergent Management of Trauma,* 2nd Ed. New York: McGraw–Hill, 2000.

Simon, Robert R., and Steven J. Koenigsknecht. *Emergency Orthopedics,* 4th Ed. New York: McGraw–Hill, 2000.

Weinzweig, Jeffrey. *Mutilated Hand.* Philadelphia: Hanley & Belfus, 2001.

PERIODICALS

Hankin, F.M., D.H. Janda, and B. Wittenberg. "Playground Equipment Contributing to a Ring Avulsion Injury." *Injury* 31, no. 8 (2000): 635–7.

Hegazi, M.M. "Hand and Distal Forearm Replantation— Immediate and Long-Term Follow-Up." *Hand Surgery* 5, no. 2 (2000): 119–24.

Levy, B.S., and D. Parker. "Children and War." *Public Health Reports* 115, no. 4 (2000): 320–5.

Moore, R.S., V. Tan, J.P. Dormans, and D.J. Bozentka. "Major Pediatric Hand Trauma Associated with Fireworks." *Journal of Orthopedic Trauma* 14, no. 6 (2000): 426–8.

ORGANIZATIONS

American Academy of Emergency Medicine. 611 E. Wells St., Milwaukee, WI 53202. (800) 884-2236. <http://www.aaem.org>.

American Academy of Physical Medicine and Rehabilitation. One IBM Plaza, Suite 2500, Chicago, IL 60611-3604. (312) 464-9700. <http://www.aapmr.org/consumers/public/amputations.htm>.

American Amputee Foundation. P.O. Box 250218, Little Rock, AR 72225-0218. (501) 666-2523.

American College of Emergency Physicians. 1125 Executive Circle, Irving, TX 75038-2522. (800) 798-1822. <http://www.acep.org>.

Amputee Coalition of America. 900 E. Hill Ave., Suite 285, Knoxville, TN 37915. (888) 267-5669. <http://www.amputee-coalition.org>.

National Amputation Foundation, 38–40 Church St., Malverne, NY 11565. (516) 887-3600. <http://www.nationalamputation.org>.

OTHER

Medical Slides Gallery. 8 August 2001. <http://allprintall.virtualave.net/Trauma_eng/2.htm> <http://allprintall.virtualave.net/Trauma_eng/4.htm>.

National Library of Medicine. 8 August 2001. <http://www.nlm.nih.gov/medlineplus/ency/article/000006.htm>.

University of Pittsburgh. 8 August 2001. <http://www.pitt.edu/~ginie/disability/calink.html>.

Wound Care Information Network. 8 August 2001. <http://medicaledu.com/kshp.htm>.

L. Fleming Fallon, Jr., MD, PhD, DrPH

Treadmill stress test *see* **Stress test**

Trench mouth *see* **Periodontitis**

Triglyceride test *see* **Lipid tests**

Triiodothyronine test *see* **Thyroid function tests**

Triple marker screen test

Definition

The triple marker screen test (also called the maternal serum screening test or multiple marker test), is a **blood** test that is performed usually between the 14th and 18th week of **pregnancy**. This screening test measures the levels of three substances, alpha-fetoprotein (AFP), human chorionic gonadotropin (hCG), and unconjugated estriol (uE3) in the maternal blood. Each level is then divided by the median concentration of that substance for the given week of pregnancy to generate a multiple of the median value (MOM). These values, along with other maternal characteristics, such as maternal age, are analyzed by a computer program to indicate the probability that the fetus has **Down syndrome**. Down syndrome is a condition that includes mental retardation, skeletal abnormalities such as upslanted eyes and cleft palate, and organ abnormalities such as **heart** disease and intestinal obstruction. Approximately 80-95% of cases are caused by a nondisjunction of chromosome 21 in the developing gamete resulting in the presence of an additional chromosome 21.

Purpose

Triple marker testing is a screening test that is used to identify the risk that a pregnant woman will give birth to an infant with Down syndrome. The test will also detect pregnancies at increased risk for Edward syndrome (trisomy 18) and Turner syndrome (monosomy X) and developmental defects associated with increased leakage of alpha fetoprotein from the fetus. The criterion used to define cutoff concentrations of the three markers is a risk for Down syndrome of one in 190. This is equal to the risk of **miscarriage** from **amniocentesis**. Women who screen "positive" (risk of 1:190 or higher) are recommended for amniocentesis. This procedure provides cells from the fetus that are cultured and analyzed to determine the number or chromosomes within each cell and detect structural chromosome abnormalities. This is the definitive method for diagnosing Down syndrome and other genetic conditions caused by an abnormal number of chromosomes (aneuploidy).

Precautions

It is very important that the correct gestational age be determined by last menstrual period dating and recorded for the risk calculation. Errors in determining the age of the fetus lead to errors when interpreting the test results. Since an AFP test is only a screening tool, an abnormal test result is not necessarily indicative of a birth defect. Accurate gestational dating lowers the false-positive and false-negative rates associated with this screening test.

The nurse or phlebotomist collecting the blood sample for these tests should observe **universal precautions** for the prevention of transmission of bloodborne pathogens.

Description

Prior to 1964, when the association between low levels of AFP and an increased risk for Down syndrome was reported risk assessment for chromosomal diseases was based upon maternal age. At age 35, the risk of carrying a Down syndrome pregnancy is approximately one in 270, and this was deemed sufficient to warrant amniocentesis. However, three of four Down syndrome pregnancies occur in women under 35 years old. When AFP testing was used along with maternal age, the rate of detection of Down syndrome increased to about 45%, but this level of sensitivity did not justify the screening of younger women because of the risk of miscarriage. The inclusion of uE3 and hCG testing has improved the detection rate to approximately 65-80% of cases for all age groups.

Alpha fetoprotein

Alpha-fetoprotein (AFP) is a glycoprotein similar in size and structure to albumin. It is made principally by the fetal **liver** and is present at very low levels after birth. In several developmental defects the most prevalent of which is an open **neural tube defect**, spina bifida, the AFP leaks from fetal **blood vessels** into the amniotic fluid. The AFP crosses the placenta and can be measured reliably in the maternal circulation by week 14. Increased maternal serum AFP also occurs in the following conditons:

- abdominal wall defects (omphalocele and gastroschisis)
- anencephaly
- Turner syndrome
- trisomy 13
- renal diseases (congenital nephrosis, polycystic **kidneys**, renal agenesis)
- oligohydramnios (decreased amount of amniotic fluid)
- more than a single fetus
- maternal **liver cancer** and other malignancies

The cutoff for a positive screen is 2.5 MOM. A positive test should be repeated, and if positive the second time, should be followed by ultrasound. If ultrasound does not explain the high level (which may be caused by twins, anancephaly, or inaccurate dating), then amniocentesis is recommended. AFP and acetylcholinesterase levels in amniotic fluid along with high resolution ultrasound are used to predict the probability of an open neural tube defect. Decreased AFP levels, below 0.75 MOM, are seen in approximately 25% of Down syndrome pregnancies. AFP is measured by double antibody sandwich radioimmunoassay or enzyme immunoassays.

Human chorionic gonadotropin and unconjugated estriol

Human chorionic gonadotropin (hCG) and unconjugated estriol are hormones. Estriol is the major estrogen of pregnancy and is produced by the placenta from dihydroepiandosterone sulfate that is made in the fetal **adrenal glands**. Estriol levels rise steadily throughout pregnancy increasing about threefold from week 24 to full term. Human chorionic gonadogropin is also made by the placenta, and it supports the corpus luteum during gestation. The corpus luteum produces progesterone, which maintains the uterus during pregnancy. Chorionic gonadotropin peaks at about 10 weeks gestation and then falls to about 20-25% of peak levels for the remainder of pregnancy. During pregnancy, both hormones diffuse from the placental membranes into the maternal blood. Abnormal levels can be indicative of potential fetal distress and stillbirth. Like AFP, uE3 is lower than normal for the time of gestation. Conversely, hCG is increased above normal by about 25% for the time of gestation. Both hormones may be measured by radioimmunoassay or fluorescent or chemiluminescent enzyme immunoassay.

When any one test exceeds the cutoff, testing should be repeated on a new sample and ultrasound should be performed in an attempt to explain the results and determine an accurate gestational age. If results are still positive and not explained by ultrasound, amniocentesis for chromosome karyotyping (chromosome counting and analysis) is recommended. When AFP, hCG, and uE3 are low for the gestational age, this may indicate trisomy 18. This condition is caused by an additional chromosome 18, and is associated with severe birth defects, mental retardation and death. The sensitivity for trisomy 18 is approximately 60-80% using cutoffs of 0.75 MOM for AFP; 0.60 MOM for uE3; and 0.55 MOM for hCG.

Preparation

There is no specific physical preparation for this test. Fasting is not required.

Aftercare

After the blood sample is drawn, pressure should be applied to the puncture site until the bleeding stops to reduce bruising, and a bandage may be applied to the site. A warm pack may be applied to the site to relieve discomfort.

KEY TERMS

Acetylcholinesterase—A chemical found only inside neural tissue. Its presence in the amniotic fluid indicates an opening in the neural tube.

Amniotic fluid—Fluid within the uterine sac in which the fetus lives until birth.

Anencephaly—A severe and usually fatal brain abnormality caused by failure of the neural tube to close at its cranial end.

Embryo—The stage of human development prior to the second month of pregnancy.

Fetus—The stage in human development from the second month of pregnancy until birth.

Karyotyping—Chromosome analysis.

Neural tube—Tube that becomes the brain and spinal cord.

Oligohydramnios—Low amniotic fluid level.

Complications

The complications associated with drawing blood are minimal, but may include bleeding from the puncture site, feeling faint or lightheaded after the blood is drawn, or blood accumulating under the puncture site (hematoma).

Results

The various immunoassays for these analytes are associated with different normal ranges because the antibody specificity and assay detection limits are somewhat different. In order to allow for interlaboratory comparison of results, the results of analytes are expressed as multiples of the median value used by the laboratory. Normal ranges expressed in concentration (e.g. ng/mL) are dependent upon gestational age, but MOMs are age adjusted and do not change. These values are used to calculate risk. If the multiple of the median value is above 2.0 MOM or 2.5 MOM (depending on the laboratory), the fetus is considered to be at a higher risk for a neural tube defect. The MOM value for amniotic fluid is then used to calculate the exact probability the fetus is affected (1:100, for example).

With respect to Down syndrome and trisomy 18, the MOM values are also used in the calculation of probability. The woman is considered to be "high risk" or "screen positive" for Down syndrome if the risk is greater than the standard risk for women who are 35 years old or older (one in 270). For trisomy 18, the cut-off is one in 150. In one study the triple marker screen test had a detection rate for Down syndrome of 67% and a false positive rate of 5%.

Health care team roles

The obstetrician orders the triple marker screen test, and explains its purpose and results to the patient. The nurse or phlebotomist collects the blood sample and transports it to the laboratory. Typically, a nurse calls the patient with her result. If abnormal, the pregnant patient is referred to a genetic counselor, who explains the test, the result, and diagnostic testing options.

Resources

BOOKS

Cunningham, Gary, et al. *Williams Obstetrics*. 20th ed. Stamford, CT: Appleton & Lange, 1997, 922-926.

Johnson, Robert, ed. *Mayo Clinic Complete Book of Pregnancy and the Baby's First Year*. NY: William Morrow and Company, 1997.

PERIODICALS

Canick, Jacob, et al. "Multiple Marker Screening for Fetal Down Syndrome." *Contemporary OB/GYN* (April 1992): 3-12.

Haddow, James, et al. "Reducing the Need for Amniocentesis in Women 35 Years of Age or Older with Serum Markers for Screening." *New England Journal of Medicine* 330 (16) (April 21, 1994): 1114-1118.

ORGANIZATIONS

American Cancer Society. 1559 Clifton Rd. NE, Atlanta, GA 30329. <http://nysernet.org/bcic/asc2/index.html>.

March of Dimes Birth Defects Foundation, National Office. 1275 Mamaroneck Ave., White Plains, NY 10605. (888) MODIMES. <http://www.modimes.org>.

National Cancer Institute. Building 31, Room 10A24, Bethesda, MD 20892. <http://www.nci.nih.gov>.

Rachael Brandt

Tube feedings

Definition

Tube feeding is a procedure used for placing food, fluids, and drugs directly into the stomach or small intestine through a tube inserted through the nose or abdomen. Tube feeding is also called enteral feeding or enteral nutrition.

Purpose

Tube feeding is used with people who have normally functioning digestive systems, but who cannot or will not take food by mouth. Common reasons to perform tube feeding include:

- stroke resulting in paralysis of the muscles involved in swallowing
- coma
- cancer of the mouth, throat, or esophagus
- trauma or burns to the mouth, throat, or esophagus
- mental illness such as anorexia or dementia that leads to refusal to eat

Most often people are fed through a nasogastric tube that goes from the nose through the esophagus and into the **stomach**. This method of tube feeding is preferred for short term feeding problems that do not last longer than about two weeks. There are two choices for tube feeding that is needed on a long term basis. One is the insertion of a nasointestinal tube that passes through the stomach and delivers nutrients directly into the small intestine. A nasointestinal tube is also used after gastric surgery, gastric trauma, or paralysis of the stomach muscles. The other option for long term feeding lasting over 30 days is a tube that is surgically placed through the abdomen directly into the small intestine. This is called a percutaneous endoscopic gastrostomy (PEG) tube. PEG tubes are often used for individuals with oral cancer as well as for elderly patients who cannot physically pass food through the mouth.

Precautions

Problems can arise in the insertion of the tube. During the actual feeding process, care must be taken to introduce the food at a manageable rate. Also, the tube must be kept clean and flushed after each use.

Description

Tube feedings can be delivered either continuously or intermittently by gravity feed or by pump. Each method has its advantages and disadvantages. The critically ill are often put on continuous feed systems. Each institution has a protocol for starting an individual on tube feedings that specifies the initial rate of flow. A nutritionist works with the physician to determine the appropriate caloric, water, and micronutrient needs of each individual. Medications can be added to the food if necessary.

In individuals needing long-term tube feeding, a PEG tube is placed through the abdominal wall during a simple surgery that lasts about 20 minutes. The tube has a valve that closes the end outside the body. When the tube is taped to the patient's stomach, it is not particularly noticeable under street clothes. Many patients with PEG tubes, or their caregivers, learn how to care for the tube and feed themselves at home. The feeding tube must be replaced about every six months.

Preparation

A nutritionist should evaluate the individual's nutrient needs before tube feeding begins. Special tube feeding diets exist for a variety of conditions such as kidney failure, liver failure, trauma, glucose intolerance, and other special needs.

Aftercare

Cleaning and maintaining the tube and feeding equipment are necessary after each use. Once the tube is removed, little aftercare is needed. After tube removal, individuals with PEG tubes will need to keep the tube site clean and covered until it heals.

Complications

Tube feeding is a relatively safe procedure. The most serious complications that occur when using a nasogastric tube involve aspiration of the nutrients. Other complications from all tube feeding can include diarrhea, changes in the absorption rate of drugs, and metabolic (fluid and electrolyte) disturbances related to the composition of the food. Many of these complications can be reduced or eliminated by working closely with a nutritionist who has expertise in tube feeding.

Results

Tube feeding is an effective way to provide nutrients, fluids, and drugs to patients who cannot take

---

KEY TERMS

Aspirate—To breathe foreign material into the lungs, as when stomach contents back up into the mouth and are breathed into the windpipe.

---

these things by mouth. The ultimate health of the patient depends largely on the reason the feeding tube was needed.

Health care team roles

A nutritionist is a key person on the health care team when caring for someone who is being tube fed. The nutritionist makes an initial needs assessment and helps the physician decide on an appropriate feeding program. Once tube feeding has begun, the nutritionist assess the results and makes recommendations to help control complications such as diarrhea. Besides the physician, other health care workers who may be involved in the care of a person being tube fed include a dietitian, nurses, and a pharmacist experienced in changes in drug metabolism caused by tube feeding. If the individual is going to be tube fed at home, a nurse will educate the patient and caregiver about tube care and feeding. A visiting nurse may follow up with a patient being tube fed at home.

Resources

BOOKS

Nuzum, Robert. "Gastrointestinal Intubation." In *Manual of Gastroenterologic Procedure*, edited by D. Drossman New York: Raven Press, 1993.

ORGANIZATIONS

American Gastroenterological Association. 4930 Del Ray Avenue Bethesda, MD 20814 (301) 654-5920. <http://www.gastro.org>.

OTHER

Dharmarajan, T.S. and D. Unnikrishnan. "Tube Feeding in the Elderly." *Postgraduate Medicine Online*. 115 (February 2004) http://www.postgradmed.com/issues/2004/02_04/dharmajan.htm (November 23, 2005).

"Nutritional Support." *The Merck Manual of Diagnosis and Therapy*. 1995-2005, Section 1, Chapter 1 http://www.merck.com/mrkshared/mmanual/section1/chapter1/1c.jsp (November 23, 2005).

Oral Cancer Foundation. "Feeding Tubes." undated http://www.oralcancerfoundation.org/dental/tube_feeding.htm (November 23, 2005).

University of Pittsburgh Medical Center. "Home Nasogastric Tube Feeding." 2003 http://

patienteducation.upmc.com/Pdf/
NasogasTubeFeed.pdf (November 23, 2005).

Tish Davidson, A.M.

Tuberculin skin test

Definition

Tuberculosis (TB) is an airborne infectious disease caused by the **bacteria** *Mycobacterium tuberculosis*. The two most common types of tests that are used to screen for this disease are the Mantoux PPD tuberculin skin test, which is generally considered the most reliable, and the TB tine test. These tests are sensitive screening tools that are designed to help identify individuals who may have been infected by tuberculosis bacteria. A diagnosis of tuberculosis is never made based on the results of a TB skin test, but requires further testing including a **sputum culture** and a **chest x ray**.

Purpose

Because TB is spread through the air, especially in poorly ventilated areas, it is more commonly found among people living in crowded conditions, such as jails, **nursing homes**, and homeless shelters. It is estimated that between 10 and 15 million people in the United States have latent tuberculosis. Many new cases of tuberculosis are multi-drug resistant making early detection of exposure a high **public health** priority. Often, a TB skin test will be given as part of a **physical examination** when an organization is hiring a new employee, particularly for those individuals seeking employment in the healthcare or food service professions.

People can be exposed to TB without showing any symptoms or necessarily developing the disease. Individuals with normally functioning immune systems generally prevent the spread of the bacteria by "walling off" or encysting the bacteria within the body. Such a structure in the **lungs** is called a "Ghon" body. Anyone who has had close contact with another person who has tuberculosis (such as a friend or family member); has been around someone with active TB; has a weakened **immune system** (immunocompromised), either from a chronic disease, such as HIV **infection**, or as a result of a tissue or organ transplant or other medical treatment designed to suppress the immune system; or displays symptoms of the disease should be tested. Symptoms of TB include a persistent cough, **fever**, weight loss, night sweats, fatigue, and loss of appetite. Often, individuals must receive the test in order to enter school or begin work.

Precautions

Although generally considered safe, it is important for the person being tested to inform a tester about any possibility of **pregnancy**, any previous positive TB test, or any active tuberculosis in the past. People who previously have had a positive TB test will probably always have a positive test and should not be tested again. Also, anyone who is known to have active TB should not be tested because the local reaction to the test may be so severe that it requires surgical care.

There are several situations when TB test results might not be accurate. These includes situations involving people who:

- Have had vaccinations (such as those for measles, polio, rubella or mumps) within the last four weeks.

- Currently have, or recently recovered from a viral infection.

- Are taking steroids.

- Have severe malnutrition.

Description

TB skin tests are usually given at a clinic, hospital, or physician's office. Sometimes the tests are given at schools or workplaces. Many cities provide free TB skin tests and follow-up care. The Mantoux PPD tuberculin skin test involves injecting 0.1 mL of PPD tuberculin standardized to a dose of five units just under the top layer of the skin (intracutaneously). Tuberculin is a mixture of antigens obtained from the culture of *M. tuberculosis*. Antigens are foreign particles or **proteins** that stimulate the immune system to produce antibodies. Two different tuberculin preparations are available, Old Tuberculin (OT) and Purified Protein Derivative (PPD). The test is usually given on the inside of the forearm about halfway between the wrist and the elbow, where a small bubble (wheal) will form as the tuberculin is injected. The skin test takes just a minute to administer and feels more like a pinprick than a shot.

After 48-72 hours, the test site must be examined by a trained person for evidence of swelling. People who have been exposed to tuberculosis will develop an **immune response**, causing a slight redness and swelling at the injection site. This is called a delayed hypersensitivity reaction, and it is mediated by immune T lymphocytes and macrophages rather than antibody.

Immune lymphocytes enter the site and release products that stimulate inflammation and the migration of macrophages into the area. This results in erthyma and accumulating cells, and cause the lesion to become hard (induration). Reactions may not peak until after 72 hours in elderly individuals or those who are being tested for the first time. If there is a lump or swelling, a health care provider will use a ruler to measure the size of the reaction.

The other method of TB skin test is called the multiple puncture test or tine test because the small test instrument has several small tines that lightly prick the skin. The small points of the instrument are either coated with dried tuberculin or are used to puncture through a film of liquid tuberculin. The test is read by measuring the size of the largest papule. Because it is not possible to precisely control the amount of tuberculin used in the tine test, a positive test should be verified using the Mantoux test. For this reason, the tine test is not as widely used as the Mantoux test and is considered to be less reliable.

It is possible that a person who has TB may receive a negative test result (called a "false negative") or a person who does not have TB may receive a positive test result (called a "false positive"). If there is some doubt, the test may be repeated or the person may be given a diagnostic test using a chest x ray or have sputum cultured to determine whether TB is present or active in the lungs. It is often recommended that a two-step PPD test be given to health care workers and persons whose response to PPD may be diminished. The test is given in the usual manner and if negative, repeated within one to three weeks. A positive reaction on the second test is considered an indication of exposure to TB even if the first result is negative.

Preparation

There is no special preparation needed before a TB skin test. A brief personal history will be taken to determine whether a person has had tuberculosis or a TB test before, has been in close contact with anyone with TB, or has any significant risk factors. Directly before the test, the skin on the arm at the injection site is cleaned with an alcohol swab and allowed to air dry. Health care workers administering the PPD injection should follow standard precautions for the prevention of exposure to bloodborne pathogens.

Aftercare

After having a TB skin test, it is extremely important to make sure that a person being tested keeps the appointment to have the test reaction read. The person is instructed to keep the test site clean, uncovered, and to not scratch or rub the area. Should severe swelling, itching, or **pain** occur, or if the person has trouble breathing, a clinic or health care provider should be contacted immediately.

Complications

The risk of an adverse reaction is very low. Occasionally, an individual who has been exposed to the TB bacteria will develop a local reaction in which the arm swells and is uncomfortable. This reaction usually disappears in two weeks. A sore may develop where the injection is given, or a fever can occur, but these are extremely rare reactions.

Results

Normal results

Among people who have not been exposed to TB, there will be little or no swelling at the test site after 48-72 hours. This is a negative test. Negative tests can be interpreted to mean that a person has not been infected with tuberculosis bacteria or that an individual has been recently infected and not enough time has elapsed for the body to react to the skin test. Persons become sensitive between two and ten weeks after the initial infection. As a result, if an individual has been in contact with someone with tuberculosis, the test should be repeated in three months. Also, because it may take longer than 72 hours for an elderly individual to develop a reaction, it may be useful to repeat the TB skin test after one week to adequately screen these people. Immunocompromised persons may be unable to react sufficiently to the Mantoux test, and either a chest x ray or sputum sample may be required.

Abnormal results

A reaction consisting of a reddened circle of 5 mm is considered positive for the following groups:

- household contacts of persons with active tuberculosis
- individuals with AIDS
- persons with old or healed tuberculosis

A reaction consisting of a reddened circle of 10 mm is considered positive in individuals with one or more of the following risk factors:

- foreign-born from Asia, Africa, or Latin America
- intravenous drug users

KEY TERMS

Antibody—A specific protein produced by the immune system in response to a specific foreign protein or particle called an antigen.

Antigen—Any foreign particle or protein that causes an immune response.

Attenuated—A live, but weakened microorganism that can no longer produce disease.

Cross-reaction—Positive reactions that occur as a result of a person's exposure to other non-tuberculosis bacteria.

Immunocompromised—A state in which the immune system is suppressed or not functioning properly.

Intracutaneous—Into the skin, in this case directly under the top layer of skin.

Mantoux or PPD test—Other names for a tuberculin skin test. PPD stands for purified protein derivative.

Percutaneous—Onto the skin; without breaking the skin.

Tuberculin—A mixture of antigens obtained from the cultured bacteria that cause tuberculosis, *Mycobacterium tuberculosis*.

- medically under-served low income populations

- residents of long-term care facilities

- individuals with certain medical conditions that increase the risk of developing tuberculosis (These medical conditions include being 10% or more below ideal body weight, chronic renal failure, **diabetes mellitus**, receiving high dose corticosteroid or other immunosuppressive therapy, some **blood** disorders such as leukemia and lymphomas, and other cancers.)

Finally, a reaction consisting of a reddened circle of 15 mm is considered positive in those with no risk factors.

A positive reaction to tuberculin may be the result of a previous natural infection with *M. tuberculosis*, infection with a variety of non-tuberculosis mycobacteria (cross-reaction), or tuberculosis **vaccination** with a live, but weakened (attenuated) mycobacterial strain. Cross-reactions are positive reactions that occur as a result of a person's exposure to other non-tuberculosis bacteria. These tend to be smaller than those caused by *M. tuberculosis*. There is no reliable way of distinguishing whether a positive TB skin test is due to a previous vaccination against tuberculosis. Generally, however, positive results are not due to vaccination exposure because few negative results convert to positive after vaccination. Reactions in vaccinated people tend to be less than 10 mm, and an individual's sensitivity to tuberculin steadily declines after vaccination. If a skin test is interpreted as positive, a chest x ray will be performed to determine whether the person has active tuberculosis or whether the body has controlled the infection.

Health care team roles

Health care team members who are involved with tuberculin skin testing include nurses or physician assistants who typically administer and read the TB test. A physician may also read the test and provide follow-up care if it is needed. Laboratory technologists culture samples of sputum and perform DNA tests which confirm the diagnosis. Radiologic technicians take chest x rays, and radiologists evaluate the films.

Resources

BOOKS

Dormandy, Thomas. *The White Death: A History of Tuberculosis.* New York, New York: University Press, 2000.

Faculty Members at The Yale University School of Medicine. "Tuberculin Skin Testing." In *The Patient's Guide to Medical Tests.* Edited by Barry L. Zaret. New York, NY: Houghton Mifflin Company, 1997.

Friedman, Lloyd N. *Tuberculosis: Current Concepts and Treatment, 2nd ed.* Boca Raton, FL: CRC Press, 2000.

Segen, Joseph C. *The Patient's Guide to Medical Tests.* New York: Facts on File, 1998.

ORGANIZATIONS

American Lung Association, 1740 Broadway, NY, NY 10019. (212)-315-8700. <http://www.lungusa.org/diseases/lungtb.html>. info@lungusa.org.

Centers for Disease Control and Prevention, 1600 Clifton Road, Atlanta, GA 30333. (404) 639-3534 or (800) 311-3435. <http://www.cdc.gov/nchstp/tb/faqs/qa.htm>.

Francis J. Curry National Tuberculosis Center, 3180 Eighteenth Street, Suite 101, San Francisco, California 94110-2028. (415) 502-4600. Fax: (415) 502-4620. <http://www.nationaltbcenter.edu/>. tbcenter@nationaltbcenter.edu.

National Tuberculosis Center, University of Medicine and Dentistry of New Jersey, 65 Bergen Street, Newark, NJ 07107-3001. (973) 972-3270. Fax: (973) 972-3268. Information Line: (800) 482-3627. <http://www.umdnj.edu/ntbcweb/>. leusmq@umdnj.edu.

OTHER

American Family Physician. "Positive Skin Tests for Tuberculosis." <http://www.aafp.org/healthinfo>.

Centers for Disease Control and Prevention: <http://www.cdc.gov/epo/mmwr/preview/mmwrhtml/rr4906a1.htm>.

"Diagnostic Standards and Classification of Tuberculosis." <http://aepo-xdv-www.epo.cdc.gov/wonder/prevguid/p0000425/body006.htm>.

State Tuberculosis Control Offices: <http://www.cdc.gov/nchstp/tb/tboffices.htm>.

World Health Organization. <http://www.who.int/gtb/>.

L. Fleming Fallon, Jr., MD, PhD, DrPH

Tuberculosis

Definition

Tuberculosis (TB) is a potentially fatal contagious disease that can affect almost any part of the body but is mainly an **infection** of the **lungs**. It is caused by a bacterial microorganism: the tubercle bacillus or *Mycobacterium tuberculosis*. Although TB can be treated and cured, and can be prevented if persons at risk take certain drugs, medical science has never succeeded in eradicating the disease. Few diseases have caused so much distressing illness for centuries and claimed so many lives.

Description

Overview

Tuberculosis was popularly known as consumption for many years. Scientists now know that it is an infection caused by *M. tuberculosis*. In 1882, one of every seven deaths in Europe was caused by TB. In that year, the microbiologist Robert Koch discovered the tubercle bacillus. Because **antibiotics** were unknown, the only means of controlling the spread of infection was to isolate patients in private sanitariums or hospitals limited to treating persons with TB. In many countries, this practice continues to this day. The net effect of this approach to treatment was to separate the study of tuberculosis from mainstream medicine. Entire organizations were set up to study not only the disease as it affected individual persons, but also its impact on society as a whole. At the turn of the twentieth century, more than 80% of the population in the United States was infected with TB before age 20, and tuberculosis was the single most common cause of death. By 1938, there were more than 700 TB hospitals in the United States.

When the industrial revolution began in the late nineteenth century, tuberculosis spread much more widely in Europe. Later, the disease began to spread throughout the United States, primarily due to the population migration to large cities that made overcrowded housing so common. When streptomycin, the first antibiotic effective against *M. tuberculosis*, was discovered in the early 1940s, the infection began to come under control. Although other, more effective anti-tuberculosis drugs were developed in the following decades, the number of cases of TB in the United States began to rise again in the mid-1980s. In part, this upsurge was again a result of overcrowding and unsanitary conditions in poor areas of large cities, prisons, and homeless shelters. Infected visitors and immigrants to the United States also contributed to the resurgence of TB. An additional factor was the emergence of acquired **immunodeficiency** syndrome (**AIDS**). Persons with AIDS are much more likely to develop tuberculosis because of their weakened immune systems than are others in the general population. As of 2001, experts estimate that between 8 and 11 million new cases of TB are reported each year throughout the world. These are estimated to cause approximately 3 million deaths. This situation is worsening. The World Health Organization estimates that by 2020, there will be 1 billion TB cases worldwide and 35 million deaths each year.

High-risk populations

THE ELDERLY. Tuberculosis is more common in elderly persons. More than one-fourth of the 19,855 cases of TB (7.4 cases per 100,000 population) reported in the United States in 1997 developed in people above the age of 65. Many elderly individuals developed the infection some years ago when the disease was more widespread. There are additional reasons for the vulnerability of older people. Those living in **nursing homes** and similar facilities are in close contact with others who may be infected. The aging process itself may weaken the body's **immune system**, which is then less able to successfully eliminate the tubercle bacillus. Finally, **bacteria** that have been dormant for some time in elderly persons may be reactivated and cause illness.

RACIAL AND ETHNIC GROUPS. TB also is more common among members of minority groups who may be likely to live under conditions that promote infection. As of 2001, approximately two-thirds of all cases of TB in the United States affect African Americans, Hispanics, Asians, and persons from the

Pacific Islands. Another one-fourth of cases affect persons born outside the United States. The risk of TB has not diminished among members of these groups.

PERSONS WITH RELEVANT LIFESTYLE FACTORS. The high risk of TB in AIDS patients extends to those infected by human immunodeficiency virus (HIV) who have not yet developed clinical signs of AIDS. Alcoholics and intravenous drug abusers are also at increased risk of contracting tuberculosis. Until the economic and social factors that influence the spread of tubercular infection are addressed and eliminated, there is no real possibility of completely eliminating the disease.

Causes and symptoms

Transmission

Tuberculosis is spread by droplet infection. This type of transmission means that when a TB patient exhales, coughs, or sneezes, tiny droplets of fluid containing tubercle bacilli are released into the air. This mist, often referred to as aerosol, can be taken into the nasal passages and lungs of a nearby susceptible person. Compared to some other infectious diseases, TB is not highly contagious. Only about one in three close contacts of a person with TB is likely to become infected. Fewer than 15% of more remote contacts are likely to become infected. As a rule, close, frequent, or prolonged contact is needed to spread the disease. Of course, if a severely infected patient emits huge numbers of bacilli, the chance of transmitting infection is much greater. Unlike many other infections, TB is not passed on by contact with a patient's clothing, bed linens, or dishes and cooking utensils. The most important exception is **pregnancy**. The fetus of an infected mother may contract TB by inhaling or swallowing bacilli that may be present in amniotic fluid.

Progression

Once inhaled, tubercle bacilli may reach the small breathing sacs in the lungs (alveoli), where they are taken up by cells called macrophages. The bacilli multiply within these cells and then spread through lymph vessels to nearby lymph nodes. Sometimes the bacilli move through **blood vessels** to distant organs. At this point they may either remain alive but inactive (quiescent), or they may cause active disease. Actual tissue damage is not caused directly by the tubercle bacillus, but by the reaction of a person's tissues to its presence. In a matter of weeks, the host develops an **immune response** to the bacillus. Cells attack the bacilli, permit the initial damage to heal, and permanently prevent future disease.

Exposure and infection does not always mean that active TB disease will develop. In fact, most people who are infected do not develop TB. At least nine out of ten people who harbor *M. tuberculosis* do not develop symptoms or physical evidence of active disease, and their x rays remain negative. They are not contagious. However, they do form a pool of infected people who may get sick at a later date and then pass their TB on to others. It is thought that more than 90% of active tuberculosis cases come from this pool. In the United States, this group numbers 10 to 15 million persons. Whether or not a particular infected person will become ill is impossible to predict with certainty. An estimated 5% of infected persons develop active cases of TB within 12-24 months of being infected. Another 5% heal initially, but after years or decades develop active tuberculosis either in the lungs or elsewhere in the body. This form of the disease is called reactivation TB, or post-primary disease. On rare occasions, a previously infected person gets sick again after a later exposure to the tubercle bacillus.

Pulmonary tuberculosis

Pulmonary tuberculosis is TB that affects the lungs. Its initial symptoms are easily confused with those of other diseases. An infected person may at first feel vaguely unwell or develop a cough blamed on smoking or a cold. A small amount of light green or yellow sputum may be coughed up when the person gets up in the morning. In time, more sputum is produced that is streaked with **blood**. Persons with pulmonary TB do not run a high **fever**, but they often have a low-grade one. They may wake up in the night drenched with cold sweat when the fever breaks. A person often loses interest in food and may lose weight. Chest **pain** is sometimes present. If the infection allows air to escape from the lungs into the chest cavity (pneumothorax) or if fluid collects in the pleural space (pleural effusion), an affected person may have difficulty breathing. If a young adult develops a pleural effusion, the probability of tubercular infection being the cause is very high. TB bacilli may travel from the lungs to lymph nodes in the sides and back of the neck. Infection in these areas can break through the skin and discharge pus. Before the development of effective antibiotics, many patients became chronically ill with increasingly severe lung symptoms, lost a great deal of weight, and developed a wasted appearance. This outcome is uncommon today—at least where modern methods of treatment are available.

Extrapulmonary tuberculosis

Although the lungs are the major site for damage caused by tuberculosis, many other organs and tissues in the body may be affected. The usual progression is for the disease to spread from the lungs to locations outside the lungs (extrapulmonary sites). In some cases, however, the first sign of disease appears outside the lungs. The many tissues or organs that tuberculosis may affect include:

- Bones. TB is particularly likely to attack the spine and the ends of the long bones. Children are especially prone to spinal tuberculosis. If not treated, the spinal bones (vertebrae) may collapse and cause **paralysis** in one or both legs.

- **Kidneys**. Along with bones, the kidneys are probably the most common site of extrapulmonary TB. There may, however, be few symptoms even though part of a kidney is destroyed. TB may spread to the bladder. In men, it may spread to the prostate gland and nearby structures.

- Female reproductive organs. The ovaries in women may become infected as TB can spread from them to the peritoneum, which is the membrane lining the abdominal cavity.

- Abdominal cavity. Tuberculous peritonitis may cause pain ranging from the vague discomfort of **stomach** cramps to intense pain that may mimic the symptoms of appendicitis.

- Joints. Tubercular infection of joints causes a form of arthritis that most often affects the hips and knees. The wrist, hand, and elbow joints also may become painful and inflamed.

- Meninges. The meninges are tissues that cover the **brain** and the **spinal cord**. Infection of the meninges by TB bacillus causes tuberculous **meningitis**, a condition that is most common in young children but is especially dangerous in the elderly. Affected people develop headaches, become drowsy, and may eventually fall into a **coma**. Permanent brain damage is the rule unless prompt treatment is given. Some people with tuberculous meningitis develop a tumor-like brain mass called a tuberculoma that can cause symptoms that resemble those of a stroke.

- Skin, intestines, **adrenal glands**, and blood vessels. All these parts of the body can be infected by *M. tuberculosis*. Infection of the wall of the body's main artery (the aorta) can cause it to rupture with catastrophic results. Tuberculous pericarditis occurs when the membrane surrounding the **heart** (the pericardium) is infected and fills up with fluid that interferes with the heart's ability to pump blood.

- Miliary tuberculosis. Miliary TB is a life-threatening condition that occurs when large numbers of tubercle bacilli spread throughout the body. Huge numbers of tiny tubercular lesions develop, causing marked weakness and weight loss, severe anemia, and gradual wasting of the body.

Diseases similar to tuberculosis

There are many forms of mycobacteria other than *M. tuberculosis*, the tubercle bacillus. Some cause infections that may closely resemble tuberculosis, but usually do so only when an infected person's immune system is defective. People who are HIV-positive are a good example. The most common mycobacteria that infect AIDS patients are a group known as *Mycobacterium avium* complex (MAC). People infected by MAC are not contagious but may develop a serious lung infection that is highly resistant to antibiotics. MAC infections typically start with an affected person coughing up mucus. The infection progresses slowly, but eventually blood is brought up and the person has trouble breathing. Among people with AIDS, MAC disease can spread throughout the body, with anemia, **diarrhea**, and stomach pain as common features. Often, these people die unless their immune systems can be strengthened. Other mycobacteria grow in swimming pools and may cause skin infections. Some of them infect **wounds** and artificial body parts such as a breast implant or mechanical heart valve. The organism that causes leprosy, *M. leprae*, is also related to TB.

Diagnosis

The diagnosis of TB is made on the basis of laboratory test results. The standard test for tuberculosis, the so-called **tuberculin skin test**, detects the presence of infection, not of active TB. Tuberculin is an extract prepared from cultures of *M. tuberculosis*. It contains substances belonging to the bacillus (antigens) to which an infected person has been sensitized. When tuberculin is injected into the skin of an infected person, the area around the injection becomes hard, swollen, and red within one to three days. Today, skin tests utilize a substance called purified protein derivative (PPD) that has a standard chemical composition and is therefore is a good measure of the presence of tubercular infection. The PPD test is also called the Mantoux test. The Mantoux PPD skin test is not, however, 100% accurate; it can produce false positive as well as false negative results. These terms have specific meanings. People who have a skin reaction and are not infected are referred to having a false positive result. Those who do not react but are in fact infected are classified as having a false negative result. The PPD test is, however, useful as a screening device. Anyone who has suspicious findings on a **chest x ray** or any condition that makes TB more likely should have a PPD test. In addition, those in close contact with someone who has active TB or persons who come from a country where TB is common should be tested, as should all healthcare personnel and those living in crowded conditions or institutions.

Because the symptoms of TB encompass a wide range of severity and affect many parts of the body, diagnosis on the basis of external symptoms is not always possible. Often, the first indication of TB is an abnormal chest x ray or other test result rather than physical discomfort. On a chest x ray, evidence of the disease appears as numerous white, irregular areas against a dark background, or as enlarged lymph nodes. The upper parts of the lungs are most often affected. A PPD test is always performed to show whether an individual has been infected by the tubercle bacillus. To verify test results, a physician obtains a sample of sputum or a tissue sample (biopsy) for culture. Three to five sputum samples should be taken early in the morning. If necessary, sputum for culture can be produced by spraying salt solution into the windpipe. Culturing *M. tuberculosis* is useful for diagnosis because the bacillus has certain distinctive characteristics. Unlike many other types of bacteria, mycobacteria can retain certain dyes even when exposed to acid. This so-called acid-fast property is characteristic of the tubercle bacillus.

Body fluids other than sputum can be used for culture. If TB has invaded the brain or spinal cord, culturing a sample of spinal fluid will make the diagnosis. If TB of the kidneys is suspected because of pus or blood in the urine, culture of the urine may reveal tubercular infection. Infection of the ovaries in women can be detected by placing a tube having a light on its end (a **laparoscope**) into the area. Samples also may be taken from the **liver** or bone marrow to detect the tubercle bacillus.

Treatment

Supportive care

In the past, treatment of TB was primarily supportive. People being treated for TB were kept in isolation, encouraged to rest, and fed well. If these measures failed, their affected lungs were collapsed surgically so that they could "rest" and heal. Today, surgical procedures still are used when necessary, but contemporary medicine relies on drug therapy as the mainstay of **home care**. Given an effective combination of drugs, individuals with TB can be treated at home as well as in a sanitorium. Treatment at home does not pose the risk of infecting other household members.

Drug therapy

Most people with TB can recover if given appropriate medication for a sufficient length of time. Three principles govern modern drug treatment of TB:

- Lowering the number of bacilli as quickly as possible. This measure minimizes the risk of transmitting the disease. When sputum cultures become negative, this has been achieved. Conversely, if the sputum cultures remain positive after five to six months, treatment has failed.

- Preventing the development of drug resistance. For this reason, at least two different drugs and sometimes three are always given at first. If drug resistance is suspected, at least two different drugs should be tried.

- Long-term, continuous treatment to prevent relapse.

Five drugs are most commonly used today to treat tuberculosis: isoniazid (INH, Laniazid, Nydrazid); rifampin (Rifadin, Rimactane); pyrazinamide (Tebrazid); streptomycin; and ethambutol (Myambutol). The first three drugs may be given in the same capsule to minimize the number of pills in the dosage. As of 2001, many persons are given isoniazid and rifampin together for six months, with pyrazinamide added for the first two months. Hospitalization is rarely necessary because most persons are no longer infectious after about two weeks of combination treatment. Follow-up involves monitoring for the presence of side effects and having monthly sputum tests. Of the five medications, isoniazid is the most frequently used drug for both treatment and prevention of TB.

Surgery

Surgical treatment of TB may be used if oral medications are ineffective. There are three surgical treatments for pulmonary TB: pneumothorax, in which air is introduced into the chest to collapse the lung; thoracoplasty, in which one or more ribs are removed; and removal of a diseased lung, in whole or in part. It is possible for individuals to survive with one healthy lung. Spinal TB may result in a severe deformity that can be surgically corrected.

Prognosis

The prognosis for recovery from TB is good for most patients, if the disease is diagnosed early and given prompt treatment with appropriate medications on a long-term regimen. Modern surgical methods have good outcomes in most cases in which they are needed. Miliary tuberculosis is still fatal in many cases but is rarely seen today in developed countries. Even in cases in which the bacillus proves resistant to all of the commonly used medications for TB, other seldom-used drugs may be tried because the tubercle bacilli have not yet developed resistance to them.

Health care team roles

Screening for tuberculosis may be conducted by nurses, physicians, physician assistants, or other trained health workers. The test is read or evaluated by a nurse, physician, or physician assistant. Treatment for TB must be prescribed and supervised by a physician. A surgeon may provide surgical intervention, often assisted by a physician assistant trained in surgery. Administration of TB medications is often supervised by nurses, although other non-medical personnel may observe TB drug ingestion. Epidemiologists collect data from many individual caregivers, and are key members of the health care team even though they do not directly provide clinical services. Pharmaceutical scientists are constantly searching for new drugs for use in treating TB.

Prevention

General measures

General measures such as avoiding overcrowded and unsanitary conditions are important aspects of prevention. Hospital emergency rooms and similar locations that are used to treat or house TB patients can be treated with ultraviolet light, which has an antibacterial effect.

Vaccination

Vaccination is one major preventive measure against TB. A vaccine called BCG (Bacillus Calmette-Guérin, named after its French developers) is made from a weakened mycobacterium that infects cattle. Vaccination with BCG does not prevent infection by *M. tuberculosis*, but it does strengthen the immune system of first-time TB patients. As a result,

KEY TERMS

Alveoli—Several small, sac-shaped cavities. In the lungs, alveoli (plural of alveolus) are found at the ends of airways, the sites where oxygen and carbon dioxide are exchanged in the blood.

Bacillus Calmette-Guérin (BCG)—A vaccine made from a damaged bacillus that is related to the tubercle bacillus, which may help prevent serious pulmonary TB and its complications.

Macrophage—A large, phagocytic cell that is found in the blood system and loose connective tissue.

Mantoux test—Another name for the PPD test.

Miliary tuberculosis—The form of TB in which the bacillus spreads through all body tissues and organs, producing many thousands of tiny tubercular lesions. Miliary TB is often fatal unless promptly treated.

Mycobacteria—A group of bacteria that includes *Mycobacterium tuberculosis*, the bacterium that causes tuberculosis, and other forms that cause related illnesses.

Peritonitis—An infection in the peritoneum (abdominal cavity).

Pleural effusion—Fluid that collects in the space normally occupied by a lung.

Pneumothorax—Air inside the chest cavity, which may cause a lung to collapse. Pneumothorax is both a complication of pulmonary tuberculosis and a means of treatment designed to allow an infected lung to rest and heal.

Pulmonary—Refers to the lungs.

Purified protein derivative (PPD)—An extract of tubercle bacilli that is injected into the skin to find out whether a person presently has or has ever had tuberculosis.

Resistance—A property of some bacteria that have been exposed to a particular antibiotic and have changed sufficiently to survive in its presence.

Sputum—Secretions produced in an infected lung and coughed up. A sign of illness, sputum is routinely used as a specimen for culturing the tubercle bacillus in a laboratory.

Tuberculoma—A tumor-like mass in the brain that sometimes develops as a complication of tuberculous meningitis.

serious complications are less likely to develop. BCG is used widely in developing countries but is not used in the United States. This is because it protects only 75% of recipients, and because everyone who receives the vaccine reacts positively to future TB screening tests. The problem is identifying the one person in four who has a false negative test result. The effectiveness of vaccination is still being studied. It is not clear whether the vaccine's effectiveness depends on the population in which it is used or on variations in its formulation.

Prophylactic use of isoniazid

Isoniazid can be given for the prevention as well as the treatment of TB. Isoniazid is effective when given daily over a period of six to 12 months to people in high-risk categories. The drug appears to be most beneficial to persons under the age of 25. Because isoniazid carries the risk of side effects (liver inflammation, nerve damage, changes in mood and behavior), it is important to administer the drug only to persons at special risk.

High-risk groups for whom isoniazid prevention may be justified include:

- Close contacts of persons with active TB, including health care workers.
- Newly infected patients whose skin test has turned positive in the past two years.
- Anyone who is HIV-positive with a positive PPD skin test. Isoniazid may be given even if PPD results are negative if there is a risk of exposure to active tuberculosis.
- Intravenous drug users, even if they are negative for HIV.
- Persons who have never been treated for TB, have positive PPD results, and show evidence of old disease on a chest x ray.
- People who have an illness or are taking a drug that can suppress the immune system.
- Persons with positive PPD results who have had intestinal surgery, have diabetes or **chronic kidney failure**, have any type of **cancer**, or are more than 10% below their ideal body weight.
- People from countries with high rates of TB who have positive PPD results.
- People from low-income groups with positive skin test results.
- Persons with a positive PPD reaction who belong to high-risk ethnic groups (African-Americans, Hispanics, Native Americans, Asians, and Pacific Islanders).

Resources

BOOKS

Dormandy, Thomas. *The White Death: A History of Tuberculosis.* New York: New York University Press, 2000.

Friedman, Lloyd N. *Tuberculosis: Current Concepts and Treatment, 2nd ed.* Boca Raton, FL: CRC Press, 2000.

Geiter, Lawrence. *Ending Neglect: The Elimination of Tuberculosis in the United States.* Washington, DC: National Academy Press, 2000.

Rom, William N. and Stewart M. Garay. *Tuberculosis.* Philadelphia: Lippincott Williams & Wilkins, 1993.

Ryan, Frank. *The Forgotten Plague: How the Battle Against Tuberculosis Was Won and Lost.* Philadelphia: Lippincott Williams & Wilkins, 1993.

PERIODICALS

Ebrahim, G.J."Multi-drug Resistant Tuberculosis." *Journal of Tropical Pediatrics* 46, no. 6 (2000): 320–1.

Hamilton, CD. "Recent Developments in Epidemiology, Treatment, and Diagnosis of Tuberculosis." *Current Infectious Disease Reports* 1, no. 1 (1999): 80–8.

Jones, T.F. and W. Moore. "The Phthisis Still With Us. Tuberculosis: The White Plague is Not Yet a Ghost of the Past." *Tennessee Medicine* 94, no. 2 (2001): 62–3.

Kochi, A. "The Global Tuberculosis Situation and the New Control Strategy of the World Health Organization." *Bulletin of the World Health Organization* 79, no. 1 (2001): 71–5.

Williamson, J. "Tuberculosis revisited or how we nearly conquered tuberculosis." *Scottish Medical Journal* 45, no. 6 (2000):183-185.

ORGANIZATIONS

American Lung Association. 1740 Broadway, New York, NY 10019. (212) 315-8700. <http://www.lungusa.org/diseases/lungtb.html>.

Centers for Disease Control and Prevention. 1600 Clifton Rd., Atlanta, GA 30333. (404) 639-3534 or (800) 311-3435. <http://www.cdc.gov/nchstp/tb/faqs/qa.htm>.

Francis J. Curry National Tuberculosis Center. 3180 18th St., Suite 101, San Francisco, CA 94110-2028. (415) 502-4600. <http://www.nationaltbcenter.edu>.

National Tuberculosis Center, University of Medicine and Dentistry of New Jersey. 65 Bergen St., Newark, NJ 07107-3001. (973) 972-3270 or (800) 482-3627. <http://www.umdnj.edu/ntbcweb>.

World Health Organization, Communicable Diseases. 20 Avenue Appia, 1211 Geneva 27, Switzerland. +41 (22) 791 4140. <http://www.who.int/gtb>.

OTHER

Centers for Disease Control and Prevention. August 2001. <http://www.cdc.gov/epo/mmwr/preview/mmwrhtml/rr4906a1.htm>.

Columbia Presbyterian Medical Center. August 2001. <http://www.cpmc.columbia.edu/tbcpp>.

Department of Health Services: Australia. August 2001. <http://www.dhs.vic.gov.au/phb/hprot/tb/tbm/tb2.html>.

State Tuberculosis Control Offices. August 2001. <http://www.cdc.gov/nchstp/tb/tboffices.htm>.

World Health Organization. August 2001. <http://www.who.int/gtb>.

L. Fleming Fallon, Jr., MD, PhD, DrPH

Tuberculosis culture *see* **Acid-fast culture**

Tumor marker tests

Definition

Tumor markers are **proteins**, hormones, enzymes, receptors, and other cellular products that are over-expressed by malignant cells. Tumor markers are usually normal cellular constituents that are present at normal or very low levels in the **blood** of healthy persons. If produced by the tumor, the substance will be increased either in the blood or in the tissue of origin.

Purpose

The majority of tumor markers are used to monitor the patient for recurrence of the tumor following treatment. In addition, some markers are associated with a more aggressive course and higher relapse rate and have value in staging and prognosis of the **cancer**. Most tumor markers are not useful for screening because levels found in early malignancy overlap those found in healthy persons. Most are elevated in conditions other than malignancy, and therefore, are not useful for the purpose or establishing a diagnosis.

Precautions

Tumor markers may be elevated in nonmalignant conditions. Not every tumor will cause an elevation of its associated marker, especially in the early stages of some cancers. When a marker is used for cancer screening or diagnosis, the physician must confirm a positive test result using imaging, biopsy, and other procedures. False positive results may occur in immunoassays when the patient has heterophile antibodies that interfere with the test. Tumor markers at very high concentrations may give erroneously low results caused by the "hook effect." This occurs when the concentration of antigen is so great that all of it cannot be bound by the antibody used in the test system.

Description

Physicians use changes in tumor marker levels to follow the course of the disease, to measure the effect of treatment, and to check for recurrence of certain cancers. Tumor markers have been identified in several types of cancer including **malignant melanoma**, multiple myeloma; and bone, breast, colon, gastric, **liver**, lung, ovarian, pancreatic, prostate, renal, and uterine cancer. Serial measurements of a tumor marker are often an effective means to monitor the course of therapy. Some tumor markers can provide physicians with information about the stage of the cancer, and some help predict the response to treatment. A decrease in the amount of the tumor marker during treatment indicates that the therapy is having a positive effect on the cancer, while an increase indicates that the cancer is growing and not responding favorably to the therapy.

There are five types of tumor markers. Many enzymes that are rich in certain tissues are found in plasma at higher levels when the cancer involves that tissue. Enzymes are usually measured by determining the rate at which they convert substrate to product, while most tumor markers of other types are measured by immunoassay. Some examples of enzymes increase in cases of malignant diseases are acid phosphatase, alkaline phosphatase, amylase, creatine kinase, gamma glutamyl transferase, lactate dehydrogenase, and terminal deoxynucleotidyl transferase.

Tissue receptors, proteins associated with the cell membrane, are another type of tumor marker. These bind to hormones and growth factors, and therefore, affect the rate of tumor growth. Some tissue receptors must be measured in biopsied tissue, while others are secreted into the extracellular fluid and may be measured in the blood. Some important receptor tumor markers are estrogen receptor, progesterone receptor, interleukin-2 receptor, and epidermal growth factor receptor.

Oncofetal antigens are proteins made by genes that are very active during **fetal development**, but which function at a very low level after birth. The genes become activated in malignancy and produce large amounts of protein. This is the largest class of tumor marker and includes the tumor associated glycoprotein antigens (designated by the letters CA). Important tumor markers of this class are alpha-fetoprotein (AFP), carcinoembryonic antigen (CEA), prostate specific antigen (PSA), cathespin-D, HER-

2/neu, CA-125, CA-19-9, CA-15-3, nuclear matrix protein, and bladder tumor-associated antigen.

Some tumor markers are the product of oncogenes. These are genes that are active in fetal development and induce tumor growth when they become active in mature cells. Some important oncogenes are BRAC-1, myc, p53, RB (retinoblastoma) gene (RB), and Ph[1] (Philadelphia chromosome).

The fifth type of tumor marker consists of hormones. This includes hormones that are normally secreted by the tissue in which the malignancy arises and those which are produced by tissues that do not normally make the hormone (ectopic production). Some hormones associated with malignancy are adrenal corticotropic hormone (ACTH), calcitonin, catecholamines, gastrin, human chorionic gonadogropin (hCG), and prolactin.

Currently, there are over 60 analytes that are measured as tumor markers. All of the enzymes and hormones mentioned above are FDA approved as tumor markers, but most of the others are not. These are designated for investigation purposes only. The following list describes the most common tumor markers approved by the Food and Drug Administration for screening, diagnosis, or monitoring of cancer.

- Alpha-fetoprotein (AFP): AFP is a glycoprotein produced by the developing fetus, but levels decline after birth. Healthy non-pregnant adults rarely have detectable levels of AFP in their blood. The AFP test is primarily used for the diagnosis of spina bifida and other abnormalities associated with cerebrospinal fluid leakage during embryonic development. In adult males and non-pregnant females, an AFP above 300 ng/L is often associated with cancer, although levels in this range may be seen in nonmalignant liver diseases. Levels above 1,000 ng/L are almost always associated with cancer. AFP is FDA-approved for the diagnosis and monitoring of patients with non-seminoma testicular cancer. It is elevated in approximately 100% of yolk sac tumors and 80% of hepatomas.

- CA125: This test is FDA-approved for the diagnosis and monitoring of women with ovarian cancer. Approximately 75% of persons with ovarian cancer shed CA-125 into the blood and have elevated levels. This includes approximately 50% of persons with Stage I disease and 90% with Stage II or higher. It is also found in approximately 20% of persons with pancreatic cancer. Other cancers detected by this marker include liver, colon, breast, lung, and digestive. **Pregnancy** and menstruation affect test results. Benign diseases detected by the test include

endometriosis, ovarian cysts, fibroids, inflammatory bowel disease, cirrhosis, peritonitis, and **pancreatitis**. CA-125 levels correlate with tumor mass, and therefore, this test is used to determine whether recurrence of the cancer has occurred following **chemotherapy**. However, in some patients, recurrence occurs without an increase in the level of CA-125.

- Carcinoembryonic antigen (CEA): A glycoprotein that is part of the normal cell membrane. CEA is shed into serum and reaches very high levels in **colorectal cancer**. Over 50% of persons with breast, colon, lung, gastric, ovarian, pancreatic, and uterine cancer have elevated levels of CEA. CEA levels in plasma are monitored in patients with CEA secreting tumors to determine if second-look surgery should be performed. CEA levels may also be elevated in inflammatory bowel disease, pancreatitis, and liver diease. CEA is also elevated in smokers, and about 5% of healthy persons have an elevated plasma level.

- Prostate specific antigen (PSA): A small glycoprotein with protease activity that is specific for prostate tissue. The antigen is present in low levels in all adult males. Therefore an elevated level may require additional testing to confirm that cancer is the cause of the elevated result. High levels are seen in **prostate cancer**, benign prostatic hypertrophy, and inflammation of the prostate. PSA is approved as a screening test for prostatic carcinoma. PSA has been found to be elevated in more than 60% of persons with Stage A and more than 70% with Stage B cancer of the prostate and has replaced the use of prostatic acid phosphatase for prostate cancer screening because it is far more sensitive. Most PSA is bound to antitrypsins in plasma but some PSA circulates unbound to protein (free PSA). Persons with a borderline total PSA (between 4-10 ng/L), but who have a low free PSA are more likely to have malignant prostate disease.

- Estrogen receptor (ER): A protein found in the nucleus of breast and uterine tissues. The level of ER in the tissue is used to determine whether a person with **breast cancer** is likely to respond to estrogen therapy with tamoxifen, which binds to the receptors blocking the action of estrogen. Women who are ER negative have a greater risk of recurrence than women who are ER positive. Tissue levels are measured using one of two methods. The tissue can be homogenized into a cytosol, and a sandwich immunoassay used to measure the concentration of ER receptor protein. Alternatively, the tissue is frozen and thin-sectioned. An immunoperoxidase stain is used to detect and measure the estrogen receptors in the tissue.

- Progesterone receptor (PR): Two proteins, like the estrogen receptor, which are located in the nuclei of both breast and uterine tissues. PR has the same prognostic value as ER, and is measured by similar methods. Tissue that does not express the PR receptors is less likely to bind estrogen analogs used to treat the tumor. Persons who test negative for both ER and PR have less than a 5% chance of responding to endocrine therapy. Those who test positive for both markers have greater than a 60% chance of tumor shrinkage when treated with hormone therapy.

- Human chorionic gonadotropin (hCG): A glycoprotein produced by cells of the trophoblast and developing placenta. Very high levels are produced by trophoblastic tumors and choriocarcinoma. About 60% of testicular cancers secrete hCG. hCG is also produced by a large number of other tumors, but at a lower frequency. Some malignancies cause an increase in alpha and/or beta hCG subunits in the absence of significant increases in intact hCG. For this reason, tests have evolved for alpha and beta hCG, and most labs use these assays as tumor marker tests. Most EIA sandwich tests for pregnancy are specific for hCG, but detect the whole molecule and are called intact hCG assays.

- Nuclear matrix protein (NMP22) and bladder tumor associated analytes (BTA): NMP22 is a structural nuclear protein that is released into the urine when bladder carcinoma cells die. Urine is tested using an immunochemical method. Approximately 70% of bladder carcinomas are positive for NMP22. BTA is comprised of type IV collagen, fibronectin, laminin, and proteoglycan, which are components of the basement membrane that are released into the urine when bladder tumor cells attach to the basement membrane of the bladder wall. These products can be detected in urine using a mixture of antibodies to the four components. BTA is elevated in about 30% of persons with low-grade bladder tumors and over 60% of persons with high-grade tumors.

Preparation

Determination of the circulating level of tumor markers involves a blood test performed by a laboratory scientist. A nurse or phlebotomist usually collects the blood by venipuncture, following standard precautions for prevention of exposure to bloodborne pathogens. Tissues are collected by a physician at the time of surgical or needle biopsy. Urine is collected by the patient using the midstream void technique.

Aftercare

Aftercare consists of routine care of the area around the puncture site. Pressure is applied for a few seconds and the wound is covered with a bandage. If a bruise or swelling develops around the puncture site, the area is treated with a moist warm compress.

Complications

Risks of venipuncture include mild dizziness, bruising, swelling, or excessive bleeding from the puncture site. As previously mentioned, results should be interpreted with caution. A single test result may not yield clinically useful information. Several results over a period of months may be needed to evaluate treatment and identify recurrence. Positive results must be interpreted cautiously because some tumor markers are increased in nonmalignant diseases and in a small number of apparently healthy persons. In addition false negative results may occur because the tumor does not produce the marker, and because levels seen in healthy persons may overlap those seen in the early stages of cancer. A false positive result occurs when the value is elevated, but cancer is not present. A false negative result occurs when the value is normal, but cancer is present.

Results

Reference ranges for tumor markers will vary from one laboratory to another because different antibodies and calibrators are used by various test systems. The values below are representative of normal values or cutoffs for commonly measured tumor markers.

- Alpha-fetoprotein (AFP): Less than 15 ng/L in men and non-pregnant women. Levels greater than 1,000 ng/L indicate malignant disease (except in pregnancy).

- CA125: Less than 35 U/mL.

- Carcinoembryonic antigen (CEA): Less than 3 μg/L for nonsmokers and less than 5 μg/L for smokers.

- Estrogen receptor: Less than 6 fmol/mg protein is negative; greater than 10 fmol/mg protein is positive.

- Human chorionic gonadotropin: Less than 20 IU/L for males and non-pregnant females. Greater than 100,00 IU/L indicates trophoblastic tumor.

- Progesterone receptor: Less than 6 fmol/mg protein is negative. Greater than 10 fmol/mg protein is positive.

- Prostate specific antigen (PSA): Less than 4 ng/L.

Health care team roles

Tumor marker tests are ordered and interpreted by a physician. In difficult cases, an oncologist may be needed. A phlebotomist, or sometimes a nurse, collects the blood, and a clinical laboratory scientist CLS(NCA)/medical technologist MT(ASCP) or clinical laboratory technician CLT(NCA)/medical laboratory technician MLT(ASCP) performs the testing.

Tumor marker tests must be correlated to other diagnostic evidence including the patient's history, physical exam, imaging, biopsy, and other laboratory results to confirm a diagnosis and provide accurate clinical staging of cancer. Consequently, many other members of the health care team, especially radiologists and radiologic technicians are often involved.

Resources

BOOKS

Burtis, C.A., and E.R. Ashwood. eds. *Tietz Fundamentals of Clinical Chemistry, 5th ed.* Philadelphia, PA: Saunders, 2001.

Cooper, Dennis L. "Tumor Markers." In *Cecil Textbook of Medicine,* edited by J. Claude Bennet and Fred Plum. Philadelphia: W.B. Saunders, 1996.

Henry, J.B., ed. *Clinical Diagnosis and Management by Lboratory Methods, 20th ed.* Philadelphia, PA: Saunders, 2001.

Shannon, Joyce Brennfleck, ed. *Medical Tests Source Book.* Detroit: Omnigraphics, Inc.

ORGANIZATIONS

National Cancer Institute. <http://www.nci.nih.gov/>.

OTHER

Abbott Laboratories. <http://www.abbottdiagnostics.com/medical_conditions/cancer/index.htm/>.

Victoria E. DeMoranville

24-hour fecal fat test *see* **Malabsorption tests**

Twin pregnancy *see* **Multiple pregnancy**

Tympanometry *see* **Audiometry**

▌Type and screen

Definition

Blood typing is a laboratory test that identifies blood group antigens (substances that stimulate an **immune response**) belonging to the ABO blood group system. The test classifies blood into four groups designated A, B, AB, and O. Antibody screening is a test to detect

---

Blood typing

Blood type	Antigen	Antibody
Group A	A	B
Group B	B	A
Group AB	A, B	None
Group O	None	A, B
Rh factor: negative	None	Rh+
Rh factor: positive	Rh	None

atypical antibodies in the serum that have been formed as a result of transfusion or **pregnancy**. An antibody is a protein produced by lymphocytes that binds to an antigen, facilitating its removal by phagocytosis or lysis. The type and screen (T&S) is performed on persons who may need a transfusion of blood products. These tests are followed by the compatibility test (cross-match). This test insures that no antibodies are detected in the recipient's serum that will react with the donor's red blood cells.

Purpose

Blood typing and screening are most commonly performed to ensure that a person who needs a transfusion will receive blood that matches (is compatible with) his or her own; and that clinically significant antibodies are identified if present. People must receive blood of the same blood type; otherwise, a severe transfusion reaction may result.

Prenatal care

Parents who are expecting a baby have their blood typed to diagnose and prevent hemolytic disease of the newborn (HDN), a type of anemia also known as erythroblastosis fetalis. Babies who have a blood type different from their mothers are at risk for developing this disease.

Determination of paternity

A child inherits factors or genes from each parent that determine his blood type. This fact makes blood typing useful in paternity testing. The blood types of the child, mother, and alleged father are compared to determine paternity.

Forensic investigations

Legal investigations may require typing of blood or such other body fluids as semen or saliva to identify criminal suspects.

Description

Blood typing and screening tests are performed in a blood bank laboratory by technologists trained in blood bank and transfusion services. The tests are performed on blood after it has been separated into cells and serum (the yellow liquid left after the blood cells are removed) Costs for both tests are covered by insurance when the tests are determined to be medically necessary.

Blood bank laboratories are usually located in blood center facilities, such as those operated by the American Red Cross, that collect, process, and supply blood that is donated, as well as in facilities, such as most hospitals, that prepare blood for transfusion. These laboratories are regulated by the United States Food and Drug Administration (FDA) and are often inspected and accredited by a professional association such as the American Association of Blood Banks (AABB).

Blood typing and screening tests are based on the reaction between antigens and antibodies. An antigen can be anything that triggers the body's immune response. The body produces a special protein called an antibody that has a uniquely shaped site that combines with the antigen to neutralize it. A person's body normally does not produce antibodies against its own antigens.

The antigens found on the surface of red blood cells are important because they determine a person's blood type. When red blood cells having a certain blood type antigen are mixed with serum containing antibodies against that antigen, the antibodies combine with and stick to the antigen. In a test tube, this reaction is visible as clumping or aggregating.

Although there are over 600 known red blood cell antigens organized into 22 blood group systems, routine blood typing is usually concerned with only two systems: the ABO and Rh blood group systems. Antibody screening helps to identify antibodies against several other groups of red blood cell antigens.

Blood typing

THE ABO BLOOD GROUP SYSTEM. In 1901, Karl Landsteiner, an Austrian pathologist, randomly combined the serum and red blood cells of his colleagues. From the reactions he observed in test tubes, he discovered the ABO blood group system. This discovery earned him the 1930 Nobel Prize in Medicine. A person's ABO blood type—A, B, AB, or O—is based on the presence or absence of the A and B antigens on his red blood cells. The A blood type has only the A antigen and the B blood type has only the B antigen. The AB blood type has both A and B antigens, and the O blood type has neither the A nor the B antigen.

By the time a person is six months old, he or she will have developed antibodies against the antigens that his or her red blood cells lack. That is, a person with A blood type will have anti-B antibodies, and a person with B blood type will have anti-A antibodies. A person with AB blood type will have neither antibody, but a person with O blood type will have both anti-A and anti-B antibodies. Although the distribution of each of the four ABO blood types varies among racial groups, O is the most common and AB is the least common in all groups.

FORWARD AND REVERSE TYPING. ABO typing is the first test done on blood when it is tested for transfusion. A person must receive ABO-matched blood because ABO incompatibilities are the major cause of fatal transfusion reactions. To guard against these incompatibilities, typing is done in two steps. In the first step, called forward typing, the patient's blood is mixed with serum that contains antibodies against type A blood, then with serum that contains antibodies against type B blood. A determination of the blood type is based on whether or not the blood clots in the presence of these sera.

In reverse typing, the patient's blood serum is mixed with blood that is known to be type A and type B. Again, the presence of clotting is used to determine the type.

An ABO incompatibility between a pregnant woman and her baby is a common cause of HDN but seldom requires treatment. This is because the majority of ABO antibodies are IgM, which are too large to cross the placenta. It is the IgG component that may cause HDN, and this is most often present in the plasma of group O mothers.

Paternity testing compares the ABO blood types of the child, mother, and alleged father. The alleged father cannot be the biological father if the child's blood type requires a gene that neither he nor the mother have. For example, a child with blood type B whose mother has blood type O requires a father with either AB or B blood type; a man with blood type O cannot be the biological father.

In some people, ABO antigens can be detected in body fluids other than blood, such as saliva, sweat, or semen. ABO typing of these fluids provides clues in legal investigations.

THE RH BLOOD GROUP SYSTEM. The Rh, or Rhesus, system was first detected in 1940 by

Landsteiner and Wiener when they injected blood from rhesus monkeys into guinea pigs and rabbits. More than 50 antigens have since been discovered that belong to this system, making it the most complex red blood cell antigen system.

In routine blood typing and cross-matching tests, only one of these 50 antigens, the D antigen, also known as the **Rh factor** or $Rh_o[D]$, is tested for. If the D antigen is present, that person is Rh-positive; if the D antigen is absent, that person is Rh-negative.

Other important antigens in the Rh system are C, c, E, and e. These antigens are not usually tested for in routine blood typing tests. Testing for the presence of these antigens, however, is useful in paternity testing, and when a technologist screens blood to identify unexpected Rh antibodies or find matching blood for a person with antibodies to one or more of these antigens.

Unlike the ABO system, antibodies to Rh antigens don't develop naturally. They develop only as an immune response after a transfusion or during pregnancy. The incidence of the Rh blood types varies between racial groups, but not as widely as the ABO blood types: 85% of whites and 90% of blacks are Rh-positive; 15% of whites and 10% of blacks are Rh-negative.

The distribution of ABO and Rh blood groups in the overall United States population is as follows:

- O Rh-positive, 38%
- O Rh-negative, 7%
- A Rh-positive, 34%
- A Rh-negative, 6%
- B Rh-positive, 9%
- B Rh-negative, 2%
- AB Rh-positive, 3%
- AB Rh-negative, 1%

In transfusions, the Rh system is next in importance after the ABO system. Most Rh-negative people who receive Rh-positive blood will develop anti-D antibodies. A later transfusion of Rh-positive blood may result in a severe or fatal transfusion reaction.

Rh incompatibility is the most common and severe cause of HDN. This incompatibility may occur when an Rh-negative mother and an Rh-positive father have an Rh-positive baby. Cells from the baby can cross the placenta and enter the mother's bloodstream, causing the mother to make anti-D antibodies. Unlike ABO antibodies, the structure of anti-D antibodies makes it likely that they will cross the placenta and enter the baby's bloodstream. There, they can destroy the baby's red blood cells, causing a severe or fatal anemia.

The first step in preventing HDN is to find out the Rh types of the expectant parents. If the mother is Rh-negative and the father is Rh-positive, the baby is at risk for developing HDN. The next step is performing an antibody screen of the mother's serum to make sure she doesn't already have anti-D antibodies from a previous pregnancy or transfusion. Finally, the Rh-negative mother is given an injection of Rh immunoglobulin (RhIg) at 28 weeks of gestation and again after delivery, if the baby is Rh positive. The RhIg attaches to any Rh-positive cells from the baby in the mother's bloodstream, preventing them from triggering anti-D antibody production in the mother. An Rh-negative woman should also receive RhIg following a **miscarriage**, abortion, or ectopic pregnancy.

OTHER BLOOD GROUP SYSTEMS. Several other blood group systems may be involved in HDN and transfusion reactions, although they are much less frequent than ABO and Rh. Some of the other groups are the Duffy, Kell, Kidd, MNS, and P systems. Tests for antigens from these systems are not included in routine blood typing, but they are commonly used in paternity testing.

Like Rh antibodies, antibodies in these systems do not develop naturally, but as an immune response after transfusion or during pregnancy. An antibody screening test is done before a cross-match to check for unexpected antibodies to antigens in these systems. A person's serum is mixed in a test tube with commercially-prepared cells containing antigens from these systems. If hemagglutination, or clumping, occurs, the antibody is identified.

Antibody screening

Antibody screening is done to look for unexpected antibodies to other blood groups, such as certain Rh (e.g. E, e, C, c), Duffy, MNS, Kell, Kidd, and P system antigens. The recipient's serum of the recipient is mixed with screening reagent red blood cells. The screening reagent red blood cells are cells with known antigens. This test is sometimes called an indirect antiglobulin or Coombs test. If an antibody to an antigen is present, the mixture will cause agglutination (clumping) of the red blood cells or cause hemolysis (breaking of the red cell membrane). If an antibody to one of these antigens is found, only blood without that antigen will be compatible in a cross-match. This sequence must be repeated before each transfusion a person receives.

Recipient's blood			Reactions with donor's red blood cells			
ABO antigens	ABO antibodies	ABO blood type	Donor type O cells	Donor type A cells	Donor type B cells	Donor type AB cells
None	Anti-A Anti-B	O				
A	Anti-B	A				
B	Anti-A	B				
A & B	None	AB				

Compatible

Not compatible

Blood typing is a laboratory test done to discover a person's blood type. If the person needs a blood transfusion, crossmatching is done following blood typing to locate donor blood that the person's body will accept. *(Illustration by Electronic Illustrators Group. The Gale Group.)*

Testing for infectious disease markers

As of 2001, pretransfusion testing includes testing blood for the following infectious disease markers:

- Hepatitis B surface antigen (HBsAg). This test detects the uter envelope of the heptatitis B virus.

- Antibodies to the core of the hepatitis B virus (Anti-HBc). This test detects an antibody to the hepatitis B virus that is produced during and after an **infection**.

- Antibodies to the hepatitis C virus (Anti-HCV).

- Antibodies to human **immunodeficiency** virus, types 1 and 2 (Anti-HIV-1, -2).

- HIV-1 p24 antigen. This test screens for antigens of HIV-1. The advantage of this test is that it can detect HIV-1 infection a week earlier than the antibody test.

- Antibodies to human T-lymphotropic virus, types I and II (Anti-HTLV-I, -II). In the United States,

HTLV infection is most common among intravenous drug users.

- Syphilis. This test is performed to detect evidence of infection with the spirochete *Treponema pallidum*.

- Nucleic acid amplification testing (NAT). NAT uses a new form of blood testing technology that directly detects the genetic material of the HCV and HIV viruses.

- Confirmatory tests. These are done to screen out false positives.

Cross-matching

Cross-matching is the final step in pretransfusion testing. It is commonly referred to as compatibility testing, or "type and cross." Before blood from a donor and the recipient are cross-matched, both are ABO and Rh typed. To begin the cross-match, a unit of blood from a donor with the same ABO and Rh

Frequency (%) of ABO and Rh blood types in U.S. population

Racial group	ABO blood type				Rh blood type	
	O	A	B	AB	Positive	Negative
Whites	45%	40%	11%	4%	85%	15%
Blacks	49%	27%	20%	4%	90%	10%

type as the recipient is selected. Serum from the patient is mixed with red blood cells from the donor. The cross-match can be performed either as a short (5–10 minutes) incubation intended only to verify ABO compatibility or as a long (45 minutes) incubation with an antihuman globulin test intended to verify compatibility for all other red cell antigens. If clumping occurs, the blood is not compatible; if clumping does not occur, the blood is compatible. If an unexpected antibody is found in either the patient or the donor, the blood bank does further testing to ensure the blood is compatible.

In an emergency, when there is not enough time for blood typing and cross-matching, O red blood cells may be given, preferably Rh-negative. O-type blood is called the universal donor because it has no ABO antigens for a patient's antibodies to combine with. In contrast, AB blood type is called the universal recipient because it has no ABO antibodies to combine with the antigens on transfused red blood cells. If there is time for blood typing, red blood cells of the recipient type (type-specific cells) are given. In either case, the cross-match is continued even though the transfusion has begun.

Autologous donation

The practice of collecting a patient's own blood prior to elective surgery for later transfusion is called autologous donation. Since the safest blood for transfusion is the patient's own, autologous donation is particularly useful for patients with rare blood types. Three to four units of blood are collected several weeks before surgery, and the patient is given **iron** supplements.

Preparation

To collect the 10 mL of blood needed for these tests, a healthcare worker ties a tourniquet above the patient's elbow, locates a vein near the the inner elbow, cleans the skin overlying the vein, and inserts a needle

into that vein. The blood is drawn through the needle into an attached vacuum tube. Collection of the sample takes only a few minutes.

Blood typing and screening must be done three days or less before a transfusion. A person does not need to change diet, medications, or activities before these tests. Patients should tell their health care provider if they have received a blood transfusion or a plasma substitute during the last three months, or have had a radiology procedure using intravenous contrast media. These can give false clumping reactions in both typing and cross-matching tests.

Aftercare

The possible side effects of any blood collection are discomfort, bruising, or excessive bleeding at the site where the needle punctured the skin, as well as dizziness or fainting. Bruising and bleeding is reduced if pressure is applied with a finger to the puncture site until the bleeding stops. Discomfort is treated with warm packs to the puncture site.

Complications

Aside from the rare event of infection or bleeding, there are no risks from the blood collection. Blood transfusions always have the risk of an unexpected transfusion reaction. These complications may include an acute hemolytic transfusion reaction (AHTR), which is most commonly caused by ABO incompatibility. The patient may complain of **pain**, difficult breathing, **fever** and chills, facial flushing, and nausea. Signs of **shock** may appear, including a drop in **blood pressure** and a rapid but weak pulse. If AHTR is suspected, the transfusion should be stopped at once.

Other milder transfusion reactions include a delayed hemolytic transfusion reaction, which may occur one or two weeks after the transfusion. It consists of a slight fever and a falling **hematocrit**, and is usually self-limited. Patients may also have allergic reactions to unknown components in donor blood.

Results

The blood type is labeled as A+, A–, B+, B–, O+, O–, AB+, or AB–, based on both the ABO and Rh systems. If antibody screening is negative, only a cross-match is necessary. If the antibody screen is positive, then blood that is negative for those antigens must be identified. The desired result of a cross-match is that compatible donor blood is found.

KEY TERMS

ABO blood type—Blood type based on the presence or absence of the A and B antigens on the red blood cells. There are four types: A, B, AB, and O.

Acute hemolytic transfusion reaction (AHTR)—A severe transfusion reaction with abrupt onset, most often caused by ABO incompatibility. Symptoms include difficulty breathing, fever and chills, pain, and sometimes shock.

Antibody—A protein produced by B-lymphocytes that binds to an antigen facilitating its removal by phagocytosis or lysis.

Antigen—Any substance that stimulates the production of antibodies and combines specifically with them.

Autologous donation—Donation of the patient's own blood, made several weeks before elective surgery.

Blood bank—A laboratory that specializes in blood typing, antibody identification, and transfusion services.

Blood type—Any of various classes into which human blood can be divided according to immunological compatibility based on the presence or absence of certain antigens on the red blood cells. Blood types are sometimes called blood groups.

Cross-match—A laboratory test done to confirm that blood from a donor and blood from the recipient are compatible. Serum from each is mixed with red blood cells from the other and observed for hemagglutination.

Gene—A piece of DNA, located on a chromosome, that determines how such traits as blood type are inherited and expressed.

Hemagglutination—The clumping of red blood cells due to blood type incompatibility.

Indirect Coombs' test—A test used to screen for unexpected antibodies against red blood cells. The patient's serum is mixed with reagent red blood cells, incubated, washed, tested with antihuman globulin, and observed for clumping.

Rh blood type—In general, refers to the blood type based on the presence or absence of the D antigen on the red blood cells. There are, however, other antigens in the Rh system.

Serum (plural, sera)—The clear, pale yellow liquid that separates from the clot when blood coagulates.

Transfusion—The therapeutic introduction of blood or a blood component into a patient's bloodstream.

Compatibility testing procedures are designed to provide the safest blood product possible for the recipient, but a compatible cross-match is no guarantee that an unexpected adverse reaction will not appear during the transfusion.

Except in an emergency, a person cannot receive a transfusion without a compatible cross-match result. In rare cases, the least incompatible blood has to be given.

Health care team roles

A physician orders the type and screen test if there is only a small chance (e.g. less than 10%) of a need for blood transfusion. The technologist types and screens the recipient (patient). If a transfusion is required, then a cross-match is performed with the patient's blood and a specific unit of donated blood. A nurse monitors the patient for signs of AHTR or other transfusion reactions during the entire procedure.

Resources

BOOKS

American Association of Blood Banks. *Technical Manual*, 13th ed. Bethesda, MD: American Association of Blood Banks, 1999.

Beadling, Wendy V., Laura Cooling, and John B. Henry. "Immunohematology." In *Clinical Diagnosis and Management by Laboratory Methods*, 20th ed., edited by John B. Henry. Philadelphia: W. B. Saunders Company, 2001.

Boral, Leonard I., Edward D. Weiss, and John B. Henry. "Transfusion Medicine." In *Clinical Diagnosis and Management by Laboratory Methods*, 20th ed. Edited by John B. Henry. Philadelphia: W. B. Saunders Company, 2001.

Daniels, Geoff. *Human Blood Groups*. Oxford: Blackwell, 1995.

Issitt, Peter D. and David J. Anstee *Applied Blood Group Serology*, 4th ed. Durham, NC: Montgomery Scientific Publications, 1998.

"Transfusion Medicine." in *The Merck Manual of Diagnosis and Therapy*, edited by Mark H. Beers, MD, and Robert Berkow, MD. Whitehouse Station, NJ: Merck Research Laboratories, 2004.

Triulzi, Darrell J., ed. *Blood Transfusion Therapy: A Physician's Handbook*, 6th ed. Bethesda: American Association of Blood Banks, 1999.

ORGANIZATIONS

American Association of Blood Banks. 8101 Glenbrook Road, Bethesda, MD 20814. (301) 907-6977. <http://www.aabb.org>.

American College of Obstetricians and Gynecologists. 409 12th Street SW, Washington, DC 20024-2188. (202) 638-5577. <http://www.acog.org>.

American Red Cross Blood Services. 430 17th Street NW, Washington, DC 20006. (202) 737-8300. <http://www.redcross.org>.

OTHER

American Association of Blood Banks. *All About Blood.* Bethesda, MD: American Association of Blood Banks, 1999.

Mark A. Best

Types I and II diabetes *see* **Diabetes mellitus**

Tzanck preparation

Definition

Tzanck preparation is a rapid test used to help physicians diagnose infections caused by herpes **viruses**. This test cannot detect the virus, but can detect the characteristic changes in cells that herpes **infection** produces.

Purpose

Herpes viruses are responsible for several superficial infections. Varicella zoster virus causes chickenpox and shingles, herpes simplex type 1 causes the **common cold** sore or **fever** blister, and herpes simplex type 2 causes the sexually transmitted disease (STD) **genital herpes**. All forms of herpes are associated with production of vesicles (blisters) and ulcers.

Physicians usually can diagnose herpes infections by looking at the type of vesicles and ulcers, and their distribution on the person's body. Sometimes laboratory evidence of herpes is needed to confirm the diagnosis. When a sample is available from a vesicular lesion, the Tzanck preparation can be done more rapidly and less expensively than other tests. It is important to note that herpes infection may be present in such lesions, and not produce a positive Tzanck test result. A positive finding is diagnostic of herpes infection, but is seen in only about 67% of herpes infections. Consequently, other laboratory tests may be required to diagnose herpes infections. Some herpes infections are present in tissues that cannot be tested by a Tzanck preparation. For example, herpes can be devastating to a newborn or a person with a weakened **immune system**. The virus may invade the **central nervous system** causing

meningitis. Laboratory culture, tests for herpes DNA, antigens, and antibodies may be needed for diagnosis in such circumstances.

Precautions

Cell collection can be performed in minutes with only minor discomfort to the patient. Health care providers should use appropriate protective measures to avoid infection when collecting the samples.

Description

Tzanck preparation is also called a Tzanck smear, herpes stain for inclusion bodies, or an inclusion bodies stain. The Tzanck preparation is performed by smearing cells taken from a fresh blister or ulcer onto a **microscope** slide. A fresh blister is opened with a scalpel or sterile needle. The physician scrapes the base of the blister with the scalpel, gathers as much cellular material as possible, and gently spreads it on a microscope slide. The cells are fixed with alcohol and stained with Giemsa stain. The cells are examined under a microscope for characteristic changes caused by herpes virus. Herpes causes formation of giant cells with multiple nuclei. The shape of each nucleus appears molded to fit together with those adjacent to it. The nuclei may also contain red inclusions characteristic of herpes infection.

Preparation

There is no special preparation required before this procedure.

Aftercare

There are no special aftercare requirements associated with this procedure.

Complications

There are no complications associated with this procedure. However, health care professionals should be careful not to expose themselves to the potentially infectious material during specimen collection.

Results

A normal smear shows no evidence of a herpes infection. However, this test may also produce false negatives. Studies have shown that the Tzanck preparation shows signs of infection in only 50–79% of people with a herpes infection. A negative Tzanck

KEY TERMS

Herpes—A family of viruses including herpes simplex types 1 and 2, and herpes zoster (also called varicella zoster). Herpes viruses cause several infections, all characterized by blisters and ulcers, including chickenpox, shingles, genital herpes, and cold sores or fever blisters.

preparation may have to be confirmed by a herpes culture or other laboratory test. A smear that shows evidence of herpes infection does not distinguish between the various infections caused by herpes virus. The physician uses the person's symptoms and other clinical findings to distinguish between these infections and will often order a culture for confirmation. Newer antigen detection tests and serologic tests are available to assist in diagnosing herpes viruses, but viral cultures are still considered the best and most cost efficient diagnostic tool available.

Health care team roles

A physician, nurse, or physician assistant collects the cell samples from the patient. The Tzanck preparation and microscopic examination may be performed by the physician, by a clinical laboratory scientist/medical technologist, or laboratory specialist with specific training in clinical diagnostic virology.

Patient education

The health care provider can be an important resource for patients with herpes infection, especially those with genital herpes. Patients with genital herpes may be embarrassed about their condition or hesitant to seek medical attention. Health care providers counsel patients, and explain prevention and treatment of sexually transmitted diseases.

Resources

BOOKS

Costello, Michael, and Margaret Yungbluth. "Viral Infections." In *Clinical Diagnosis and Management by Laboratory Methods*. 20th ed., edited by John Bernard Henry. Philadelphia: W. B. Saunders Company, 2001, pp.1045-1052.

Parker, Frank. "Diagnostic Tests and Aids in Examination of the Skin." In *Cecil Textbook of Medicine*. 21st ed., edited by Lee Goldman and J. Claude Bennett. Philadelphia: W. B. Saunders Company, 2000, p.2271.

PERIODICALS

Emmert, David H. "Treatment of Common Cutaneous Herpes Simplex Virus Infections." *American Family Physician* 61 (March 15, 2000): pp.1697-1708.

ORGANIZATIONS

American Social Health Association. PO Box 13827, Research Triangle Park, NC 27709. (919) 361-8400. <http://www.ashastd.org>.

Division of Sexually Transmitted Diseases, National Center for HIV, STD and TB Prevention, Centers for Disease Control and Prevention. 1600 Clifton Road NE, Atlanta, GA 30333. (800) 311-3435. <http://www.cdc.gov>.

Linda D. Jones, B.A., PBT (ASCP)

Tzanck smear *see* **Tzanck preparation**

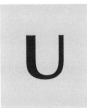

Ultrasonic encephalography

Definition

Ultrasonic encephalography, or echoencephalography, is the use of ultrasound to produce a noninvasive diagnostic image of the **brain** and its structures, including the alignment down the midline, the size of ventricles, and the presence of bleeding or tumors.

Purpose

Ultrasonic encephalography is a noninvasive way to create images of the brain. Also called intracranial ultrasound or head ultrasound, the test is most commonly used on children under the age of two to diagnose hemorrhage or hydrocephalus (enlargement of the head due to accumulation of fluid). It is particularly useful in the neonatal intensive care unit to provide bedside monitoring of premature babies who are at higher risk for hemorrhage. A series of tests are commonly ordered for babies born earlier than 34 weeks of gestation.

Ultrasonic encephalography can also detect the swelling inside the head (cerebral **edema**), as shown by an increase in the size of the lateral ventricles, sometimes seen in diabetic children. The test can be used in adults to monitor the size of the ventricles or to determine a shift in the structure of the brain from midline due to swelling or a tumor. However, for adults and older children, this test has been largely replaced by computed tomography (CT).

Precautions

There are no contraindications to ultrasonic encephalography.

Description

Ultrasonic encephalography uses ultrasound to produce diagnostic images of the brain. Ultrasonic waves are sound in the range above what normally can be heard by the human ear, anything above 20,000 Hertz (cycles per second) in frequency. Ultrasonic encephalography generally uses high frequency sounds waves, in the ranges of 5 to 10 MHz.

Sound waves can produce an image of the brain because of the different densities present in the tissue of the brain, **blood**, or tumor and the cerebrospinal fluid within the ventricles. Matter of different density reflects, or echoes, the sound waves differently, allowing the machine to distinguish between the structures.

The fineness of the distinguishing process is known as resolution. Resolution is affected by the frequency of sound waves used. As frequency increases, resolution increases. However, an increase in frequency reduces the ability of the sound waves to penetrate into the brain. Because of this relationship, successful ultrasonic encephalograms often zero in on the structures of interest, maximizing the resolution by using the highest frequency that penetrates sufficiently into the head.

A main reason why ultrasonic encephalography is used in newborns and children under the age of two is the presence of the anterior and posterior fontanelle, triangular structures at the top and back of the head where bones of the **skull** have not yet fused. As bone is a poor conductor of ultrasonic waves, the fontanelles provide convenient conduits into and out of the brain for the ultrasound pulses. Once the bones have fused together, the resolution of the ultrasound is greatly reduced by having to pass through bone in order to visualize the brain.

Ultrasonic encephalography involves sending ultrasonic waves through the top of the head, bouncing them off the brain structures, and recording the resulting echo. The results of the test can be produced in a plotted graphic form, known as an A-mode echo or in a two-dimensional mode. In A-mode, one axis represents the time required for the return of the echo and the other corresponds to the strength of the echo. A 2-D echo produces a cross-sectional image of the brain. As of mid-2000, 3-D imaging of the neonatal brain was still in experimental stages, with poor visualization as compared to 2-D images.

The **ultrasound unit** used for echoencephalography includes a TV monitor (cathode ray tube or CRT), a transducer for sending and receiving the ultrasonic waves, the transmitter, the receiver, the amplifier, and recording devices. The transducer is a hand-held instrument that is generally used both to transmit sound waves and to receive the echoes. The transducer includes the element, electrode connections to the transmitter and the receiver, backing material, a matching layer, and a protective face.

The element is the core of the transducer, the material that actually produces the sound waves. Elements are built around piezoelectric ceramic (e.g. barium titanate or lead zirconate titanate) chips. (Piezoelectric refers to electricity that is produced when pressure is put on certain crystals such as quartz.) These ceramic chips react to electric pulses by producing sound waves (they are transmitting waves) and react to sound waves by producing electric pulses (receiving). Bursts of high-frequency electric pulses supplied to the transducer by the transmitter cause it to produce the scanning sound waves. The transducer then receives the returning echoes, translates them back into electric pulses, and sends them to the receiver. The backing material helps to focus the sound energy into the element, while the matching layer helps to reduce reflection of the sound from the transducer surface. The protective face shields the internal components of the transducer. Electrodes connect the transmitter and the receiver to the transducer. The amplifier boosts the returning signals and prepares them to be displayed on the TV monitor (CRT).

Preparation

The patient who is undergoing an ultrasonic encephalogram is laid on his or her back or side and must be still during the test. It is suggested that children two months to one year of age not eat or drink for three hours before the test, so a bottle can be drunk during the exam. Particular care must be taken if the child is connected to a respirator. Warmed conducting gel is placed on the head to ensure an air-free contact between the transducer and the head (air is a very poor conductor of ultrasound) and to allow the transducer to slide easily.

The area that provides the least amount of interference with the ultrasound waves is called the acoustic window. For infants and young children, the best acoustic windows are transfontanelle, that is, through either the posterior or anterior fontanelle. Some standard views from the anterior fontanelle include midline sagittal (viewed from the side, through the midline, or middle of the head), lateral sagittal (viewed from the side, displaced from the midline), and coronal views (viewed from the front, angled toward the back, middle, and front). Axial views (across the temple) can be used, despite the reverberation artifacts caused by the skull, to follow lateral ventricle size.

An ultrasonic encephalogram is noninvasive, causes no **pain**, and takes about 20–30 minutes.

Aftercare

After the test, the patient can return to regular daily activities and meals.

Complications

There are no complications or side effects of ultrasonic encephalography.

Results

Ultrasonic encephalograms are mainly performed for the diagnosis and follow-up of neonatal hemorrhage, hydrocephalus, and congenital malformations. **Premature infants** often develop bleeding in the germinal matrix of the caudate nucleus. The caudate nucleus is an elongated, arched gray mass in the center of the brain next to the lateral ventricles, and the germinal matrix is a group of brain cells in that area that is still developing. Bleeding can also occur in the choroid plexus (spongy tissue of the ventricles) and rarely, the cerebellum. If the bleeding is severe it can leak into the ventricle, a problem known as intraventricular hemorrhage (IVH). All of these bleeding problems can be seen initially as echogenic areas (white areas) that later can be replaced by fluid-filled cysts that scan as dark areas.

Bleeding in the neonate is sometimes associated with the later development of **cerebral palsy**, although other risk factors, such as bronchopulmonary dysplasia (BPD) appear to be equally predictive.

When looking for hydrocephalus, measurements of the ventricles are done. On a lateral sagittal view, the distance from the curve of the choroid plexus to the tip of the occipital horn generally should not be more than 16 mm. Using a coronal view, the body of the lateral ventricle should generally not be more than 3 mm. Finally, an axial view is often used to

KEY TERMS

Acoustic window—Area through which ultrasound waves move freely.

Congenital malformation—A deformity present at birth.

Echogenic—Highly reflective of ultrasound waves; these tissues show as a white area in the scan.

Hemorrhage—Bleeding, the escape of blood from the vessels.

Hydrocephalus—A congenital or acquired condition characterized by an increase in size of the cerebral ventricles. Without treatment it can cause enlargement of the head, brain shrinkage, mental deterioration, and convulsions.

Intracranial—Inside the skull.

Ventricle—A small cavity in the brain. Humans have two lateral ventricles, a third ventricle, and a fourth ventricle.

determine the lateral ventricular ratio, which is the lateral ventricular width divided by the hemispheric width (both widths measured from the outer border to the midline). The ratio is compared to previous measurements to see if swelling is developing.

There are many congenital malformations of the brain that can be either diagnosed or the severity determined with ultrasonic encephalography. Some representative examples include microcephaly, holoprosencephaly, Dandy-Walker Syndrome, and encephalocele. These conditions can have serious prognoses, so ultrasound is an effective means of determining what treatment, such as placement of a shunt or surgery, should take place.

Health care team roles

Ultrasonic encephalograms are often produced by specially trained ultrasound technologists. Training for such a position usually involves study at a two-year college or vocational program. A typical program would include:

- elementary principles of ultrasound
- ultrasound transducers
- pulse-echo principles & instrumentation
- ultrasound image storage & display
- artifacts (erroneous results)

- quality assurance
- bioeffects and safety

Certification of ultrasound technologists specializing in neurological work such as ultrasonic encephalography is available through the American Registry of Diagnostic Medical Sonographers as a registered diagnostic medical sonographer with a specialty in neurosonology. Certification requires passing both a general and a specialized test.

A physician such as pediatrician, neonatologist, or radiologist does the final review and diagnosis based on the results of an ultrasonic encephalogram. The doctor can be present for the exam or may review saved images.

Resources

BOOKS

Barkovich, A. James "Brain and Spine Injuries."
    In *Pediatric Neuroimaging*. Philadelphia: Lippincott
    Williams & Wilkins, 2000, p. 189.
"Neonatal and Infant Brain Imaging." In *Diagnostic
    Ultrasound*, edited by Carol M. Rumack, et al.
    St. Louis, MO: Mosby, 1998, p. 1443.

PERIODICALS

Kitabchi, Abbas E., et al. "Management of Hyperglycemic
    Crises in Patients With Diabetes." *Diabetes Care*
    (January 2001): 131.
Salerno, C.C., et al. "Three-dimensional Ultrasonographic
    Imaging of the Neonatal Brain in High-risk Neonates:
    Preliminary Study." *Journal of Ultrasound Medicine* 19
    (August 2000): 549–55.

OTHER

Harrison, Helen "Ultrasound of Premature Infants and Risk
    Factors for Cerebral Palsy and Developmental
    Problems." *Observations on Prematurity*. <http://
    www.comeunity.com/premature/research/
    helen-brainscans.html> (April 23, 2001).

Michelle L. Johnson, M.S., J.D.

Ultrasound technology *see* **Diagnostic medical sonography**

Ultrasound unit

Definition

An ultrasound unit is a noninvasive medical device used to produce images of body tissues and organs from differential reflections of ultrasonic sound waves. The technique of diagnostic imaging performed by

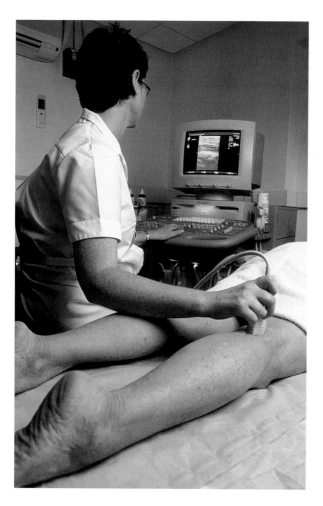

Patient undergoing a Doppler ultrasound (angiodynography) scan to study blood flow and explore potential deep vein thrombosis. The display (upper right) shows the area being studied. The transducer being held against the leg sends high frequency sound waves and picks up their echoes. *(James King-Holmes / Photo Researchers, Inc. Reproduced by permission.)*

ultrasound units is called ultrasonography. Ultrasonic waves are sound waves of a higher frequency than the human ear can detect. The frequency of a sound wave is the number of times per second that it cycles, and the number of cycles is measured in hertz (Hz). For example, one kilohertz (kHz) is one thousand cycles per second. Human **hearing** can detect sound in the range between 20 hertz to about 20 kilohertz (20kHz), or 20,000 cycles per second. Ultrasound images are generally produced using sound waves in the range between 1.6 to 10 million megahertz (MHz). Body tissues of different density reflect, or echo, sound waves differently, allowing the sonographer to distinguish between the structures.

Purpose

The first account of diagnostic ultrasound was published in 1942 by Dr. Karl Dussik, an Austrian psychiatrist. Dr. Dussik used ultrasound to locate **brain** tumors. Although ultrasound is better known as a technique of diagnostic imaging, it is also used at present in a variety of therapeutic applications.

Diagnostic applications

Ultrasonographic imaging can be used to visualize most soft-tissue organs. Dr. Dussik used ultrasound to visualize the cerebral ventricles in his pioneering use of the technique. Ultrasound is now used routinely to examine the **kidneys** or **liver** for the presence of tumors or cysts. The gall bladder can be checked for gallstones. Ultrasonography can also be used to examine **blood vessels** in the abdomen, extremities, or neck for evidence of swelling or blockage. One of the best-known diagnostic applications of ultrasound is its use during **pregnancy** to monitor the development, position, sex, and number of babies present in the mother's uterus.

Diagnostic ultrasound units are used to guide instruments during such invasive treatments as needle biopsies. Intraoperative sonography is used during many other procedures and even in combination with other medical imaging techniques. For example, intraoperative ultrasound is used during neurosurgery to detect brain tissue movement that can compromise the use of other more detailed imaging systems, such as computed tomography (CT) or **magnetic resonance imaging** (MRI).

Therapeutic applications

Ultrasonography also has therapeutic applications, although the frequencies used for therapy are usually in different frequency ranges than those used in diagnostic ultrasound.

BODY FLUID SAMPLING. A technique developed at MIT uses ultrasound to draw samples of tissue fluid through the skin without the use of needles. Ultrasound waves disorganize the fatty layers in the outer layer of human skin, thus increasing the skin's permeability sufficiently to allow molecules of tissue fluid to travel through into a vacuum cylinder. The researchers apply ultrasound to the skin at 20 kHz frequency for two minutes. This frequency is much lower than that used to visualize fetuses in the womb. The technique shows promise as a noninvasive way for diabetics to monitor their **blood** sugar levels.

PHYSIOTHERAPY. Ultrasound waves produce heat as well as sound echoes. The low levels of heat produced by ultrasound appear to speed up wound healing, first by facilitating the release of histamine, a chemical that attracts white blood cells to the injured tissue. Second, ultrasound stimulates fibroblasts to secrete collagen, a fibrous protein found in connective tissue that increases the strength of the healing tissue. Ultrasound can also be applied to the area around the wound to provide mild heat in order to stimulate blood circulation in the area. A frequency of 3 MHz is used for most skin **wounds**, 1 MHz for deeper wounds or the area around the wound.

A British study indicates that ultrasound therapy applied to the wrist provides good short-term relief of mildly to moderately severe **carpal tunnel syndrome**. The beneficial effects of the treatment last for at least six months. It is thought that the ultrasound waves relieve the symptoms of the syndrome by relieving inflammation.

TUMOR DETECTION AND TREATMENT. Ultrasound can be used to scan for endometrial **cancer** in post-menopausal women without the need for a surgical biopsy. The ultrasound captures a detailed image of the lining of the uterus, which allows not only for immediate evaluation of the results, but is also more accurate than a biopsy.

Focused high-intensity ultrasound is being tested as a technique for destroying cancerous tumors within the body. The high-intensity beam, which is about 10,000 times as powerful as the ultrasound beams used to monitor pregnancies, appears to work by heating the cancer cells to nearly the temperature of boiling water. The cancer cells die within seconds. In 1999, the FDA granted approval for the use of focused ultrasound to treat enlarged prostate glands in men.

Description

An ultrasound unit includes a television monitor (cathode ray tube or CRT), a transducer for sending and receiving the ultrasonic waves, a transmitter, receiver, amplifier, and a strip chart recorder.

The transducer

The transducer, which is also called a probe, is a hand-held instrument used to both generate the sound waves and receive the echoes. The transducer typically functions as a generator about 10% of the time and as a receiver the other 90%. The transducer includes an element, electrode connections to the transmitter and the receiver, backing material, a matching layer, and a protective face.

The element is the core of the transducer—the material that actually produces the sound waves. Elements are usually made of such ceramic materials as barium titanate or lead zirconate titanate. These materials change shape when electrical current is applied, which produces the ultrasonic waves. When ultrasonic waves are absorbed by the element, electrical energy is produced. The transducer of a real-time scanner typically contains over 300 crystals arranged in a row, each emitting and receiving an ultrasound beam in rapid succession.

The remaining parts of the transducer help to focus the sound waves for most effective function. The backing material directs the sound energy into the element, while the matching layer reduces reflection of the sound from the transducer surface. The protective face shields the internal components of the transducer.

There are three fundamental types of transducer used in medical applications: convex, linear, and phased array. Transducers come in different shapes and sizes for use in different scanning applications. Obstetrical scans often use a convex probe that is shaped like a curved soap bar. Probes for vaginal scans are long and slender. There are specially designed probes that couple biopsy needles with the transducer, so that the ultrasound can be easily used to guide the needle.

Remaining parts of the unit

The remaining parts of the ultrasound unit initiate or receive the signals collected by the transducer or are involved in reconstructing the electronic signals into an image. The transmitter creates the impulses sent to the transducer to generate the sound energy. The receiver accepts the electric current generated in the transducer by returning sound energy. Electrodes connect the transmitter and the receiver to the transducer. The amplifier boosts the returning signals and prepares them for display on the monitor (CRT).

One of the advantages of ultrasound is the compactness of the actual unit. Although most portable units are stored on a wheeled cart, completely portable ultrasounds weighing just over 5 lbs (2 kg) and carried by a handle built into the unit, are also available.

The compactness and portability of ultrasound has made it the diagnostic method of choice for isolated medical settings. Remote linkups can allow doctors to review ultrasound images taken many miles away. The space shuttle is equipped with an ultrasound, both for monitoring the effects of weightlessness on astronauts and experimental animals and for emergency use.

Ultrasound modes

The ultrasound monitor is used to display the images produced. Depending on the kind of transducer, the monitor has several basic modes of display, including A-mode, B-mode, M-mode, and Doppler. A-mode is the simplest form of ultrasound; it analyzes a single beam. The A-mode display is a series of peaks indicating the distance of the structure being scanned from the transducer as time elapses. Isolated use of A-scans is now rare, but this display mode can be used to ensure that the time-gain compensation is set correctly and to check the accuracy of the distance measurements between echoes.

B-mode is the image that results from converting the peaks of A-mode into dots whose brightness varies with the strength of the signal. Stronger signals appear more nearly white and weaker signals more nearly black. In a real-time system, B-mode scans repeat about 30 times a second, thus capturing such movements within the patient as the beating of the **heart** or a fetus sucking its thumb.

M-mode displays B-mode dots on a moving-time basis. Before the development of real-time systems, M-mode was used to monitor the opening and closing of heart valves. It is still useful in determining the precise timing of valve opening as well as coordinating valve motion with **electrocardiography**, phonocardiography (the study of heart sounds), and Doppler.

Doppler ultrasound depicts the movement of fluid, usually blood, within the body. The technique is based on the fact that sound waves change in frequency when bounced off a moving target, called a sample volume. If the sample volume is moving away from the transducer, the frequency of the bounced sound wave is increased after the echo, while the frequency is decreased if the sample volume is moving toward the transducer. There are two kinds of Doppler analysis, pulsed wave (PW) and continuous wave (CW). Pulsed wave has proved very useful for analyzing blood flow in a particular area of the heart or group of vessels, while continuous wave is better suited for evaluation of a single valve or vessel. Doppler output is often enhanced with a color display. With most of these systems, shades of red indicate that blood is flowing toward the transducer, while shades of blue represent flow away from the transducer.

Operation

To perform an ultrasound scan, the patient is placed on an examination table with the area to be imaged uncovered. A gel, warmed for comfort, is applied to the skin to prevent air bubbles between the transducer and the body. The sonographer sweeps the transducer across the area of interest, keeping contact with the patient's skin.

In order to obtain the best possible images, the sound waves are sent within a particular area called the acoustic window. For example, a commonly used acoustic window for an echocardiograph (ultrasound of the heart) is the left parasternal approach, which allows visualization of all the valves and chambers. Acoustic windows avoid bone and such air-filled organs as the **lungs**, as both bone and air are poor media for ultrasonic waves.

The level of detail of the imaging process is known as resolution. Resolution is affected by the frequency of sound waves used. As frequency increases, resolution increases. Increase in frequency, however, reduces the sound waves' depth of penetration into body tissue. Because of this inverse relationship, sonographers usually focus on the structures of interest, maximizing the resolution by using the highest frequency that will penetrate the tissue to the required depth.

Settings

The settings of an ultrasound unit include the power output (gain or attenuation) and the time gain compensation (gain curve or swept gain), controlled by four variables: the slope rate (slope), the slope start (delay), and the near and far gain (initial gain). Each of these controls affects the way the echoes are sent or received. The power output alters the echoes throughout the ultrasonic field by varying the amount of sound sent (gain) or the strength of the signal after it comes back to the transducer (attenuation), measured in decibels. Excessive gain can produce too many echoes and differentiation between tissues can be lost.

One major source of interference is echoes from the skin and subcutaneous tissues. These can be eliminated by altering the slope delay value by 0.8–1.2 in (2–3 cm). Near gain alters the power of the echoes in the near field. This value is adjusted so that enough information about the near field is present in the image, but not so much as to swamp out signals from small structures farther from the transducer. Far gain governs the strength of the echoes from distant structures, and must be adjusted to ensure all parts of the organ or structure being studied are well represented in the image.

Preprocessing and postprocessing controls can be used to clarify an image for a more detailed look at a particular section. Preprocessing controls assign values to returning echoes before they are displayed and can help accentuate borders between structures. Postprocessing assigns values to echoes after they have been displayed, thus helping to accentuate low-level echoes.

Real-time scanners have such special controls as calipers (to measure distances); cineloop (a replay function to help select an image for a photo); frame rate; freeze frame; and record (to videotape the image).

Doppler ultrasound units have an additional set of controls. The range gate cursor is used to indicate the depth and area placement of the sample volume, overlaid on a B-scan. A second control is inversion, which allows flow away from the transducer to become a positive rather than negative value for easier viewing. Velocity scale allows changes for different rates of cardiac output; sweep speed changes the rate at which the information is displayed. Wall filter settings are used to eliminate signal noise and artifacts caused by the patient's movement. The angle correct bar aligns the blood flow and the ultrasound beam because the angle must be no greater than 60 degrees. The size of the angle is important because the smaller the angle between beam and flow, the greater the Doppler shift. Finally, Doppler gain adjustments ensure that the image of color flow is set so that variations are seen within the vessel and any artificial flow outside the vessel is eliminated.

Safety

Ultrasound appears to be one of the safest imaging technologies as well as one of the least expensive. As of 2001, there were no confirmed biological effects on patients or instrument operators with exposure to ultrasound for the time periods and frequencies used in diagnostic procedures. The current position of the American Institute of Ultrasound in Medicine (AIUM) is that the benefits to patients with diagnostic ultrasound outweigh any known risks—although the possibility always exists that adverse biological effects may be identified in the future.

Ultrasound during pregnancy is regarded as appropriate when performed to help the physician determine the baby's health and due date. Ultrasound examination can also determine the baby's position in the womb or the existence of a **multiple pregnancy**. Ultrasound also may be used to detect some birth defects. The AIUM, however, does not condone the use of ultrasound solely to determine fetal sex.

Maintenance

Maintenance of ultrasound equipment is performed by specially trained technicians who may belong to the hospital engineering staff or an outsource company. Maintenance includes visual inspections, periodic cleaning, and system performance checks. Performance checks ensure that all power supply voltages are within tolerance and image performance is maintained.

Health care team roles

Ultrasound units are operated by specially trained ultrasound technologists. Nurses assist with patient preparation and education about the procedure. A physician, who may be a radiologist, surgeon, internist, or gynecologist performs the final review and diagnosis based on the results of the ultrasound. The physician may be present during the examination or may make the final review and diagnosis based on saved images.

KEY TERMS

Acoustic window—The area through which ultrasound waves move freely.

Attenuation—Reduction of the strength of the sound signal as it travels through body tissues.

Decibel—A unit used to express differences in acoustic power. A decibel (dB) is equal to 10 times the common logarithm of the ratio of two sound signals.

Frequency—The number of cycles per second of a sound wave, measured in hertz. One thousand cycles per second is equal to one kilohertz (kHz).

Gain—The strength of the ultrasound signal as it leaves the transducer.

Hertz—A unit of measurement of the frequency of sound waves, equal to one cycle per second. It is named for Heinrich R. Hertz (1857-1894), a German physicist.

Real-time—A type of ultrasound that involves computerized images that respond immediately to user input, in order to record movement.

Sample volume—The area of blood flow analyzed by Doppler ultrasound.

Sonographer—A technician who operates ultrasound units.

Transducer—The handheld part of the ultrasound unit that produces the ultrasound waves and receives the echoes.

Ultrasonography—A diagnostic imaging technique that utilizes reflected ultrasonic waves to delineate, examine, or measure internal body tissues or organs.

Ultrasound—Sound above what can be heard by the human ear, generally above 20,000 Hz (cycles per second).

Training

Ultrasound technologists have usually completed a training program in a two-year college or vocational program. A typical course list includes:

- elementary principles of ultrasound
- ultrasound transducers
- pulse-echo principles and instrumentation
- ultrasound image storage and display
- artifacts (erroneous results)
- quality assurance
- bioeffects and safety

The American Registry of Diagnostic Medical Sonographers certifies ultrasound technologists as registered diagnostic medical sonographers (RDMS); registered diagnostic cardiac sonographers (RDCS); registered vascular technologists (RVT); and registered ophthalmic ultrasound biometrists. Specialty areas within these credentials include abdominal sonography, neurosonology, obstetrics and gynecology, and ophthalmology (RDMS); adult and pediatric **echocardiography** (RDCS); and noninvasive vascular technology (RVT).

Resources

BOOKS

Allan, Paul L. et al. *Clinical Doppler Ultrasound*. London: Churchill Livingstone, 2000.

Rumach, Carol M. et al., eds. *Diagnostic Ultrasound*. St. Louis, MO: Mosby, 1998.

Sanders, Roger C. *Clinical Sonography: A Practical Guide*. Boston: Little, Brown and Company, 1998.

Segan, Joseph C., and Joseph Stauffer. *The Patient's Guide to Medical Tests*. New York: Facts On File, Inc., 1998.

PERIODICALS

"Drawing Blood Could Become History with MIT Ultrasound Technique." *MIT News* (February 28, 2000).

Ebenbichler, G.R., et al. "Ultrasound treatment for treating the carpal tunnel syndrome: Randomised 'sham' controlled trial." *British Medical Journal* 316 (March 7, 1998): 731-735.

Galen, Barbara A. "Diagnostic Imaging: An Overview." *Primary Care Practice* 3 (September/October 1999).

ORGANIZATIONS

American Institute of Ultrasound in Medicine, 14750 Sweiter Lane, Suite 100, Laurel, MD 20707-5906. (301) 498-4100 or (800) 638-5352. <http://www.aium.org>.

American Registry of Diagnostic Medical Sonographers (ARDMS), 600 Jefferson Plaza, Suite 360, Rockville, MD 20852-1150. (301) 738-8401 or (800) 541-9754. <http://www.ardms.org>.

OTHER

McCulloch, Joseph, PhD. *Ultrasound in Wound Healing*. <http://www.medicaledu.com/ultrasnd.htm>.

Michelle L. Johnson, M.S., J.D.

Universal precautions

Definition

Universal precautions are safety procedures established by the Centers for Disease Control and Prevention (CDC) and the American Dental Association (ADA).

Purpose

These precautions are used in medical and dental offices to prevent the transmission of infectious diseases to patients and health care workers.

Description

Universal precautions are standards of **infection control** practices designed to reduce the risk of transmission of bloodborne infections.

Personal protective equipment

Protective equipment includes gloves, gowns, masks, and eyewear worn by health care workers to reduce the risk of exposure to potentially infectious materials.

Examination gloves are used for procedures involving contact with mucous membranes. They reduce the incidence of contamination to the hands, but they cannot prevent penetrating injuries from needles or other sharp instruments. Gloves are changed after each patient and discarded, and must never be washed or disinfected for reuse. Washing with surfactants may cause wicking (the enhanced penetration of liquids through undetected holes in the glove). Disinfecting agents may cause deterioration of the gloves. Petroleum jelly may also break down latex. Utility gloves may be used when handling contaminated instruments and cleaning of the treatment area or sterilization room.

Fluid-resistant gowns, laboratory coats, or uniforms should be worn when clothing is likely to be soiled with **blood** or other bodily fluids. Reusable protective clothing should be washed separately from other clothes, using a normal laundry cycle. Protective clothing should be changed daily or as soon as visibly soiled. They should be removed before personnel leave areas of the dental office used for laboratory or patient-care activities.

Masks and protective eyewear, or chin-length, plastic face shields should be worn when splashing or spattering of blood or other body fluids is likely. A mask should be changed between patients or during patient treatment if it becomes wet or moist. A face shield or protective eyewear should be washed with appropriate cleaning agents when visibly soiled.

Careful handling and disposal of sharps

Sharp disposable items, such as needles, saliva ejectors, rubber prophy cups and scalpels that cannot be sterilized and are contaminated with blood or other body fluids need to be discarded in puncture resistant containers. Special delivery companies pick up the containers once they are full and replace them with empty containers.

Careful handling and cleaning of contaminated equipment

Dental instruments must be cleaned and sterilized after each use. Recommended sterilization methods include autoclaving or using a dry heat oven or ''chemiclave,'' a unit that cleans with the use of chemicals. Sterilization equipment is commonly found in a special area of the building away from the treatment areas.

Cleaning and disinfecting of all surfaces such as lights, drawer handles, and countertops is accomplished by a chemical solution formulated to kill infectious **bacteria**, spores, and **viruses** after each patient is seen. Medical facilities follow specific heat sterilization procedures, which are outlined by the CDC. Plastic barriers cover items that are not easily disinfected by chemical spray, such as light handles, chair control buttons, and instrument trays. Many offices and hospitals have seamless floors with linoleum or a laminate surface so that spills can be contained and cleaned quickly.

Non-critical items that cannot be heat sterilized are sterilized by chemical immersion formulated to kill infectious bacteria and viruses.

Universal precautions are intended to supplement rather than replace recommendations for routine **infection** control, such as hand washing.

Preparation

Proper planning and management of supplies needed for universal precautions are essential in reducing the occupational risk of infectious diseases. Such measures should include, but are not limited to:

- risk assessment
- setting of standards and protocols
- risk reduction
- post-exposure measures
- first aid

Complications

Complications include the possible increase of medical and dental fees to the patient to offset costs associated with the equipment, disinfectants, and sterilization procedures needed for universal precautions.

Results

Universal precautions are designed to result in the reduction of the transmission of infectious diseases to patients and health care workers.

Health care team roles

Universal precautions require all medical and dental staff personnel involved in patient care to use appropriate personal protective equipment. Guidelines for health care settings for discarding of waste material are under a separate code by individual state agencies and governmental departments.

The environment in which health care is provided is greatly affected by universal precautions, both for the patient and care providers. Measures that promote a safe work environment include:

- education of employees about occupational risks and methods of prevention of HIV and other infectious diseases
- provision of protective equipment
- provision of appropriate disinfectants to clean up spills of blood or other body fluids
- easy accessibility of puncture-resistant sharps containers
- maintaining appropriate staffing levels
- measures that reduce and prevent **stress**, isolation, and burnout
- controlling shift lengths
- providing post-exposure counseling, treatment, and follow-up

The U.S. Department of Labor Occupational Safety and Health Administration (OSHA) requires employers in the medical and dental fields to make hepatitis B virus (HBV) vaccines available without cost to employees who may be exposed to blood or other infectious materials. In addition, the CDC recommends that all workers be vaccinated against HBV, as well as **influenza**, measles, mumps, rubella, and tetanus, both for the protection of personnel and patients.

Resources

PERIODICALS

OSHA News Release. *Prevention is the Best Medicine.* May 9, 2001. <http://www.osha.gov/media/oshnews/may01/national-20010509.html>.

ORGANIZATIONS

American Dental Association 211 East Chicago Ave., Chicago, IL 60611. (312) 440-2500. <http://www.ada.org>.

Centers for Disease Control and Prevention 1600 Clifton Rd., Atlanta, GA 30333 (404) 639-3311. <http://www.cdc.gov>.

U.S. Department of Labor Occupational Safety and Health Administration (OSHA) 200 Constitution Avenue, N.W., Washington, DC 20210. <http://www.osha.gov>.

World Health Organization (WHO) 20, via Appia, Geneva 27, Switzerland (44) 22 791 4701. <http://www.who.int/>.

OTHER

Laundry. CDC. <http://www.cdc.gov/ncidod/hip/Sterile/laundry.htm>.

Waste Disposal. CDC. <http://www.cdc.gov/ncidod/hip/BLOOD/Waste.htm>.

Universal Precautions. ADA frequently asked questions; <http://ada.org/public/faq/infection.html#precautions>.

Cindy F. Ovard, RDA

Upper GI exam

Definition

An upper GI examination is a fluoroscopic examination (a type of x-ray imaging) of the upper gastrointestinal tract, including the esophagus, **stomach**, and upper **small intestine** (duodenum).

Purpose

An upper GI series is frequently requested when a patient experiences unexplained symptoms of abdominal **pain**, difficulty in swallowing (**dysphagia**), regurgitation, **diarrhea**, or unexplained weight loss. It is used to help diagnose disorders and diseases of, or related to, the upper gastrointestinal tract, including cases of hiatal hernia, diverticula, ulcers, tumors, obstruction, enteritis, gastroesophageal reflux disease, **Crohn's disease**, abdominal pain, and pulmonary aspiration.

Precautions

Because of the risks of radiation exposure to the fetus, pregnant women are advised to avoid this procedure. In addition, children having to undergo this exam must be shielded with lead, when possible. Patients with an obstruction or perforation in their bowel should not ingest barium (a radiopaque substance used to visualize the GI tract) for an upper GI, but may still be able to undergo the procedure if a water-soluble contrast medium is substituted for the barium.

Glucagon, a medication sometimes given prior to an upper GI procedure, may cause nausea and dizziness. It is used to relax the natural movements of the stomach, which will enhance the overall study.

Description

An upper GI series takes place in a hospital or clinic setting and is performed by an x-ray technologist and a radiologist. Before the test begins, the patient is sometimes administered an injection of glucagon, a medication which slows stomach and bowel activity, to allow the radiologist to get a clearer picture of the gastrointestinal tract. In order to further improve the clarity of the upper GI pictures, the patient may be given a cup of fizzing crystals to swallow, which distend the stomach by producing gas.

Once these preparatory steps are complete, the patient stands against an upright x-ray table, and a fluoroscopic screen is placed in front of him. The patient will be asked to drink from a cup of flavored barium sulfate, a thick and chalky-tasting liquid that allows the radiologist to see the digestive tract, while the radiologist views the esophagus, stomach, and duodenum on the fluoroscopic screen. The patient will be asked to change positions frequently in order to coat the entire surface of the gastrointestinal tract with barium, to move overlapping loops of bowel to isolate each segment, and to obtain multiple views of each segment. The technician or radiologist may press on the patient's abdomen in order to spread the barium thought the folds within the lining of the stomach. The x-ray table will also be moved several times throughout the procedure. The radiologist will ask the patient to hold his breath periodically while exposures are being taken. After the radiologist completes his or her portion of the exam, the technologist will take several additional films of the GI tract. The entire procedure takes approximately 30 minutes.

In addition to the standard upper GI series, a doctor may request a detailed small bowel follow-through (SBFT), which is a timed series of films. After the preliminary upper GI series is complete, the patient will be given some additional barium sulfate to drink, and escorted to a waiting area while the barium moves through the small intestines. X rays are taken at 15-minute intervals until the barium reaches the colon (the only way to be sure the terminal ileum is fully seen is to see the colon or ileocecal valve). Then the radiologist will obtain additional views of the terminal ileum (the most distal segment of the small bowel, just before the colon). This procedure can take from one to four hours.

Esophageal radiography, also called a barium esophagram or a barium swallow, is a study of the esophagus only, and is usually performed as part of the upper GI series (though sometimes only a barium swallow is done). It is commonly used to diagnose the cause of difficulty in swallowing (dysphagia) and for detecting hiatal hernia. A barium sulfate liquid and sometimes pieces of food covered in barium are given to the patient to drink and eat while a radiologist examines the swallowing mechanism on a fluoroscopic screen. The test takes approximately 30 minutes.

Preparation

Patients must not eat, drink, or smoke for eight hours prior to undergoing an upper GI examination. Longer dietary restrictions may be required, depending on the type and diagnostic purpose of the test. Patients undergoing a small bowel follow-through exam may be asked to take **laxatives** the day prior to the test. Upper GI patients are required to wear a hospital gown, or similar attire, and to remove all jewelry, so the camera has an unobstructed view of the abdomen.

Aftercare

No special aftercare treatment or regimen is required for an upper GI series. The patient may eat and drink as soon as the test is completed. The barium sulfate may make the patient's stool white for several days, and can cause constipation; therefore patients are encouraged to drink plenty of water in order to eliminate it from their system.

Complications

Because the upper GI series is an x-ray procedure, it does involve minor exposure to ionizing radiation. Unless the patient is pregnant, or multiple radiological or fluoroscopic studies are required, the small dose of radiation incurred during a single procedure poses little risk. However, multiple studies requiring fluoroscopic exposure that are conducted in a short time period have been known, on very rare occasions, to cause skin death (necrosis) in some individuals. This risk can be minimized by careful monitoring and documentation of cumulative radiation doses administered to these patients.

Results

A normal upper GI series shows a healthy, normally functioning, and unobstructed digestive tract. Hiatal hernia, obstructions, inflammation, including ulcers, polyps of the esophagus, stomach, or small intestine, or irregularities in the swallowing mechanism are just a few of the possible abnormalities that may show up on an upper GI series. Additionally, abnormal peristalsis, or digestive movements of the stomach and intestines can often be visualized on the fluoroscopic part of the exam, and in the interpretation of the SBFT.

Health care team roles

The radiologist and technologist are a team, in the compliance and completion of an optimal upper GI study. The well-prepared technologist will promote efficiency of the radiologist's portion of the exam. Having all supplies available and being ready to handle a variety of situations are essential in doing barium studies.

KEY TERMS

Crohn's disease—A chronic, inflammatory bowel disease usually affecting the ileum, the colon, or both.

Diverticula—Pouchline herniations through the muscular wall of an organ such as the stomach, small intestine, or colon.

Enteritis—Inflammation of the mucosal lining of the small intestine.

Gastroesophageal reflux disease—A painful, chronic condition in which stomach acid flows back into the esophagus causing heartburn and, in time, erosion of the lining of esophagus.

Hiatal hernia—Protrusion of the stomach up through the diaphragm.

Patient education

The technologist, and to some degree the radiologist, can ease a patient through this exam by giving the patient a brief overview of what he or she will need to do and what to expect while having this exam. Although the exam is painless and simple, there will still be some concern by the patient who is unfamiliar with the procedure. Keeping the positioning directions simple makes it easy for the patient to comply, and creates for a positive experience for all concerned.

Training

The technologist will have had a minimum of two years training in **radiologic technology**, and extensive experience in barium studies, as this is one area that a student radiographer will show early competence in. The technologist is also fully educated on the anatomy and physiology of the gastrointestinal tract, and must demonstrate this on written exams, as well as a clinical evaluation prior to completing the program.

Resources

BOOKS

Ross, Linda, ed. *Gastrointestinal Diseases and Disorders Sourcebook*, Vol. 16. Detroit: Omnigraphics, 1996.

PERIODICALS

Newman, J. "Radiographic and Endoscopic Evaluation of the Upper GI Tract." *Radiology Technology* 69 (Jan-Feb 1998): 213-26.

Debra Novograd, B.S.,R.T.(R)(M)

Upper limb orthoses

Definition

An orthosis is a device that is applied to the body in order to protect and stabilize body parts, to prevent or correct scarring and deformities, or to aid in performance of certain functions. Upper limb orthoses are applied to the shoulder, elbow, arm, wrist, or hand. These devices may be called orthoses, orthotic devices, or splints.

Purpose

Upper limb orthoses can be used for a wide variety of purposes. Some of the more common uses include:

- stabilizing **fractures** or unstable joints
- immobilizing joints to promote healing
- preventing or correcting joint contractures
- correcting subluxation of joints or improper alignment of tendons
- preventing formation of burn scar tissue
- maintaining correct joint alignment
- assisting movement of joints
- reducing muscle tone in spastic muscles

Description

Materials and construction

Although ready-made orthoses are available for some applications, many are custom made to fit the specific needs of each patient. Orthoses can be constructed of plaster, wood, metal, cloth, or plastic. Since the 1960s, most orthoses have employed lightweight thermoplastic materials, which are plastics that become pliable when they are heated and retain their shape once they cool. They come in sheets of varying thickness, and they can be composed of any of several polymer compounds. The thermoplastic sheets can be molded to fit body parts exactly, and some can be reshaped repeatedly as the treated body part changes shape. The resulting orthotic device is lightweight and relatively easy to use and maintain.

Thermoplastic materials are usually classified into high- and low-temperature types, based on the temperature at which they become pliable. High-temperature thermoplastic materials must be molded at a temperature that is too high to come in contact with human skin. These materials must be molded over a plaster model of the body part, but have the advantage of being stronger and more durable than low-temperature thermoplastics. They are used in situations where the orthosis will undergo a lot of stress or will be used for a long time. High-temperature thermoplastics require special tools for cutting and shaping, and orthoses made from these materials are usually constructed by an orthotist, a technician who specializes in constructing these devices.

Many upper limb orthoses are constructed of low-temperature thermoplastics. This material becomes pliable below 180 °F (80 °C), and it can be molded directly against the body. It is relatively easy to cut and shape, and many therapists construct orthoses using these materials. Precut shells made from low-temperature thermoplastics are also available. The therapist can use a precut thermoplastic shell as the base for a device and then modify it to fit by trimming and adding pads and straps. Orthoses made from low-temperature thermoplastics are commonly used in situations in which the orthosis will receive relatively little stress or is intended for temporary use. These orthoses are especially important when a device is needed quickly, such as in postsurgical or trauma treatment.

Both high- and low-temperature orthoses must be attached to the body. Most modern orthoses use straps made of hook-and-loop tape for this purpose. This material is lightweight, durable, and readily adjustable, and it comes in a variety of widths and colors. Orthoses can also include padding to cushion sensitive areas, as well as specialized linings. Patients often use a separate interface that absorbs perspiration and protects the skin, and which can be washed or replaced as needed.

Types of orthoses

The upper limbs comprise a complex system of muscles, joints, ligaments, and tendons, which are capable of a number of distinct movements. For this reason, a wide variety of upper limb orthoses have come into existence. These devices often go by multiple names, reflecting the name of the manufacturer, the name of the person who developed the device, or the anatomy and function it serves. No single naming system has become dominant. Most authors today refer to the devices in terms of anatomy or function rather than using more obscure historical names, but users must be careful to distinguish one device from another.

Orthoses are usually classified as either static or dynamic, depending on the amount of joint movement each device allows. Static orthoses hold a body part in a fixed position and do not allow joint movement.

Some static orthoses do not contain joints, as with fracture orthoses that stabilize the long bones of the arm after a fracture. Most others simply maintain the joint at a particular angle, providing support and proper positioning. For example, a static wrist orthosis can be used to hold the wrist in a neutral position to promote healing and prevent injury during activities. Sometimes static orthoses include attachments that help patients perform functional activities. For example, a hand-wrist orthosis may include an attachment for pens or eating utensils.

Static orthoses sometimes serve the function of promoting eventual joint movement. Serial or progressive orthoses loosen joints that have become frozen due to contractures or arthritis. Serial orthoses involve several similar devices used in a series, with each successive device gradually increasing the range of motion of the affected joint by providing a gentle stretching action. Progressive orthoses accomplish similar goals, but do so by allowing adjustments in the device so that it gradually increases the amount of stretch created in the joint. Serial and progressive orthoses must be designed and used carefully to provide the correct amount of stretching in the joint. Excessive stretching can damage the tissues, and inadequate stretching will be ineffective.

Dynamic orthoses allow or create joint movement. These devices hold the joint in the proper position while assisting movement using springs, rubber bands, or other mechanical features. Dynamic orthoses are useful for patients who have weakened muscles or limited neuromuscular control, because they allow the patient to perform actions that would be difficult or impossible without assistance. These devices promote independence in patients who have handicapping conditions, and they are common in rehabilitation settings. Since no single device can perform all the movements that the human hand can perform, the patient may need to use several different dynamic devices in order to carry out activities of daily living.

Operation

Although there is a wide variety of upper limb orthoses, most of these devices operate on similar principles. The general goal of most orthoses is to provide stability and support while allowing as much motion as possible. Immobilizing joints for long periods has proven deleterious for most patients. Muscles atrophy, joints stiffen, skin tightens, and the healing process is ultimately slowed. By allowing movement while restricting motion that would create stress on joints, muscles, or tendons, orthotic devices allow healing and preserve range of motion and function.

Exact fit is a key element for many upper limb orthoses. In order to work properly, the orthosis must hold the body part in an exact position. If the orthosis does not fit exactly, it may not work and could actually cause harm. This can become a problem in situations where the patient has experienced swelling and may require a new fitting for the orthosis once the swelling has resolved. Poor fit can also lead to discomfort and the development of pressure sores.

Dynamic orthoses usually operate with the aid of attached outriggers. These provide a place to attach rubber bands, springs, or other materials that assist motion. They also provide leverage and help to ensure that the joint stays in proper position during movement. These devices require exact fit, as well as adjustment to ensure that the device works properly.

Many upper limb orthoses require a period of training for the patient to learn how to use the device properly. This is especially true with devices that assist motion, because the patient must initiate the motion properly in order for the orthosis to work. Patients with a long history of **paralysis** or immobilization may require considerable time in order to learn how to use the device.

It is very important to consider the patient's motivation and attitude toward the orthosis as part of the treatment plan. Since most upper limb orthoses are removable, patients can choose whether or not to use these devices. Patients may object to orthoses because of discomfort, unattractive appearance, or restrictiveness of the device. Health care professionals must work closely with the patient to ensure that the patient will accept the orthosis and use it properly.

Maintenance

Many upper limb orthoses require little or no maintenance. This is especially true for static orthoses and for those intended for temporary use. The plastic shell can be wiped clean, and materials worn underneath the orthosis can be washed or replaced. The patient may need to be checked periodically to ensure that the orthosis fits. Dynamic orthoses may require adjustments and replacement of worn springs, rubber bands, and the like.

Health care team roles

Creating and employing upper limb orthoses often involves a team approach, especially in rehabilitation settings. A physician who specializes in physical

medicine and rehabilitation may prescribe the orthosis, which is then built by an orthotist. An occupational therapist or physical therapist may help the patient learn to use the orthosis. In other instances, the physician may refer the patient to an occupational therapist, who then determines that an orthosis would be helpful. Many occupational therapists design and build orthoses themselves, but they may also recommend ready-made devices or refer the patient to an orthotist. Physicians from other disciplines, especially orthopedics, may employ orthoses, as do physical therapists. These professionals may refer the patient for a custom-made device or prescribe a ready-made one.

Training

Health care professionals who create and fit upper limb orthoses must have a good understanding of the anatomy and physiology of the upper limbs. They must also understand the mechanics and forces involved in making various body movements, and they must be familiar with the materials and tools involved in constructing orthoses. Certified orthotists are specialists who focus exclusively on fitting and building orthoses. Certification as an orthotist requires a baccalaureate degree in the field of orthotics and **prosthetics**, or a degree in another field followed by a six-month to one-year certificate training program. Orthotists must also pass a certification exam.

Resources

BOOKS

Lunsford, Tom. "Upper-Limb Orthoses." In *Physical Medicine and Rehabilitation: The Complete Approach,* edited by Martin Grabois, Susan J. Garrison, Karen A. Hart, and L. Don Lehmkuhl. Malden, Massachusetts: Blackwell Science, 2000, pp. 530-543.

McKee, Pat, and Leanne Morgan. *Orthotics in Rehabilitation: Splinting the Hand and Body.* Philadelphia: F.A.Davis, 1998.

Redford, John B., John V. Basmajian, and Paul Trautman. *Orthotics: Clinical Practice and Rehabilitation Technology.* New York: Churchill Livingstone, 1995.

PERIODICALS

Schutt, Ann H. "Upper extremity and Hand Orthotics," *Physical Medicine and Rehabilitation Clinics of North America* 3 (1992): 223-241.

ORGANIZATIONS

American Academy of Orthotists and Prosthetists. 526 King St., Ste. 201, Alexandria, VA 22314. (703) 836-0788. <http://www.oandp.org>.

National Rehabilitation Information Center. 1010 Wayne Ave., Ste. 800, Silver Spring, MD 20910. (800) 346-2742. <http://www.naric.com>.

OTHER

Grant, Dorothy. "Orthotist and Prosthetist." *American Medical Association Website* 2001. <http://www. ama-assn.org/ama/pub/category/4356.html> (June 11, 2001).

Denise L. Schmutte, Ph.D.

Upper limb prostheses

Definition

A prosthesis is an artificial device that substitutes for a missing part of the body. Upper limb prostheses can be applied anywhere from the shoulder joint through the fingers, including the fingers, the hand, the wrist, the forearm, the elbow, the upper arm, and the shoulder.

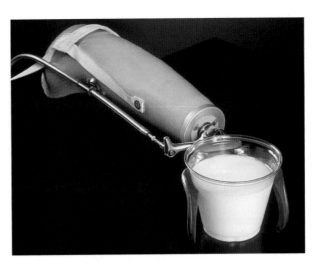

Individuals who have lost an upper limb can relearn basic functions with the help of arm and hand prostheses. *(SIU BioMed/Custom Medical Stock Photo. Reproduced by permission.)*

Purpose

Most patients require prostheses as the result of amputation. The affected body part must be removed due to severe damage or disease that threatens the patient's survival or is too damaged to be repaired. Amputations of upper limbs are usually due to accidents, particularly in industrial settings. Victims tend to be younger and in good health otherwise, and often have a normal life expectancy. It is particularly important for them to regain substantial upper-limb function to maintain independence. Upper limb prostheses are also important for those who are missing upper limbs due to congenital conditions. This group includes children, who may use prostheses from very early in life and require regular refitting and revision of their prostheses as they grow.

Patients use upper limb prostheses for two general purposes: to improve their appearance and to increase their ability to perform tasks. Unfortunately, these two purposes often conflict with one another. Prostheses that look like normal hands are often limited in their functionality, while highly functional devices may look unattractive. Many patients use two different prostheses: one for situations in which appearance is most important, and another for situations in which adequate function is desired.

The most important goal for function-oriented upper limb prostheses is reproducing actions performed by the hands. The human hand is capable of many distinct and complex actions, which are often crucial for independent functioning. The patient must be able to grasp and manipulate objects of varying sizes and shapes in order to carry out basic activities such as dressing, grooming, and eating, as well as work-related activities. Most prosthetic devices can perform only one or two distinct actions, and so a large number of specialized prostheses have come into being, each designed for a particular purpose. These include devices designed for particular work functions, such as using tools, and also devices intended for leisure activities, such as holding a golf club or throwing a bowling ball. New developments in the field of **prosthetics** are raising hopes for a "bionic hand" that is capable of multiple actions, but devices of this type are still experimental.

Description

Materials and construction

Upper limb prostheses can be constructed of a variety of materials, depending on the purpose of the prosthesis. Prostheses used for cosmetic purposes are usually constructed of lightweight plastics, and are designed to match the color and shape of the patient's intact hand. Prostheses used to perform work usually need to be much more durable. These devices usually include components made out of different materials, such as soft plastic or silicon for the socket that fits the device to the patient's body, hardened plastic or wood for the body of the device, and metal for joints and the functional tool at the end of the prosthesis.

Prostheses can be classified as endoskeletal or exoskeletal. Endoskeletal prostheses consist of a hard inner core covered by a soft outer material. These devices tend to be lightweight, but they are usually less durable than exoskeletal prostheses. Cosmetic prostheses are often constructed with an endoskeletal design. Exoskeletal prostheses have a hard outer shell, which can usually withstand considerable force. Exoskeletal designs are usually preferred for prostheses designed to perform work.

Amputations are usually classified according to the point at which the limb is removed. In general, amputations below the elbow require simpler devices than those that occur above the elbow, because above-the-elbow prostheses require some sort of substitute for the elbow joint. Amputations at or above the shoulder joint add yet another level of complexity to the prosthesis.

TERMINAL DEVICES. Virtually all upper limb prostheses involve some sort of terminal device, which is the most distal part (farthest from the patient's trunk). The simplest terminal devices include a hook, a cosmetic hand, or some other element that has no moving parts, and are referred to as passive terminal devices.

Active terminal devices, which involve moving parts, are much more common. These devices can be shaped like a hook, a hand, or any specialized tool. They often involve one stationary part and one moving part. The patient controls the moving part using a body control device or a myoelectric control, allowing the patient to grasp things between the stationary part and the moveable part. Some devices allow the patient to have voluntary control over closing the device, while others allow voluntary control over opening the device. Patients are able to perform a variety of work-related and self-care activities using these devices.

CONTROLS. The most common control system is the body-powered or mechanical system. With this system, the user operates the terminal device by flexing a muscle near the stump of the amputated limb. The energy from the user's movement is transferred to the prosthesis by means of a stainless steel cable. Body-powered prostheses are popular and are used by about 90 percent of amputees who use a prosthesis. These devices are simple, durable, and easy to use. These systems are also preferred because they provide some feedback to the user, who can detect the action of the terminal device through the cable.

An alternative control system involves myoelectric control of the terminal device. Myoelectric devices detect the electrical potential of contracting muscles and use the potential to control an electric motor that operates the terminal device. Myoelectric devices allow a stronger grip than body-powered devices, and they also provide the ability to regulate the amount of force in the grip. Despite these advantages, myoelectric systems are less popular than body-powered systems. They are expensive, they break down more easily, and they force the user to rely on battery power. These systems also provide less feedback to the user, who must rely on **vision** to regulate his or her activity. Technological improvements are making these devices more reliable, and they may become more popular in the future. Some devices combine myoelectric controls for the terminal device with body-powered controls for the elbow joint.

SOCKETS AND HARNESSES. The fit between the prosthesis and the body is an important element in assuring that the prosthesis is comfortable and functional. Most upper limb prostheses have a pliable socket that is custom molded over the stump to assure an exact fit. Many above-the-elbow systems depend on a harness to hold the prosthesis in place and provide an attachment point for control devices. Harnesses are usually made of Dacron straps that fit over the shoulders or around the upper arm. Some upper limb prostheses can be attached without a harness.

Operation

Fitting

Prompt fitting is very important. Research has shown that patients are more likely to reject an upper limb prosthesis if it is fitted more than 30 days after amputation surgery. Early fitting also helps control swelling and **pain** in the stump. If the patient's surgeon feels it is appropriate, the mold for a temporary prosthesis can be made immediately after surgery. The patient can begin adjusting to the prosthesis and can begin to make decisions about the features he or she wants in a permanent device. The patient may wear the temporary prosthesis for several weeks while the size and shape of the stump are stabilizing.

Patient adaptation

Patients require considerable time and training in order to accept and use upper limb prostheses. They must learn to detect and control fairly subtle movements in or near the stump in order to control the prosthesis. They must also learn how to care for the stump and how to prevent pressure sores. Finally, they must adjust to the changes in their lives brought about by the loss of an upper limb. Training usually takes place over the course of several weeks, during which the patient increases wearing time and begins to use the prosthesis for functional activities. The training and adjustment period can be lengthy, and it is important for the patient to have a continuing relationship with supportive therapists.

Use

Patients can use upper limb prostheses to perform a variety of functions, but motivation is often a limiting factor. The biggest obstacle to using the prosthesis may be the patient's reliance on the intact hand. If the patient becomes used to doing things with one hand, it will be much more difficult to adjust to using a prosthesis. Patients who refuse an upper limb prosthesis may eventually suffer from overuse injuries in the intact limb. Patients with bilateral amputations are forced to rely on prostheses in order to perform the functions of daily living, and tend to accept the prostheses readily, since they are a means of restoring function.

Maintenance

The maintenance needs for upper limb prostheses vary with the complexity of the device. Devices that incorporate electric motors require regular battery changes and tend to need more maintenance than

---

> ## KEY TERMS
>
> **Body-powered prosthesis**—A prosthesis that is controlled by mechanical action. The user flexes a muscle and the energy from this action is transferred to the prosthesis by means of a cable.
>
> **Endoskeletal prosthesis**—A prosthesis that is constructed with a hard core and a soft outer covering.
>
> **Exoskeletal prosthesis**—A prosthesis that is constructed with a hard outer layer.
>
> **Myoelectric prosthesis**—A prosthesis that is controlled by electrical impulses. The patient flexes a muscle and the electrical potential of the activity is used to control an electric motor that operates the prosthesis.
>
> **Prosthetist**—A technician who specializes in the fitting and building of prosthetic devices.
>
> **Terminal device**—A device attached to the distal end of a prosthesis. The patient uses the terminal device to perform functional activities.

body powered or passive devices. Cosmetic gloves that are used to make the prosthesis look more like a hand also require maintenance. The gloves can become stained or torn and may need frequent cleaning and replacement. Patients also need periodic adjustments to their prostheses to ensure that they work and fit properly.

Health care team roles

The process of creating and employing upper limb prostheses involves several health care professionals. Physicians who specialize in physical medicine and rehabilitation usually prescribe the prostheses, and patients learn to use the devices in a rehabilitation setting. Prostheses are fitted and custom-built by prosthetists, who are specially trained technicians in this field. Occupational therapists help patients learn to perform adaptive tasks using the prostheses. Patients tend to respond best when the professionals involved work as a team and provide the patients with ongoing support.

Training

Prosthetics is a specialized field with a complex body of knowledge. Certification as a prosthetist requires a baccalaureate degree in the field of orthotics and prosthetics, or a degree in another field, followed by a six-month to one-year certificate training program. Prosthetists must also pass a certification exam, and may require additional certification in order to fit certain specialized devices.

Resources

BOOKS

Murdoch, George, and A. Bennett Wilson, Jr. *A Primer on Amputations and Artificial Limbs.* Springfield, Illinois: Charles C. Thomas, 1998.

Spires, M. Catherine, Linda Miner, and Miles O. Colwell. "Upper-Extremity Amputation and Prosthetic Rehabilitation." In *Physical Medicine and Rehabilitation: The Complete Approach,* edited by Martin Grabois, Susan J. Garrison, Karen A. Hart, and L. Don Lehmkuhl. Malden, Massachusetts: Blackwell Science, 2000, pp. 549-582.

PERIODICALS

Fillon, Mike. "The New Bionic Man." *Popular Mechanics* 176 (February, 1999):50.

Uellendahl, Jack E. "Upper Extremity Myoelectric Prosthetics." *Physical Medicine and Rehabilitation Clinics of North America* 11 (August, 2000): 639-652.

ORGANIZATIONS

American Academy of Orthotists and Prosthetists. 526 King St., Ste. 201, Alexandria, VA 22314. (703) 836-0788. <http://www.oandp.org>.

National Rehabilitation Information Center. 1010 Wayne Ave., Ste. 800, Silver Spring, MD 20910. (800) 346-2742. <http://www.naric.com>.

OTHER

Grant, Dorothy. "Orthotist and Prosthetist." *American Medical Association Website* 2001. <http://www.ama-assn.org/ama/pub/category/4356.html> (June 11, 2001).

Denise L. Schmutte, Ph.D.

Upper respiratory infection *see* **Common cold**

Uric acid tests *see* **Kidney function tests**

Urinalysis

Definition

A urinalysis is a group of manual and/or automated qualitative and semi-quantitative tests performed on a urine sample. A routine urinalysis usually includes the following tests: color, transparency, specific gravity, pH, protein, glucose, ketones, **blood**, bilirubin, nitrite,

---

Common drugs that may affect urine color

Generic and brand names	Urine color
Anisindione (Miradon)	Red-orange in alkaline urine
Cascara sagrada	Red in alkaline urine; yellow-brown in acid urine
Chloroquine (Aralen)	Rusty yellow or brown
Chlorzozazone (Paraflex)	Orange or purple-red
Docusate calcium (Doxidan, Surfak)	Pink to red to red-brown
Furazolidone (Furoxone)	Brown
Iron preparations (Ferotran, Imferon)	Dark brown or black on standing
Levodopa	Dark brown on standing
Methylene blue (Urolene Blue)	Blue-green
Nitrofurantoin (Macrodantin, Nitrodan)	Brown
Phenazopyridine (Pyridium)	Orange to red
Phenindione (Eridione)	Red–orange in alkaline urine
Phenolphthalein (Ex-Lax)	Red or purplish pink in alkaline urine
Phenothiazines (e.g., prochlorperazine [Compazine])	Red-brown
Phenytoin (Dilantin)	Pink, red, red-brown
Riboflavin (vitamin B)	Intense yellow
Rifampin	Red-orange
Sulfasalazine (Azulfidine)	Orange-yellow in alkaline urine
Triamterene (Dyrenium)	Pale blue fluorescence

SOURCE: Pagana, K.D. and T.J. Pagana. *Mosby's Diagnostic and Laboratory Test Reference.* 3rd ed. St. Louis: Mosby, 1997.

---

urobilinogen, and leukocyte esterase. Some laboratories include a microscopic examination of urinary sediment with all routine urinalysis tests. If not, it is customary to perform the microscopic exam, if transparency, glucose, protein, blood, nitrite, or leukocyte esterase is abnormal.

Purpose

Routine urinalysis is performed for several reasons:

- general health screening to detect renal and metabolic diseases

- diagnosis of diseases or disorders of the **kidneys** or urinary tract

- monitoring of patients with diabetes

In addition, quantitative urinalysis tests may be performed for diagnosis of many specific disorders, such as endocrine diseases, bladder **cancer, osteoporosis**, and phorphyrias. This often requires the use of a timed urine sample. Examples include the d-xylose absorption test for malabsorption, creatinine clearance test for glomerular function, the 24-hour urinary metanephrine test for pheochromocytoma, and the microalbumin test. The urinary microalbumin test measures the rate of albumin excretion in the urine using immunoassay. This test is used to monitor the renal vascular function of persons with **diabetes mellitus**. In diabetics, the excretion of greater than 200 μg/mL albumin is predictive of impending glomerular disease.

Precautions

Voided specimens

All patients should avoid intense athletic training or heavy physical work before the test, as these activities may cause small amounts of blood to appear in the urine. Many urinary constituents are labile, and samples should be tested within one hour of collection or refrigerated. Samples may be stored at 36-46 °F (2-8°C) for up to 24 hours for chemical urinalysis tests; however, the microscopic exam should be performed within four hours, if possible. To minimize sample contamination, women who require a urinalysis during menstruation should insert a fresh tampon before providing a urine sample.

Over two-dozen drugs are known to interfere with various chemical urinalysis tests. These include:

- ascorbic acid
- chlorpromazine
- L-dopa
- nitrofurantoin (Macrodantin, Furadantin)
- penicillin
- phenazopyridine (Pyridium)
- rifampin (Rifadin)
- tolbutamide

Preservatives used to prevent loss of glucose and cells may affect biochemical test results. The use of preservatives should be avoided whenever possible.

Description

Routine urinalysis consists of three testing groups, physical characteristics, biochemical tests, and microscopic evaluation.

Physical tests

Physical tests are color, transparency (clarity), and specific gravity. In some cases, volume (daily output) may be measured. Color and transparency are determined from visual observation.

COLOR. Normal urine is straw to amber in color. Abnormal colors include bright yellow, brown, black (gray), red, and green. These pigments may result from medications, dietary sources, or diseases. For example, red urine may be caused by blood or hemoglobin, beets, medications, and some **porphyrias**. Black-gray urine may result from melanin (melanoma) or homogentisic acid (alkaptonuria). Bright yellow urine may be caused by bilirubin. Green urine may be caused by biliverdin or medications. Orange urine may be caused by some medications or excessive urobilinogen. Brown urine may be caused by excessive amounts of prophobilin, or urobilin.

TRANSPARENCY. Normal urine is transparent. Cloudy or turbid urine may be caused by both normal or abnormal processes. Normal conditions giving rise to turbid urine include precipitation of crystals (usually urates or phosphates), mucus, or vaginal discharge. Abnormal causes of turbidity include the presence of blood cells, yeast, and **bacteria**. Turbidity is typically graded by visual comparison to standard solutions of barium sulfate.

SPECIFIC GRAVITY. The specific gravity of urine is a measure of the concentration of dissolved solutes, and it reflects the ability of the renal tubules to concentrate the urine (conserve water). It is usually measured by determining the refractive index of a urine sample (refractometry) or by chemical analysis. Specific gravity varies with fluid and solute intake. It will be increased (above 1.035) in persons with diabetes mellitus and persons taking large amounts of medication. It will also be increased after radiologic studies of the kidney owing to the excretion of x-ray contrast dye. Consistently low specific gravity (1.003 or less) is seen in persons with diabetes insipidus. In renal failure, the specific gravity remains equal to that of the plasma (1.008-1.010) regardless of changes in salt and water intake. Urine volume below 400 mL per day is termed oliguria, and may occur in persons who are dehydrated and those with glomerular disease owing to reduced glomerular filtration. Volume in excess of 2 liters per day is termed polyuria and is common in persons with diabetes mellitus and diabetes insipidus.

Biochemical tests

Biochemical testing of urine is performed using dry reagent strips, often called dipsticks. A urine dipstick consists of a white plastic strip with absorbent microfiber cellulose pads attached to it. Each pad contains dried reagents needed for a specific test.

When performing dry reagent strip testing, health professionals should adhere strictly to the manufacturer's instructions. General instructions for performing the test manually are as follows:

- Mix the sample by inverting the container several times.

- Insert the reactive portion of the dipstick, completely, but briefly.

- Remove the dipstick from the container by sliding the back of the dipstick along the rim to remove excess urine.

- Adhere to the reaction time stated on the package insert; and note that not all the tests are to be read at the same time.

- Compare the color of the test areas on the dipstick with the color chart on the bottle label by holding the strip close to the color blocks.

- Record the results for each test using the concentration given by the closest color match.

A dry reagent strip reader may be used as an alternative to visual comparison of color reactions. This device consists of a special colorimeter that measures the optical density of each reagent pad by reflectance. All reactions are read at the precise timed interval, resulting in greater precision than visual interpretation of color intensity.

Additional tests are available to measure bilirubin, protein, glucose, ketones, and urobilinogen in urine. In general, these individual tests provide greater sensitivity, and therefore, permit detection of a lower concentration of the respective substance. A brief description of the most commonly used dry reagent strip tests follows.

1. pH: A combination of pH indicators (methyl red and bromthymol blue) react with hydrogen ions (H^+) to produce a color change over a pH range of 5.0 to 8.5. pH is useful in determining metabolic or respiratory disturbances in acid-base balance. For example, kidney disease often results in retention of H^+ (reduced acid excretion). pH varies with a person's diet, tending to be acidic in those who eat meat but more alkaline in vegetarians. It is also useful for the classification of urine crystals. Crystals commonly found in acid urine are uric acid, urate, and oxalate, while those commonly found in alkaline urine include phosphates and carbonates.

2. Protein: Based upon a phenomenon called the "protein error of indicators," this test uses a pH indicator, such as tetrabromphenol blue, that changes color (at constant pH) when albumin is present in the urine. The protein affects the ionization constant (pKa) of the dye, making it behave as if it were exposed to a more alkaline solution. The test for protein is far more sensitive to albumin than to globulins. Albumin is important in determining the presence of glomerular damage. The glomerulus is the network of capillaries that filters low molecular weight solutes such as urea, glucose, and salts, but normally prevents passage of protein or cells from blood into filtrate. Albuminuria occurs when the glomerular membrane is damaged, a condition called glomerulonephritis.

3. Glucose: Glucose is measured by the glucose oxidase reaction. Glucose oxidase catalyzes the oxidation of glucose by oxygen. This produces hydrogen peroxide and gluconic acid. The peroxide reacts with potassium iodide or another chromogen, producing iodine or other colored product. The glucose test is used to monitor persons with diabetes. When blood glucose levels rise above 160 mg/dL, glucose will be detected in urine. Consequently, glycosuria may be the first indicator that diabetes or another hyperglycemic condition is present. **Copper** sulfate tests should not be used to test urine for glucose because the reagent reacts with many nonglucose-reducing substances. The copper sulfate test may be used to screen newborns for galactosuria and other disorders of carbohydrate **metabolism** that cause urinary excretion of a sugar other than glucose.

4. Ketones: At alkaline pH, sodium nitroprusside or ferricyanide forms a violet-colored complex with acetoacetic acid and acetone. These ketones are produced in excess in disorders of carbohydrate metabolism, especially Type 1 diabetes mellitus. In diabetes, excess ketoacids in the blood may cause life-threatening acidosis and **coma**. These ketoacids and their salts spill into the urine causing ketonuria. Ketones are also found in the urine in several other conditions including **fever**, **pregnancy**, glycogen storage diseases, and in persons on a carbohydrate restricted diet.

5. Blood: Hemoglobin (also myoglobin) is capable of catalyzing the reduction of hydrogen peroxide. In the presence of hemoglobin, hydrogen peroxide will oxidize a dye such as benzidine to form a colored product. Red cells and hemoglobin may enter the urine from the kidney or lower urinary tract. This test detects abnormal levels of either, which may be caused by excessive red cell destruction, glomerular disease, kidney or urinary tract **infection**, malignancy, or urinary tract injury.

6. Bilirubin: Bilirubin is a breakdown product of hemoglobin. Most of the bilirubin produced is conjugated by the **liver** and excreted into the bile, but a very small amount of conjugated bilirubin is reabsorbed by the portal circulation and reaches the

general circulation to be excreted in the urine. Normally, the level of urinary bilirubin is below the detection limit of the test. Bilirubin reacts with a diazonium salt to form azobilirubin, which is violet. Bilirubin in the urine is derived from the liver, and a positive test indicates hepatic disease or hepatobiliary obstruction.

7. Specific gravity: Solutes in the urine promote ionization of malic acid bound to a polyelectrolyte. As the malic acid residues ionize, H^+ is released; this changes the color of a pH indicator, bromthymol blue. High ionic strength causes the indicator to behave as if the solution were more acidic, and the indicator becomes green. Specific gravity is a measure of the concentrating ability of the kidneys.

8. Nitrite: Some bacteria including the lactose positive *Enterobactericeae, Staphylococcus, Proteus, Salmonella,* and *Psuedomonas* are able to reduce nitrate in urine to nitrite. A positive test for nitrite indicates bacteruria. Nitrite reacts with p-arsenilic acid or sulfanilamide to form a diazonium compound. The diazo group reacts with a quinoline dye to form a red product.

9. Urobilinogen: Urobilinogen reacts with p-dimethylaminobenzaldehyde (Ehrlich's reagent) or methoxybenzene-diazonium tetrafluoroborate at an acid pH to form a red or orange color. Urobilinogen is formed in the gastrointestinal tract by the bacterial reduction of conjugated bilirubin. Increased urinary urobilinogen occurs in prehepatic **jaundice** (hemolytic anemia), hepatitis, and other forms of hepatic necrosis that impair the enterohepatic circulation. The test is helpful in differentiating these conditions from obstructive jaundice which results in decreased production of urobilinogen. The Watson-Schwartz test is used to confirm the presence of urobilinogen or differentiate between urobilinogen and porphobilinogen. This is a quantitative test using Ehrlich's reagent and a timed urine sample. Urobilinogen is differentiated from porphobilinogen based upon its solubility in chloroform.

10. Leukocytes: Nonspecific esterases in polymorphonuclear white blood cells (neutrophils) will hydrolyze a pyrole ester of alanine or indoxycarbonic acid to form a pyrole alcohol. The product reacts with a diazonium compound forming a purple azo complex. The presence of white blood cells in the urine usually signifies a urinary tract infection, such as cystitis, or renal disease, such as pyelonehritis or glomerulonephritis.

Microscopic examination

The urine may contain cells that originated in the blood, the kidney, and lower urinary tract, and the microscopic examination of urinary sediment can provide valuable clues regarding many diseases and disorders involving these systems. The microscopic exam is performed after concentrating a 12 mL volume of urine by centrifugation. The supernatant is poured off and the sediment resuspended in a small volume of residual supernatant. A drop of the sediment is placed on a glass slide and a cover glass is applied. Alternatively, a special centrifuge tube and plastic slide may be used to achieve uniform concentration and chamber depth. The sediment is examined under low power for casts, crystals, and mucus threads. Casts are deposits of gelled protein that form in the renal tubules and are washed into the filtrate over time. The number and type of casts per low power field is recorded, and the amount and type of crystals and mucus are graded semi-quantitatively. The magnification is increased to high power (400 x) in order to count the number of red blood cells, white blood cells, and epithelial cells per field. Bacteria, yeast, and trichomonads are identified at high power, and are reported in semi-quantitative terms (e.g., small, moderate, large).

The presence of bacteria or yeast and white blood cells differentiates a urinary tract infection from possible contamination in which case the WBCs are not seen. The presence of cellular casts (casts containing RBCs, WBCs, or epithelial cells) identifies the kidneys (versus the lower urinary tract) as the source of such cells. Cellular casts and renal epithelial cells signify the presence of renal disease. The microscopic exam also identifies both normal and abnormal crystals in the sediment. Abnormal crystals are those formed as a result of an abnormal metabolic process and are always clinically significant. These include bilirubin, cystine, tyrosine, leucine, and cholesterol crystals. Normal crystals are formed from normal metabolic processes, but may be implicated in formation of urinary tract stones (calculi).

Routine urinalysis including microscopic exam may be fully automated using the Yellow Iris workstation. This instrument uses a dry reagent strip reader, harmonic oscillation (for specific gravity), and flow-focused image analysis to perform all of the steps of the urinalysis.

Preparation

A urine sample is collected in an unused disposable plastic cup with a tight-fitting lid. A randomly voided sample is suitable for routine urinalysis although the first-voided morning urine is most concentrated and therefore, preferred. The best sample is one collected in a sterile container after the external genitalia have been cleansed using the midstream void (clean-catch) method. This sample may be cultured, if findings indicate bacteriuria.

- Females should use a clean cotton ball moistened with lukewarm water (or antiseptic wipes provided with collection kits) to cleanse the external genital area, before collecting a urine sample. To prevent contamination with menstrual blood, vaginal discharge, or germs from the external genitalia, they should release some urine before beginning to collect the sample. A urine specimen obtained this way is called a midstream or clean-catch sample.

- Males should use a piece of clean cotton, moistened with lukewarm water or antiseptic wipes to cleanse the head of the penis and the urethral meatus. They should draw back the foreskin, if not circumcised. After the area has been thoroughly cleansed, they should use the midstream void method to collect the sample.

- For infants, a parent or health care worker should cleanse the child's outer genitalia and surrounding skin. A sterile collection bag should be attached to the child's genital area and left in place until the child has urinated. It is important to not touch the inside of the bag, and to remove it as soon as a specimen has been obtained.

Urine samples can also be obtained via bladder catheterization, a procedure used to collect uncontaminated urine when the patient cannot void. A catheter is a thin flexible tube that a health care professional inserts through the urethra into the bladder to allow urine to flow out. To minimize the risk of infecting the patient's bladder with bacteria, many clinicians use a Robinson catheter, which is a plain rubber or latex tube that is removed as soon as the specimen is collected. If urine for culture is to be collected from an indwelling catheter, it should be aspirated from the line using a syringe and not removed from the bag in order to avoid contamination by urethral flora.

Suprapubic bladder aspiration is a collection technique sometimes used to obtain urine from infants younger than six months or urine directly from the bladder for culture. The doctor withdraws urine from the bladder into a syringe through a needle inserted through the skin.

Aftercare

The patient may return to normal activities after collecting the sample and may start taking medications that were discontinued before the test.

KEY TERMS

Acidosis—A condition of the blood in which bicarbonate levels are below normal.

Alkalosis—A condition of the blood and other body fluids in which bicarbonate levels are higher than normal.

Cast—An insoluble gelled protein matrix that takes up the form of the renal tubule in which it deposited. Casts are washed out by normal urine flow.

Catheter—A thin flexible tube inserted through the urethra into the bladder to allow urine to flow out.

Clean-catch specimen—A urine specimen that is collected from the middle of the urine stream after the first part of the flow has been discarded.

Cystine—An amino acid normally reabsorbed by the kidney tubules. Cystinuria is an inherited disease in which the reabsorption of cystine and some other amino acids is defective. Cystine crystals form in the kidney leading to obstructive renal failure.

Ketones—Substances produced during the breakdown of fatty acids. They are produced in excessive amounts in diabetes and certain other abnormal conditions.

pH—A chemical symbol used to describe the acidity or alkalinity of a fluid, ranging from 1 (more acid) to 14 (more alkaline).

Porphobilinogen—An intermediary product in the biosynthesis of heme.

Urethra—The tube that carries urine from the bladder to the outside of the body.

Urinalysis (plural, urinalyses)—The diagnostic testing of a urine sample.

Voiding—Another word for emptying the bladder or urinating.

Complications

There are no risks associated with voided specimens. The risk of bladder infection from catheterization with a Robinson catheter is about 3%.

Results

Normal urine is a clear straw-colored liquid, but may also be slightly hazy. It has a slight odor and some laboratories will note strong or atypical odors on the urinalysis report. It may contain some normal crystals, squamous or transitional epithelial cells from the bladder, lower urinary tract, or vagina. Urine may contain transparent (hyaline) casts especially if collected after vigorous **exercise**. However, the presence of hyaline casts may signify renal disease when the cause cannot be attributed to exercise, running, or medications. Normal urine contains a small amount of urobilinogen, and may contain a few RBCs and WBCs. Normal urine does *not* contain detectable glucose or other sugars, protein, ketones, bilirubin, bacteria, yeast cells, or trichomonads. Normal values representative of many laboratories are given below.

- Glucose: negative (quantitative less than 130 mg/day or 30 mg/dL).
- Bilirubin: negative (quantitative less than 0.02 mg/dL).
- Ketones: negative (quantitative 0.5-3.0 mg/dL).
- pH: 5.0-8.0.
- Protein: negative (Quantitative 15-150 mg/day, less than 10 mg/dL).
- Blood: negative.
- Nitrite: negative.
- Specific gravity: 1.015-1.025.
- Urobilinogen: 0-2 Ehrlich units (quantitative 0.3-1.0 Ehrlich units).
- Leukocyte esterase: negative.
- Red blood cells: 0-2 per high power field.
- White blood cells: 0-5 per high power field (0-10 per high power field for some standardized systems).

Health care team roles

Doctors, nurses, or laboratory scientists may provide the patient with instructions for sample collection. Laboratory scientists most often perform the tests, though in a physician's office, the doctor, nurse, or physician assistant may perform the visual examination of the sample and the dipstick test.

Resources

BOOKS

Chernecky, Cynthia C, and Berger, Barbara J. *Laboratory Tests and Diagnostic Procedures*. 3rd ed. Philadelphia, PA: W. B. Saunders Company, 2001.

Kee, Joyce LeFever. *Handbook of Laboratory and Diagnostic Tests*, 4th ed. Upper Saddle River, NJ: Prentice Hall, 2001.

PERIODICALS

Gantzer, Mary Lou. "The Value of Urinalysis: An Old Method Continues to Prove Its Worth." *Clinical Laboratory News* (1998).

ORGANIZATIONS

American Association of Kidney Patients. 100 S. Ashley Drive, Suite 280, Tampa, FL 33260. (800)749-2257.

American Kidney Fund. 6110 Executive Blvd., Suite 1010, Rockville, MD 20852. (301)881-3052. <http://www.arbon.com/kidney>.

National Kidney and Urologic Diseases Information Clearinghouse. 3 Information Way, Bethesda, MD 20892-3580.

OTHER

ARUP Laboratories. <http://www.arup-lab.com/>.

The University of Iowa. Virtual Hospital. <http://secundus. vh.org/Providers/CME/CLIA/UrineAnalysis/ UrineAnalysis.html> (July 20, 1999).

Victoria E. DeMoranville

Urinary catheterization, female *see* **Catheterization, female**

Urinary catheterization, male *see* **Catheterization, male**

Urinary system

Definition

The urinary system consists of organs, muscles, tubes, and nerves that are responsible for producing, transporting, and storing urine. The major structures of the urinary system include the **kidneys**, the ureters, the bladder, and the urethra.

Description

The kidneys

The two kidneys are located lateral (to each side) to the spinal column, along the posterior (back) wall of the abdominal cavity. Each kidney is bean-shaped and approximately the size of one's fist (4 to 5 in, or 10 to 13 cm in length). The hilus is the indentation found along the medial side (the side closest to the midline of the body) of the kidney and is the point at which **blood vessels** (the renal artery and renal vein), nerves, and the ureter enter and exit the organ. The outer layer of the kidney is called the renal cortex, and the inner region of the organ is called the renal medulla.

The individual filtering unit of the kidney is called a nephron, of which there are approximately one million in each kidney. Each nephron extends from the renal cortex into the renal medulla and empties into the funnel-like reservoir of the kidney called the

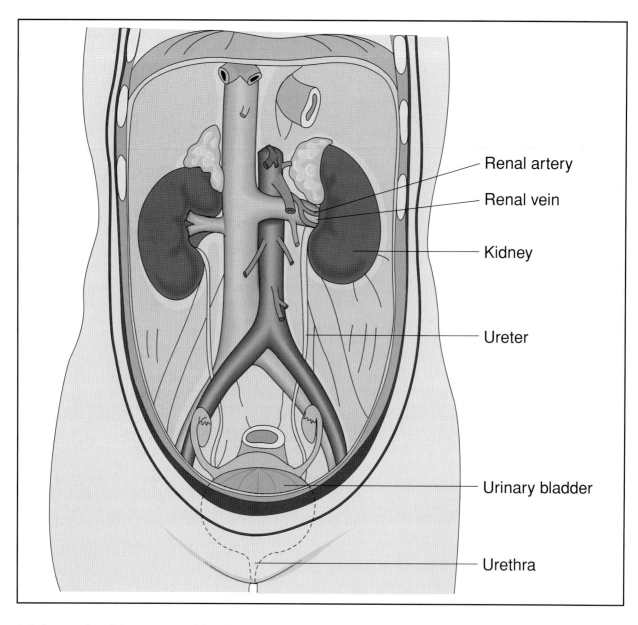

Renal artery

Renal vein

Kidney

Ureter

Urinary bladder

Urethra

Anterior overview of the structures of the urinary system. *(Delmar Publishers, Inc. Reproduced by permission.)*

renal pelvis. There are three major components of the nephron: Bowman's capsule, the glomerulus (plural, glomeruli), and the renal tubule. Bowman's capsule is a structure that contains the glomerulus, a cluster of capillaries that is the main filtering device of the nephron. The afferent arteriole brings **blood** from the branches of the renal artery into Bowman's capsule, where fluid is filtered through the glomerulus. Blood exits the glomerulus by way of the efferent arteriole, passing through the persitubular capillaries and eventually entering the renal vein. The renal tubule has four main sections: the proximal tubule, the loop of Henle, the distal tubule, and the collection tubule. The end closest to Bowman's capsule is called the proximal tubule. The loop of Henle extends

from the proximal tubule in the renal cortex to the medulla and back to the cortex, into the distal tubule. The distal tubule empties into a collecting duct which in turn empties into the renal pelvis.

The ureters

Urine is transported from the renal pelvis of each kidney to the urinary bladder by way of a thin muscular tube called the ureter. The ureter of an adult is typically 8 to 10 in. (21 to 26 cm) long and approximately 0.25 in. (0.75 cm) in diameter. The walls of the ureter are muscular and help to force urine toward the bladder, away from the kidneys.

The bladder

The urinary bladder is a hollow organ with flexible, muscular walls; it is held in place with ligaments attached to the pelvic bones and other organs. Its primary function is to store urine temporarily until urination occurs, when urine is discharged from the body. When the bladder is empty, its inner wall retracts into many folds that expand as the bladder fills with fluid. The bladder of a healthy adult can typically hold up to 2 cups (0.5 l) of urine comfortably for two to five hours. Circular muscles called sphincters are found at bladder openings—from the ureters and to the urethra—and control the flow of urine out of the bladder by closing tightly around the opening.

The urethra

The urethra is a tube that leads from the bladder to the body's exterior. In females, the urethra is typically about 1.5 in. (4 cm) in length and carries only urine; its opening is found anterior (in front of) the opening to the vagina. In males, however, the urethra is much longer—approximately 8 in. (20 cm) in length—and extends from the bladder to the tip of the penis. It passes through the prostate gland; semen is directed into the urethra via the ejaculatory ducts of the prostate. The male urethra therefore alternately transports urine (during urination) and semen (during ejaculation).

Function

Production and transport of urine

Urine is a fluid composed of water and dissolved substances that are in excess of what the body needs to function, as well as various wastes that are by-products of **metabolism**, such as urea, a nitrogen-based waste. These substances are transported into the bloodstream, which enters the kidney by way of the afferent arteriole, a branch of the renal artery.

The blood is filtered from there through the glomerulus, where glucose, **minerals**, urea, other soluble substances, and water pass through to the renal tubule. This fluid is called filtrate. Filtered blood leaves the glomerulus through the efferent arteriole, which branches into the renal vein. The filtrate is transported through the renal tubule where, under normal circumstances, most of the water (about 99%), glucose, and other substances are reabsorbed into the bloodstream through the peritubular capillaries. Urine is what remains at the distal end of the renal tubule.

KEY TERMS

Cystitis—Inflammation of the urinary bladder.

Dialysis—A medical procedure in which waste products are filtered from the bloodstream by a machine.

Filtrate—The fluid that results when blood is filtered through the glomerulus; a precursor to urine.

Hilus—The indentation found along the medial side of the kidney; the point at which blood vessels (the renal artery and renal vein), nerves, and the ureter enter and exit the organ.

Nephritis—Inflammation of the kidney.

Nephron—The individual filtering unit of the kidney; consists of Bowman's capsule, the glomerulus, and the renal tubule.

Renal cortex—The outer layer of the kidney.

Renal medulla—The inner region of the kidney.

Renal pelvis—The funnel-like reservoir of a kidney that empties to the ureter.

Sphincters—Circular muscles that control the flow of urine in/out of openings to/from the bladder.

The urine is transported from the distal and collections tubule to a collection duct and into the renal pelvis. It enters the ureter and is transported to the bladder; a small amount of urine is carried from the renal pelvis to the bladder via the ureter every 10 to 15 seconds. As the bladder fills with urine, pressure from the accumulating fluid stimulates nerve impulses causing the muscles in the wall of the bladder to tighten. Simultaneously, the sphincter muscle at the opening to the urethra is signaled to relax, and urine is forced out of the bladder through the urethra.

Role in human health

Kidney diseases and other urinary system disorders affect millions of Americans to some degree. An estimated 8.4 million new urinary conditions occur each year, including infections of the kidneys, urinary tract, bladder, and others. Urinary tract stones prompt over 1.3 million visits annually to the doctor's office with over 250,000 hospital stays. Urinary incontinence is estimated to affect 13 million adults in the United States. In 1998, approximately 398,000 individuals were diagnosed with end-stage renal disease (ESRD), of which over 63,000 died. In that same year, 245,910 patients utilized dialysis services—a medical procedure in which waste products are filtered from the bloodstream by a machine.

Common diseases and disorders

- Nephritis (also called glomerulonephritis): Nephritis is an inflammation of the kidneys. It may be caused by a bacterial **infection** (pyelonephritis) or an abnormal **immune response**. Chronic nephritis may result in extensive damage to the kidneys and eventual kidney failure.

- Urinary tract infection (UTI): This broad term includes infections of the urethra and/or bladder (lower UTI) or the kidneys and/or ureters (upper UTI). UTIs may be caused by **bacteria**, **fungi**, **viruses**, or parasites.

- Cystitis: More commonly known as a bladder infection, cystitis is common in women and may be caused by bacteria introduced into the urethra from the vagina. Cystitis in males may result from a prostate infection. It can be treated successfully with antibiotics.

- Urinary incontinence: This is defined as involuntary urination. Urinary incontinence may involve an urgent desire to urinate followed by involuntary urine loss (urge incontinence); an uncontrolled loss of urine following actions such as laughing, sneezing, coughing, or lifting (**stress** incontinence); loss of small amounts of urine from a full bladder (overflow incontinence); continual leakage of urine (total incontinence); or a combination of problems (mixed incontinence).

- Kidney/urinary tract cancers: **Cancer** may develop in any of the structures of the urinary system. Kidney cancer accounts for approximately 2% of cancers diagnosed in adults, more often affecting males than females. Bladder cancer may also occur, with smoking being the most significant risk factor.

- Urinary tract stones: Urinary calculi or urinary tract stones may also be called **kidney stones** or bladder stones, depending on the site of their formation. They may form because of an excess of salts or a lack of stone-formation inhibitors in the urine. Urinary tract stones may cause bleeding, **pain**, urine obstruction, or infection.

Resources

BOOKS

Tortora, Gerard, and Sandra Grabowski. Chapter 26. In *Principles of Anatomy and Physiology,* 8th ed. New York: John Wiley, 1996.

PERIODICALS

Johnson, Sarah T. "From incontinence to confidence." *American Journal of Nursing* (February 2000): 69–74.

ORGANIZATIONS

American Foundation for Urologic Disease. 1128 N. Charles Street, Baltimore, MD 21201. (800) 242-2383. <http://www.afud.org>.

National Institute of Diabetes and Digestive and Kidney Diseases. 31 Center Drive, MSC 2560, Bethesda, MD 20892-2560. <http://www.niddk.nih.gov>.

National Kidney Foundation. 30 East 33rd Street, New York, NY 10016. (800) 622-9010. <http://www.kidney.org>.

OTHER

Berkow, Robert, Mark H. Beers, Andrew J. Fletcher, and Robert M. Bogin, eds. "Section 11: Kidney and Urinary Tract Disorders." *The Merck Manual: Home Edition.* 2000. <http://www.merck.com/pubs/mmanual_home/sec11/122.htm>.

Fadem, Stephen Z. "How the Kidney Works." *The Nephron Information Center.* 2000. <http://nephron.com/htkw.html>.

"Kidney and Urologic Disease Statistics for the United States." *National Kidney and Urologic Diseases Information Clearinghouse.* June, 1999. <http://www.niddk.nih.gov/health/kidney/pubs/kustats/kustats.htm>.

"Your urinary system and how it works." *National Kidney and Urologic Diseases Information Clearinghouse.* 1 May, 1998. <http://www.niddk.nih.gov/health/urolog/pubs/yrurinar/index.htm>.

Stephanie Islane Dionne

Urine culture

Definition

A urine culture is a diagnostic laboratory test performed to detect the presence of **bacteria** in the urine (bacteriuria).

Purpose

Urine cultures are performed to isolate and identify the pathogenic microorganism(s) responsible for causing a urinary tract **infection** (UTI). Urinary tract infections are more common in females and in children than in adult males. UTI is associated with discomfort (usually burning) on urination, and may be accompanied by **fever**, malaise, and lower abdominal or back **pain**. All of the urinary structures except the urethra are normally sterile. Most organisms reach the bladder, ureters, and **kidneys** by ascending the urethra. The most commonly encountered urinary tract pathogen is *E. coli*. *Enterococcus faecalis* is the most common gram positive organism to cause UTI. Infections with *Klebsiella, Proteus,* and other *Enterobacteriaceae* are also common. Some organisms not as commonly encountered such as *Candida albicans, Haemophilus influenzae, Mycobacterium tuberculosis, Salmonella spp.,* and *Staphylococcus aureus* usually enter the **urinary system** via the **blood** or lymphatics.

Description

There are several different methods used to collect a urine sample for culture. The most common is the midstream clean-catch technique. Hands should be washed before beginning. For females, the external genitalia are washed two or three times with a cleansing agent and rinsed with water. In males, the external head of the penis is similarly cleansed and rinsed. The patient is then instructed to begin to urinate, and the urine is collected midstream into a sterile container. In infants, a urinary collection bag (plastic bag with an adhesive seal on one end) is attached over a girl's labia or a boy's penis to collect the specimen.

Another method is the catheterized urine specimen in which a lubricated catheter (thin rubber tube) is inserted into the bladder. This avoids contamination from the urethra or external genitalia. If the patient already has a urinary catheter in place, a urine specimen may be collected by clamping the tubing below the collection port and using a sterile needle and syringe to obtain the urine sample; urine cannot be taken from the drainage bag, as it is not fresh and has had an opportunity to grow bacteria at room temperature. On rare occasions, the physician may collect a urine sample by inserting a needle directly into the bladder (suprapubic aspiration). Bladder puncture is warranted when repeated efforts to culture the urine grow contaminants from the urethra. This is especially common in infants. Suprapubic tap is also indicated when anaerobic UTI is suspected.

The urine must be cultured within one hour of collection if not refrigerated. However, refrigerated samples may be stored for up to 24 hours before plating the sample. Urine culture is a quantitative procedure. A calibrated inoculating loop that holds 0.01 or 0.001 mL of urine is inserted vertically into the urine sample and used to transfer the urine to a sterile agar plate. If urine is obtained by bladder puncture, 0.1 mL is transferred to the plate using a sterile pipet. The urine is spread evenly across the plate with a glass rod as opposed to streaking the plate with the loop. This procedure is usually performed on plates of 5% sheep blood agar, which detects growth of most organisms, and on a plate of MacConkey agar or other selective and differential medium for isolation of gram-negative organisms. Additionally, some labs plate urine on colistin-nalidixic acid agar (CNA) or other selective medium for gram-positive bacteria. The plates are incubated at 36°C for 18 to 24 hours and read for growth. The number of colonies is multiplied by the appropriate factor to give the colony count per mL urine. Some organisms, such as *Mycobacterium tuberculosis,* may be isolated from urine and require special culture media and growth conditions.

Plates that show no growth at 24 hours are incubated another day and read again. Growth of more than three species indicates contamination, and the culture should be repeated with a new specimen. For one to three species, plates are held and a partial identification (e.g. gram-negative rod, lactose positive) is reported when there is less than 10,000 colony forming units (CFU) per mL. Usually, when less than 10,000 CFU/mL are recovered the organism is considered a contaminant from the urethra. Exceptions are the presence of *Staphylococcus aureus* and organisms isolated from a catheter sample or suprapubic aspiration. Common urethral contaminants include coagulase negative staphylococci, diptheroids, and lactobaccilli. Each colony type giving 10,000 or more CFU/mL is identified and antibiotic susceptibility testing is performed. UTI is diagnosed when a species produces greater than 100,000 CFU/mL. Counts between 10,000 and 100,000 may be significant depending on the organism and patient-specific conditions (e.g. urine collected from a catheter or a patient receiving antibiotic treatment).

Preparation

Drinking a glass of water 15-20 minutes before the test is helpful if there is no urge to urinate.

Aftercare

There are no other special preparations or aftercare required for the test.

Complications

There are no risks associated with the culture test itself. If insertion of a urinary catheter is required to obtain the urine, there is a slight risk of introducing infection from the catheter. Patients receiving antibiotic treatment prior to collection may have negative culture results.

Results

Urine is normally sterile, and there should be no growth. Greater than 100,000 CFU/mL of any single colony type is considered evidence of UTI. Any growth from a catheter or suprapubic sample or growth of *S. aureus* is considered significant. Greater than 10,000 CFU/mL may be significant in some patient populations and clinical settings.

Health care team roles

The patient collects his or her own sample with the aid of instructions provided by the physician or nurse. A clinical laboratory scientist, NCA(CLS)/medical technologist, MT(ASCP) usually performs the culture and sensitivity testing. A physician makes the diagnosis and treatment decision based upon the colony count, organism(s) identified, antibiotic susceptibility profile, **urinalysis** results, and patient-specific findings.

Resources

BOOKS

Chernecky, Cynthia C, and Berger, Barbara J. *Laboratory Tests and Diagnostic Procedures,* 3rd ed. Philadelphia, PA: W. B. Saunders Company, 2001.

Finegold, S.M., and E.J. Baron. *Bailey and Scott's Diagnostic Microbiology,* 10th ed. Philadelphia: Mosby, 1998.

Kee, Joyce LeFever. *Handbook of Laboratory and Diagnostic Tests,* 4th ed. Upper Saddle River, NJ: Prentice Hall, 2001.

Malarkey, Louise, and Mary Ellen McMorrow. *Nurse's Manual of Laboratory Tests and Diagnostic Procedures.* Philadelphia: W. B. Saunders, 1996.

ORGANIZATIONS

American Foundation for Urologic Disease. 300 West Pratt Street, Suite 401, Baltimore, MD 21201.

National Kidney and Urologic Diseases Information Clearinghouse. Information Way, Bethesda, MD 20892-3580. (301)654-4415. nkudic@aerie.com.

OTHER

"Urine culture." <http://www.healthanswers.com> (Feb. 27, 1998).

"Urine culture." <http://www.thriveonline.com> (Feb. 25, 1998).

Victoria E. DeMoranville

Urine specimen collection

Definition

The urine specimen collection is a procedure used to obtain a sample of urine from a patient. The sample is used for diagnostic tests.

Purpose

The purpose of obtaining a urine sample is to test for any abnormalities that may be present, such as **bacteria**, ketones, or drugs.

Precautions

The skin of the genital area should be cleansed with a mild disinfectant to prevent contamination of the urine specimen or irritation of the delicate membranes of the area.

Description

A urine specimen is sometimes called a clean-catch, **urine culture**, or midstream specimen of urine, and is a method of collecting a quantity of urine for testing.

Preparation

The procedure and the reasons for it are explained to the patient. Able patients may be allowed to collect the urine sample, following the guidelines explained by the nurse.

Nurses who collect the urine sample should be sure to wash and dry their hands carefully. The items required for the procedure are as follows:

- a sterile urine cup for children and adults
- a sterile urine bag for infants
- a bedpan or urinal for patients unable to use the toilet
- sterile swabs
- sterile towels
- sterile gloves

For females, the area around the vulva is wiped and dried thoroughly with the sterile swabs and towels, working from front to back, with the nurse wearing sterile gloves. If the patient is unable to use the toilet, the bedpan is placed beneath her. When the urine begins to flow, the first part is allowed to pass into the toilet or bedpan. Then the sterile container is

placed in position and filled with the mid-stream portion of the urine. The remainder of the urine is then allowed to pass into the toilet or bedpan. The lid is placed securely on the cup.

For males, the area around the penis and urethra is wiped and dried thoroughly with the sterile swabs and towels, working from front to back, with the nurse wearing sterile gloves. If the patient is uncircumcised, the foreskin should be held back during the complete procedure to prevent the skin contaminating the sample. The patient then begins to pass urine into the toilet or a urinal. Then, the sterile container is placed in position and filled with the mid-stream portion of the urine, taking care that the penis does not touch the sides of the container. The remainder of the urine is then allowed to pass into the toilet or urinal. The lid is placed securely on the cup.

For infants, the genitals are cleansed and dried thoroughly using the sterile wipes and towels. A sterile urine collection bag is placed over the area, with the adhesive tape firmly stuck onto the baby's skin. A fresh diaper is put on the child over the collecting bag and checked frequently for the child having passed urine into the bag. When the specimen is obtained, it is poured into a sterile container and sent immediately for testing.

Aftercare

The patient should be made comfortable.

All swabs, towels, and gloves should be disposed of in appropriate containers. The nurse should again wash and dry the hands thoroughly.

The specimen should be sent for testing as quickly as possible. Speed in testing the sample is essential in order to obtain an accurate result.

Complications

If there is a delay in sending the specimen for testing, some organisms present in the urine may die while others multiply, resulting in a false reading.

Patients should inform medical staff of any medications currently being taken as elements of the drugs may be present in the urine.

Results

Normal urine is free from bacteria and is a clear, amber color. It is slightly acidic.

KEY TERMS

Genitals—The reproductive organs.

Ketones—Substances that are present in the blood and urine and occur in large amounts in diseases such as diabetes.

Membrane—A thin layer of tissue lining a part of the body.

Urethra—The tube through which urine flows from the bladder to the outside genitalia.

Vulva—The visible external female genitalia.

Health care team roles

The nurse should be aware of the qualities of normal urine, and note if the patient has any difficulties in passing urine.

Resources

ORGANIZATIONS

American Nurses Association. 600 Maryland Ave. SW, Suite 100 West, Washington, DC 20024. (202) 651-7000. <http://www.ana.org>.

OTHER

"Urine Culture: Clean–Catch." *Medline Medical Encyclopedia.* National Library of Medicine Web site. 8 August 2001. <http://www.nlm.nih.gov/medlineplus/ency/article/003751.htm>.

"Urine Sample." *General Health Encyclopedia.* Health Central Website. 8 August 2001. <http://www.healthcentral.com/mhc/top/003751.cfm>.

Margaret A. Stockley, RGN

Urobilinogen test *see* **Urinalysis**

Urography *see* **Intravenous urography**

Urticaria *see* **Hives**

Uterine stimulants

Definition

Uterine stimulants (uterotonics) are medications that cause, or increase the frequency and intensity of, uterine contractions. These drugs are used to induce (start) or augment (stimulate) labor, facilitate uterine contractions following a **miscarriage**, induce abortion, or reduce hemorrhage following **childbirth**

---

or abortion. The three uterotonics used most frequently are oxytocins, prostaglandins, and ergots. Depending upon the type of drug, uterotonics may be given intravenously (IV), intramuscularly (IM), as a vaginal gel or suppository, or in oral form.

Purpose

Uterine stimulants are used to induce, or begin, labor in certain circumstances when the mother has not begun labor naturally. These circumstances may include if the mother is post-dates, that is, gestation is over 40 weeks—especially if tests indicate a decrease in amniotic fluid volume. They may be used in cases of premature rupture of the membranes, preeclampsia (elevated **blood pressure** in the late stage of **pregnancy**), diabetes, and intrauterine growth retardation (IUGR) when these conditions require delivery before labor has begun. They may be recommended if the expectant mother lives a great distance from the healthcare facility and there is concern for either her or her baby's safety if she were unable to reach the facility once labor begins. They are also used in the augmentation of existing contractions to increase strength and frequency when labor is not progressing well.

According to the American College of Obstetrics and Gynecology (ACOG), the 1990s saw an increase in the rate of induced labor—from 9% to 18%. In a May 31, 2001, statement, the ACOG reported that the increase in the cesarian rate seen over the same period of time was not due to the induction process but to other factors, such as the condition of the cervix at the time of induction and whether or not the pregnancy was the woman's first.

Oxytocin and prostaglandin (PG) are naturally occurring hormones used to induce labor. They are also available in synthetic form (Pitocin and Syntocinon are the synthetic counterparts of oxytocin). PG is also used to ripen the cervix prior to induction, which is sometimes sufficient to stimulate labor, and the woman needs no further medication for labor to progress. There are many forms of PGs, but those of greatest interest are PGE_1, PGE_2, and $PGF2_{alpha}$. Research is investigating which are the most effective for which process. For example, PGE_2 in the form of dinoprostone (Cervidil and Prepidil) has proven superior to the PGF series in cervical ripening. Misoprostol (Cytotec), a synthetic PGE_1, also is effective in cervical ripening and labor induction, while the $PGF2_{alpha}$ analog, carboprost (Prostin 15-M, or Hemabate), is the preferred PG uterine stimulant. The ergots, which significantly increase uterine activity, have severe side effects in many women. Only one ergot,

methylergonovine maleate (Methergine) is now used in the United States, and is used only to control postpartum hemorrhage (PPH).

Oxytocin is also used in a contraction stress test (CST). This is done prior to the onset of labor to evaluate the fetus's ability to handle uterine contractions. To avoid the possibility of exogenous (introduced) oxytocin putting the woman into labor, she may instead be asked to stimulate her nipples to cause the release of natural oxytocin. A negative, or normal, test is one in which there are three contractions in a 10-minute period, with no abnormal slowing of the fetal **heart** rate (FHR). False positives of the CST do occur, however. Also, the expectant mother should remain in the health care setting for about half an hour after a negative test to make sure the test did not stimulate labor.

If a woman has a miscarriage, oxytocin may be used to bring on contractions to assure that all the products of conception (POC) are expelled from the uterus. If the fetus died but was not expelled, prostaglandin (PGE_2) may be used to ripen the cervix to facilitate a dilatation and evacuation, and/or to encourage more uterine contractions. In this case, prostaglandin may be used either in gel form or as a vaginal suppository.

In a routine delivery, oxytocin may be ordered after the placenta has been delivered in order to increase uterine contractions and minimize bleeding. Oxytocin (Pitocin) also may be used to treat uterine hemorrhage. While hemorrhage occurs in about 4% of vaginal deliveries and 6% of cesarian deliveries, it accounts for about 35% of maternal deaths due to bleeding during pregnancy. The role of oxytocin is to bring on and strengthen uterine contractions. If the hemorrhage stems from the placental detachment site, contractions help to close off the **blood vessels** and thereby stop the excessive bleeding. Additional medications may be used, including $PGF2_{alpha}$ (Hemabate), misoprostol (Cytotec), or the ergot methylergonovine (Methergine). If the uterus is contracted but bleeding continues, the cause may be retained placenta, genital tract laceration, or uterine rupture. Large clots that remain in the lower part of the uterus can inhibit the uterus from contracting, leading to uterine atony (lack of tone or tension), a leading cause of postpartum hemorrhage. Uterine contractions also help to expel large clots and placental fragments.

Precautions

It is important to establish a clear baseline of **vital signs** before a woman is given any medication to induce labor. Consistent reevaluation and documentation of vital signs allow for faster recognition of an abnormal change in a woman's condition. Also, a clear labor and delivery record will assist the postpartum nurse in monitoring for changes as well. Documentation includes time and dosage of any medications given, as well as any side effects that might occur. Proper documentation will help avoid the chance of medication doses being given too close together. An increasing pulse and a decreasing **blood** pressure signal a potential hemorrhage. When oxytocin is given by IV, it must be diluted in IV fluid and never given as a straight IV. PGs should not be given if there is any question about fetal well-being, for example, an abnormal FHR tracing. The ergot Methergine should never be given via IV and never to a woman with **hypertension**.

Description

Oxytocin

Oxytocin's major functions are in labor and **lactation**. In vitro, production and secretion of oxytocin is stimulated by the **pituitary gland**. Just what happens to initiate labor remains a mystery, although much research has focused on this area. The hormone estrogen appears to increase the number of oxytocin receptors as the gestation period increases. The degree to which uterine muscles are sensitive to oxytocin's action appears linked to the number of oxytocin receptors. Oxytocin levels increase as labor progresses, and the fetus also secretes oxytocin during labor, increasing the amount of circulating oxytocin.

In a normally progressing labor, contractions become more frequent, more intense, and last longer. In a dysfunctional labor, contractions may weaken, become further apart, or even stop. A prolonged labor puts the mother at risk of fatigue, which can increase the likelihood of a cesarian delivery or fetal distress. Oxytocin may be given to augment the labor. Some women may need only a very small amount in order to "jump start" labor once again. For others it may be necessary to continue the oxytocin in small increments. Oxytocin increases the strength, duration, and frequency of contractions, so care must be taken to prevent the contractions from becoming too strong or too frequent. If the mother has an **infection**, labor may not progress as usual. Oxytocin is less effective in such cases.

Naturally occurring oxytocin plays a role in breastfeeding by facilitating both milk ejection and the letdown reflex. When the neonate suckles at the breast, the nipple stimulation sends a message to the pituitary gland to release oxytocin. Oxytocin then causes the milk gland cells to constrict, pushing the milk forward towards the nipples. Breastfeeding immediately after delivery encourages oxytocin production and causes uterine contractions, helping the uterus to become firm and close off the blood vessels at the placental detachment site. This process limits the amount of blood lost after childbirth. Because the release of oxytocin is inhibited by fear, **pain**, embarrassment, and distraction, providing the new mother with a calm environment in which she can focus on her infant will facilitate breastfeeding and the production of oxytocin.

Prostaglandins

Prostaglandins play a major role in the stimulation of uterine contractions that begin the labor process. Research indicates that PGs also facilitate the mother's transition between phases of the labor process. Some PGs promote vasoconstriction while others promote vasodilation. One function of PGs is to promote cervical effacement and dilation during labor. Oxytocin plays a role in stimulating the release of PGs. Infection stimulates their release, also, which appears to be a factor in the initiation of up to 30% of cases of **preterm labor**. PGs serve a function in immunosuppression, but the exact mechanism is unclear. They also may be a major factor in regulating umbilical blood flow by keeping the ductus arteriosus open during fetal life.

Ergots

Ergots are produced by a fungus that forms primarily on rye grain. Because of its potentially harmful side effects, one form (Ergonovine, or Ergotrate) was taken off the market in 1993 and methylergonovine maleate (Methergine) is now the only form used, and is used only as a uterine stimulant to control PPH. (There is no evidence that Methergine used as a prophylactic decreases the risk of PPH.) Even so, because of the complications it can cause, and because its use is contraindicated in a large number of women, Methergine has been replaced by the PGs as the second-line uterotonic of choice.

Preparation

Before any procedure is begun or medication administered, it is important for the nurse to review the information with the pregnant woman to ensure that she understands what will take place and the potential side effects of the medication. Any **allergies** to medication need to be reviewed, as well as any prior response the mother may have had to the medications. The mother may be anxious about induction or augmentation, fearing that the contractions will come too fast or that she will feel out of control of the process. The nurse needs to address her concerns, as well as those of her partner.

Aftercare

Close supervision of the mother during induction or cervical ripening must take place. The FHR and uterine contractions are usually monitored for an hour after induction. Frequent checks of vital signs alert the nurse to any potential complications.

Complications

Oxytocin

The effect of IV oxytocin is rapid following administration. The individual response to oxytocin can vary considerably, and administration is usually increased slowly and incrementally. Hyperstimulation of the uterus, which can result from oxytocin augmentation, can place the fetus at risk for asphyxia. Hyperstimulation is defined as more than five contractions in 10 minutes, contractions lasting longer than 60 seconds, and increased uterine tonus either with or without significant decrease in FHR. Uterine rupture has also been linked to oxytocin administration, particularly for periods longer than four hours. Oxytocin has a small antidiuretic effect that is usually dose related and that can lead to water intoxication (hyponatremia). Onset occurs gradually and may go unnoticed. Signs may include reduced urine output, confusion, nausea, convulsions, and **coma**. Mothers receiving oxytocin need to have their blood pressure monitored closely, as both hypotension and hypertension can occur, and—although the subject remains controversial—evidence suggests oxytocin increases the incidence of **neonatal jaundice**. Although oxytocin may put women with a classical cesarian section scar from a prior delivery at increased risk of uterine rupture, contraindications to the use of the drug are virtually the same as contraindications for labor. Other side effects of oxytocin include nausea, vomiting, cardiac arrhythmias, and fetal bradycardia. When used judiciously, oxytocin is a very effective medication for the progression of labor.

Prostaglandins

Significant systemic side effects are associated with the use of PGs. These include headache, nausea, **diarrhea**, tachycardia, vomiting, chills, **fever**, sweating, hypertension, and hypotension. There is also increased incidence of uterine hyperstimulation and

---

KEY TERMS

Atony—In uterine atony, the uterus fails to contract after delivery, remaining relaxed. This flaccid condition can lead to hemorrhage, and puts the mother at risk of shock and death.

Augment—Drugs to augment labor are given after labor has begun, but fails to progress, or when the contractions have slowed down and are weak or ineffective, prolonging labor unnecessarily.

Hemorrhage—The loss of an excessive amount of blood in a short period of time. After childbirth, a loss of more than 500 mL over a 24-hour period is considered postpartal hemorrhage. The blood loss may be sudden and swift, or slow and continuous.

Induce, induction—To begin or start.

Post-dates—Gestation longer than approximately 40 weeks. Up to 42 weeks may still be still considered normal.

---

potential for uterine rupture. $PGF2_{alpha}$ (carboprost—Prostin 15-M or Hemabate) can cause hypotension, pulmonary **edema**, and—in women with asthma—intense bronchospasms. Because it stimulates the production of steroids, carboprost may be contraindicated in women with adrenal gland disease. When used for abortion, it may result in sufficient blood loss to cause anemia, necessitating a transfusion. Medical problems (or history) of diabetes, epilepsy, heart or blood vessel disease, **jaundice**, kidney disease, or **liver** disease should be brought to the attention of the health care practitioner before the patient is given carboprost. Also, in rare instances, ophthalmic pressure has increased in women with **glaucoma** with the use of this PG.

Ergots

Ergots have an alpha adrenergic action with a vasoconstricive effect. They can cause hypertension, cardiovascular changes, **cyanosis**, muscle pain, tingling, other symptoms associated with decreased blood circulation, and severe uterine cramping. The health care professional should be well aware of other medications being taken by the patient. The presence or history of medical problems such as angina, hypertension, stroke, infection, kidney and liver disease, and Raynaud's phenomenon may be contraindications to the use of this drug.

Results

Anticipated outcomes for uterine stimulants are either to prepare the cervix for childbirth, induce or stimulate uterine contractions to produce a safe delivery of a newborn, encourage a complete spontaneous or induced abortion, eliminate blood clots or other POC debris from the uterus, and decrease or stop hemorrhage following childbirth or abortion. Normal results would meet these outcomes without significant side effects—either for the mother or, in the case of childbirth, the infant.

Heath care team roles

Nurses play a major role in preparing the patient for and administering uterine stimulants, and monitoring the patient and fetus during the labor process. Because the choice of drug, its form of administration, and its side effects vary, knowledge of uterine physiology is an important aspect of caring for women and their fetuses undergoing treatment with these drugs. Nurses must be aware of potential complications and side effects, as well as dosing requirements, criteria assessment, and contraindications to these drugs. They should take a complete medical history of the patient, including prescription and over-the-counter medications, illnesses, and disease. In most instances a gynecologist or other qualified physician will perform the actual delivery, although this may occasionally be facilitated by a midwife. A pediatrician or family health care practitioner will examine the newborn infant and administer treatment if required. The nurse can be an important source of information and comfort to women facing induction of labor or abortion, and to new mothers facing the initial responsibility of parenthood.

Resources

BOOKS

Creasy, Robert K., and Robert Resnik. *Maternal-Fetal Medicine,* 4th ed. Philadelphia: W. B. Saunders Company, 1999.
Rakel, Robert A. *Conn's Current Therapy 2000.* Philadelphia: W.B. Saunders Company, 2000.
Scott, James. *Danforth's Obstetrics and Gynecology,* 8th ed. Philadelphia: Lippincott Williams & Wilkins, 1999.

OTHER

American College of Obstetricians and Gynecologists (ACOG). 409 12th St. SW, PO Box 96920, Washington, DC 20090-6920. <http://www.acog.com>.

Esther Csapo Rastegari, R.N., B.S.N., Ed.M.

Uterus x rays *see* **Hysterosalpingography**

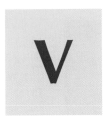

Vaccination

Definition

Vaccination is the use of vaccines to produce immunity to specific diseases.

Purpose

Many diseases that once caused widespread illness, disability, and death now can be prevented through the use of vaccines. Vaccines are medicines that contain weakened or dead **bacteria**, **viruses**, or pollen antigens. When a person takes a vaccine, his or her **immune system** responds by producing antibodies—substances that weaken or destroy disease-causing organisms. When the person is later exposed to live bacteria or viruses of the same kind that were in the vaccine, the antibodies prevent those organisms from making the person sick. In other words, the person becomes immune to the disease the organisms normally cause. The process of building up immunity by taking a vaccine is called immunization.

Vaccines are used in several ways. Some, such as the rabies vaccine, are given only when a person is likely to have been exposed to the virus that causes the disease, such as through a dog bite, for example. Others are given to travelers planning to visit countries where certain diseases are common. Vaccines such as the **influenza** vaccine, or "flu shot," are given mainly to specific groups of people—older adults and others whose health is at high risk if they develop influenza or its complications. Then, there are vaccines that are given to almost everyone, such as the one that prevents diphtheria.

Children routinely have a series of vaccinations that begin at birth. The American Academy of Pediatrics recommends that children be fully immunized before the age of two years in order for them to be protected during their most vulnerable period. Given according to a specific schedule that is issued every year by the Department of Health, these vaccinations protect against hepatitis B, diphtheria, tetanus, pertussis, measles, mumps, rubella, varicella (chickenpox), polio, and *Hemophilus influenza* type B (HiB). This series of vaccinations is recommended by the American Academy of Family Physicians, the American Academy of Pediatrics, and the Centers for Disease Control and Prevention and is required in all states before children can enter school. All states will make exceptions for children who have medical conditions such as **cancer** that prevent them from having vaccinations, and some states also will make exceptions for children whose parents object for religious or other reasons.

Vaccines are also available for preventing anthrax, cholera, hepatitis A, Japanese encephalitis, meningococcal **meningitis**, plague, pneumococcal **infection**, **tuberculosis**, typhoid **fever**, and yellow fever.

Some vaccines are combined in one injection, such as the measles-mumps-rubella (MMR) or diphtheria-pertussis-tetanus (DPT) combinations.

Precautions

Vaccines are not always effective, and there is no way to predict whether a vaccine will "take" in any particular person. To be most effective, vaccination programs depend on whole communities participating. The more people who are vaccinated, the lower everyone's risk of being exposed to a disease. Even people who do not develop immunity through vaccination are safer when their friends, neighbors, children, and coworkers are immunized.

Like most medical procedures, vaccination has risks as well as substantial benefits. Anyone who takes a vaccine should make sure that he or she is fully informed about both the benefits and the risks. Any questions or concerns should be discussed with a physician or other health care provider. The Centers for Disease Control and Prevention, located in Atlanta, Georgia, is a good source of information.

Vaccines may cause problems for people with certain **allergies**. For example, people who are allergic to

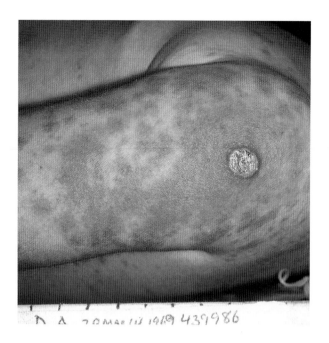

N A 70MAR III 1919 439986

An allergic reaction to a vaccination shot. *(Photograph by Lester V. Bergman, Corbis Images. Reproduced by permission.)*

the **antibiotics** neomycin or polymyxin B should not take rubella vaccine, measles vaccine, mumps vaccine, or the combined measles-mumps-rubella (MMR) vaccine. Anyone who has had a severe allergic reaction to baker's yeast should not take the hepatitis B vaccine. Patients who are allergic to antibiotics such as gentamicin sulfate, streptomycin sulfate, or other aminoglycosides should check with their physicians before taking influenza vaccine, as some influenza vaccines contain these drugs. Also, some vaccines, including those for influenza, measles, and mumps, are grown in the fluids of chick embryos and should not be taken by people who are allergic to eggs. In general, anyone who has had an unusual reaction to a vaccine in the past should let his or her physician know before taking the same kind of vaccine again. The physician also should be told about any allergies to foods, medicines, preservatives, or other substances.

People with certain other medical conditions should be cautious about taking vaccines. Influenza vaccine, for example, may reactivate Guillain-Barre syndrome in people who have had it before. This vaccine also may worsen illnesses that involve the **lungs**, such as bronchitis or **pneumonia**. Vaccines that cause fever as a side-effect may trigger seizures in people who have a history of seizures caused by fever.

Certain vaccines are not recommended for use during **pregnancy**, but some may be given to women at especially high risk of getting a specific disease such as polio. Vaccines also may be given to pregnant women to prevent medical problems in their babies. For example, vaccinating a pregnant woman with tetanus toxoid can prevent her baby from getting tetanus at birth.

Women should avoid becoming pregnant for three months after taking rubella vaccine, measles vaccine, mumps vaccine, or the combined measles-mumps-rubella (MMR) vaccine as these could cause problems in the unborn baby.

Women who are breastfeeding should check with their physicians before taking any vaccine.

Description

Vaccinations can also be called shots or immunizations. Most vaccines are given as injections, but a few, such as the oral polio vaccine, are given by mouth.

The time involved in administering vaccinations is minimal; however, the nurse should allow time before and after the procedure for answering questions and for monitoring the patient for potential side-effects up to 30 minutes following a vaccination.

Most insurance companies cover routine vaccinations. The patient should be advised to check with their provider for their current list.

Recommended dosage

The recommended dosage depends on the type of vaccine and may be different for different patients. The health care professional who administers the vaccine will decide on the proper dose.

A vaccination health record will help parents and health care providers keep track of a child's vaccinations. The record should be started when the child has his or her first vaccination and should be updated with each additional vaccination. While most physicians follow the recommended vaccination schedule, parents should understand that some flexibility is allowed. For example, vaccinations that are scheduled for age two months may be given anytime between six and 10 weeks. When possible, follow the schedule. However, slight departures will not prevent the child from developing immunity, as long as all the vaccinations are given at around the right times. The child's physician is the best person to decide when each vaccination should be given.

Anyone planning a trip to another country should check with a health care provider to find out what vaccinations are needed. Some vaccinations must be given as much as 12 weeks before the trip, so getting this information early is important. Many major hospitals and medical centers have travel clinics that can provide this information. The Traveler's Health Section of the Centers for Disease Control and Prevention also has information on vaccination requirements.

Complications

Most side-effects from vaccines are minor and easily treated. The most common are **pain**, redness, and swelling at the site of the injection. Some people may also develop a fever or a rash. In rare cases, vaccines may cause severe allergic reactions, swelling of the **brain**, or seizures. Anyone who has an unusual reaction after receiving a vaccine should get in touch with a physician right away.

Results

Immunity to a particular disease is expected after one or more vaccinations, depending on the formula of the vaccine used. This immunity is usually permanent, but follow-up doses are required with certain diseases such as tetanus, which requires a booster every ten years.

Vaccines may interact with other medicines and medical treatments. When this happens, the effects of the vaccine or the other medicine may change or the risk of side effects may be greater. For example, radiation therapy and cancer drugs may reduce the effectiveness of many vaccines or may increase the chance of side-effects. Anyone who takes a vaccine should inform their physician about other medicines he or she is taking and should ask whether the possible interactions could interfere with the effects of the vaccine or the other medicines.

Health care team roles

Vaccinations are the best way to be protected from life-threatening diseases. Because of the widespread use of vaccines, most of these illnesses are rarely seen in the United States. It is important that the nursing staff remain up-to-date with the current trends in immunization as outlined by the Department of Health. The immunization rates in the health department should be looked at for improvement to ensure that children and patients at risk are fully immunized. The nurse should be able to provide an overview of the principles of vaccination, general vaccination recommendations, routine vaccinations for travelers, and questions on impending flu epidemics. In addition, the nurse should explain the procedure to the patient and answer questions regarding a vaccine's efficacy and its possible side-effects. Brochures may also be available to give to patients to inform them about the reasons for vaccination as well as the risk of potential side-effects.

KEY TERMS

Anthrax—An infectious disease caused by a type of bacterium. The disease can be passed from animals to people and usually is fatal. Symptoms include sores on the skin.

Antibody—A type of protein produced in the blood or in the body tissues that helps the body fight infection.

Cholera—An infection of the small intestine caused by a type of bacterium. Drinking water or eating seafood or other foods that have been contaminated with the feces of infected people can spread the disease. It occurs in parts of Asia, Africa, Latin America, India, and the Middle East. Symptoms include watery diarrhea and exhaustion.

Encephalitis—Inflammation of the brain, usually caused by a virus. The inflammation may interfere with normal brain function and may cause seizures, sleepiness, confusion, personality changes, weakness in one or more parts of the body, and even coma.

Guillain-Barre syndrome—A disease of the nerves with symptoms that include sudden numbness and weakness in the arms and legs, sometimes leading to paralysis. The disease is serious and requires medical treatment, but most people recover completely.

Pertussis—Whooping cough.

Rubella—German measles.

Tuberculosis—An infectious disease that usually affects the lungs, but may also affect other parts of the body. Symptoms include fever, weight loss, and coughing up blood.

Typhoid fever—An infectious disease caused by a type of bacterium. People with this disease have a lingering fever and feel depressed and exhausted. Diarrhea and rose-colored spots on the chest and abdomen are other symptoms. The disease is spread through poor sanitation.

Yellow fever—An infectious disease caused by a virus. The disease, which is spread by mosquitoes, is most common in Central and South America and Central Africa. Symptoms include high fever; jaundice (yellow eyes and skin); and dark-colored vomit, a sign of internal bleeding. Yellow fever can be fatal.

If a child is being vaccinated, the parent can bring along a favorite toy to help distract the child and make him or her more at ease if there is a delay in being seen. Seeing the same health care provider regularly will enable familiarity to become established, and a parent can hold the child in the lap while the vaccination is being given, making the situation less traumatic.

Needle-free jet injectors, which force the vaccine serum through the skin using a blast of air, are also available in some clinics. They are slightly faster than a needle and could be less painful for the patient, while eliminating the risk of needlestick injuries.

Resources

ORGANIZATIONS

National Immunization Information Hotline. Centers for Disease Control and Prevention. (800) 232-2522.

OTHER

Centers for Disease Control National Immunization Program. <http://www.cdc.gov/nip>.

Global Alliance for Vaccines and Immunization (GAVI). <http://www.vaccinealliance.org>.

National Vaccine Injury Compensation Program. Parklawn Building, Room 8A-46 5600 Fishers Lane, Rockville, MD 20857. <http://www.bhpr.hrsa.gov/vicp>.

Margaret Stockley

Vaccines *see* **Vaccination**

Vaginal medicine administration

Definition

Vaginal medicines are topical agents prepared specifically for insertion into a woman's vagina. They are compounded in the form of a cream, foam, gel, tablet, or suppository, and are absorbed through the vaginal mucousa. Vaginal medicine in the form of a cream, foam, gel, or tablet is administered using a specific applicator that is provided by the manufacturer. Suppositories have the medicine suspended in wax and are shaped like a small bullet. They are inserted into the vagina with the index finger. Vaginal medicines are most often administered at bedtime, as the reclined position enhances medication absorption.

Purpose

Vaginal medicines are most commonly used to combat **infection**, inflammation, or dryness of the vaginal mucousa. Other types of vaginal medicines include spermicides (i.e., to prevent conception), **chemotherapy** (i.e., for **cancer** treatment), and aborticides (i.e., for inducing labor).

Precautions

Vaginal tissue can be traumatized by the forceful use of applicators or fingernails during medicine administration, so medications should be introduced into the vagina gently. Patients should be encouraged to relax, as this will decrease resistance to the mode of insertion. One should not attempt to insert vaginal medication when a patient is confused and combative.

Medicine should not be delivered via the vagina if it is not labeled for vaginal use. Vaginal medicine should not be taken orally.

Description

A female staff member must be present in the room when a male nurse administers a vaginal medication. The patient should be positioned on her back, with knees bent. Her legs should be drawn up toward the hips, and the heels should be flat on the bed. A sheet across the abdomen and upper legs, falling just over the knees, will decrease the patient's feeling of exposure. Directions for filling the applicator should followed. At this point, the patient should be advised to drop her knees apart. The nurse should wash his or her hands and put on disposable gloves. Using one hand, the nurse should spread the labia and expose the vaginal opening. If there is drainage or exudate, the nurse should cleanse the area with warm, soapy water, using cotton balls or a clean washcloth. The vaginal opening should be rinsed and allowed to air dry. A small amount of water-soluble lubricant should then be placed on the tip of the applicator or suppository, the labia spread, and the suppository or applicator tipped into the vaginal opening. The suppository or applicator should be moved gently down, toward the posterior (i.e., back) wall of the vagina, toward the spine 2–4 inches (5-10 cm), or until resistance is felt. The suppository or applicator should then be angled upward. When using an applicator to deliver cream or gel, the plunger should be gently pushed to deliver the medicine. The nurse should then remove his or her finger and/or the applicator from the vagina. The disposable latex gloves should be disposed of properly.

Preparation

Before beginning to administer vaginal medicines, the door to the room should be closed to ensure privacy. (A female staff member must already be present if the nurse is a male.) The patient should empty her bladder just before administration. The nurse should check the medication label each time medicine is given; this will avoid medication errors. The medication must be checked to confirm that it is the right medicine, the right dose (i.e., strength), the right time, the right patient, and the right method of administration. The expiration date on the label should be checked; outdated medication should never be used. If the nurse has not yet put on disposable gloves, it should be done at this time. His or her hands should be washed, and gloves should be put on.

Aftercare

The used applicator should be placed on a clean paper towel to prevent the spread of microorganisma. The patient should be covered and encouraged to maintain a reclined position, with knees up, for at least 10 minutes (30 minutes after a suppository). This will allow time for medicine absorption. If the applicator is reusable, it should be washed in warm soapy water, thoroughly rinsed, air dried, and placed back in the medicine box or a plastic bag until the next use. The used gloves and disposable applicator should be put into a trash bag, which can be sealed and discarded. The nurse should wash his or her hands. The patient should be given a mini-pad (or small sanitary napkins) to protect her underwear from medicine that may leak out.

The patient should be instructed not to use tampons after vaginal medicine administration; they will absorb the medicine more rapidly than the vaginal mucousa, and the full effect of the drug will not be achieved.

Complications

Tissue irritation or allergic reactions can result from vaginal medications. If irritation, swelling, or redness of the tissue is apparent, or if the patient complains of **pain** or burning, the next dose of medicine should not be given until the physician has been consulted.

Results

Most vaginal medicines will produce the desired effects within several days to one week. Spermicides and aborticide vaginal medicines act more rapidly when used as directed. If the patient experiences vaginal pain at the time of medicine instillation, or the condition does not improve, the physician should be contacted.

Health care team roles

Vaginal medicines are administered by a licensed nurse (R.N. or L.P.N.) in the health care setting. An alert and cooperative patient may be allowed to administer the medicine under the direction of the nurse. The nurse should, however, assess the site and the effectiveness of the medicine. The patient or members of the patient's family can be taught to administer vaginal medicines in the home setting.

BOOKS

Medication Administration, Nurse's Clinical Guide, Pennsylvania: Springhouse Corporation, 2000.

OTHER

"Gyno-Trosyd vaginal cream/tabs." Medicine Info, *E-Doc Online*. October 1999. <http://www.edic.ci.za/nedukubj/oridycts/1072.html>.

"Medaspor vaginal cream." Medicine Info, *E-Doc Online*. October 1999. <http://www.edoc.co.za/medilink/products/1347.html>.

"Procedure For Medication Administration, Procedure 61." *University of Arkansas Online*. December 2000. <http://www.uams.edu/nursingmanual/procedures/procedure61.htm>.

Stanford, Elizabeth K., M.D. "Vaginitis." Virtual Medical Library, *Journal of Family Medicine Online*. April 2001. <http://www.ccspublishing.com/journals/secure/gynecol/secure/vaginitis.htm>.

"Sulfonamides (Vaginal)." Medlineplus, *National Institutes of Health Online*. Micromedex, Inc. January 2001. <http://www.nlm.nih.gov/medlineplus/druginfo/sulfonamidesvaginal202541.html>.

"Vaginal Yeast Infections." Information From Your Family Doctor. *American Academy of Family Physicians Online*. August 2000. <http://familydoctor.org/handouts/206.html>.

Mary Elizabeth Martelli, R.N., B.S.

Varicose veins

Definition

Varicose veins are dilated, tortuous, elongated superficial veins that are usually seen in the legs.

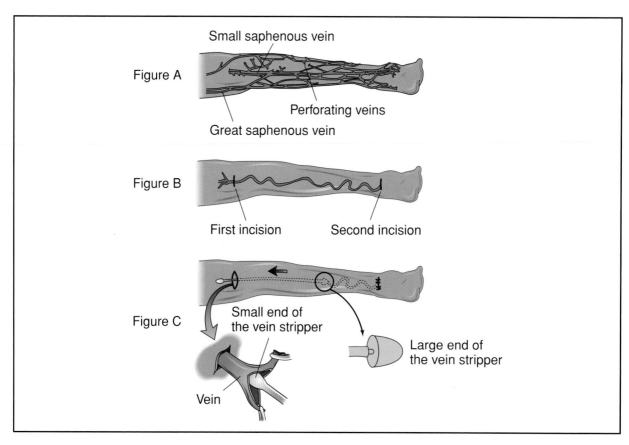

Figure A
Small saphenous vein
Perforating veins
Great saphenous vein

Figure B
First incision
Second incision

Figure C
Small end of the vein stripper
Large end of the vein stripper
Vein

Varicose veins may be removed from the body surgically when they are causing pain and when hemorrhaging or recurrent thrombosis appear. Surgery involves making an incision through the skin at both ends of the section of vein being removed (figure B). A flexible wire is inserted through one end and extended to the other. The wire is then withdrawn, pulling the vein out with it (figure C). *(Illustration by Electronic Illustrators Group. The Gale Group.)*

Description

Varicose veins, also called varicosities, are seen most often in the legs, although they can be found in other parts of the body. Most often, they appear as lumpy, winding vessels just below the surface of the skin. There are three types of veins: superficial veins that are just beneath the surface of the skin, deep veins that are large **blood vessels** found deep inside muscles, and perforator veins that connect the superficial and deep veins. The superficial veins are the **blood** vessels most often affected by varicose veins and are the veins first seen when the varicose condition has developed.

The inside walls of veins have valves that open and close in response to blood flow. When the left ventricle of the **heart** pushes blood out into the aorta, it produces the high pressure pulse of a heartbeat and pushes blood throughout the body. Between heartbeats, there is a period of low **blood pressure**. During the low pressure period, blood in the veins is affected by gravity and tends to flow backward. The valves in the veins prevent this from happening. Varicose veins

start when one or more valves fail to close. The blood pressure in that section of vein increases, causing additional valves to fail. This allows blood to pool and stretch the veins, further weakening the walls of the veins. The walls of the affected veins lose their elasticity in response to increased blood pressure. As the vessels weaken, more and more valves are unable to close properly. The veins become larger and wider over time and begin to appear as lumpy, winding chains underneath the skin. Varicose veins can also develop in the deep veins. Varicose veins in the superficial veins are called primary varicosities, while varicose veins in the deep veins are called secondary varicosities.

Liver disease can cause the appearance of varicose veins in the esophagus or on the surface of the abdomen. These appear in response to increased pressure of blood that is unable to move through a diseased liver. Varicose veins in the esophagus are called esophageal varicosities. Varicose veins on the surface of the abdomen often resemble a spider or the head (caput) of the mythological character Medusa.

Causes and symptoms

The predisposing causes of varicose veins are multiple. Lifestyle and hormonal factors play a role. Some families seem to have a higher incidence of varicose veins, indicating that there may be a genetic component to this disease. Varicose veins are progressive. As one section of a vein weakens, it causes increased pressure on adjacent sections. These sections often develop varicosities. Varicose veins can appear following **pregnancy**, thrombophlebitis, congenital blood vessel weakness, or **obesity**, but are not limited to these conditions. **Edema** of the surrounding tissue, ankles, and calves, is not usually a complication of primary (superficial) varicose veins and, when seen, usually indicates that the deep veins may have varicosities or clots.

Varicose veins are a common problem. Approximately 15% of the adult population in the United States has varicose veins. Women have a much higher incidence of this disease than men. The symptoms can include aching, **pain**, itchiness, or burning sensations, especially when standing. In some cases, with chronically bad veins, there may be a brownish discoloration of the skin or ulcers (open sores) near the ankles. A condition that is frequently associated with varicose veins is spider-burst veins. Spider-burst veins are very small veins that are enlarged. They may be caused by back-pressure from varicose veins, but can be caused by other factors. They are frequently associated with pregnancy, and there may be hormonal factors associated with their development. They are primarily of cosmetic concern and do not present any medical concerns.

Diagnosis

Varicose veins can usually be seen. In cases where varicose veins are suspected, but cannot be seen, a physician may frequently detect them by palpation (pressing with the fingers). X rays or ultrasound tests can detect varicose veins in the deep and perforator veins and rule out blood clots in the deep veins.

Treatment

There is no cure for varicose veins. Treatment falls into two classes: relief of symptoms and removal of the affected veins. Symptom relief includes such measures as wearing support stockings, which compress the veins and hold them in place. This keeps the veins from stretching and limits pain. Other measures are sitting down, using a footstool when sitting, avoiding standing for long periods of time, and raising the legs

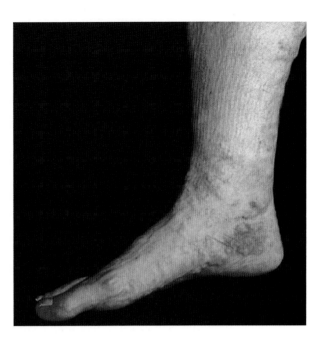

Varicose veins on a man's leg. *(Photograph by Keith, Custom Medical Stock Photo. Reproduced by permission.)*

whenever possible. These measures work by reducing the blood pressure in leg veins. Prolonged standing allows the blood to collect under high pressure in the varicose veins. **Exercise** such as walking, biking, and swimming, is beneficial. When the legs are active, the leg muscles help pump the blood in the veins. This limits the amount of blood that collects in the varicose veins and reduces some of the symptoms. These measures reduce symptoms, but do not stop the disease.

Surgery is also used to remove varicose veins from the body. It is recommended for those that cause pain or are very unsightly and when hemorrhaging or recurrent thrombosis appear. Surgery involves making an incision through the skin at both ends of the section of vein being removed. A flexible wire is inserted through one end and extended to the other. The wire is then withdrawn, pulling the vein out with it. This is called "stripping" and is the most common method to remove superficial varicose veins. As long as the deeper veins are still functioning properly, a person can live without some of the superficial veins. Because of this, stripped varicose veins are not replaced.

Injection therapy is an alternate therapy used to seal varicose veins. This prevents blood from entering the sealed sections of the vein. The veins remain in the body, but no longer carry blood. This procedure can be performed on an out-patient basis and does not require anesthesia. It is frequently

KEY TERMS

Congenital—Existing at or before birth; a condition that developed while the fetus was in utero or as a consequence of the birth process.

Edema—Swelling caused by a collection of fluid in a tissue or body cavity.

Hemorrhage—Bleeding from blood vessels.

Palpation—The process of examining a person using the sense of touch.

Thrombosis—Blockage of a blood vessel due to a clot or thrombus.

used if people develop more varicose veins after surgery to remove the larger varicose veins and to seal spider-burst veins for people concerned about cosmetic appearance. Injection therapy is also called sclerotherapy. At one time, a method of injection therapy was used that did not have a good success rate. Veins did not seal properly and blood clots formed. Modern injection therapy is improved and has a much higher success rate.

Prognosis

Untreated varicose veins become increasingly large and more obvious with time. Surgical stripping of varicose veins is successful for most people. Most do not develop new, large varicose veins following surgery. Surgery does not decrease a person's tendency to develop varicose veins. Varicose veins may develop in other locations after stripping.

Health care team roles

Family physicians or gynecologists often make a initial referral to a vascular surgeon for treatment. Nurses may instruct patients in practices to prevent worsening of the condition, if surgery is not warranted.

Prevention

Varicose veins in the legs can be minimized by maintaining good physical condition and engaging in exercise throughout life. This is especially important for women during pregnancy. Persons who are at risk of developing varicose veins can wear support hosiery. Refraining from standing for long periods of time is helpful. If standing is inevitable, flexing the muscles of the calf every minute or two will help to prevent blood pooling.

Resources

BOOKS

Goldman, Michael P., Robert A. Weiss, and John J. Bergan. *Varicose Veins and Telangiectasias: Diagnosis and Treatment.* 2nd ed. New York: Matthew Medical Books, 1999.

Hull, Russell. "Peripheral Venous Disease." In *Cecil Textbook of Medicine*, 21st ed. Ed. Lee Goldman and J. Claude Bennett. Philadelphia: W.B. Saunders, 2000.

Sadick, Neil S. *Manual of Sclerotherapy.* Philadelphia: Lippincott Williams & Wilkins, 2000.

Townsend, Courtney M. *Sabiston Textbook of Surgery: The Biological Basis of Modern Surgical Practice.* 16th ed. Philadelphia: Saunders, 2001.

Tretbar, L. L. *Venous Disorders of the Legs: Principles and Practice.* New York: Springer Verlag, 1999.

PERIODICALS

de Cossart, L. "Varicose Veins and Pregnancy." *British Journal of Surgery* 88, no. 3 (2001): 323-324.

Foldi, M., and G. Idiazabal. "The Role of Operative Management of Varicose Veins in Patients with Lymphedema and/or Lipedema of the Legs." *Lymphology* 33, no. 4 (2001): 167-171.

Guex, J. J., and M. N. Isaacs. "Comparison of Surgery and Ultrasound Guided Sclerotherapy for Treatment of Saphenous Varicose Veins: Must the Criteria for Assessment be the Same?" *International Journal of Angiology* 19, no. 4 (2000): 299-302.

Tessari, L., A. Cavezzi, and A. Frullini. "Preliminary Experience with a New Sclerosing Foam in the Treatment of Varicose Veins." *Dermatological Surgery* 27, no. 1 (2001): 58-60.

ORGANIZATIONS

American Association for Vascular Surgery. 13 Elm Street, Manchester, MA 01944-1314. (978) 526-8330. <http://www.vascsurg.org/doc/842.html>.

Peripheral Vascular Surgery Society. 824 Munras Avenue, Suite C, Monterey, CA 93940. (831) 373-0508. <http://www.pvss.org> suzanne@DMCcompanies.com.

OTHER

Merck Manual. <http://www.merck.com/pubs/mmanual/section16/chapter212/212h.htm>.

National Library of Medicine. <http://www.nlm.nih.gov/medlineplus/varicoseveins.html>.

University of Michigan School of Medicine. <http://www.med.umich.edu/1libr/topics/circ03.htm>.

L. Fleming Fallon, Jr., MD, DrPH

Vascular headache *see* **Migraine headache**

Vascular sonography

Definition

Vascular sonography, also called vascular ultrasound, is a diagnostic procedure that uses sound waves to produce images of the **blood vessels** and **blood** flow.

Purpose

Vascular sonography is used to evaluate blood flow in the arteries and veins. This test has many applications, including diagnosis of deep vein thrombosis (DVT), claudication, atherosclerosis, and congenital vascular malformations. In addition to its diagnostic capabilities, vascular sonography can be used to determine whether a patient is a good candidate for a vascular procedure such as **angioplasty**. It can also be used to evaluate the success of a surgical procedure such as bypass surgery or graft transplantation (adequate blood flow to the graft would indicate a successful graft transplantation). Furthermore, vascular sonography may be used to determine the blood flow to tumors and chronic **wounds** in order to aid in treatment planning.

Finally, vascular sonography can be used to identify blood clots and other blockages to blood flow. The test can reveal blood clots requiring anticoagulant therapy, blood clots that may embolize (travel) to other organs (including the **lungs**), and blockages to blood flow in the **brain** that might result in a stroke.

Vascular sonography is usually performed in a hospital's radiology department, or its vascular laboratory, which focuses on vascular imaging and evaluation. However, because vascular ultrasound units are portable, vascular sonography can be performed at the bedside of patients in the emergency room, or anywhere else in the hospital, if necessary.

Vascular sonography may be recommended by a primary care physician after detecting sounds of abnormal blood flow (usually via **stethoscope**). It may be performed in patients with suspected narrowing of the carotid arteries in the neck (who are at increased risk of stroke), or in patients with suspected abnormalities in the superficial blood vessels in the arms and legs. It may also be used to detect narrowing of the deeper abdominal vessels (such as the renal arteries and superior mesenteric artery), or to rule out bleeding in the abdomen following trauma.

Precautions

Because smoking can cause constriction of blood vessels, patients should not smoke before vascular sonography.

Description

Medical ultrasound scanning works in a manner similar to sonar and radar. Vascular sonography relies on ultrasonic sound waves transmitted at high frequencies (approximately 2 to 10 megahertz) beyond the level of human **hearing**. The sound waves are aimed at the area of interest. Depending on the tissue or liquid the sound waves encounter, different echoes return to the scanner. The scanner then interprets these echoes to produce an image.

Vascular sonography may be performed using a handheld portable ultrasound scanner or a larger mobile scanner, both of which have an ultrasound probe with a transducer, and a computer that processes the echoed sound waves into an image. Larger scanners are usually equipped with a videotape recorder or digital image acquisition system to record the examination, as well as a medical image printer for hard copies.

For vascular sonography, the patient is positioned on a bed or table so that the area to be imaged can be easily accessed. A special gel, called acoustic coupling gel, is placed on the skin over the area to be imaged to enhance the transmission of sound waves. The probe is held over the area of interest and occasionally moved. The ultrasound probe's transducer emits sound waves that are transmitted through the body and reflected back as echoes, which are then converted into an image. The probe can be positioned along the vessel for a longitudinal scan or across the vessel for a transverse scan. During an abdominal or neck examination, the patient may be asked to hold the breath or stop swallowing. Examinations of the arms and legs may require that the limb be elevated or compressed.

Vascular ultrasound images can be acquired and displayed as gray-scale or Doppler images. Gray-scale images use different shades of gray to indicate differences in the strength of echoes; echoes from blood are of lower strength and appear darker than surrounding tissue. Gray-scale images can depict the layers of the vessel wall and show real-time arterial motion.

Doppler imaging uses the frequency shift caused by the Doppler effect to produce images of blood flow. The Doppler effect is a principle of physics involving light and sound; relative to an observer, the frequency of any light or sound wave will vary as the source of the wave approaches or moves away. Ultrasound scanners with Doppler imaging capability detect and calculate the changes in frequency of the speed of blood flow relative to a computer marker placed by the sonographer. Color Doppler imaging superimposes color over moving structures on the gray-scale images. For example, red and yellow in a blood vessel image indicates flow away from the probe, while blue and green indicates flow toward the probe. Color Doppler imaging can be used to identify areas of arterial narrowing.

When areas of vessel narrowing or obstruction are detected, the sonographer can use the ultrasound scanner to take measurements and make calculations. The scanner's computer allows cursors to be placed on areas to be measured and automatic measurements to be recorded.

Preparation

If the abdominal vessels are being imaged, then the patient is required to fast for six to eight hours before the test, since bowel activity and gas can interfere with the quality of the ultrasound study. Otherwise, no special preparation is necessary.

Aftercare

There is no special aftercare for this examination.

Complications

Because vascular sonography is a noninvasive procedure that does not use radiation, there are no known complications associated with it.

Results

Normal results show normal blood flow in the area under examination.

Abnormal results show abnormalities in blood flow. The sonogram can identify obstructions and abnormalities in vessels, including blood clots, arterial plaques, and stenoses (narrowing). The results might indicate a diagnosis of DVT, internal bleeding (in the abdomen), or inadequate blood flow to a grafted area. Appropriate therapy or surgery is then performed.

Health care team roles

Vascular sonography is performed by an ultrasonographer with special training in vascular ultrasound techniques. The sonographer should be a registered

---

KEY TERMS

Angioplasty—A procedure that seeks to increase blood flow through narrow or occluded vessels.

Atherosclerosis—"Hardening of the arteries"; a build-up of plaque in the arteries that results in vessel narrowing or blockage.

Claudication—A chronic condition caused by narrowing of the arteries to the legs characterized by pain or cramping while walking, primarily in the calf.

Deep vein thrombosis (DVT)—A blood clot in one of the deep veins of the arms or legs characterized by symptoms of pain, redness, and swelling over the affected veins; may result in pulmonary embolism (a clot in the lungs), which can be life threatening.

Graft—Grafts are tissues (or organs) which have been taken from one location and surgically transplanted to another. Grafts may be taken from one person and given to another (for example, organ tranplants), or may be taken from one part of a person and placed on another part (for example, burn victims may have some unaffected skin surgically removed and then placed on the burned area). Other types of grafts also exist.

Renal arteries—The arteries that supply blood to the kidneys.

Superior mesenteric artery—One of the arteries that supplies blood to the abdominal organs.

---

vascular technologist, and the vascular lab should be accredited by the Intersocietal Commission for the Accreditation of Vascular Laboratories (ICAVL). A radiologist or other physician experienced in vascular imaging techniques interprets the ultrasound examination results. During some examinations, the sonographer may print out images for consultation with the radiologist, or the radiologist may perform some of the examination.

Resources

PERIODICALS

Kosoff, George. "Basic Physics and Imaging Characteristics of Ultrasound." *World Journal of Surgery* 24 (February 2000):134-142.

Lunt, Michael John. "Review of Duplex and Colour Doppler Imaging of Lower-Limb Arteries and Veins."

Worldwide Wounds (September 2000). <http://www.worldwidewounds.com/2000/sept/Michael-Lunt/Doppler-Imaging.html>.

Phillips, Gareth W.L. "Review of Arterial Vascular Ultrasound." *World Journal of Surgery* 24 (February 2000): 232-240.

Phillips, Gareth W.L. "Review of Venous Vascular Ultrasound." *World Journal of Surgery* 24 (February 2000): 241-248.

ORGANIZATIONS

American Institute of Ultrasound in Medicine (AIUM). 14750 Sweitzer Lane, Suite 100, Laurel, MD 20707-5906. (301) 498-4100. <http://www.aium.org>.

American Registry of Diagnostic Medical Sonographers (ARDMS). 600 Jefferson Plaza, Suite 360, Rockville, MD 20852-1150. (800) 541-9754. <http://www.ardms.org>.

American Society of Radiologic Technologists (ASRT). 15000 Central Avenue SE, Albuquerque, NM 87123-2778. (800) 444-2778. <http://www.asrt.org>.

Society of Diagnostic Medical Sonography (SDMS). 12770 Coit Road, Suite 708, Dallas, TX 75251-1319. (972) 239-7367. <http://www.sdms.org>.

Society of Vascular Technology(SVT). 4601 Presidents Drive, Suite 260, Lanham, MD 20706. (301) 459-7550. <http://www.svtnet.org>.

OTHER

Dombro, Andy. "Vascular Problems of the Lower Extremities." <http://www.americasdoctor.com>.

Vascular Ultrasound Imaging. <http://www.radiologyinfo.org/content/ultrasound-vascular.htm>.

Jennifer E. Sisk, M.A.

Vascular study *see* **Angiography**

Vasodilatory shock *see* **Shock**

Vasovagal faint *see* **Syncope**

Veganism

Definition

Veganism is a system of dietary and lifestyle practices that seeks to promote health and peace while reducing the suffering of both people and animals. Vegans (pronounced vee-guns) are vegetarians who do not eat any foods (eggs, dairy products, meat, etc.) derived from animal sources. Most vegans also do not use products that require for their production the death or suffering of animals, such as leather, fur, wool, and certain cosmetics.

Origins

The word "vegetarian" was coined in England in 1847 by the founders of the Vegetarian Society of Great Britain. "Vegetarian" has been used to describe people who do not eat meat, but do consume dairy products and eggs. The Vegan Society was founded in England in 1944 by Donald Watson and others who believed that vegetarians should strive to exist without eating or using any animal products at all. Watson stated that the crisis of World War II may have been a motivation behind his founding of the Vegan Society, because he saw so much turmoil and suffering in the world around him. The Vegan founders believed that the first step to creating a better world would be to develop a diet that did not cause the death or suffering of any living beings. The term "vegan" is derived from the Latin word *vegetus*, which means "full of life," which the founders hoped their system would be. "Vegan" also starts with the same three letters as "vegetarian," and ends with the last two, as its founders believed they were starting with vegetarian ideas and taking them to their logical conclusion.

The American Vegan Society (AVS) was founded in 1960 by Jay Dinshah. The same year, the AVS began to publish a journal called *Ahimsa*, which is a Sanskrit word that means "not causing harm" and "reverence for life." Dinshah and others conceived veganism to be a philosophy of living that has nonviolence, peace, harmony, honesty, service to the world, and knowledge as its goals. In 1974, the AVS became affiliated with the North American Vegetarian Society, which was formed to bring together all of the vegetarian groups in North America.

Since the 1970s, there has been a vast amount of research concerning **nutrition** and diet. It has been discovered that diets that are centered around meat and dairy products, such as the typical American diet, are high in cholesterol and saturated fat but low in fiber. These diets have been linked to many health problems, including **heart** disease, strokes, and diabetes, which together cause 68% of all the deaths in the United States. Thus, the interest in diets that reduce or eliminate foods that contribute to these conditions has grown considerably. In 1992, the *Vegetarian Times* magazine took a poll that estimated that 13 million Americans, or 5% of the population, consider themselves vegetarian. Of the vegetarians, 4% are vegans, which amounts to nearly 520,000 Americans.

Benefits

Vegan diets are often recommended as dietary therapy for heart disease, high cholesterol, diabetes, strokes, **cancer**, **obesity**, arthritis, **allergies**, **asthma**, environmental illness, **hypertension**, **gout**, gallstones, **kidney stones**, ulcers, colitis, digestive disorders, premenstrual syndrome, **anxiety**, and depression. At present, however, no studies exist that define the efficacy of vegan diets in treating these conditions. Nevertheless, a well-designed vegan diet is an effective weight-loss diet, and is an economical and easy preventive health practice.

Description

Veganism can be better understood by considering the ethical, ecological, and health reasons that motivate vegans.

Ethical considerations

A vegan lifestyle seeks to promote awareness, compassion, and peace. Veganism is an ethical system as well as a diet. Ethics refers to rules of conduct or the ways in which people interact with others and the world. One poll in England showed that 83% of vegans listed ethical reasons as their main consideration in their practices. Vegans believe that health encompasses not only individuals' bodies, but also includes healthy relationships between people and their actions towards other living things, the earth, and the environment. Vegans believe that as long as animals are treated cruelly and are killed for meat, then the world's ethical and spiritual health will suffer. Vegans believe that people should become aware of how their food choices are creating suffering and affecting the health of the world as a whole. For instance, it has been estimated that the grain that goes to feed livestock in America could feed 1.3 billion people, which would relieve a large measure of the **pain** and suffering in the world.

Vegans claim that egg and dairy production may cause animals just as much suffering as killing them for meat, because modern factory farming treats animals as unfeeling machines instead of as living beings. Eggs are produced by keeping chickens in small cages and in painful and unsanitary conditions. Vegans claim that dairy cattle are subjected to cruel treatment as well, being bred artificially and caged for much of their lives. Dairy cattle are also injected with hormones that make them produce unnaturally high quantities of milk while weakening their immune systems and making them sick and unhealthy. Large amounts of **antibiotics** need to be used on weakened cows, which in turn affects the health of humans and creates diseases that are resistant to medicine. Dairy farming causes death to cows as well because undesirable or old cows are slaughtered for meat.

Other animal products are avoided by vegans as well. Leather, wool, and fur are not used because they result in the suffering of animals from their production. Some vegans do not use honey because they believe that the collection of honey is harmful to bees. Many vegans avoid using sugar, because some sugar is made by using charcoal from the bones of dead cattle. Vegans also do not use products that have been tested on animals, and vegans are active in resisting the use of animals for dissection and medical experiments. Vegans are typically outspoken against hunting and the cruel treatment of animals in zoos or for entertainment (e.g., cockfighting and bullfighting).

Helping the Earth

Vegans believe that their dietary and lifestyle practices would contribute to a healthier world ecology. Vegans can cite many statistics that show that the American meat-centered diet is contributing to environmental problems. The main thrust of vegans' ecological position is that it takes many more resources to produce meat than it does to provide a grain-based diet, and people can be fed better with grain than with meat. For instance, it takes 10 lbs (4.5 kg) of grain to make 1 lb (0.45 kg) of beef. On one acre of land, 20,000 lbs (9,000 kg) of potatoes can be grown compared to 125 lbs (57 kg) of beef during the same time. In America, livestock consume six and a half times as much grain as the entire population. Different dietary habits here could improve the world, vegans argue. Environmental problems caused by the inefficient production of livestock include topsoil loss, water shortages and contamination, deforestation, toxic waste, and air pollution.

Health considerations

People who eat vegetarian diets are at lower risk for many conditions, including heart disease, certain cancers, diabetes, obesity, high **blood pressure**, gallstones, and kidney stones. A vegan diet contains no cholesterol, because cholesterol is found only in animal products. Diets high in cholesterol and saturated fat are responsible for heart disease. American men overall have a 50% risk of having a heart attack, while vegans have only a 4% risk. Vegans consume as much as four times the amount of fiber as the average person, and high fiber intake is believed to reduce the risk of heart disease, diabetes, cancer, and digestive tract problems. Vegan diets are also high in protective nutrients that are found in fruits and vegetables, such as antioxidants.

A vegan diet can also reduce exposure to chemicals that are found in meat and dairy products, such as pesticides and synthetic additives such as hormones. Chemicals tend to accumulate in the tissue of animals that are higher in the food chain, a process called bioaccumulation. By not eating animal products, vegans can avoid the exposure to these accumulated toxins, many of which are believed to influence the development of cancer. It is important, however, for vegans to eat organically produced vegetables and grains, as vegans who eat nonorganic food get high doses of pesticides. One study showed that DDT, a cancer-causing pesticide, was present in significant levels in mother's milk for 99% of American women, but only 8% of vegetarian women had significant levels of the pesticide. The risks of women getting **breast cancer** and men contracting **prostate cancer** are nearly four times as high for frequent meat eaters as for those who eat meat sparingly or not at all. High consumption of dairy products has been linked to diabetes, anemia, **cataracts**, and other conditions.

Vegan diets may also be beneficial for those with allergic or **autoimmune disorders** such as asthma, allergies, and rheumatoid arthritis. Animal products cause allergic reactions in many people, and studies have shown that allergic responses and inflammation may be improved by eliminating animal products from the diet. Furthermore, vegan diets are effective weight loss diets, because the high levels of fiber and low levels of fat make it possible for dieters to eat until they are full and still take in fewer calories than other diets.

Preparations

Those considering veganism may wish to adopt the diet gradually to allow their bodies and lifestyles time to adjust to different eating habits. Some nutritionists have recommended "transition" diets to help people change from a meat-centered diet in stages. Many Americans eat meat products at nearly every meal, and the first stage of a transition diet is to substitute just a few meals a week with wholly vegetarian foods. Then, particular meat products can be slowly reduced and eliminated from the diet and replaced with vegetarian foods. Red meat can be reduced and then eliminated, followed by poultry and fish. For vegans, the final step would be to substitute eggs and dairy products with other nutrient-rich foods. Individuals should be willing to experiment with transition diets, and be patient when learning how to combine veganism with such social activities as dining out.

Vegans should become informed on healthful dietary and nutrition practices as well. Sound nutritional guidelines include decreasing the intake of fat, increasing fiber, and emphasizing fresh fruits, vegetables, legumes, and whole grains in the diet, while avoiding processed foods and sugar. Vegans can experiment with meat substitutes, foods that are high in protein and essential nutrients. Tofu and tempeh are soybean products that are high in protein, **calcium**, and other nutrients. There are "veggie-burgers" that can be grilled like hamburgers, and vegan substitutes for turkey and sausage with surprisingly realistic textures and **taste**. Furthermore, there are many vegan cookbooks on the market, as cooking without meat or dairy products can be challenging for many people.

Vegans should also become familiar with food labels and food additives, because there are many additives derived from animal sources that are used in common foods and in such household items as soap. Vegans may also find social support at local health food stores or food cooperatives.

Precautions

Vegans should be aware of particular nutrients that may be lacking or need special attention in non-animal diets. These include protein, **vitamin B$_{12}$**, **riboflavin**, **vitamin D**, calcium, **iron**, **zinc**, and essential fatty acids. Furthermore, pregnant women, growing children, and people with certain health conditions have higher requirements for these nutrients.

Vegans should be sure to get complete **proteins** in their diets. A complete protein contains all of the essential amino acids, which are essential because the body cannot make them. Meat and dairy products generally contain complete proteins, but most vegetarian foods such as grains and legumes contain incomplete proteins since they lack one or more of the essential amino acids. Vegans can easily obtain complete proteins by combining particular foods. For instance, beans are high in the amino acid lysine but low in tryptophan and methionine. Rice is low in lysine and high in tryptophan and methionine. Thus, a combination of rice and beans makes a complete protein. In general, combining legumes such as soy, lentils, beans, and peas with grains like rice, wheat, or oats forms complete proteins. Nuts or peanut butter with grains such as whole wheat bread also forms complete proteins. Proteins do not necessarily need to be combined in the same meal, but should generally be combined over a period of a few days.

Getting enough vitamin B_{12} is an issue for vegans because meat and dairy products are its main sources. Vegans are advised to take vitamin supplements containing B_{12}. Spirulina, a nutritional supplement made from algae, is used as a vegetarian source of this vitamin, as are fortified soy products and nutritional yeast. The symptoms of vitamin B_{12} deficiency include muscle twitching and irreversible nerve damage; weakness; numbness and tingling in the extremities; and a sore tongue.

Riboflavin (vitamin B_2) is also generally found in high amounts in animal sources, so vegans should be aware of this fact and take a supplement if necessary. Vegetable sources of riboflavin include brewer's yeast, almonds, mushrooms, whole grains, soybeans, and green leafy vegetables.

Vitamin D can be obtained from vitamin supplements, fortified foods, and sunshine. Calcium can be obtained from enriched tofu, seeds, nuts, legumes, and dark green vegetables, including broccoli, kale, spinach, and collard greens. Iron is found in raisins, figs, legumes, tofu, whole grains (particularly whole wheat), potatoes, and dark green leafy vegetables, and by cooking with iron skillets. Iron is absorbed more efficiently by the body when iron-containing foods are eaten with foods that contain **vitamin C**, such as fruits, tomatoes, and green vegetables. Zinc is abundant in nuts, pumpkin seeds, legumes, whole grains, and tofu. Getting enough omega-3 essential fatty acids may be an issue for vegans. These are found in walnuts, canola oil, and such supplements as flaxseed oil. Vegans should consider purchasing organically grown food when possible, to avoid exposure to pesticides and to contribute to sound agricultural practices.

Research and general acceptance

Scientists have analyzed **vegetarianism** more frequently, mainly because there are higher numbers of lacto-ovo vegetarians around the world than there are vegans. Studies have repeatedly shown many benefits of plant-based diets.

A significant study of veganism was published in 1985 in the *Journal of Asthma*, which used a vegan diet to treat asthma. After one year, 92% of patients exhibited significant improvement in asthma symptoms and in such measurements as lung capacity and cholesterol levels. People on the diet also experienced fewer episodes of colds and **influenza**. Researchers concluded that the vegan diet was helpful for asthma because it

---

KEY TERMS

Bioaccumulation—The process in which toxic chemicals collect in the tissues of humans and other animals toward the top of the food chain.

Cholesterol—A steroid fat found in animal foods that is also produced in the body from saturated fat for several important functions. Excess cholesterol intake is linked to many diseases.

Complex carbohydrates—Carbohydrates that are broken down by the body into simple sugars for energy. They are found in grains, fruits, and vegetables. Complex carbohydrates are generally recommended by nutritionists over refined sugar and honey, because they are a better source of energy and often contain fiber and nutrients as well.

Legume—A group of plant foods that includes beans, peas, and lentils. Legumes are high in protein, fiber, and other nutrients.

Organic food—Food grown without the use of synthetic pesticides and fertilizers.

Saturated fat—A fat that is usually solid at room temperature. Saturated fats are found mainly in meat and dairy products but also in such vegetable sources as some nuts, seeds, and avocados.

Unsaturated fat—A type of fat found in plant foods that is typically liquid at room temperature. Unsaturated fats can be monounsaturated or polyunsaturated, depending on their chemical structure. They are the most frequently recommended dietary fats.

---

reduced food allergies, which are commonly caused by animal products. Scientists theorized that the animal-free diet also may have altered the patients' prostaglandin levels. Prostaglandins are hormone-like substances responsible for many body processes including allergic reactions. Finally, researchers proposed that the high quantity of antioxidants and plant nutrients in the vegan diet may have contributed to strengthened immune systems.

Resources

BOOKS

Barnard, Neal, M.D. *Food For Life*. New York: Harmony, 1993.

Stepaniak, Joanne. *The Vegan Sourcebook*. Los Angeles: Lowell House, 1998.

PERIODICALS

Ahimsa. American Vegan Society (AVS). 56 Dinshah Lane. PO Box H. Malaga, NY 08328. (609) 694-2887.

Vegetarian Journal. Vegetarian Resource Group (VRG). PO Box 1463. Baltimore, MD 21203.

ORGANIZATIONS

Vegan Outreach. 211 Indian Drive. Pittsburgh, PA 15238. (412) 968-0268.

Douglas Dupler

Vegetarianism

Definition

Vegetarianism is the voluntary abstinence from eating meat. Vegetarians refrain from eating meat for various reasons, including religious, health, and ethical ones. Lacto-ovo vegetarians supplement their diet with dairy (lactose) products and eggs (ovo). Vegans (pronounced vee-guns) do not eat any animal-derived products at all.

Origins

The term vegetarian was coined in 1847 by the founders of the Vegetarian Society of Great Britain, but vegetarianism has been around as long as people have created diets. Some of the world's oldest cultures advocate a vegetarian diet for health and religious purposes. In India, millions of Hindus are vegetarians because of their religious beliefs. One of the ancient mythological works of Hinduism, the *Mahabharata*, states that, "Those who desire to possess good **memory**, beauty, long life with perfect health, and physical, moral and spiritual strength, should abstain from animal foods." The **yoga** system of living and health is vegetarian, because its dietary practices are based on the belief that healthy food contains *prana*. Prana is the universal life energy, which yoga experts believe is abundant in fresh fruits, grains, nuts and vegetables, but absent in meat because meat has been killed. Yogis also believe that spiritual health is influenced by the practice of *ahimsa*, or not harming living beings. The principle of *ahimsa* (non-violence) appears in the Upanishads (Vedic literature) from c. 600–300 B.C. Taking of animal life or human life under any circumstances is sinful and results in rebirth as a lower organism. It became a fundamental element of Jainism, another religion of India. Some Buddhists in Japan and China are also vegetarian because of spiritual beliefs. In the Christian tradition, the Trappist Monks of the Catholic Church are vegetarian, and some vegetarians argue that there is evidence that Jesus and his early followers were vegetarian. Other traditional cultures, such as those in the Middle East and the Mediterranean regions, have evolved diets that frequently consist of vegetarian foods. The Mediterranean diet, which a Harvard study declared to be one of the world's healthiest, is primarily, although not strictly, vegetarian.

The list of famous vegetarians forms an illustrious group. The ancient Greek philosophers, including Socrates, Plato, and Pythagoras, advocated vegetarianism. In modern times, the word to describe someone who likes to feast on food and wine is "epicure," but it is little known that Epicurus, the ancient philosopher, was himself a diligent vegetarian. Other famous vegetarians include Leonardo da Vinci, Sir Isaac Newton, Leo Tolstoy, Ralph Waldo Emerson, and Henry Thoreau. This century's celebrated vegetarians include Gandhi, the physician Albert Schweitzer, writer George Bernard Shaw, musician Paul McCartney, and champion triathlete Dave Scott. Albert Einstein, although not a strict vegetarian himself, stated that a vegetarian diet would be an evolutionary step for the human race.

Vegetarianism in America received a lot of interest during the last half of the nineteenth century and the beginning of the twentieth century, during periods of experimentation with diets and health practices. Vegetarianism has also been a religious practice for some Americans, including the Seventh-day Adventists, whose lacto-ovo vegetarian diets have been studied for their health benefits. Vegetarianism has been steadily gaining acceptance as an alternative to the meat-and-potatoes bias of the traditional American diet. In 1992, *Vegetarian Times* magazine performed a poll that showed that 13 million Americans, or 5% of the population, identified themselves as vegetarians.

Several factors contribute to the interest in vegetarianism in America. Outbreaks of **food poisoning** from meat products, as well as increased concern over the additives in meat such as hormones and **antibiotics**, have led some people and professionals to question meat's safety. There is also an increased awareness of the questionable treatment of farm animals in factory farming. But the growing health consciousness of Americans is probably the major reason for the surge in interest in vegetarianism. **Nutrition** experts have built up convincing evidence that there are major problems with the conventional American diet, which is centered around meat products that are high in cholesterol and saturated fat and low in fiber. **Heart** disease, **cancer**, and diabetes, which cause 68% of all deaths in America, are all believed to be influenced by this diet. Nutritionists have repeatedly shown in studies that a healthy diet consists of plenty of fresh vegetables and fruits, complex **carbohydrates** such as whole grains, and foods that are high in fiber and low in cholesterol and saturated fat. Vegetarianism, a diet that fulfills all these criteria, has become part of many healthy lifestyles. In alternative medicine, vegetarianism is a cornerstone dietary therapy, used in Ayurvedic medicine, detoxification treatments, macrobiotics, the Ornish diet for heart disease, and in therapies for many chronic conditions.

Benefits

Vegetarianism is recommended as a dietary therapy for a variety of conditions, including heart disease, high cholesterol, diabetes, and stroke. Vegetarianism is a major dietary therapy in the alternative treatment of cancer. Other conditions treated with a dietary therapy of vegetarianism include **obesity**, **osteoporosis**, arthritis, **allergies**, **asthma**, environmental illness, **hypertension**, **gout**, gallstones, hemorrhoids, **kidney stones**, ulcers, colitis, premenstrual syndrome, **anxiety**, and depression. Vegetarians often report higher energy levels, better digestion, and mental clarity. Vegetarianism is an economical and easily implemented preventative practice as well.

Preparations

Some people, particularly those with severe or chronic conditions such as heart disease or cancer, may be advised by a health practitioner to become vegetarian suddenly. For most people, nutritionists recommend that a vegetarian diet be adopted gradually, to allow people's bodies and lifestyles time to adjust to new eating habits and food intake.

Some nutritionists have designed transition diets to help people become vegetarian in stages. Many Americans eat meat products at nearly every meal, and the first stage of a transition diet is to substitute just a few meals a week with wholly vegetarian foods. Then, particular meat products can be slowly reduced and eliminated from the diet and replaced with vegetarian foods. Red meat can be reduced and then eliminated, followed by pork, poultry, and fish. For those wishing to become pure vegetarians or vegans, the final step would be to substitute eggs and dairy products with other nutrient-rich foods. Individuals should be willing to experiment with transition diets, and should have patience when learning how to combine vegetarianism with social activities such as dining out.

The transition to vegetarianism can be smoother for those who make informed choices with dietary practices. Sound nutritional guidelines include decreasing the intake of fat, increasing fiber, and emphasizing fresh fruits, vegetables, legumes, and whole grains in the diet while avoiding processed foods and sugar. Everyone can improve their health by becoming familiar with recommended dietary and nutritional practices, such as reading labels and understanding basic nutritional concepts such as daily requirements for calories, protein, fat, and nutrients. Would-be vegetarians can experiment with meat substitutes, foods that are high in protein and essential nutrients. Thanks to the growing interest in vegetarianism, many meat substitutes are now readily available. Tofu and tempeh are products made from soybeans that are high in protein, **calcium**, and other nutrients. There are "veggie-burgers" that can be grilled like hamburgers, and vegetarian substitutes for turkey and sausage with surprisingly authentic textures and **taste**. There are many vegetarian cookbooks on the market as well.

Precautions

In general, a well-planned vegetarian diet is healthy and safe. However, vegetarians, and particularly vegans who eat no animal products, need to be aware of particular nutrients that may be lacking in non-animal diets. These are amino acids, **vitamin B_{12}**, **vitamin D**, calcium, **iron**, **zinc**, and essential fatty acids. Furthermore, pregnant women, growing children, and those with health conditions have higher requirements for these nutrients.

Vegetarians should be aware of getting complete proteins in their diets. A complete protein contains all of the essential amino acids, which are the building blocks for protein essential to the diet because the body cannot make them. Meat and dairy products generally contain complete **proteins**, but most vegetarian foods such as grains and legumes contain incomplete proteins, lacking one or more of the essential amino acids. However, vegetarians can easily overcome this by combining particular foods in order to create complete proteins. For instance, beans are high in the amino acid lysine but low in tryptophan and methionine, but rice is low in lysine and high in tryptophan and methionine. Thus, combining rice and beans makes a complete protein. In general, combining legumes such as soy, lentils, beans, and peas with grains like rice, wheat, or oats forms complete proteins. Eating dairy products or nuts with grains also makes proteins complete. Oatmeal with milk on it is complete, as is peanut butter on whole wheat bread. Proteins do not necessarily need to be combined in the same meal, but generally within four hours.

Getting enough vitamin B_{12} may be an issue for some vegetarians, particularly vegans, because meat and dairy products are the main sources. Vitamin supplements that contain vitamin B_{12} are recommended. Spirulina, a nutritional supplement made from algae, is also a vegetarian source, as are fortified soy products and nutritional yeast.

Vitamin D can be obtained by **vitamins**, fortified foods, and sunshine. Calcium can be obtained in enriched tofu, seeds, nuts, legumes, dairy products, and dark green vegetables including broccoli, kale, spinach, and collard greens. Iron is found in raisins, figs, legumes, tofu, whole grains (particularly whole wheat), potatoes, and dark green leafy vegetables. Iron is absorbed more efficiently by the body when iron-containing foods are eaten with foods that contain **vitamin C**, such as fruits, tomatoes, and green vegetables. Zinc is abundant in nuts, pumpkin seeds, legumes, whole grains, and tofu. For vegetarians who don't eat fish, getting enough omega-3 essential fatty acids may be an issue, and supplements such as flax-seed oil should be considered, as well as eating walnuts and canola oil.

Vegetarians do not necessarily have healthier diets. Some studies have shown that some vegetarians consume large amounts of cholesterol and saturated fat. Eggs and dairy products contain cholesterol and saturated fat, while nuts, oils, and avocados are vegetable sources of saturated fat. To reap the full benefits of a vegetarian diet, vegetarians should be conscious of cholesterol and saturated fat intake. Vegetarians may also consider buying organic foods, which are grown without the use of synthetic chemicals, as another health precaution.

Research and general acceptance

A vegetarian diet has many well-documented health benefits. It has been shown that vegetarians have a higher life expectancy, as much as several years, than those who eat a meat-centered diet. The U.S. Food and Drug Administration (FDA) has stated that data has shown vegetarians to have a strong or significant probability against contracting obesity, heart disease, **lung cancer**, colon cancer, **alcoholism**, hypertension, diabetes, gallstones, gout, kidney stones, and ulcers. However, the FDA also points out that vegetarians tend to have healthy lifestyle habits, so other factors may contribute to their increased health besides diet alone.

A vegetarian diet, as prescribed by Dr. Dean Ornish, has been shown to improve heart disease and reverse the effects of atherosclerosis, or hardening of the arteries. It should be noted that Dr. Ornish's diet was used in conjunction with **exercise**, **stress** reduction, and other holistic methods. The Ornish diet is lacto-ovo vegetarian, because it allows the use of egg whites and non-fat dairy products.

Vegetarians have a resource of statistics in their favor when it comes to presenting persuasive arguments in favor of their eating habits. Vegetarians claim that a vegetarian diet is a major step in improving the health of citizens and the environment. Americans eat over 200 lbs (91 kg) of meat per person per year. The incidence of heart disease, cancer, diabetes, and other diseases has increased along with a dramatic increase in meat consumption during the past century. Many statistics show significantly smaller risks for vegetarians contracting certain conditions. The risks of women getting **breast cancer** and men contracting prostrate cancer are nearly four times as high for frequent meat eaters as for those who eat meat sparingly or not at all. For heart attacks, American men have a 50% risk of having one, but the risk drops down to 15% for lacto-ovo vegetarians and to only 4% for vegans. For cancer, studies of populations around the world have implied that plant-based diets have lower associated risks for certain types of cancer.

Vegetarians claim other reasons for adopting a meat-free diet. One major concern is the amount of pesticides and synthetic additives such as hormones that show up in meat products. Chemicals tend to accumulate in the tissue of animals that are higher in the food chain, a process called bioaccumulation. Vegetarians, by not eating meat, can avoid the exposure to these accumulated toxins, many of which are known to influence the development of cancer. One study showed that DDT, a cancer-causing pesticide, was present in significant levels in mother's milk for 99% of American women, but only 8% of vegetarian women had significant levels of the pesticide. Women who eat meat had 35 times higher levels of particular pesticides than vegetarian women. The synthetic hormones and antibiotics added to American cattle has led some European countries to ban American beef altogether. The widespread use of antibiotics in livestock has made many infectious agents more resistant to them, making some diseases harder to treat.

KEY TERMS

Cholesterol—A steroid fat found in animal foods that is also produced in the body from saturated fat for several important functions. Excess cholesterol intake is linked to many diseases.

Complex carbohydrates—Complex carbohydrates are broken down by the body into simple sugars for energy, are found in grains, fruits, and vegetables. They are generally recommended in the diet over refined sugar and honey, because they are a more steady source of energy and often contain fiber and nutrients as well.

Legume—Group of plant foods including beans, peas, and lentils, which are high in protein, fiber, and other nutrients.

Organic food—Food grown without the use of synthetic pesticides and fertilizers.

Saturated fat—Fat that is usually solid at room temperature, found mainly in meat and dairy products but also in vegetable sources such as some nuts, seeds, and avocados.

Unsaturated fat—Fat found in plant foods that is typically liquid (oil) at room temperature. They can be monounsaturated or polyunsaturated, depending on the chemical structure. Unsaturated fats are the most recommended dietary fats.

Vegetarians resort to ethical and environmental arguments as well when supporting their food choices. Much of U.S. agriculture is dedicated to producing meat, which is an expensive and resource-depleting practice. It has been estimated that 1.3 billion people could be fed with the grain that America uses to feed livestock, and starvation is a major problem in world health. Producing meat places a heavy burden on natural resources, as compared to growing grain and vegetables. One acre of land can grow approximately 40,000 lbs (18,000 kg) of potatoes or 250 lbs (113 kg) of beef, and it takes 50,000 gal (200,000 l) of water to produce 1 lb (0.45 kg) of California beef but only 25 gal (100 l) of water to produce 1 lb (0.45 kg) of wheat. Half of all water used in America is for livestock production. Vegetarians argue that the American consumption of beef may also be contributing to global warming, by the large amounts of fossil fuels used in its production. The South American rainforest is being cleared to support American's beef consumption, as the United States yearly imports 300 million lbs (136 million kg) of meat from Central and South America.

The production of meat has been estimated as causing up to 85% of the loss of topsoil of America's farmlands.

Despite the favorable statistics, vegetarianism does have its opponents. The meat industry in America is a powerful organization that has spent millions of dollars over decades advertising the benefits of eating meat. Vegetarians point out that life-long eating habits are difficult to change for many people, despite research showing that vegetarian diets can provide the same nutrients as meat-centered diets.

Resources

BOOKS

Akers, Keith. *A Vegetarian Sourcebook*. New York: Putnam, 1993.

Null, Gary. *The Vegetarian Handbook*. New York: St. Martins, 1987.

Robbins, John. *Diet for a New America*. Walpole, New Hampshire: Stillpoint, 1987.

PERIODICALS

Vegetarian Journal. Vegetarian Resource Group (VRG). PO Box 1463, Baltimore, MD 21203.

Vegetarian Nutrition and Health Letter. 1707 Nichol Hall, Loma Linda, CA 92350. (888) 558-8703.

Vegetarian Times. 4 High Ridge Park, Stamford, CT 06905. (877) 321-1796.

ORGANIZATIONS

North American Vegetarian Society (NAVS). PO Box 72, Dolgeville, NY 13329. (518) 568-7970.

Douglas Dupler

Venography *see* **Phlebography**

Venous Doppler ultrasound

Definition

Venous Doppler ultrasound, also called sonography and ultrasonography, is a noninvasive, painless procedure used to evaluate blood flow in major veins in the arms and legs. It uses high frequency sound waves that are above the level of human hearing (ultrasound). In Doppler ultrasound, these sound waves are transmitted through the body and are echoed back to produce images of blood flow in body tissues and organs.

Purpose

Venous Doppler ultrasound is used to assess the direction, velocity, and turbulence of blood flow through major veins in the patient's arms, legs, and neck. A Doppler study of blood flow can be used to diagnose many conditions, such as blood clots, incompetent valves in leg veins, which cause fluid to accumulate (venous insufficiency) or deep vein thrombosis. A blood clot forms when blood changes from a flowing liquid into a solid mass. A clot located in the heart or a blood vessel is a called a thrombus. Clots are usually found in veins. These clots can cause thrombosis, which is the obstruction of blood flow through the blood vessel. Deep vein thrombosis is a condition caused when a clot develops in the large vein. This condition usually occurs in the legs and arms.

The Doppler exam is also used to diagnose varicose veins. Varicose leg vein symptoms include swelling of the legs, twisted or enlarged leg veins, and leg discomfort. The test is also used to map a patient's veins. This provides information about portions of damaged veins that may need to be removed. Doppler ultrasound can be used to evaluate and diagnose tumors with vascular involvement and aids in the placement of a catheter, a narrow tube placed in a blood vessel. Venous Doppler ultrasound is done as an alternative to venography, which is an invasive procedures with greater risks to the patient than Doppler ultrasound. Diagnostic Doppler ultrasound can also be performed on arteries (see arterial Doppler ultrasound).

Precautions

Venous Doppler ultrasonography is harmless, as it uses no ionizing (x-ray) radiation, and there are no known harmful effects. It is a safe procedure for pregnant women and does not affect cardiac pacemakers, metal implants or metal fragments lodged in the body.

Although the ultrasound test is not painful, the transducer is pressed on the skin and may cause discomfort in a patient already experiencing pain from conditions such as swollen limbs.

Cigarette smoking may alter the results of the test, as nicotine can cause arteries in the extremities to constrict.

Description

Ultrasound is the medical use of sound waves with frequencies too high to be heard by humans. Ultrasound waves used for medical imaging are usually in the range of 2 to 10 megahertz (MHz). During this procedure, an instrument called a transducer converts electrical signals into ultrasound waves, directs the high-frequency sound waves to the vein being tested, and then converts the returning ultrasound waves that bounce off the body tissue back into electrical signals. These electrical signals can be converted into images by a computer. Computer images may be preserved as recorded movement or as still pictures.

Doppler ultrasound takes advantage of the Doppler effect, a physics principle that states that relative to an observer, the frequency of any sound or light wave will vary as the source of the wave approaches or moves away. For example, the pitch of a siren changes as a police car moves toward, past, and then away from the listener. When used to evaluate blood flow, sound waves increase in frequency when they echo from red blood cells moving toward the transducer and decrease in frequency when they move away from the transducer. The change in frequency is related to the velocity of the moving red blood cells and can be measured to determine the velocity of the blood flow. Flowing blood also makes a sound that can be heard with Doppler ultrasound.

Doppler ultrasound tests usually take between 30 and 60 minutes. Exam length is based on factors such as the location of the area to be scanned and the difficulty in obtaining images. The procedure begins with the patient being positioned for the scan. The patient may recline or stand. The health professional applies a water-soluble gel to the skin over the area to be scanned. The health care worker then places the transducer on the area covered by gel and moves the device on the skin.

Diagnostic information from the transducer is relayed in several ways:

- Continuous-wave Doppler is the simplest mode. Information is received from all of the moving reflectors in the path of the beam.

- In pulsed-wave Doppler, the transducer sends a series of short sound pulses into the body, with pauses between each pulse to allow for the detection of the returning sounds that are echoing back from the red blood cells. Pulsed-wave Doppler allows the operator to select a specific area of interest for flow analysis.

- The duplex Doppler ultrasound scan is also known as 2-D or two-dimensional ultrasound. The duplex procedure uses two types of ultrasound at the same time. Information from the scan is relayed to a computer, which creates an image of blood vessels and organs. The images change continuously and may be filmed or taped. The computer also transforms the reflected sound into a graph that charts information about the direction and velocity of blood flow.

- The color Doppler ultrasound produces a two-dimensional image of a blood vessel. The test also transforms reflected sound into colors that are displayed on the a computer monitor. These colors indicate the velocity and direction of blood flow. For example, red and blue indicate that the flow is away from the transducer, while blue and green indicate that the blood is flowing towards the transducer. The colors can be superimposed on the image of the blood vessel.

- The power Doppler ultrasound scan is more sensitive than the color Doppler ultrasound. The sensitivity of this scan allows evaluation of areas that are unscannable by other ultrasound methods. The power Doppler scan is useful in examining small blood vessels.

The fee for venous Doppler ultrasound tests varies. Cost factors include the type of tests needed and the areas to be scanned. Medical insurance usually covers a portion of the test cost.

Preparation

Patients are advised to dress comfortably for the venous Doppler ultrasound test. Clothing, jewelry, and other items must be removed from the area to be scanned. The health care provider should be informed of any medications that the patient is taking, especially blood pressure and vascular medications that could interfere with interpretation of results. If a scan of the abdomen is planned, the patient may be instructed to fast six or more hours before the test.

Aftercare

No aftercare is required.

Complications

As of late 2005, there were no known complications related to the venous Doppler ultrasound test.

Results

Normal results for venous Doppler ultrasound show healthy vessels and unobstructed blood flow. Abnormal results revealed by Doppler ultrasound include the presence of blood clots in veins, closed

---

KEY TERMS

Artery—A blood vessel that carries blood away from the heart to the rest of the body.

Blood clot—A solid substance that develops in arteries or veins that can block the flow of blood and have serious health effects.

Blood vessel—A tube in which blood circulates. Arteries, arterioles capillaries, venules, and veins are blood vessels.

Varicose vein—An enlarged, twisted vein usually located in the leg.

Vein—A blood vessel that carries blood from a part of the body back toward the heart.

---

veins, deep vein thrombosis and arterial conditions including arteriosclerosis, and arterial occlusion.

Health care team roles

A venous Doppler ultrasound examination may be performed by a physician, radiologist, or technologist. The radiologist is a physician and can interpret the test results. The primary-care physician usually discusses test results with the patient and if needed will prescribe treatment for conditions revealed by the test.

The technologist is an allied health professional with special training to perform ultrasound tests (a sonographer). Education for technologists and sonographers ranges from one to four years of training. The length of the program depends on factors such as whether the person is earning a degree or a professional certificate and what other ultrasound tests they are learning to perform.

Patient education consists of informing the patient about the test procedure. This can be done in advance by providing the patient with printed material about the venous Doppler ultrasound exam.

Resources

BOOKS

Evans, David and W. Norman McDicken. *Doppler Ultrasound: Physics, Instrumentation and Signal Processing*. Hoboken, NJ: John Wiley & Sons, 2000.

Kremkau, Frederick, James Eckenhoff, and Leroy Vandam. *Diagnostic Ultrasound: Principles and Instruments*. Philadelphia: Elsevier Health Sciences, 2005.

Ridgway, Donald P. *Introduction to Vascular Scanning: A Guide for the Complete Beginner*. Pasadena, CA: Davies Publishing, Inc., 2004.

PERIODICALS

Kyrle, Paul A; Eichinger, Sabine. "Deep Vein Thrombosis." *The Lancet* 365 (March 26, 2005): 1163.

ORGANIZATIONS

American College of Radiology. 1891 Preston White Dr., Reston, VA 20191-4397. (703) 648-8900. http://www.acr.org.

Radiological Society of North America. Jorie Blvd., Oak Brook, IL 60523-2251. (800) 381-6660. http://www.rsna.org.

Society for Vascular Ultrasound. 4601 Presidents Dr., Suite 260, Lanham, MD 20706-4831. (301) 459-7550. http://www.svunet.org.

OTHER

Johnson, Steve. "Mining Waves to Treat Varicose Veins." *Knight-Ridder/Tribune News Service* (Sept. 13, 2005) http://www.mercurynews.com.

Liz Swain

Ventilation assistance

Definition

Ventilation assistance includes a variety of methods designed to help restore or improve breathing function in patients who are unable to adequately breathe on their own. These methods range from at-home **oxygen therapy** for patients with chronic obstructive pulmonary disease (COPD) to mechanical ventilation for patients with acute **respiratory failure**. Ventilation assistance therapies usually include the following categories:

• oxygen therapy
• continuous positive airway pressure (CPAP)
• hyperbaric oxygen therapy
• mechanical ventilation
• newborn life support

Purpose

Ventilation assistance is used for disease or injury that causes progressive or sudden respiratory failure. It may also be used after surgery until patients recover enough to breathe adequately on their own. Physicians choose the therapy based on the type and stage of the disease process, as well as on the results of **blood** and pulmonary function tests that indicate the oxygenation status of the patient.

Oxygen therapy

Home oxygen therapy is commonly ordered for patients with COPD, and is usually started when a patient's pulse oximetry (amount of hemoglobin saturated with oxygen) is below 90% on room air. Oxygen therapy is also used in the hospital to support a patient's respiratory status after illness, injury, or surgery.

Continuous positive airway pressure (CPAP)

One of the most common uses of CPAP is for patients with sleep apnea. It may also be used for both infants and adults with **respiratory distress syndrome**, collapse of lung tissue (atelectasis), or abnormalities of the lower airways.

Hyperbaric oxygen therapy

Hyperbaric oxygen therapy is used when there is an immediate need for greater blood oxygen saturation. Divers with **decompression sickness** (the bends), climbers with altitude sickness, patients suffering from severe **carbon monoxide poisoning**, and children or adults in acute respiratory distress may require hyperbaric oxygenation. In recent years, physicians have also used this therapy to assist in burn and wound healing, since the pressure under which the oxygen is delivered can reach areas that have an inadequate blood supply under normal conditions.

Mechanical ventilation

Mechanical ventilation is used for patients with acute respiratory distress, temporarily after surgery, or while sedated or pharmacologically paralyzed. Most patients can be weaned off of mechanical ventilation and resume breathing on their own. Some patients require long-term mechanical ventilation (i.e., quadriplegia) and, in some cases, mechanical ventilation is considered life-support for patients who would otherwise die.

Newborn life support

Newborn babies, particularly those who are born premature, may require ventilation assistance immediately after birth, since their **lungs** may not be fully developed. Some newborns may have serious respiratory problems or complications from birth, such as respiratory distress syndrome, neonatal wet lung syndrome, apnea of prematurity, or persistent fetal circulation (delayed closure of the ductus arteriosis and foramen ovale).

Precautions

Ventilation assistance can be beneficial during acute illness and it may provide a higher quality of life if the patient has end-stage COPD. However, oxygen is not a benign substance, and precautions must be used with any of these therapies.

Oxygen therapy

Oxygen is an extremely flammable gas, so patients who smoke should not have oxygen therapy prescribed. If there are family members who smoke, they must avoid smoking in the area of oxygen use.

Continuous positive airway pressure (CPAP)

Although CPAP can be very helpful in alleviating the symptoms of sleep apnea, it can also be uncomfortable because patients must wear a tight-fitting mask over their nose and the oxygen is pushed into their airway with considerable force. Patients who are unable or unwilling to comply with the physician's instructions regarding the use of CPAP are not likely to have it prescribed.

Hyperbaric oxygen therapy

Hyperbaric oxygen therapy involves administering 100% oxygen at three times the normal atmospheric pressure. This creates a high risk for fire and explosive decompression, as well as a risk for pulmonary and neurological toxicity. The benefits must be weighed against the potential complications. All patients, particularly children, must be carefully monitored while in the hyperbaric chamber.

Mechanical ventilation

The use of mechanical ventilation can cause pulmonary damage from high pressures. It is often frightening for patients because they are hooked up to an endotracheal or tracheostomy tube that prevents them from speaking and may make them feel like they are breathing through a straw. Usually, patients require sedation or even pharmacological **paralysis** to prevent accidental removal of the tube and to keep them from fighting against the ventilator.

Newborn life support

Not all infants with breathing problems require mechanical ventilation. The physician makes the determination based on the maturity and respiratory condition of the infant. Bronchopulmonary dysplasia is a chronic pulmonary disease that can develop in **premature infants** from high pressures and high oxygen levels delivered during mechanical ventilation.

Description

Oxygen therapy

Supplemental oxygen may be ordered for a patient who has pulse oximetry values below 90% on room air. The primary purpose of oxygen therapy is to prevent damage to vital organs caused by inadequate oxygen supply. Since there is a risk of oxygen toxicity, the lowest possible level of oxygen (measured in liters/minute) is ordered to maintain the patient's pulse oximetry at an acceptable level. The oxygen is administered via nasal cannula, mask, or tracheostomy.

Patients with chronic hypoxemia often receive long-term oxygen therapy at home. A physician must prescribe home oxygen and the patients' pulse oximetry is monitored to ensure that they are receiving the correct amount of oxygen. Some patients require oxygen therapy only at night or when exercising.

The type of home oxygen system chosen varies depending on availability, cost, and the mobility of the patient. Patients who are ambulatory, especially those who work, need a system with a small portable tank. Frequent oxygen delivery and refilling of portable tanks is necessary.

In the case of respiratory distress in both newborns and adults, oxygen therapy may be attempted before mechanical ventilation since it is noninvasive and less expensive. Oxygen is also effective in treating patients with other diseases such as **cystic fibrosis**, chronic congestive **heart failure**, or other lung diseases.

Continuous positive airway pressure (CPAP)

Sleep apnea is caused by the collapse of the upper airway. CPAP administers a constant pressure during both inhalation and exhalation, which prevents a collapse. CPAP is usually administered through a tight-fitting mask as humidified oxygen. (When CPAP is administered through an endotracheal or tracheostomy tube, it is not used for sleep apnea). Patients receiving CPAP in a hospital setting must have continuous vital sign monitoring, along with periodic sampling of blood gas values.

Hyperbaric oxygen therapy

Hyperbaric oxygen therapy delivers pure oxygen under pressure that is three times that of normal atmospheric pressure. This treatment is especially effective for treating decompression sickness in scuba divers. The oxygen is delivered inside of a plastic cylinder-shaped chamber that is large enough for the patient to lie down in. The therapy usually lasts one hour, although it can take up to five hours. Before the patient exits the chamber, the pressure is gradually lowered back to normal atmospheric level.

Mechanical ventilation

In general, mechanical ventilation replaces or supports the normal ventilatory lung function of the patient. Although mechanical ventilation is usually used for acute illness or injury in an intensive care setting, patients who require long-term mechanical ventilation can receive it at home under the supervision of a physician and home health agency. The patient must have a tracheostomy for long-term therapy.

There are several modes of mechanical ventilation, each offering different advantages and disadvantages. Many can be used in conjunction with one another.

CONTROL VENTILATION (CV). CV delivers the preset volume or pressure regardless of the patient's own inspiratory efforts. This mode is used for patients who are unable to initiate a breath. If it is used with spontaneously breathing patients, they must be sedated and/or pharmacologically paralyzed so they do not breathe out of synchrony with the ventilator.

ASSIST-CONTROL VENTILATION (A/C) OR CONTINUOUS MANDATORY VENTILATION (CMV). Both A/C and CMV deliver the preset volume or pressure in response to the patient's inspiratory effort, but will initiate the breath if the patient does not do so within the set amount of time. This mode is used for patients who can initiate a breath but who have weakened respiratory muscles. The patient may need to be sedated to limit the number of spontaneous breaths as hyperventilation can occur in patients with high respiratory rates.

SYNCHRONOUS INTERMITTENT MANDATORY VENTILATION (SIMV). SIMV delivers the preset volume or pressure and preset respiratory rate while allowing the patient to breathe spontaneously. The vent initiates each breath in synchrony with the patient's breaths. SIMV is used as a primary mode of ventilation as well as a weaning mode. (During weaning, the preset rate is gradually reduced, allowing patients to slowly regain breathing on their own.) The disadvantage of this mode is that it may increase the work of breathing and respiratory muscle fatigue. Breathing spontaneously through ventilator tubing has been compared to breathing through a straw.

POSITIVE-END EXPIRATORY PRESSURE (PEEP). PEEP is positive pressure that is applied by the ventilator at the end of expiration. This mode does not deliver breaths but is used as an adjunct to CV, A/C, and SIMV to improve oxygenation by opening collapsed alveoli at the end of expiration. Complications from the increased pressure can include decreased cardiac output, lung rupture, and increased intracranial pressure.

PRESSURE SUPPORT VENTILATION (PSV). PSV is preset pressure that augments the patient's spontaneous inspiration effort and decreases the work of breathing. The patient completely controls the respiratory rate and tidal volume. PSV is used for patients with a stable respiratory status and is often used with SIMV during weaning.

INTERMITTENT POSITIVE PRESSURE BREATHING (IPPB). IPPB is a form of assisted ventilation in which compressed oxygen is delivered under positive pressure into the patient's airway until a preset pressure is reached. Exhalation is passive. The cycle is repeated for the ordered number of breaths. IPPB is often used for a short time after a patient is weaned off of a ventilator to promote maximal lung expansion and to help clear secretions.

Newborn life support

Premature infants, particularly those born before the 28th week of gestation, have underdeveloped breathing muscles and immature lungs. These infants require respiratory support either by oxygen hood or through mechanical ventilation. The length of time that support is needed depends on the infant's gestational age and respiratory effort. CPAP can be delivered through a nasal or endotracheal tube by a ventilator that is specifically designed for neonates. As the infant's respiratory status improves, the ventilator can be weaned off.

Preparation

In an acute situation, preparation for any of these treatments includes gathering equipment and educating the patient and/or family about the treatment. At-home oxygen therapy or mechanical ventilation requires education and cooperation with a home health agency and respiratory therapist. Blood and pulmonary function tests are done to assist in individualizing the treatment for the patient.

Aftercare

Blood and pulmonary function tests are performed to verify that the treatment was successful or to monitor and adjust treatments if the therapy is long term. Mechanical ventilation requires frequent oral, nasal, or **tracheostomy care** for the area surrounding the insertion site of the breathing tube.

Complications

Ventilation assistance can be life saving, but these therapies also create their own set of complications and side effects.

Oxygen therapy

At-home oxygen therapy carries risk if patients or their families do not handle the oxygen in a safe manner. Patients and their families should not smoke near the oxygen supply and they should keep the tank and tubing away from any source that could cause electrical spark, flames, or intense heat.

Continuous positive airway pressure (CPAP)

The effectiveness of CPAP for sleep apnea may be limited if patients do not apply the mask properly or if they do not wear it while sleeping. Possible complications of CPAP include skin abrasions from the mask, nasal congestion, nasal or oral dryness, and discomfort from the pressure of oxygen delivery.

Hyperbaric oxygen therapy

Hyperbaric oxygen therapy is painless; however, the high atmospheric pressure can lead to pulmonary and neurological oxygen toxicity. As with any oxygen therapy, there is the risk of flammability or explosion.

Mechanical ventilation

One complication of mechanical ventilation may be patients' dependence on the ventilator and the inability to wean them off. The physician should carefully select the mode of ventilation and monitor each patient's progress to prevent this complication. Intubation and mechanical ventilation are frightening and uncomfortable for many patients and they may fight the ventilator. If this occurs, the patient should be sedated, and pharmacologically paralyzed if needed, to promote optimal ventilation. However, prolonged sedation and paralysis can cause complications as well. Intubation may cause irritation to the trachea and larynx, and a tracheostomy can be associated with a risk of bleeding, pneumothorax (punctured lung), local **infection**, and increased incidence of aspiration.

Newborn life support

Mechanical ventilation in neonates can result in bronchopulmonary dysplasia from lung injury caused by high oxygen concentrations and high pressures. It also increases the risk of infection in premature babies. Complications of PEEP or CPAP can include pneumothorax and decreased cardiac output.

Results

Oxygen therapy

In the case of COPD, oxygen therapy does not treat the disease but can prolong life, increase quality of life, and delay the onset of more serious symptoms. Effective oxygen therapy for any patient should lead to improved or sustained levels of oxygen in arterial blood.

Continuous positive airway pressure (CPAP)

Successful CPAP should result in a reduction in periods of apnea for patients with sleep apnea. Hospitalized patients on CPAP should show improvement in blood gas values and pulse oximetry.

Hyperbaric oxygen therapy

After one or two treatments, scuba divers undergoing emergency treatment in a hyperbaric chamber should exhibit immediate improvement in oxygen levels throughout the body, regardless of blood flow restrictions. Patients receiving oxygen chamber therapy for difficult **wounds** may receive treatments daily for several weeks before satisfactory results are reached. Patients with carbon monoxide **poisoning** should show improvement in neurologic function. Results of hyperbaric oxygen therapy depend largely on how quickly the patient was transported to the chamber, as well as on the severity of the initial condition.

Mechanical ventilation

Successful mechanical ventilation should result in a gradual decrease in dependence on the ventilator, with eventual complete restoration of

KEY TERMS

Aspiration—Accidental suction of fluids or vomit into the respiratory system.

Endotracheal tube—Tube inserted into the trachea via either the oral or nasal cavity for the purpose of providing a secure airway and delivery of mechanical ventilation.

Hypoventilation—Reduced gas exchange in the lungs resulting in low oxygen levels and high carbon dioxide levels.

Hypoxemia—Deficient oxygen supply in the blood.

Pharmacological paralysis—Paralysis induced by medication to promote optimal mechanical ventilation.

Pneumothorax—Air in the plerual space that can exert pressure on the heart and opposite lung, leading to decreased cardiac and pleural function.

Pulse oximetry—Measure of the percent of hemoglobin saturated with oxygen.

Tracheostomy—Surgically created opening in the trachea for the purpose of providing a secure airway and long term ventilation assistance.

patient's respiratory status and the level of effectiveness of the treatments. The respiratory therapist generally makes any ventilator changes ordered by the physician and sets up equipment required for treatment. Both the nurse and respiratory therapist are responsible for documenting their assessment of the patient's respiratory status. Both are also responsible for teaching the patient and family about the chosen treatment.

The nurse, respiratory therapist, or lab personnel may be responsible for drawing arterial **blood gases**, but the results are obtained by lab personnel. The nurse may need to inform the physician of the results, as changes in treatment may need to be made. The respiratory therapist often administers pulmonary function tests and reports the results to the physician.

Resources

BOOKS

Norris, June, ed. *Critical Care Skills: A Nurse's Photo Guide.* Springhouse, PA: Springhouse Corporation, 1996.

Porth, C. *Pathophysiology: Concepts of Altered Health States.* Philadelphia, PA: Lippincott, 1998.

Thelan, Lynne, et al. *Critical Care Nursing: Diagnosis and Management.* St. Louis, MO: Mosby, 1998.

ORGANIZATIONS

American Lung Association. 800-LUNG-USA or 800-586-4872. <http://www.lungusa.org>.

Hyperbaric Research and Treatment Center. <http://www.hyperbaricrx.com>.

Abby Wojahn, R.N., B.S.N., C.C.R.N.

spontaneous respiration. A COPD exacerbation may be successfully treated with mechanical ventilation, and the patient may return to home oxygen therapy. Pediatric patients on long-term mechanical ventilation at home should demonstrate normal growth and development. Some patients in a hospital intensive care unit may be unable to breathe again without the ventilator; if the ventilator is the only thing keeping them alive, families and physicians may have to make hard decisions about continuing life support.

Newborn life support

Ventilation assistance is considered successful when the infant's respiratory rate is reduced by 30–40%, **chest x ray** and oxygen levels are improved, and the infant is able to breathe spontaneously.

Health care team roles

The nurse and respiratory therapist are responsible for carrying out the physician's orders for any type of ventilation assistance. The nurse monitors the

Ventilation management

Definition

Ventilation management involves providing optimal mechanical ventilation in order to promote the patient's recovery and to reestablish spontaneous breathing.

Purpose

Mechanical ventilation is used when a patient is unable to breathe adequately on their own. The purpose of ventilation management is to "breathe for them" until they are sufficiently recovered to initiate respiration. This process is usually a gradual one, and is referred to as weaning. During the ventilatory weaning process, the modes of mechanical ventilation are gradually changed to allow the patient to initiate more breaths while the ventilator provides less.

Precautions

Ventilatory weaning should not be attempted until the patient's respiratory status is stable and they are arousable and able to follow commands. If the patient is unstable or unarousable, attempting to wean may cause unnecessary physical **stress** and may delay recovery.

Description

The ventilatory weaning process is accomplished by decreasing the number of breaths supplied by the ventilator, as well as by changing the way in which those breaths are delivered to the patient. The process also depends on the reason why the patient requires mechanical ventilation. For example, post-operative cardiac bypass patients are generally weaned within a few hours after surgery. However, a patient with extensive lung disease may require days or weeks to wean.

There are three primary methods used to wean patients from the ventilator. These include T-piece, synchronized intermittent mandatory ventilation and pressure support ventilation. A short description of each of these is included here. The method chosen depends on the patient's respiratory status and on how long they have been on the ventilator.

T-piece trials consist of alternating intervals of time on the ventilator with intervals of spontaneous breathing. To facilitate spontaneous breathing, the patient is removed from the ventilator and a T-shaped tube is attached to the endotracheal tube or tracheostomy tube. One end of this tubing is attached to an oxygen flowmeter and the other end is open. The amount of oxygen to be used is ordered by the physician. The patient on a T-piece doesn't have the ventilator as back-up if they can't breathe, so they must be monitored closely. If they tire out or their respiratory status becomes unstable, they should be reconnected to the ventilator. The goal of this method of weaning is to gradually increase the amount of time spent off the ventilator.

Synchronized intermittent mandatory ventilation (SIMV) is a ventilator mode that delivers a preset number of breaths to the patient but coordinates them with the patient's spontaneous breaths. Thus, the ventilator may be set to deliver 12 breaths per minute but the patient's respiratory rate may be 16 (12 ventilator-initiated breaths plus four patient-initiated breaths.) The goal of SIMV weaning is to gradually decrease the number of breaths delivered by the ventilator, which allows the patient to take more breaths of their own. The ventilator rate is usually decreased by one to three breaths at a time and an arterial **blood** gas (ABG) is obtained 30 minutes after the change to assess the patient's respiratory status. The benefits of SIMV weaning are that the patient has the ventilator for back-up if they fail to take a breath and the ventilator alarms will sound if they are not tolerating weaning. However, the patient should still be closely monitored for signs of respiratory fatigue.

Pressure support ventilation (PSV) augments the patient's spontaneous inspiration with a positive pressure "boost." This decreases the resistance created from breathing through ventilator tubing and is used with the SIMV mode to decrease the work of breathing.

If the patient tolerates SIMV weaning, the ventilator mode may be changed to constant positive airway pressure (CPAP) as a final trial of spontaneous breathing prior to removing the endotracheal tube. In this mode, patients will breathe on their own but have the benefit of the ventilator alarms if they have difficulty. CPAP maintains constant positive pressure in the airways, which facilitates **gas exchange** in the alveoli. PSV is often used with the CPAP mode to further decrease the work of breathing. If the patient tolerates CPAP, the endotracheal tube is removed and a face mask with humidified oxygen is applied for a short time. If the patient remains stable, a nasal cannula may be used to deliver oxygen.

If the patient has a tracheostomy, the weaning process is the same as with a endotracheal tube, with the exception that after the ventilator is disconnected, a tracheostomy collar may be used to deliver humidified oxygen instead of a face mask or nasal cannula. This is simply a mask-like device that fits loosely over the tracheostomy and is held in place by an elastic band around the neck.

Preparation

As discussed earlier, the patient's respiratory status must be stable and they must be arousable and able to follow commands prior to initiating weaning. Patients who require mechanical ventilation are often kept sedated or even paralyzed with drugs to facilitate optimal ventilation. These drugs must be tapered off prior to weaning.

Weaning criteria should be done to determine the patient's readiness to wean. The best indicators include a vital capacity of at least 10-15 cc/kg and a negative inspiratory fraction of greater than -30 cm H$_2$O, however, many other factors are also measured. The patient should be suctioned prior to any weaning attempt, both orally and via the endotracheal tube or tracheostomy. A **pulse oximeter** and **cardiac monitor** should be applied if they are not already present. Weaning should be done when there is adequate staffing so the patient can be closely monitored.

Aftercare

The patient's respiratory status should be assessed after any period of weaning. The ventilator should be securely reconnected and the patient made comfortable and reassured if necessary.

Complications

The greatest risk of ventilator weaning (especially premature weaning) is respiratory distress. The patient must be closely monitored and the weaning stopped before the respiratory distress becomes too great to control. Patients may also have **anxiety** or fear about weaning, which can complicate their respiratory distress.

Results

The goal of ventilation management is to wean the patient from mechanical support and to reestablish spontaneous respiration.

Health care team roles

The nurse and respiratory therapist share equal roles in ventilator management. Both are responsible for suctioning and monitoring the patient during weaning periods. Since the nurse is at the bedside the most, they have the primary monitoring role and are often able to predict the best time for a weaning trial. It is the nurse's responsibility to communicate with the respiratory therapist in planning when weaning trials will occur. The respiratory therapist is generally responsible for making the actual ventilator changes. Both the nurse and respiratory therapist document the ventilator change and their assessment of the patient's respiratory status before, during, and after the weaning period. Both are responsible for teaching and reassuring the patient and family regarding the weaning process.

Patients may be fearful about weaning because it is difficult for them to communicate around the endotracheal tube or tracheostomy. They may be afraid no one will know if they're having difficulty breathing. The nurse should explain all procedures before

---

KEY TERMS

Alveoli—Saclike structures in the lungs where oxygen and carbon dioxide exchange takes place.

Endotracheal tube—Tube inserted into the trachea via either the oral or nasal cavity for the purpose of providing a secure airway.

Negative inspiratory fraction—The amount of force used to draw air into the lungs during maximal inspiration.

Pulse oximeter—Noninvasive machine that measures the amount of hemoglobin that is saturated with oxygen.

Tracheostomy—Surgically created opening in the trachea for the purpose of providing a secure airway. This is used when the patient requires long term ventilatory assistance.

Ventilator—Device used to provide assisted respiration and positive pressure breathing.

Vital capacity—Maximum volume of air that can be expelled from the lungs after a maximal inspiration.

---

performing them, reassure the patient that they will be closely monitored, and ensure that the patient's call light is within reach. It is important that the patient actually see the nurse enter the room frequently, as this is the only way they will know they are being monitored.

Resources

BOOKS

Thelan, Lynne, et al. *Critical Care Nursing: Diagnosis and Management*. St. Louis, MO: Mosby, 1998.

PERIODICALS

Hanneman, H. "Weaning from Short Term Mechanical Ventilation" *Critical Care Nurse* 19, no. 5 (1999): 86-89.

Abby Wojahn, RN, BSN, CCRN

Ventilators

Definition

A ventilator is a device used to provide assisted respiration and positive-pressure breathing.

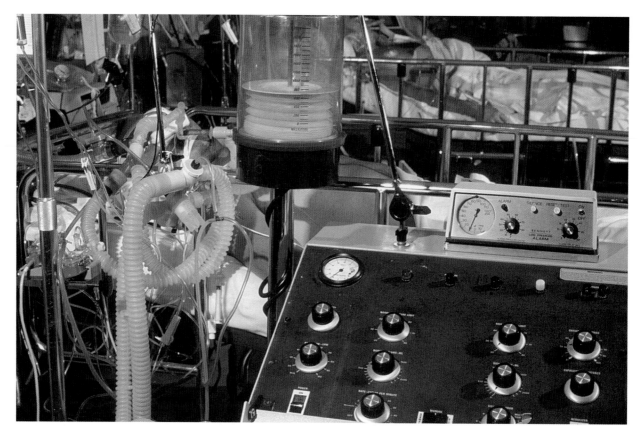

Ventilators assist with respiration for patients who cannot breathe on their own due to respiratory failure from trauma, paralysis, or other causes. *(M. English, MD/Custom Medical Stock Photo. Reproduced by permission.)*

Purpose

Ventilators are used to provide mechanical ventilation for patients with **respiratory failure** who cannot breathe effectively on their own. They are also used to decrease myocardial gas consumption or intracranial pressure, provide stability of the chest wall after trauma or surgery, and when a patient is sedated or pharmacologically paralyzed.

Description

Different types of ventilators can be programmed to provide several modes of mechanical ventilation. A brief overview of each type and mode follows.

Negative-pressure ventilators

The original ventilators used negative pressure to remove and replace gas from the ventilator chamber. Examples of these include the iron lung, the Drinker respirator, and the chest shell. Rather than connecting to an artificial airway, these ventilators enclosed the body from the outside. As gas was pulled out of the ventilator chamber, the resulting negative pressure caused the chest wall to expand, which pulled air into the **lungs**. The cessation of the negative pressure caused the chest wall to fall and exhalation to occur. While an advantage of these ventilators was that they did not require insertion of an artificial airway, they were noisy, made nursing care difficult, and the patient was not able to ambulate.

Positive-pressure ventilators

Postive-pressure ventilators require an artificial airway (endotracheal or tracheostomy tube) and use positive pressure to force gas into a patient's lungs. Inspiration can be triggered either by the patient or the machine. There are four types of positive-pressure ventilators: volume-cycled, pressure-cycled, flow-cycled, and time-cycled.

VOLUME-CYCLED VENTILATORS. This type delivers a preset tidal volume then allows passive expiration. This is ideal for patients with acute **respiratory distress syndrome** (ARDS) or bronchospasm, since the same tidal volume is delivered regardless of the amount of airway resistance. This type of ventilator is the most commonly used in critical care environments.

PRESSURE-CYCLED VENTILATORS. These ventilators deliver gases at a preset pressure, then allow passive expiration. The benefit of this type is a decreased risk of lung damage from high inspiratory pressures, which is particularly beneficial for neonates who have a small lung capacity. The disadvantage is that the tidal volume delivered can decrease if the patient has poor lung compliance and increased airway resistance. This type of ventilation is usually used for short-term therapy (less than 24 hours). Some ventilators have the capability to provide both volume-cycled and pressure-cycled ventilation. These combination ventilators are also commonly used in critical care environments.

FLOW-CYCLED VENTILATORS. Flow-cycled ventilators deliver oxygenation until a preset flow rate is achieved during inspiration.

TIME-CYCLED VENTILATORS. Time-cycled ventilators deliver oxygenation over a preset time period. These types of ventilators are not used as frequently as the volume-cycled and pressure-cycled ventilators.

Modes of ventilation

Mode refers to how the machine will ventilate the patient in relation to the patient's own respiratory efforts. There is a mode for nearly every patient situation; plus, many different types can be used in conjunction with each other.

CONTROL VENTILATION (CV). CV delivers the preset volume or pressure regardless of the patient's own inspiratory efforts. This mode is used for patients who are unable to initiate a breath. If it is used with spontaneously breathing patients, they must be sedated and/or pharmacologically paralyzed so they don't breathe out of synchrony with the ventilator.

ASSIST-CONTROL VENTILATION (A/C) OR CONTINUOUS MANDATORY VENTILATION (CMV). A/C or CMV delivers the preset volume or pressure in response to the patient's inspiratory effort, but will initiate the breath if the patient does not do so within a preset amount of time. This mode is used for patients who can initiate a breath but who have weakened respiratory muscles. The patient may need to be sedated to limit the number of spontaneous breaths, as hyperventilation can occur in patients with high respiratory rates.

SYNCHRONOUS INTERMITTENT MANDATORY VENTILATION (SIMV). SIMV delivers the preset volume or pressure and preset respiratory rate while allowing the patient to breathe spontaneously. The vent initiates each breath in synchrony with the patient's breaths. SIMV is used as a primary mode of ventilation as well as a weaning mode. (During weaning, the preset rate is gradually reduced, allowing the patient to slowly regain breathing on their own.) The disadvantage of this mode is that it may increase the effort of breathing and cause respiratory muscle fatigue. (Breathing spontaneously through ventilator tubing has been compared to breathing through a straw.)

POSITIVE-END EXPIRATORY PRESSURE (PEEP). PEEP is positive pressure that is applied by the ventilator at the end of expiration. This mode does not deliver breaths but is used as an adjunct to CV, A/C, and SIMV to improve oxygenation by opening collapsed alveoli at the end of expiration. Complications from the increased pressure can include decreased cardiac output, lung rupture, and increased intracranial pressure.

CONSTANT POSITIVE AIRWAY PRESSURE (CPAP). CPAP is similar to PEEP, except that it works only for patients who are breathing spontaneously. The effect of CPAP (and PEEP) is compared to inflating a balloon but not letting it completely deflate before inflating it again. The second inflation is easier to perform because resistance is decreased. CPAP can also be administered using a mask and CPAP machine for patients who do not require mechanical ventilation but who need respiratory support (for example, patients with sleep apnea).

PRESSURE SUPPORT VENTILATION (PSV). PS is preset pressure which augments the patient's spontaneous inspiration effort and decreases the work of breathing. The patient completely controls the respiratory rate and tidal volume. PS is used for patients with a stable respiratory status and is often used with SIMV during weaning.

INDEPENDENT LUNG VENTILATION (ILV). This method is used to ventilate each lung separately in patients with unilateral lung disease or a different disease process in each lung. It requires a double-lumen endotracheal tube and two ventilators. Sedation and pharmacologic **paralysis** are used to facilitate optimal ventilation and increase comfort for the patient on whom this method is used.

HIGH FREQUENCY VENTILATION (HFV). HFV delivers a small amount of gas at a rapid rate (as much as 60-100 breaths per minute). This is used when conventional mechanical ventilation would compromise hemodynamic stability, during short-term procedures, or for patients who are at high risk for lung rupture. Sedation and/or pharmacologic paralysis are required.

INVERSE RATIO VENTILATION (IRV). The normal inspiratory:expiratory ratio is 1:2, but this is reversed during IRV to 2:1 or greater (the maximum is 4:1). This method is used for patients who are still hypoxic, even with the use of PEEP. Longer inspiratory time increases the amount of air in the lungs at the end of expiration (the functional residual capacity) and improves oxygenation by reexpanding collapsed alveoli. The shorter expiratory time prevents the alveoli from collapsing again. This method requires sedation and therapeutic paralysis because it is very uncomfortable for the patient.

Ventilator settings

Ventilator settings are ordered by a physician and are individualized for the patient. Ventilators are designed to monitor most components of the patient's respiratory status. Various alarms and parameters can be set to warn healthcare providers that the patient is having difficulty with the settings.

RESPIRATORY RATE. The respiratory rate is the number of breaths the ventilator will deliver to the patient over a specific time period. The respiratory rate parameters are set above and below this number, and an alarm will sound if the patient's actual rate is outside the desired range.

TIDAL VOLUME. Tidal volume is the volume of gas the ventilator will deliver to the patient with each breath. The usual setting is 5-15 cc/kg. The tidal volume parameters are set above and below this number and an alarm sounds if the patient's actual tidal volume is outside the desired range. This is especially helpful if the patient is breathing spontaneously between ventilator-delivered breaths since the patient's own tidal volume can be compared with the desired tidal volume delivered by the ventilator.

OXYGEN CONCENTRATION (FIO$_2$). Oxygen concentration is the amount of oxygen delivered to the patient. It can range from 21% (room air) to 100%.

INSPIRATORY:EXPIRATORY (I:E) RATIO. As discussed above, the I:E ratio is normally 1:2 or 1:1.5, unless inverse ratio ventilation is desired.

PRESSURE LIMIT. Pressure limit regulates the amount of pressure the volume-cycled ventilator can generate to deliver the preset tidal volume. The usual setting is 10-20 cm H$_2$O above the patient's peak inspiratory pressure. If this limit is reached the ventilator stops the breath and alarms. This is often an indication that the patient's airway is obstructed with mucus and is usually resolved with suctioning. It can

also be caused by the patient coughing, biting on the endotracheal tube, breathing against the ventilator, or by a kink in the ventilator tubing.

FLOW RATE. Flow rate is the speed with which the tidal volume is delivered. The usual setting is 40-100 liters per minute.

SENSITIVITY/TRIGGER. Sensitivity determines the amount of effort required by the patient to initiate inspiration. It can be set to be triggered by pressure or by flow.

SIGH. The ventilator can be programmed to deliver an occasional sigh with a larger tidal volume. This prevents collapse of the alveoli (atelectasis) which can result from the patient constantly inspiring the same volume of gas.

Operation

Many ventilators are now computerized and have a user-friendly control panel. To activate the various modes, settings, and alarms, the appropriate key need only be pressed. There are windows on the face panel which show settings and the alarm values. Some ventilators have dials instead of computerized keys, e.g., the smaller, portable ventilators used for transporting patients.

The ventilator tubing simply attaches to the ventilator on one end and to the patient's artificial airway on the other. Most ventilators have clamps that prevent the tubing from draping across the patient. However, there should be enough slack so that the artificial airway isn't accidentally pulled out if the patient turns.

Ventilators are electrical equipment so they must be plugged in. They do have battery back up, but this is not designed for long-term use. It should be ensured that they are plugged into an outlet that will receive generator power if there is an electrical power outage. Ventilators are a method of life-support. If the ventilator should stop working, the patient's life will be in jeopardy. There should be a bag-valve-mask device at the bedside of every patient receiving mechanical ventilation so they can be manually ventilated if needed.

Maintenance

When mechanical ventilation is initiated, the ventilator goes through a self-test to ensure it is working properly. The ventilator tubing should be changed every 24 hours and another self-test run afterwards. The **bacteria** filters should be checked for occlusions or tears and the water traps and filters should be checked for condensation or contaminants. These should be emptied and cleaned every 24 hours and as needed.

Health care team roles

The respiratory therapist is generally the person who sets up the ventilator, does the daily check described above, and changes the ventilator settings based on the physician's orders. The nurse is responsible for monitoring the alarms and the patient's respiratory status. The nurse is also responsible for notifying the respiratory therapist when mechanical problems occur with the ventilator and when there are new physician orders requiring changes in the settings or the alarm parameters. The physician is responsible for keeping track of the patient's status on the current ventilator settings and changing them when necessary.

Training

Training for using and maintaining ventilators is often done via hands-on methods. Critical care nurses usually have a small amount of class time during which they learn the ventilator modes and settings. They then apply this knowledge while working with patients on the unit under the supervision of a nurse preceptor. This preceptorship usually lasts about six weeks (depending upon the nurse's prior experience) and includes all aspects of critical care. Nurses often learn the most from the respiratory therapists, since ventilator management is their specialty.

Respiratory therapists complete an educational program that specifically focuses on respiratory diseases, and equipment and treatments used to manage those diseases. During orientation to a new job, they work under the supervision of an experienced respiratory therapist to learn how to maintain and manage the ventilators used by that particular institution. Written resources from the company that produced the ventilators are usually kept in the **respiratory therapy** department for reference.

Physicians generally do not manage the equipment aspect of the ventilator. They do, however, manage the relation of the ventilator settings to the patient's condition. They gain this knowledge of physiology during medical school and residency.

KEY TERMS

Alveoli—Saclike structures in the lungs where oxygen and carbon dioxide exchange takes place.

Bag-valve-mask device—Device consisting of a manually compressible bag containing oxygen and a one-way valve and mask that fits over the mouth and nose of the patient.

Endotracheal tube—Tube inserted into the trachea via either the oral or nasal cavity for the purpose of providing a secure airway.

Hemodynamic stability—Stability of blood circulation, including cardiac function and peripheral vascular physiology.

Hypoxic—Abnormal deficiency of oxygen in the arterial blood.

Intracranial pressure—The amount of pressure exerted inside the skull by brain tissue, blood, and cerebral-spinal fluid.

Peak inspiratory pressure—The pressure in the lungs at the end of inspiration.

Pharmacologically paralyzed—Short-term paralysis induced by medications for a therapeutic purpose.

Tracheostomy tube—Surgically created opening in the trachea for the purpose of providing a secure airway. This is used when the patient requires long-term ventilatory assistance.

Weaning—The process of gradually tapering mechanical ventilation and allowing the patient to resume breathing on their own.

Resources

BOOKS

Marino, P. *The ICU Book.* Baltimore: Williams & Wilkins, 1998.

Thelan, Lynne, et al. *Critical Care Nursing: Diagnosis and Management.* St. Louis: Mosby, 1998.

OTHER

Puritan-Bennett 7200 Series Ventilator System Pocket Guide. Booklet. Mallinckrodt, 2000.

Abby Wojahn, R.N., B.S.N., C.C.R.N.

Ventilatory weaning process *see* **Ventilation management**

Vertebral column

Definition

The vertebral column is a flexible column, formed by a series of bones called vertebrae. It is part of the axial skeleton and consists of seven cervical, 12 thoracic, five lumbar, five sacral, and four coccygeal vertebrae. Its major function is to enclose and protect the **spinal cord** and provide structural support to the head and trunk.

Description

The vertebral column—or spinal column—is composed of a series of 33 separate bones known as vertebrae. It is located in the trunk of the body and extends from the base of the **skull** to the pelvis. It belongs to the axial skeleton, meaning that portion of the skeleton associated with the **central nervous system** that also includes the bones of the cranium, ribs, and breastbone. The vertebral column consists of seven cervical—or neck—vertebrae, twelve thoracic vertebrae, and five lumbar vertebrae, followed by the sacrum, composed of five fused vertebrae, and by four coccygeal vertebrae which are sometimes fused together and called the coccyx. The coccyx—or tailbone—is the last bone of the vertebral column.

Vertebrae are stacked on top of one another from the first cervical vertebra, called C1 or the atlas, to the sacrum. Only the first 24 vertebrae are considered movable. Both the superior and inferior surfaces of each vertebra are covered by a thin layer of cartilage joined to disk-shaped pads of fibrous cartilage, called intervertebral disks, that cushion the vertebrae and stabilize the vertebral column while allowing it to move. Each disk has a jelly-like core, the nucleus pulposus surrounded by a ring of tough fibrous tissue, the annulus fibrosus. The vertebrae are also bound together by two strong ligaments running the entire length of the vertebral column and by smaller ligaments between each pair of connecting vertebrae. Several groups of muscles are also attached to the vertebrae, providing additional support as well as movement control. The length of the vertebral column depends on the height of the vertebrae and the thickness of the intervertebral disks.

There are four normal curvatures in the vertebral column of the adult that align the head with a straight line through the pelvis. In the region of the chest and sacrum, they curve inwards and each is known as a kyphosis. In the lower back and neck regions, they curve outward and each is known as a lordosis.

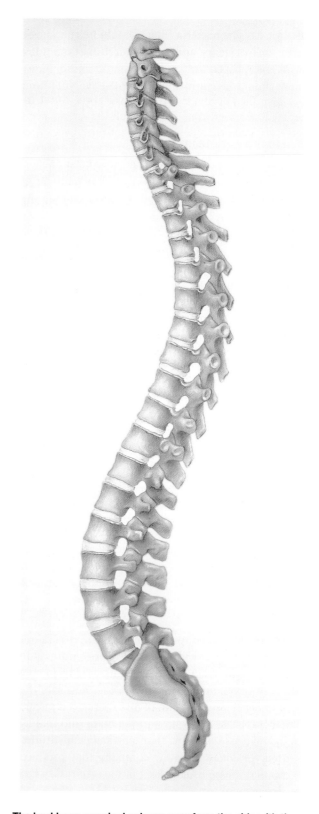

The backbone or spinal column seen from the side with the front of the spine at left. The spine is a flexible column of small compact bones called vertebrae. It extends from the base of the skull to the small of the back and encloses and protects the spinal cord. *(Michel Gilles / Photo Researchers, Inc. Reproduced by permission.)*

All vertebrae have common features. A typical vertebra consists of two parts: an arch that encloses an opening called a vertebral foramen; and a body. Since the vertebrae are all stacked on top of one another, the foramina form the vertebral canal that houses the spinal cord from which the spinal nerves emerge. The body of a vertebra is a round, stocky part on the surface of which the intervertebral disk lies and it has two projections, called pedicles, that connect around the foramen to similar bony projections on the arch called facets. Besides enclosing the foramen with its facets, an arch also has three bony spikes, a spinous process located directly opposite the body and two transverse processes on each side of the foramen. These bony elements serve as important sites of attachment for deep back muscles. There are also differences between vertebrae, depending on their location in the column:

- The cervical vertebrae. The seven cervical vertebrae are numbered C1 to C7. Together, they make up the bony axis of the neck. Typical cervical vertebrae have large vertebral foramina, and oval-shaped vertebral bodies. They are the smallest vertebrae of the column, but their bone density is higher than that of all the other vertebrae. The transverse processes of the cervical vertebrae are special because they also contain transverse foramina, which are passageways for arteries leading to the **brain**. The two first cervical vertebrae are special, because they provide a seat for the head. C1 directly supports and balances the skull. It has practically no body and looks like a ring with two transverse processes. On its upper surface, C1 also has two kidney-shaped facets that link it to the skull. The other special cervical vertebra is C2. It forms an axis which bears a tooth-like odontoid process on its body. This bony spike projects upward and lies in the ring of C1. As the head is turned from side to side, C1 thus pivots around the odontoid process of C2.

- The thoracic vertebrae. The thoracic vertebrae are numbered T1 to T12 and are located in the chest area. They are larger than the cervical vertebrae. They have round foramina and long, pointed spinous processes that slope downward. Thoracic vertebrae have a unique feature, additional facets on the sides of their bodies that join them with the ribs. Starting with T3 and moving down, their bodies increase in size.

- The lumbar vertebrae. The lumbar vertebrae are numbered L1 to L5. They feature large, massive bodies, triangular foramina, and robust spinous and transverse processes. Their facets are oriented so as to favor a wide range of bending flexibility. Lumbar vertebrae also contain small extra bony processes on their bodies that serve as sites of attachment for back muscles.

- The sacrum. In the adult, the sacrum consists of five vertebrae that are fused together. It has a characteristically wide body curved upon itself and a triangular foramen. It is shorter and wider in the female than in the male. It links with L5 above and the coccyx below and it articulates on each side with the bones of the pelvis forming the sacroiliac joints with the iliac bones on either side. In addition to its characteristic shape, it contains two additional foramina through which spinal nerves pass.

- The coccyx. The tailbone is a small triangular bone consisting of four fused rudimentary vertebrae. The number of coccygeal vertebrae may be five or three. They all lack pedicles and spinous processes, but a primitive body and transverse processes can be recognized in each of the first three vertebrae. The last vertebra is a mere small nodule of bone.

Function

The vertebral column has several major functions. It protects the sensitive spinal cord, which it encloses. It functions as a strong and flexible rod that allows movement of the trunk. It supports the head and acts as a pivot. It is also a point of structural attachment for the ribs.

Role in human health

The vertebral column plays a major protective role in human health because it encloses the spinal cord, that delicate bundle of nerve tissue which carries nerve impulses between the brain and the rest of the body. The vertebral column also plays another important role, not only in providing structural support for the chest, but also in maintaining the posture of the body and in locomotion.

Common diseases and disorders

Injuries to the vertebral column are common and are usually caused by one of three types of severe pressure: longitudinal compression, hinging, or shearing. Longitudinal compression usually occurs as a result of a fall from a height, and it crushes one vertebra lengthwise against another. Hinging can occur in **whiplash** injuries: it subjects the vertebral column to sudden and violent acceleration and recoil motions.

Annulus fibrosus—Peripheral ring of fibrous tissue in an intervertebral disk.

Atlas—The atlas is the first cervical vertebra, C1, the one upon which the base of the skull rests. Along with C2, it provides the pivot assembly around which the skull rotates.

Axial skeleton—The skeleton associated with the central nervous system and that consists of the cranium, all the bones of the vertebral column, the ribs, and the sternum. Those portions of the skeleton not associated with the central nervous system are associated with the appendicular skeleton or the skeleton of the extremities, such as the arms and legs.

Central nervous system (CNS)—One of two major divisions of the nervous system. The CNS consists of the brain, the cranial nerves and the spinal cord.

Cervical vertebrae—The seven vertebrae of the neck.

Coccyx—The last bone of the vertebral column just below the sacrum, also called the tailbone.

Condyle—A rounded enlargement that has an articulating surface.

Foramen—A hole in a bone usually for the passage of blood vessels and/or nerves.

Foramen magnum—Large opening at the base of the skull that allows passage of the spinal cord.

Ilium—The upper and largest part of the bony pelvic girdle, also called the iliac wing.

Intervertebral disk—Disk-shaped pads of fibrous cartilage interposed between the vertebrae of the vertebral column that provide cushioning and join the vertebrae together.

Nervous system—This is the entire system of nerve tissue in the body. It includes the brain, the brainstem, the spinal cord, the nerves and the ganglia and is divided into the peripheral nervous system (PNS) and the central nervous system (CNS).

Nucleus pulposus—Jelly-like core of an intervertebral disk.

Pelvis—The basin-shaped cavity that contains the bladder and reproductive organs of the body.

Process—A general term describing any marked projection or prominence on a bone.

Sacroiliac joints—Joints that allow the sacrum and the ilium to articulate.

Sacrum—The triangular-shaped bone found between the fifth lumbar vertebra and the coccyx. It consists of five fused vertebrae and it articulates on each side with the bones of the pelvis (ilium), forming the sacroiliac joints.

Skull—All of the bones of the head.

Spinal cord—Elongated part of the central nervous system (CNS) that lies in the vertebral canal of the vertebral column and from which the spinal nerves emerge.

Vertebra—Flat bones that make up the vertebral column. The spine has 33 vertebrae.

Vertebral canal—Hollow part of the vertebral column formed by the vertebral foramina of all vertebrae. It encloses the spinal cord.

Vertebral foramen—The opening formed in vertebrae that allows passage of the spinal cord.

Shearing, which can occur when a person is knocked over with great force, combines both hinging and twisting forces. Any of these forces can dislocate the vertebrae, fracture them, or rupture the ligaments that bind them together. Damage to the vertebrae and ligaments usually causes severe **pain** and swelling in the injured area. In severe cases, the spinal cord may be affected as well, and thus sensory and/or motor nerve functions. Other common disorders and diseases of the vertebral column include:

- Degenerative disc disease (DDD). DDD affects the vertebral discs. As each disc is under constant pressure during flexion and extension of the vertebral column, the discs begin to wear and tear with age.

- Discitis. Discitis, or disc space **infection**, is an inflammation of the intervertebral disc that occurs in adults but more commonly in children. Its cause is believed to be infectious.

- Facet joint syndrome. The facet joints can get inflamed following injury or arthritis and cause pain and stiffness. It affects more commonly the facet joints of the cervical vertebrae and typically causes pain in this area as well headaches and difficulty rotating the head.

- Hyperlordosis. Hyperlordosis, also simply called lordosis, refers to an exaggerated lordosis of the lumbar vertebrae. It can be caused by **pregnancy** or obesity.

- Lumbar herniated disc. This condition represents a common cause of low back and leg pain. A herniated intervertebral disc is a ruptured disk. Symptoms may include dull or sharp pain, muscle spasm or cramping, and leg weakness or loss of leg function.

- **Osteoarthritis**. Osteoarthritis is a degenerative form of arthritis, it is a progressive joint disease associated with aging. In the vertebral column, osteoarthritis can affect the facet joints, which allow the body to bend and twist.

- Scheuermann's kyphosis. Scheuermann's kyphosis refers to an exaggerated kyphosis of the thoracic vertebrae. It can be caused by rickets or poor posture.

- Scoliosis. Abnormal sideways curvature of the vertebral column.

- Spondylolisthesis. A forward displacement of one vertebra on another, usually in the lower back region due to either a traumatic or a congenital defect.

- Vertebral osteomyelitis. Vertebral osteomyelitis is the infection of the bones of the vertebral column. It may be caused by either a **bacteria** or a fungus. Bacterial or pyogenic vertebral osteomyelitis is the most common form.

Resources

BOOKS

Bryan, Glenda J. *Skeletal Anatomy*. Philadelphia: W. B. Saunders Co., 1996.

Simon, Seymour. *Bones: Our Skeletal System (Human Body)*. New York: Morrow (Harper-Collins), 1998.

OTHER

"The Vertebral Column." *Bartleby.com edition of Gray's Anatomy of the Human Body.* <http://www.bartleby.com/107/19.html>.

Monique Laberge, Ph.D.

Vincent's infection *see* **Periodontitis**

Viral loading test *see* **AIDS tests**

Viral meningitis *see* **Meningitis**

Viruses

Definition

A virus is an infectious agent, often highly host-specific, consisting of genetic material surrounded by a protein coat.

Description

Viruses infect virtually every life form, including humans, animals, plants, **fungi**, and **bacteria**. So small that they cannot be seen by a light **microscope**, viruses range in size from about 30 nanometers (about 0.000001 in) to about 450 nanometers (about 0.000014 in) and are between 100 to 20 times smaller than bacteria. As of the seventh report of the International Committee on Taxonomy of Viruses (ICTV), published in September 2000, known viruses have been assigned to 1550 species in 53 different families. Hundreds of other viruses remain unclassified due to lack of information.

All standard viruses share a general structure of genetic material, or viral genome, and a protein coat, called a capsid. The viral genome is made of either deoxyribose nucleic acid (DNA), the genetic material found in plants and animals, or ribonucleic acid (RNA), a compound plant and animal cells use in protein synthesis. The protein capsid is made of repeating, often-identical subunits known as capsomeres. Viruses are not strictly free-living, as they cannot reproduce on their own. Instead, they use host cell machinery to make both the viral genome and capsids of the newly formed viruses, or virions.

The broad category of viruses also includes unusual infective agents that are missing one or more components of standard viruses. These unconventional viruses include viroids, which exist as circular RNA molecules that are not packaged, and prions, infective particles that contain protein and little or no nucleic acids.

Some viral infections can cause damage to the host cell, resulting in disease to the organism. Other viral infections appear to make the host cells divide uncontrollably, causing the development of **cancer**. However, many viral infections are asymptomatic and do not result in disease. There are no cures for viral infections, due in part to the difficulty of developing drugs that adversely affect only the virus and not the host. Accordingly, preventative measures such as vaccines play an important role in the treatment of viral diseases.

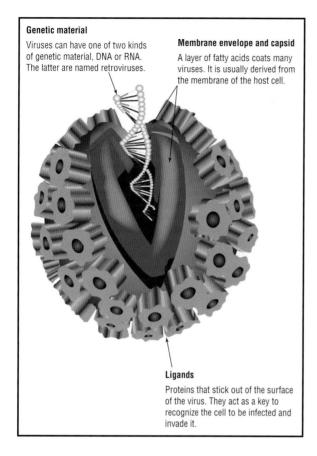

Genetic material
Viruses can have one of two kinds of genetic material, DNA or RNA. The latter are named retroviruses.

Membrane envelope and capsid
A layer of fatty acids coats many viruses. It is usually derived from the membrane of the host cell.

Ligands
Proteins that stick out of the surface of the virus. They act as a key to recognize the cell to be infected and invade it.

The structure of a virus. (Illustration by GGS Information Services, Inc. The Gale Group.)

Function

The primary function of a virus is to infect host cells and create more viruses. The virus does this by taking over the host cell's protein and genetic material-making processes, forcing it to produce the new viruses. Exactly how viruses function in this manner is best understood by examining general viral structure, classification, and reproductive strategies.

Structure and classification

There are three basic structures for standard viral capsids: icosahedral, helical, and complex. Icosahedral capsids are 20-sided, made of triangular capsomere subunits. The points of the triangular subunits join at 12 vertices about the shape. Although exact structure varies from virus type to virus type, a common arrangement is five or six neighboring triangular subunits at each vertex. Some viruses show more than one capsomere arrangement within the capsid. An example of a virus having an icosahedral structure is adenovirus, the virus that can cause acute respiratory disease or viral **pneumonia** in humans.

The helical viruses have protein subunits that curve about a central axis running the length of the virus. The fanlike arrangement of protein forms a three-dimensional ribbon-shaped structure that covers the viral genome. Some of these capsid structures are stiff and rodlike, while other helical viruses are more flexible. The **influenza** virus is an example of a virus with a helical capsid structure.

The third type of virus capsid structure is called complex. Although the structure is regular from virus to virus of the same type, the symmetry is not patterned enough to be fully understood. For example, poxvirus, the virus that causes smallpox in humans, has a complex capsid structure of over 100 **proteins**. Virologists are still trying to determine the exact arrangement of these proteins.

The combination of the capsid and the viral genome is known as a nucleocapsid. Some nucleocapsids are infective in this form and are known as naked viruses. Others require a surrounding lipid membrane derived from the host cell to be infective. The membrane envelope can encompass one or more nucleocapsids and usually contains on its surface at least one viral protein in addition to the host cell components. Viruses of this type are called enveloped or coated viruses.

Viruses are classified according to structural characteristics such as whether the virus genome is made of DNA or RNA. Both of these nucleic acids can form ladder-like structures where each side of the ladder is known as a strand. Viruses are differentiated by whether the DNA or RNA is single or doubled-stranded. The type of capsid structure and whether the virus is naked or enveloped are also considered. A few viral classifications take into account differences in replication strategy.

Replication

The generalized replication cycle for standard viruses begins with the absorption of the virus by the host cell. Absorption involves an interaction between the viral particle and the potential host cell. This is often mediated by a viral protein that is recognized by a binding protein located on the surface of the host cell. Whether the host cell recognizes the viral protein often determines whether a particular cell can or cannot function as a host for a particular virus. For example, the hemagglutin protein of the influenza virus, a viral protein found within the lipid envelope of this coated virus, interacts with a receptor found on the surface of the epithelial cells that line the human respiratory tract.

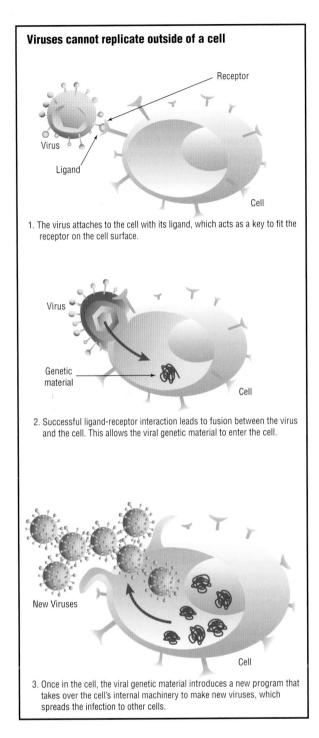

Viruses cannot replicate outside of a cell

1. The virus attaches to the cell with its ligand, which acts as a key to fit the receptor on the cell surface.

2. Successful ligand-receptor interaction leads to fusion between the virus and the cell. This allows the viral genetic material to enter the cell.

3. Once in the cell, the viral genetic material introduces a new program that takes over the cell's internal machinery to make new viruses, which spreads the infection to other cells.

(Illustration by GGS Information Services, Inc. The Gale Group.)

The next step in the virus replication cycle is penetration and, if necessary, the uncoating of the virus in the host cell. With some coated viruses, the envelope membrane fuses directly with the host membrane, allowing movement of nucleocapsid into the cell's cytoplasm. Other coated viruses are brought into the cell using endosomes, small vesicles of cellular membrane that bud inwardly and are used to move materials into the cell. Due to the lower pH environment of the endosome, the virus coat can fuse with the endosomal membrane to gain access to the cell cytoplasm. Naked viruses are sometimes small enough to move without help through the host cellular membrane, while others use the endosome system.

Once inside the cell, the virus takes over the host cell's protein and nucleic acid production, directing it to produce viral proteins and genomes. For many viruses having a DNA genome, the viral nucleic acid is inserted or integrated directly into the host cell's own DNA, that make up the cell's chromosomes. RNA viruses tend to keep the genome independent from the host cell's genetic material. In either case, the host cell is fooled into using the viral genetic material as the instructions for the production of new infectious virions. In order to ensure that new virions will be formed, viruses often have mechanisms that speed up the protein formation of the host cell. Sometimes the mechanism will be specific for increased production of viral proteins, while others speed up all protein formation.

A special method of producing new virions is employed by retroviruses, such as the human **immunodeficiency** virus (HIV). These viruses carry their genomes as RNA, but upon entry into the host cell a viral enzyme known as reverse transcriptase converts the viral RNA into DNA, and that molecule is integrated into the host genome. The enzyme is called reverse transcriptase because generally genetic information moves from DNA to RNA copies rather than this reverse process. The integrated DNA is known as a provirus and will be replicated when the host cell divides, to be inherited by the two resulting daughter cells.

After production of the viral proteins and genomes by the host cellular machinery, the capsid is assembled around the genetic material and, for some viruses, a maturation step occurs that is necessary for infectivity. Finally, the new virions are released from the cell. Some coated viruses leave the cell by budding and do not cause the death of the host cell. The budding process is how the virus acquires its lipid membrane envelope. Other viruses lyse, or break down, the host cell membrane. Lysis kills the host cell.

Because of the ability of viruses to carry genetic material into and out of a cell during the reproduction cycle, viruses can function as vectors in **genetic engineering**. This is done by inserting foreign genetic material into viral genomes and allowing the material to be

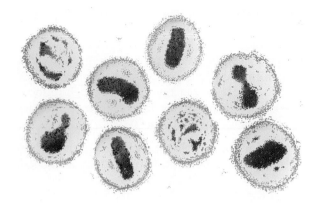

This color-enhanced transmission electron micrograph (TEM) shows the Hanta virus, Bunyaviridae. *(Chris Bjornberg / Photo Researchers, Inc. Reproduced by permission.)*

integrated and expressed in bacteria and animal cells. Viral vectors are often the basis for gene therapies that in their simplest form attempt to cure genetic defects by providing non-mutated copies of a damaged gene to an organism.

Role in human health

Viruses that infect humans cause damage to the infected cells, resulting in outward symptoms seen as human disease. Human viruses gain entry into the body using various routes. Some viruses are transmitted through skin-to-skin contact, such as herpes simplex 1, the virus that causes cold sores. Others are transmitted through exposure to infected **blood**, the mode of transmission of the hepatitis B virus. Some of the most easily caught viruses, such as varcella-zoster, the virus that causes chicken pox, are transmitted through water droplets suspended in the air. The virus is transmitted when the droplets are breathed in and come in contact with the respiratory tract of the new host.

Gastrointestinal viruses are transmitted through exposure to waste products containing virus particles that has contaminated water or food, and entry into the host's digestive tract through the mouth. Rotavirus, a cause of a diarrheal illness common in children, is transmitted in this manner. Sexually transmitted viruses move from host to host through sexual contact and enter the body by the genitourinary route. HIV and human papilloma virus (HPV) are examples of viruses that are sexually transmitted.

After gaining entry into the host, the response at a cellular level to the viral **infection** varies with the type of virus and the virulence of the strain. Thus, the response can vary from no apparent change, to detectable changes in the cell, known as cytopathic effects (CPE), to loss of growth control or malignancy. Virulence refers to the ability of a virus to cause disease in a host. Some viruses are highly virulent, causing disease with almost every infection. Measles, rabies, and influenza are virulent viruses. Other less virulent viruses, such as Epstein-Barr virus, which causes mononucleosis, only rarely results in disease symptoms.

Viral infections follow patterns that are specific to the virus. Some infections are localized, that is, restricted to a particular cell type or organ, while others are disseminated throughout the body. Disseminated infections are often propagated through the nervous system or the bloodstream. Infections can be acute, where the patient's **immune system** self-limits the disease and recovers, or chronic, where the infection continues for a long period of time.

Some viruses have the ability to cause an initial disease state upon infection and then establish a latent or dormant infective state. For example, herpes viruses cause blisters on the skin as a result of their lytic replication, but then establish a latent infection in nerve cells. Upon a stimulus such as exposure to the sun or **stress** the virus switches back to a lytic cycle, again producing blisters at the site of infection. In this way, the infection can persist for months or even years.

Several viruses, such as human papilloma viruses and Epstein-Barr virus, have been strongly associated with human cancers. The exact role of viruses in malignancy is not yet understood, as environmental and host genetic factors also seem to contribute to the development of tumors. However, it is highly probable that viruses are key triggers for a number of human cancers.

Another effect of viruses on human health is infection by zoonotic viruses, that is, viruses that can be transmitted from an animal host of another species to humans. Some of these viruses are transmitted through a blood-sucking insect intermediary, such as a mosquito, while others are transmitted directly from the infected animal to humans. Many of these viruses raise important **public health** concerns. An example of a mosquito-transmitted virus is flavivirus that causes West Nile encephalitis in humans. A strain of hantavirus was discovered in 1993 that infects rodents and transmits directly to humans, causing a respiratory illness.

Although most infect plants and animals, a few unconventional viruses cause human disease. The only know human viroid is the delta virus (hepatitis D) that requires co-infection with hepatitis B to be infective. The combined infection of hepatitis B and D causes more severe symptoms than B alone. An example of a human prion-mediated disease is Cruetzfeldt-Jakob disease (CJD), which causes neurological symptoms and is fatal. Of significant concern is a possible variant of CJD reported in Great Britain that affects younger individuals. Although cause and effect has not been conclusively shown, there is suspicion that this disease results from eating beef contaminated with the prion that causes bovine spongiform encephalopathy, or mad cow disease.

Immunological response

When challenged by a viral infection, the human body responds with both antibodies and cell-mediated responses to counteract the virus. Antibodies, produced by B lymphocytes, are specific for surface proteins of the virus. When acting as a target for antibodies, such viral proteins are known as antigens. The binding of the antibodies to the viruses can inactive them or target them as foreign for destruction by other components of the immune system. Antibodies can also bind to viral proteins seen in the membrane of infected cells, directing their elimination by the immune system. Antibodies mediate the immunity to reinfection by the same virus. Unfortunately, many viruses have high rates of mutation that alter the surface antigens, rendering the host again susceptible to infection. This process is the reason that one cold does not make a person immune to all rhinoviruses, a virus with at least 95 different serotypes (a characteristic of a virus based on the antibodies that are produced against the surface antigens upon infection).

Non-specific cell-mediated responses are also important to the body's fight against viruses. The production of interferons and cytokines, in particular, is known to help control viral infections. However, the side effects of these molecules, including **fever**, malaise, fatigue and muscle pains, significantly contribute to the physical symptoms of viral infections.

Diagnosis

In general there are three methods of diagnosing viral disease in humans. Some viruses can be identified clinically, as the infection causes unmistakable outward signs. The blistery pox of the varicella-zoster or chicken pox virus is a good example of a clinically diagnosed viral disease. Viral diseases can also be diagnosed epidemiologically, through known exposure to certain viruses or virus-harboring hosts.

However, many virus infections cannot be diagnosed definitively without diagnostic testing.

Diagnostic testing can involve direct detection, using electron microscopy, light microscopy of CPE seen in host cells, detection of viral antigen in patient samples, or detection of the viral genome using the polymerase chain reaction (PCR) test. Effective tests for some viral infections involve indirect detection, generally using cell culture systems to grow the virus *in vitro* (outside the organism). A final method of diagnosing viral illnesses is serological testing that involves the detection of antibodies against the virus antigen in samples taken at presentation and during convalescence. A serious drawback to traditional serological testing is the amount of time needed to obtain the results. New techniques are being developed, however, that may speed serological tests and make them more useful.

Treatment

Most viral diseases have no cure, so treatment involves easing symptoms and allowing the body's immune system to eliminate the virus. Viruses are not affected by **antibiotics**, which target bacteria. However, a handful of anti-viral drugs have been developed and many more are in the developmental and drug trial stage. In general, the development of anti-viral drugs has been hampered by the parasitic relationship between viruses and their hosts. It has been difficult to find pharmacological means to kill the virus without harming the host. The speed of viral infection has also been a problem, as viral numbers are so high by the time the infection has symptoms, the drugs have little effect.

Amantadine and rimantiadine are two drugs that have been used successfully against influenza A. These drugs appear to inhibit the absorption of the influenza virus into the epithelial cells of the respiratory tract and, accordingly, are administered prior to infection as a prophylaxis.

Herpes simplex and varicella-zoster infections can be treated with acyclovir, valacyclovir, and famciclovir. Cytomegalovirus infection can be treated with ganciclovir, foscarnet, and cidofovir. All of these drugs are converted into a chemical that interferes with the production of the viral genome. As a viral enzyme produces the genome for these viruses, the chemical does not interfere with the production of genetic material for the host cell.

A number of drugs that inhibit reverse transcriptase have been developed for treatment of HIV. The best known of these is Zidovudine (AZT). The other major target for antiviral HIV drugs is the viral protease, an enzyme that cleaves both viral structural proteins and enzymes apart after formation by the host cell. Because the virus is noninfective if these cleavages do not occur, drugs inhibiting the protease action are effective antivirals. As advances in this field happen quickly, the International **AIDS** Society/USA Panel provides periodic recommendations as to what drugs given in what combinations have proven to be most effective inn the treatment of AIDS.

Finally, genetically engineered interferon has been used with some success against hepatitis B and C and human papillovirus. However, the severe side effects of this protein, in particular nausea and vomiting, have hampered its usefulness.

Prevention

The most effective method of treatment of viral diseases is prevention of the infection. Vaccines, where the immune system is exposed to non-infective viral antigens to allow the development of protective antibodies, have proven effective in controlling many viral illnesses. Vaccines are made of inactivated (killed) virus, attenuated (weakened) virus, or isolated viral proteins, that are known as subunit vaccines. Vaccines are available for the viruses that cause measles, mumps, rubella, poliomyelitis, rabies, hepatitis A and B, influenza, varicella-zoster (chicken pox) and yellow fever. Many other vaccines are in the developmental or clinical trial stages.

The greatest drawback to vaccines is the inability of the protection to counter the same virus that has altered its antigens through mutation. Thus, viruses that undergo rapid mutation are difficult to control using **vaccination**. One solution used for influenza is to create a new vaccine every season against the viruses that are predicted to be responsible for upcoming flu outbreaks. Although this is an imperfect system, influenza vaccination is instrumental in shortening epidemics and protecting the populations most at risk for complications, including the chronically ill, the elderly, and health care workers (primarily to prevent transmitting infection to those as risk).

A second preventative measure is the avoidance of infection by blocking transmission at the point of viral entry. This is done through the isolation of infected patients and avoiding contact with infected biological material such as lesions, blood, and airborne particles through the use of gloves, masks, and other barriers. Health care providers must practice careful hygiene of patients, including immediate removal of vomit or **diarrhea**, and thorough hand washing. These measures are taken equally to avoid patient-to-provider and provider-to-patient transmission of viruses. For

---

KEY TERMS

Capsid—The protein structure of a virus.

Capsomere—The protein subunits of the capsid.

Endosome—A membrane-mediated means of transporting materials from outside to inside the cell.

Genome—The genetic material encoding the genes of an organism.

Nucleocapsid—The combination of the capsid and viral genome.

Prion—An unconventional virus that is made almost entirely of protein.

Reverse transcriptase—A retroviral enzyme that produces DNA copies of genetic information encoded by RNA.

Virion—A single infectious virus particle.

Viroid—An unconventional virus that is made of uncoated RNA.

Zoonotic—A type of virus that primarily infects an insect or animal, but can be transmitted to humans.

---

zoonotic viruses, transmission can be reduced through pesticide control of the insect or animal reservoir of the disease.

Common diseases and disorders

Several hundred different viruses infect humans. The viruses that occur chiefly in humans can be categorized as respiratory, enteric, exanthematous, hepatitis, or persistent. The most common respiratory viruses include the rhinoviruses (the **common cold**) and the influenza viruses. Common enteric viruses include polioviruses (now rare because of vaccination), coxsachie viruses (herpangina), and epidemic gastroenteritis viruses such as rotaviruses. Rubeola (measles) and rubella (German measles) are two common exanthematous viruses.

Hepatitis viruses type A through E are known, with type A most often responsible for epidemics of the disease. Many of the persistent viruses are quite widespread and include cytomegalovirus (usually asymptomatic), Epstein-Barr virus (mononucleosis), Herpes simplex virus (cold sores and **genital herpes**), human herpes virus type 6 (roseola), human papilloma virus (warts), and varicella-zoster virus (chicken pox and shingles).

Zoonotic viruses, that chiefly infect insects or animals, with humans as minor or accidental host, are generally rarer. The diseases caused by these viruses are limited to areas that can support the insect or animal host as well as humans. Rabies is the most widespread of these diseases. Flaviviruses (yellow and dengue fever), bunyaviruses (California encephalitis and Hantavirus pulmonary syndrome), and filoviruses such as ebola (hemorrhagic fever) are other examples of zoonoitic viruses that cause human disease.

Human disease caused by nonconventional viruses is very rare. The most common is CJD, a prion-mediated disease that occurs in one in a million individuals. Hepatitis D is the only known human viroid, and it requires co-infection with hepatitis B. Other diseases caused by nonconventional viruses are kuru and Gerstmann-Sträussler-Scheinker syndrome (GSS), both caused by prions.

Resources

BOOKS

Brooks, George F. et al. "General Properties of Viruses" and "Pathogenesis & Control of Viral Disease." In *Medical Microbiology*. Appleton & Lange, 1998.

Collier, Leslie and John Oxford. *Human Virology*. New York: Oxford University Press, 2000.

PERIODICALS

Carpenter, Charles et al. "Antiretroviral Therapy in Adults" *JAMA* 283 (January 2000): 381–90.

Mahoney, M.C. "Adult immunization—influenza vaccine" *American Family Physician* 69 (May 2000): 2901–2902.

"Provider-to-Patient Transmission" *American Journal of Nursing* 99 (May 1999): 17.

OTHER

"Virology." *On-line Textbook of Microbiology and Immunology*. University of South Carolina School of Medicine, Department of Microbiology. <http://www.med.sc.edu:85/book/welcome.htm> (March 15, 2001).

Michelle L. Johnson, M.S.

Vision

Definition

Vision is sight, the act of seeing with the eyes. Sight conveys more information to the **brain** than either **hearing**, touch, **taste**, or **smell**, and contributes enormously to **memory** and other requirements for normal human functioning.

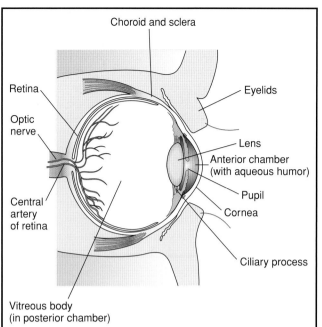

Structures of the eye. *(Delmar Publishers, Inc. Reproduced by permission.)*

Description

Because humans see objects with two eyes simultaneously, vision is binocular, and therefore stereoscopic. Vision begins when light enters the eye, stimulating photoreceptor cells in the retina called rods and cones. The retina forms the inner lining of each eye and functions in many ways like film in a camera. The photoreceptor cells produce electrical impulses which they transmit to adjoining nerve cells (**neurons**), which converge at the optic nerve at the back of the retina. The visual information coded as electrical impulses travels along nerve tracts to reach each visual cortex in the posterior of the brain's left and right hemispheres. Each eye conveys a slightly different, two-dimensional image to the brain, which decodes and interprets these images into a colorful, three-dimensional view of the world. The speed of the completion of this task is sensitive enough that it can be registered only on scientific equipment, rather than by human observation.

Function

Because human eyes are separated by about 2.6 in (6.5 cm), each eye has a slightly different horizontal view. This phenomenon is called binocular displacement. The visual images reaching each eye's retina are two-dimensional and flat. In normal binocular vision, the blending of these images into one single image is called stereopsis.

Monocular stereopsis, or depth perception, is also available. For example, even with one eye closed, a nearby car will appear much larger than the same sized car a mile away. The ability to unconsciously and instantaneously assess depth and distance allows humans to move without continually bumping into objects, also providing eye/hand coordination.

Ocular dominance

Studies strongly indicate there is a critical period during which normal development of the visual system takes place and environmental information is permanently encoded within the brain. Although the exact time frame is not clear, it is believed that by age six or seven years, visual maturation is complete. Animal studies show that if one eye is covered during the critical period, neurons in the visual pathway and brain connected to the covered eye do not develop to optimal performance. When that eye is uncovered, only neurons relating to the unrestricted eye function in the visual process. This is an example of "ocular dominance," when cells activated by one eye dominate the cells of the other. It is not an abnormal development.

Memory

The same way in which vision plays an important role in memory, memory plays an important role in vision. The brain accurately stores visual data which it draws upon every time the eyes look at something.

Electrochemical messengers

The entire visual pathway—from the retina to the visual cortex—is paved with millions of neurons. From the time light enters the eye until the brain forms a visual image, vision relies upon the process of electrochemical communication between neurons. Each neuron has a cell body with branching fibers called dendrites and a single long, cylindrical fiber called an axon. When a neuron is stimulated it sends chemicals called neurotransmitters, which cause the release of electrical impulses along the axon. The point where information passes from one cell to the next is a gap called a synapse, and neurotransmitters affect the transmission of electrical impulses on to an adjacent cell. This synaptic transmission of impulses is repeated until the message reaches the appropriate location in the brain. In the retina, approximately 125 million rods and cones transmit information to approximately 1 million ganglion cells. As a result, that many rods and cones must converge onto one single ganglion cell. At the same time, however, information from each single rod and cone "diverges" on to more than one ganglion cell. This complicated phenomenon of convergence and divergence occurs along the entire optic pathway. The brain must transform all this stimulation into useful information and respond to it by sending messages back to the eye and other parts of the brain before we are able to see.

Although the pupil regulates to some degree the amount of light entering the eye, the rods and cones ennable vision to adapt to extremes. Vision ennabled by rods begins in dim light. Cones function in bright light and are responsible for color vision and visual activity.

When light hits the surface of an object, it is absorbed, reflected, or passes through it. The amount of light absorbed by an object is determined by the amount of pigment contained in that object. The more heavily pigmented the object, the darker it appears because it absorbs more light. A sparsely pigmented object, which absorbs little light and reflects a lot of back, appears lighter.

Color vision

Humans have three types of eye pigments: blue, green, and red. This combination, the primary colors, composes every impression of colors for humans. Human color vision extends 30 degrees from the macula, and after that distance, red and green are indistinguishable. That occurs due to the fact that in the periphery of the retina only a few cones are present that detect motion. Because rods are present, the periphery cannot determine colors. For example, a red object that is brought closer from the periphery will at first appear colorless. When the object is moved closer, the eyes will eventually pick up the red pigment.

Perception of color is dependent on three conditions. First, whether people have normal color vision; second, whether an object reflects or absorbs light; and third, whether the source of light transmits wavelengths within the visible spectrum. Rods contain only one pigment which is sensitive to very dim light, and which facilitates night vision but not color. Cones are activated by bright light and let us see colors and fine detail. There are three types of cones containing different pigments that absorb wavelengths in the short (S), middle (M), or long (L) ranges. The peak wavelength absorption of the S (blue) cone is approximately 430 nm; the M (green) cone 530 nm; and the L (red) cone 560 nm.

The range of detectable wavelengths for all three types of cones overlap, and two of them—the L and M cones—respond to all wavelengths in the visible spectrum. Most of the light we see consists of a mixture of all visible wavelengths which results in "white" light, like that of sunshine. Cone overlap and the amount of stimulation they receive from varying wavelengths produces the vivid colors and gentle hues present in normal color vision.

Optic pathway

Only about 10% of the light which enters the eye reaches the photoreceptors in the retina. This is because light must pass first through the cornea aqueous, pupil, lens, and vitreous humors (the liquid and gel-like fluids inside the eye), the **blood vessels** of the lining of the eye, and then through two layers of nerve cells (ganglion and bipolar cells in the retina).

Visual discrimination

The retina has the ability to distinguish between visual stimuli, and the greater this ability, the greater the sensitivity in making such distinctions. The retina distinguishes visual stimuli in three ways: light discrimination (brightness sensitivity), spatial discrimination (ability to recognize shapes and patterns) and temporal (sensations) discrimination. Human temporal discrimination is limited. For example, this allows people to watch television without noticing the wavy lines that would distort the picture.

Optic chiasma

Vision functions in the brain are divided into two areas: the afferent (sensory) system and the efferent (motor) system. Synaptic transmission of impulses from retinal cells follows the optic nerve (an extension of the brain) to the optic chiasma, also referred to as the optic chiasm, an x-shaped junction in the brain where half the fibers from each eye cross to the other side of the brain. Consequently, visual information from the right half of each retina travels to the right visual cortex, and visual information from the left half of each retina travels to the left visual cortex. Information from the right half of our environment is processed in the left hemisphere of the brain, and vice versa. Damage to the optic pathway or visual cortex in the left brain—perhaps from a stroke—can cause loss of the right visual field. As a result, only information entering the eye from the left side of our environment is processed, even though information still enters the eye from both visual fields.

Visual cortex

Each visual cortex is about 2 in (5 cm) square and contains about 200 million nerve cells which respond to elaborate stimuli. In primates, there are about 20 different visual areas in the visual cortex, the largest being the primary, or striate, cortex. The striate cortex sends information to an adjacent area which in turn transmits to at least three other areas about the size of postage stamps. Each of these areas then relays the information to several other remote areas called accessory optic nuclei.

Visual acuity

Visual acuity, keenness of sight, and the ability to distinguish small objects develops rapidly in infants between the age of three and six months, and decreases rapidly as people approach middle age. Optometrists and ophthalmologists test visual acuity during a routine examination, and poor acuity is often correctable with glasses, **contact lenses**, or refractive **laser surgery**. Visual acuity is highly complex and is influenced by many factors.

Retinal eccentricity

The area of the retina on which light is focused influences visual acuity, which is sharpest when the object is projected directly onto the central fovea—a tiny indentation at the back of the retina comprised entirely of cones. Acuity decreases rapidly toward the retina's periphery, as well as the number of cones. Studies have indicated recently that this may result from the decreasing density of ganglion cells toward the retina's periphery.

Luminance

Luminance is the intensity of light reflecting off an object, and influences visual acuity. Dim light activates only rods, and visual acuity is poor. As luminance increases, more cones become active and acuity levels rise. Pupil size also affects acuity. When the pupil expands, it allows more light into the eye. However, because light is then projected onto a wider area of the retina, optical irregularities can occur. Two issues are key regarding pupil size: light to the retina—more is better, up to a point; and, whether or not the light is hitting the rods or the the cones—for example, with bright illumination, the pupil naturally constricts because only cones are stimulated and thus increase visual acuity. A very narrow pupil can reduce acuity because it greatly reduces retinal luminance; but a small pupil (for example, a "pinhole") will increase acuity in people

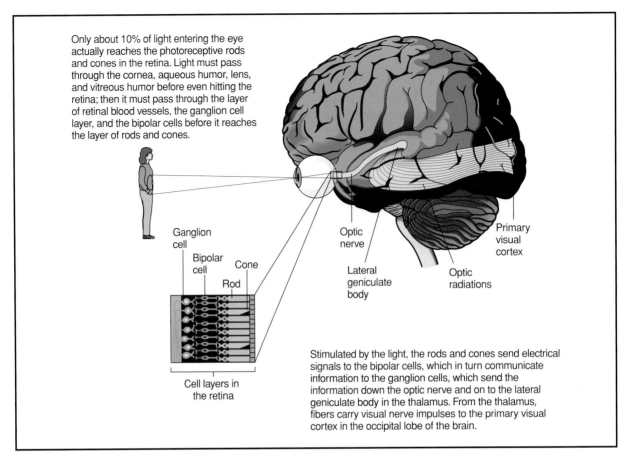

Only about 10% of light entering the eye actually reaches the photoreceptive rods and cones in the retina. Light must pass through the cornea, aqueous humor, lens, and vitreous humor before even hitting the retina; then it must pass through the layer of retinal blood vessels, the ganglion cell layer, and the bipolar cells before it reaches the layer of rods and cones.

Ganglion cell
Bipolar cell
Cone
Rod

Cell layers in the retina

Optic nerve
Lateral geniculate body
Optic radiations
Primary visual cortex

Stimulated by the light, the rods and cones send electrical signals to the bipolar cells, which in turn communicate information to the ganglion cells, which send the information down the optic nerve and on to the lateral geniculate body in the thalamus. From the thalamus, fibers carry visual nerve impulses to the primary visual cortex in the occipital lobe of the brain.

The anatomy of vision. *(Illustration by Hans & Cassidy. The Gale Group.)*

with refractive errors. Optimal acuity seems to occur with an intermediate pupil size, but the optimum size varies depending on the degree of external luminance.

Accommodation

Accommodation is the eye's ability to adjust its focus in order to bring about sharp images of both far and near objects. Accommodation begins to decline around age 20 and is so diminished by the mid-50s that sharp close-up vision is seldom possible without corrective lenses. This condition, called **presbyopia**, is the most common vision problem in the world.

Role in human health

Human memory and mental processes rely heavily on sight. There are more neurons in the nervous system dedicated to vision than to any other of the five senses, indicating vision's importance. The almost immediate interaction between the eye and the brain in producing vision makes even the most intricate computer program pale in comparison. Although sighted individuals might seldom pause to imagine

life without sight, vision is considered to be the most desirable of all human senses. Without it, a person's relationship to the surrounding world and the ability to interact with the environment, is considered seriously diminished.

Common diseases and disorders

Color-blindness

Approximately 8% of all human males experience abnormal color vision, or color "blindness" or deficiency. Women who experience color-deficiency will pass the X-linked recessive gene to any son, and each will be color-blind. Color-blindness is caused when one of the pigments in a person's photoreceptors is abnormal. Red deficient individuals are easier to categorize because that wavelength has minimal overlap with the other primary colors.

Various diseases and conditions can also cause color-blindness. These defects usually occur in one eye and can be intermittent, while congenital defects are present in both eyes and remain constant.

Strabismus

Strabismus is the condition whereby visualization of two images occurs when viewing a single object. This results from a lack of parallelism of the visual axes of the eyes. In one form (known colloquially as cross-eyes) one or both eyes turn inward toward the nose. In another form, (known colloquially as wall-eyes), one or both eyes turn outward. A person with strabismus does not usually see a double image—particularly if onset was at a young age and remained untreated. This occurs due to the brain's suppressesion of the image from the weaker eye, causing neurons associated with the dominant eye (ocular dominance) take over.

Amblyopia (known colloquially as lazy eye) is the most common visual problem associated with strabismus. Amblyopia involves severely impaired visual acuity, and is the result of suppression and ocular dominance; it affects an estimated 4 million people in the United States and is a common cause of blindness in younger people.

Strabismus appears to be hereditary, and is often obvious soon after birth. In many cases, strabismus is correctable. The critical period extends until a child reaches the ages of six or seven. It is involved in normal neuronal development of vision thus rendering it crucial that the problem be detected and treated as early as possible.

Other common visual problems

Slight irregularities in the shape or structure of the eyeball, lens, or cornea cause imperfectly focused images on the retina. Resulting visual distortions include **hyperopia** (far-sightedness, or the inability to focus on close objects), **myopia** (near-sightedness, in which distant objects appear out of focus), and **astigmatism** (which causes distorted visual images) and presbyopia. These distortions can usually be rectified with corrective lenses or refractive surgery.

Resources

BOOKS

Billig, Michael D., Gary H. Cassel, and Harry G. Randall. *The Eye Book: A Complete Guide to Eye Disorders and Health*. Baltimore and London: The Johns Hopkins University Press, 1998.

Hart, William M., Jr., ed. *Adler's Physiology of the Eye*. St. Louis, Baltimore, Boston, Chicago, London, Philadelphia, Sydney, Toronto: Mosby Year Book, 1992.

Lent, Roberto, ed. *The Visual System-From Genesis to Maturity*. Boston, Basel, Berlin: Birkhauser, 1992.

KEY TERMS

Accommodation—The eye's ability to focus clearly on both near and far objects.

Cones—Photoreceptors for daylight and color vision are found in three types, each type detecting visible wavelengths in either the short, medium, or long, (blue, green, or red) spectrum.

Ganglion cells—Neurons in the retina whose axons form the optic nerves.

Ocular dominance—When cells in the striate cortex respond more to input from one eye than from the other.

Optic pathway—The neuronal pathway leading from the eye to the visual cortex. It includes the eye, optic nerve, optic chiasm, optic tract, geniculate nucleus, optic radiations, and striate cortex.

Rods—Photoreceptors which allow vision in dim light but do not facilitate color.

Stereopsis—The blending of two different images into one single image, resulting in a three-dimensional image.

Suppression—A "blocking out" by the brain of unwanted images from one or both eyes. Prolonged, abnormal suppression will result in underdevelopment of neurons in the visual pathway.

Synapse—Junction between cells where the exchange of electrical or chemical information takes place.

Visual acuity—Keenness of sight and the ability to focus sharply on small objects.

Visual field—The entire image seen with both eyes, divided into the left and right visual fields.

Zinn, Walter J., and Herbert Solomon. *Complete Guide to Eyecare, Eyeglasses & Contact Lenses*, 4th ed. Hollywood, FL: Lifetime Books, 1996.

ORGANIZATIONS

National Eye Institute of the National Institute of Health. 9000 Rockville Pike, Bethesda, MD 20892. (301) 496-5248. <http://www.nei.nih.gov>.

The Lighthouse National Center for Education. 111 E. 59th Street. New York, NY 10022. (800) 334-5497. <http://www.lighthouse.org>.

Mary Bekker

Visual disorders

Definition

Visual disorders are an impairment in **vision**, the ability to see. Total blindness is the inability to tell light from dark, or the total lack of vision. Visual impairment or low vision is a severe reduction in vision that cannot be corrected with standard glasses or **contact lenses**, and reduces a patient's ability to function at certain tasks. Legal blindness, defined as a severe visual impairment, refers to a best-corrected central vision of 20/200 or worse in the better eye, best corrected, or a visual acuity of better than 20/200 but with a visual field no greater than 20°—for example, side vision that is so reduced that it appears as if the person is looking through a tunnel.

Description

Vision is measured, as a rule, using a Snellen chart. A Snellen chart has letters of different sizes that are read, one eye at a time, from a distance of 20 ft (6.1 m). People with normal vision are able to read the 20 ft line at 20 ft—20/20 vision—or the 40 ft (12.2 m) line at 40 ft, the 100 ft (30.5 m) line at 100 ft, and so forth. If at 20 ft the smallest readable letter is larger, vision is designated as the distance from the chart over the size of the smallest letter that can be read.

Eye care professionals measure vision in many ways. Vision clarity indicates the strength of an individual's central visual status. The diopter is the unit of measure for refractive errors such as nearsightedness, farsightedness, and **astigmatism**, and indicates the strength of corrective lenses needed. Patients do not just see straight ahead; the entire vision area is called the visual field. Some patients see clearly but have areas of reduced vision or blind spots in parts of their visual field. Others have good vision in the center but poor vision around the edges (peripheral visual field). Patients with very poor vision may be unable to view any letters on the eye chart; they then will be asked to count fingers at a given distance from their eyes. This distance becomes the measure of their ability to see.

The World Health Organization (WHO) defines impaired vision in five categories:

- Low vision 1 is a best corrected visual acuity of 20/70.
- Low vision 2 starts at 20/200.
- Blindness 3 is below 20/400.
- Blindness 4 is worse than 5/300.

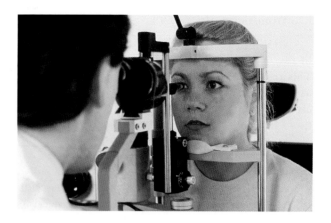

Optometrist administering a glaucoma test to a female patient. *(Custom Medical Stock Photo. Reproduced by permission.)*

- Blindness 5 is no light perception at all.
- A visual field between 5° and 10° (compared with a normal visual field of about 120°) enters category 3; less than 5° into category 4, even if the tiny spot of central vision is perfect.

Color blindness represents the reduced ability to perceive certain colors, usually red and green. It is a hereditary defect and affects few tasks. Contrast sensitivity describes the ability to distinguish one object from another. Patients with reduced contrast sensitivity may have problems seeing things in the fog, for instance, due to decreased contrast between the object and the fog.

According to the WHO over 40 million people worldwide have vision that is category 3 or worse, 80% of whom live in developing countries. Half of the blind population in the United States is older than 65.

Causes and symptoms

The leading causes of blindness include:

- **macular degeneration**
- **glaucoma**
- **cataracts**
- **diabetes mellitus**

Other possible etiologies include infections, injury, or poor **nutrition**.

Infections

Most infectious eye diseases have been eliminated in the industrialized nations through sanitation, medication, and **public health** measures. Viral infections are the main exception to this statement. Some infections that may lead to visual impairment include:

- Herpes simplex keratitis. A viral **infection** of the cornea. Repeated occurrences may lead to corneal scarring.

- Trachoma. Trachoma is caused by an incomplete bacterium, *Chlamydia trachomatis*, that is easily treated with standard **antibiotics**. It is transmitted directly from eye to eye, mostly by flies. The chlamydia gradually destroy the cornea. This disease accounts worldwide for six to nine million of the third of a billion documented cases of blindness.

- Leprosy (Hansen's disease). This bacterial disease has a high affinity for the eyes. It can be effectively treated with medicines.

- River blindness. Much of the tropics of the Eastern Hemisphere are infested with *Onchocerca volvulus*, a worm that causes "river blindness." This worm is transmitted by fly bites and can be treated with a drug called ivermectin. Twenty-eight million people suffer from the disease, and 40% of those have incurred blindness as a result.

Other causes

When a pregnant woman is exposed to certain diseases, such as rubella or toxoplasmosis, congenital eye problems can occur in her child. Also, eye injuries can result in blindness. **Brain** disease or disease in the optic nerves account for a minimal amount of blindnesses. **Multiple sclerosis** and similar nervous system diseases, brain tumors, eye socket diseases, and head injuries are also rare causes of blindness.

Nutrition

Vitamin A deficiency is a widespread cause of corneal degeneration in children in developing nations. As many as five million children develop xerophthalmia from this deficiency each year. Five percent become blind.

Diagnosis

A low vision examination differs from a general examination. In many cases, the patient already has had a complete eye exam and is referred to a low vision specialist. These specialists can be either optometrists (O.D.s) or ophthalmologists (M.D.s). Case history, visual status, and eye health evaluation are common to both examinations, but other elements vary.

Because the low vision examination often results from a general examination, the specialists focus more intensely on the specific complaints detailing a patient's daily visual demands. Examiners must determine the exact source and outcome of the patient's visual challenges. Because many of these patients are elderly and may not want to complain about poor vision, it is crucial that the physician or ophthalmic assistant document the patient's complaints by asking specific questions. For example, one question might be whether the patient is experiencing difficulty reading a phone book or street signs. Examiners might also give patients a "take-home test." Sometimes patients can see and read the charts easily in the physician's office. However, the difference between an acuity chart in the doctor's office and a newspaper read in poor lighting at someone's dining room table could be a key to understanding what problems the person is experiencing on a daily basis, and how best to address them.

Tests may include depth perception, color vision, and contrast sensitivity. Eye charts, with a larger range of letters than a Snellen eye chart, will be used. Testing distance will vary depending on the patient's ability to see. Refraction is facilitated with the use of a trial frame. Patients with poor vision may not be able to distinguish between lenses in the phoropter. The take-home test is more "real-life" in that it ennables the patient to utilize his or her side vision as well.

Treatment

There are many options for patients with visual impairment. There are optical and nonoptical aids. Optical aids include:

- Telescopes. May be used to read street signs, watch television, and attend plays and sporting events.

- Hand magnifiers. May be used to read labels on items at the store, and menus.

- Stand magnifiers. May be used to read books, magazines, and other material.

- Prisms. Are utilized to move the image onto a healthy part of the retina, providing a helpful technique for vision only in eye diseases in which the healthy part of the retina exists.

- Closed circuit television (CCTV). For large magnification (for example, for reading fine print).

Nonoptical aids include special illumination, large print books and magazines, check-writing guides, large print dials on the telephone, and more. Special computer software is also used to provide low vision patients usable access—access which enables the individual to read what is being accessed—to computer programs.

Ophthalmic occupational therapists or rehabilitation specialists usually work in tandem with low vision specialists to help patients use these devices properly. Many times these professionals will make visits to the patient's home to ensure correct use of these aids and answer any questions about low vision. Patients sometimes will be able to use the device correctly in the physician's office, but may be unable to do so at home. This inability can be due to forgetfulness; more often it is due to a low vision plan that has not been correctly adapted to the person's home environment. Home visits are crucial for effective treatment.

In some geographic areas as of 2001, **Medicare** has paid for part of the low vision therapy and rehabilitative services. However, low vision aids were not reimbursed by Medicare.

For those who are blind, extensive resources are available to improve the quality of life. For the legally blind, financial assistance for help may be possible from state and private organizations. Braille and audio books are increasingly available. Books-on-tape are provided free of charge from the Library of Congress to those who qualify as legally blind; and the service is usually arranged through the local public library. Guide dogs provide well-trained eyes and independence. Occupational therapists and rehabilitation specialists can provide orientation and mobility training. Special schools for blind children exist throughout the United States, as well as access to disability support through Social Security and private institutions.

Prognosis

The prognosis is often determined by the severity of the impairment and the ability of the aids to correct it. It also depends on the patient's ability and willingness to learn how to utilize the devices. The benefits of a thorough low vision examination include presentation of the most current low vision aids.

Health care team roles

Skilled ophthalmic nurses, technicians, and assistants help the O.D.s and M.D.s diagnose low vision by assisting with testing. These professionals log the patient history and perform many of the preliminary tests. Highly skilled technicians perform visual field tests and refractions.

Occupational therapists and rehabilitation specialists play an important role in treating low vision patients. They answer questions about low vision aids and instruct them on the devices' proper uses. They also help provide a sense of independence to these patients who may have previously been restricted in their activities by a total lack of or limited vision.

These therapists and specialists also help totally blind patients adjust to daily life by providing orientation and mobility training. They evaluate home and job environments and make recommendations for adaptation. These professionals also consult with family members to ensure effective care methods. Especially with older adults, a total care plan that includes family and caretakers is essential to the success of offsetting the negative effects or trauma of decreased vision.

Patient education

Low vision specialists, the referring O.D.s and M.D.s, and ophthalmic staff need to make sure their patients fully understand their conditions. Many elderly patients are confused by the diagnosis and need to be carefully told what their condition means and what treatment options they can utilize. Some practitioners use a video explaining macular degeneration, for example, to further emphasize the disease's impact. Large-print brochures also are helpful. Occupational therapists and rehabilitation specialists need to make sure they emphasize the correct use of visual aids so patients can receive the maximum benefit from them.

Prevention

Regular eye exams are important to detect silent eye problems (for example, glaucoma). Left untreated, glaucoma can result in blindness.

Corneal infections can be treated with effective antibiotics. When a cornea has become opaque beyond recovery it must be transplanted.

Cataracts should be removed when they interfere with a person's quality of life.

Primary prevention addresses the causes before they begin to cause eye damage. In those climates and environments where it is an issue for eye diseases, fly control can be accomplished by simple sanitation methods. Public health measures can reduce the incidence of many infectious diseases. Vitamin A supplementation, when appropriate, will eliminate xerophthalmia completely. Isome studies show that protecting the eyes against ultraviolet (UV) light will reduce the incidence of cataracts, macular degeneration, and some other eye diseases. UV coatings can be placed on regular glasses, sunglasses, and ski goggles.

Protective goggles should also be worn during certain activities for protection.

Secondary prevention addresses treating established diseases before they cause irreversible eye damage. Regular general physical examinations can also detect systemic diseases such as diabetes or high **blood pressure**. Diabetes control is a crucial factor in preserving sight in people affected by the disease.

Resources

BOOKS

"Neuro-ophthalmology." *Cecil Textbook of Medicine.* Edited by J. Claude Bennett and Fred Plum. Philadelphia, PA: W. B. Saunders, 1996.

ORGANIZATIONS

American Academy of Ophthalmology. P.O. Box 7242, San Francisco, CA 94120-7242. (415) 561-8500. <http://www.eyenet.org>.

American Foundation for the Blind. 11 Penn Plaza, Suite 300, New York, NY 10001. (800) 232-5463. <http://www.afb.org>.

Guide Dogs for the Blind. P.O. Box 1200, San Rafael, CA 94915. (415) 499-4000. <http://www.guidedogs.org>.

International Eye Foundation. 7801 Norfolk Avenue, Bethesda, MD 20814. (301) 986-1830.

The Lighthouse National Center for Education. 111 E. 59th Street. New York, NY 10022. (800) 334-5497. <http://www.lighthouse.org>.

National Association for the Visually Handicapped. 22 West 21st Street, New York, NY 10010. (212) 889-3141.

National Center For Sight. (800) 221-3004.

National Children's Eye Care Foundation. One Clinic Center, A3-108, Cleveland, OH 44195. (216) 444-0488.

National Eye Institute of the NIH. 9000 Rockville Pike, Bethesda, MD 20892. (301) 496-5248. <http://www.nei.nih.gov>.

Mary Bekker

Visual evoked potential study *see* **Evoked potential studies**

Vital capacity test *see* **Pulmonary function test**

Vital signs

Definition

Simply stated, vital signs are "signs of life." Temperature, beat of the **heart** (pulse), respiratory rate, and **blood pressure** signal that a person is alive. All of these vital signs can be observed, measured, and

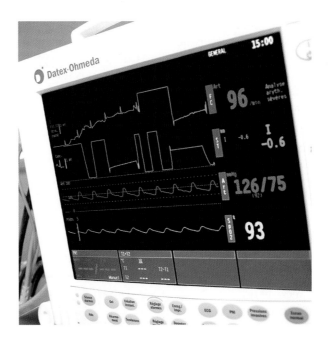

This monitor shows a patient's vital signs, including heart rate, temperature, blood pressure, blood oxygenation, and exhaled carbon dioxide. *(AJPhoto / Photo Researchers, Inc. Reproduced by permission.)*

monitored. This will enable the assessment of the level at which the individual is functioning. Normal ranges of measurements of vital signs change with a person's age and medical condition.

Purpose

To establish a baseline on admission to a hospital or clinic, the nurse should take the patient's vital signs. It is his or her responsibility to detect any abnormalities from the patient's normal state, and to establish if current medication(s) is having the desired effect.

Precautions

As there may be no knowledge of the patient's previous vital signs for comparison, it is important that the nurse be aware that there is a wide range of normal values that can apply to patients of different ages. The nurse should take as detailed a medical history from the patient as possible; any known medical or surgical history, prior measurements of vital signs, and details of current medication(s) should be recorded on the patient's chart. Any physical exertion prior to measurement of vital signs, such as climbing stairs, may affect the measurements. Thirty minutes prior to the taking of one's vital signs, the patient should not have consumed tobacco, caffeinated drinks, or alcohol.

Blood pressure is taken using a cuff that is the correct size for the patient; this will provide the most accurate reading. The reading can be 10 to 50 millimeters (mm) Hg too high with a cuff that is too small; a false reading of **hypertension** (high blood pressure) may result.

All types of sphygmomanometers—a cuff that can be filled with air, a hollow rubber bulb that pumps the air, and a glass tube that contains a column of mercury—should be calibrated annually by a trained technician. This will ensure that equipment remains accurate.

Description

Vital signs are recorded from once hourly to four times hourly, and as required by the patient's condition.

Temperature is recorded to check for pyrexia (a febrile condition) or to monitor the degree of hypothermia. The body's normal temperature, taken orally, is 98.6 °F (37 °C), with a range of 97.8 to 99.1 °F (36.5-37.2 °C). A **fever** is a temperature of 101 °F (38.3 °C) or higher in an infant younger than three months or above 102 °F (38.9 °C) for older children and adults. Hypothermia is recognized as a temperature below 96 °F (35.5 °C).

The pulse is checked for any abnormalities of the heart by measuring the rate, rhythm, and regularity of the beat, as well as the strength and tension of the beat against the arterial wall. The strength of the beat is raised during conditions such as fever and lowered by conditions such as **shock** and intracranial pressure. The average rate for older children (age 12 and up) and adults is 72 beats per minute (bpm). Tachycardia is a pulse rate over 100 bpm, while bradycardia is a pulse rate of under 60 bpm.

Respirations are quiet, slow, and shallow when the adult is asleep, and rapid, deeper, and noisier during and after activity.

Average respiration rates at rest are:

- infants, 34 to 40 per minute

- children five years of age, 25 per minute

- older children and adults, 16 to 20 per minute

Tachypnea is rapid respiration above 20 per minute.

Blood pressure is recorded for older children and adults. A normal blood pressure reading is 120/70.

Preparation

The patient should be sitting down or lying comfortably to ensure that the readings are taken in a similar position each time. There should be little excitement, which can affect the results. The equipment required is a watch with a second hand, an electronic or mercury **thermometer**, an electronic or manual **sphygmomanometer** with an appropriate sized cuff, and a **stethoscope**.

Manufacturer's guidelines should be followed when taking a temperature with an electronic thermometer. The result displayed on the LCD screen should be read, then recorded in the patient's chart. Electronic temperature monitors do not have to be cleaned after use. They have protective guards that are disposed of after each use; these ensure that infections are not spread.

A mercury thermometer can be used to monitor a temperature by three methods:

- Axillary, under the armpit.

- Orally, under the tongue. This method is never used with infants or very young children. Very young children might accidentally bite or break them. They also have difficulty holding oral thermometers under their tongues long enough for their temperatures to be accurately measured.

- Rectally, inserted into the rectum. This method is the gold standard for recording the temperature of infants. Although somewhat controversial because of potential discomfort and trauma to the baby, the investigators of a Harvard Medical School study, published in *Archives of Pediatrics and Adolescent Medicine*, discovered that rectal thermometers were more accurate than ear thermometers in detecting high fevers. With the ability to detect low-grade fevers, rectal thermometers can be useful in discovering serious illnesses, such as **meningitis** and **pneumonia**. The tip of the thermometer is usually blue to distinguish it from the silver tip of an oral/axillary thermometer.

To record the temperature using a mercury thermometer, one should shake down the thermometer by holding it firmly at the clear end and flicking it quickly a few times, with the silver end pointing downward. The health care provider who is taking the temperature should confirm that the mercury is below a normal body temperature.

The silver tip of the thermometer should be placed under the patient's right armpit. The arm clamps the thermometer into place, against the chest. The thermometer should stay in place for three to four minutes. After the appropriate time has elapsed, the thermometer should be removed and held at eye level. During this waiting period, the body temperature will be measured. The mercury will have risen to a mark that indicates the temperature of the patient.

To record the oral temperature, the axillary procedure should be followed, except that the silver tip of the thermometer should be placed beneath the tongue for three to four minutes, then read as described previously.

In both cases, the thermometer is wiped clean with an antiseptic and stored in an appropriate container to prevent breakage.

The rectal thermometer, used to take accurate temperatures in infants, should be shaken down, as discussed previously. A small amount of water-based lubricant should be placed on the colored tip of the thermometer. With the infant lying on his or her stomach, the nurse must hold the child securely in place. The tip of the thermometer should then be inserted into the child's rectum carefully to avoid discomfort and possible injury—no more than one-half inch, or 2 cm—and held there for two to three minutes. After the thermometer is removed, it should be read (as described previously), and wiped clean with an antibacterial wipe. It should then be stored in an appropriate container to prevent breakage.

The pulse can be recorded anywhere that a surface artery runs over a bone, but the radial artery in the wrist is the most common point. To take the pulse, one should place his or her index, middle, and ring fingers over the radial artery. It is located above the wrist, on the anterior surface of the thumb side of the arm. Gentle pressure should be applied, taking care to avoid obstructing the patient's blood flow. The rate, rhythm, strength, and tension of the pulse should be noted. If there are no abnormalities detected, the pulsations can be counted for half a minute, and the result doubled. However, any irregularities discerned indicate that the pulse should be recorded for one minute. This will eliminate the possibility of error.

The fingers should be kept on the wrist, while the frequency of respirations in one minute is recorded. Every effort should be made to prevent patients from becoming aware that their breathing is being checked; if the patients were to realize this, they might consciously alter the rate at which they breathe. Both pulse and respiration results should be noted in the patient's chart.

Blood pressure is taken using a cuff that is the correct size for the patient. This will ensure the most accurate reading possible. With an electronic unit, the cuff is placed level with the heart and, if possible, wrapped around the upper left arm. Following the manufacturer's guidelines, the cuff is inflated and then deflated automatically, and the health care provider records the reading. If blood pressure is monitored manually, a cuff is placed level with the heart and wrapped around the upper arm. Placing a stethoscope over the brachial artery in front of the elbow with one hand and listening through the earpiece, the cuff should be inflated until the artery is occluded, and no sound is heard. The cuff should then be inflated a further 10 mm Hg above the last sound heard. Opening the valve in the pump slowly—no faster than 5 mm Hg per second—pressure in the cuff is deflated until a sound is detected over the brachial artery. This point is noted as the systolic pressure. The pressure is further deflated until a soft muffled sound is heard. This allows the diastolic pressure to be taken. As in the case with children, sounds will continue to be heard as the cuff deflates to zero.

The results are charted, with the systolic pressure being recorded first, and then the diastolic pressure. An entry in the patient's chart might appear as 120/70 (systolic/diastolic).

Aftercare

The patient should be made comfortable and reassured that recording vital signs is part of normal health checks, and that it is necessary to ensure that his or her health is being correctly monitored. Any abnormalities in the vital signs must be reported to the medical staff.

Complications

There is a nationwide initiative to ban the sale of mercury thermometers and promote mercury-free devices for monitoring blood pressure. Health activists are concerned about mercury contaminating the environment after it has been discarded. Several states have banned the use of products containing mercury and stores such as Wal-Mart, CVS, and Kmart have already stopped selling mercury thermometers. According to a study by the Mayo Clinic in March 2001, mercury-free devices can monitor information without compromising accuracy. The Environmental Protection Agency's October 1999 report, "Reducing Mercury Use in Health Care," advises using alternative mercury products to avoid the future need for increased regulations and to protect human health and wildlife by reducing unnecessary exposure to mercury.

Results

The vital signs are recorded and compared with normal ranges for the patient's age and medical condition. Based on these results, it is decided whether any further action needs to be taken.

Health care team roles

Patients may ask questions about specific concerns they have regarding their vital signs, or even about a particular disease. The nurse can counsel on the prevention of illness, but can direct the patient to the physician for specific questions.

Resources

PERIODICALS

"Eleven of the Nation's Leading Retailers and Manufacturers Give Mercury Fever Thermometers the Heave-Ho." *PRNewswire via COMTEX/-Health Care Without Harm*. Accessed September 27, 2000.

ORGANIZATIONS

American Nurses Association, 600 Maryland Avenue, SW, Suite 100 West, Washington, DC 20024. (202) 651-7000.

OTHER

"About Blood Pressure." American Heart Association, National Center, 7272 Greenville Avenue, Dallas, TX 752311. (800) AHA-USA1.

Associated Press. "Best Way to Take Baby's Temperature? Bottoms Up!" Chicago. <http://www.abclocal.go.com/wtvd/health/031401_NH_thermometers.html>. Accessed June 29, 2001.

Environmental Protection Agency. <http://www.epa.gov/bns/merchealth>.

Franklin Institute Online. "Vital Signs." Accessed June 17, 2001. <http://www.sln.fi.edu>.

"High Blood Pressure." Mayoclinic.com. September 28, 2000. <http://www.mayoclinic.com>.

"Home Monitoring of High Blood Pressure." American Heart Association, National Center, 7272 Greenville Avenue, Dallas, TX 752311. (800) AHA-USA1.

Rathe, Richard. "Vital Signs." *University of Florida*. Accessed December 19, 2000. <http://www.medinfo.ufl.edu/yea1/bcs/clist/vitals.html>.

"Vital Signs." *University of Maryland Medicine*. <http://www.umm.drkoop.com>. June 24, 2001.

"What is High Blood Pressure?" American Heart Association, National Center, 7272 Greenville Avenue, Dallas, TX 752311. (800) AHA-USA1.

Margaret A. Stockley, RGN

Vital signs in children

Definition

Vital signs are the observation of temperature, pulse, respiration, and **blood pressure**. Vital signs may be different in children than in adults or the elderly.

Purpose

The goal of obtaining a child's vital signs is to establish a baseline on admission and detect any abnormalities from the normal state.

Precautions

As there may be no prior knowledge of the patient's previous vital signs for comparison, it is important that the nurse be aware of the wide range of normal values that apply to children of different ages.

Description

Vital signs are recorded hourly to every four hours and as needed based on the patient's condition.

Temperature is recorded to check for pyrexia or monitor the degree of hypothermia. The body's normal temperature is 98.6 °F (37 °C). A **fever** is a body temperature two standard deviations greater than 98.6 °F (37 °C) taken orally, or 100.4 °F (38 °) taken rectally or above 102 °F (38.9 °C) for older children. Hypothermia is recognized by a temperature below 96 °F (35.5 °C).

The rate and rhythm of the pulse is checked to detect any abnormalities of the **heart**; the beat of the pulse reflects the strength and tension of the beat against the arterial wall. The strength of the beat increases, for example, with fever; it is lowered by conditions such as **shock** and inter-cranial pressure.

Respirations are quiet, slow, and shallow when the child is asleep; rapid, deeper, and noisier respirations are heard during and after activity. Average rates of respiration:

- infants: 34 to 40 per minute
- children aged one to five years: 25 per minute
- children older than five years: 16 to 20 per minute

Preparation

Have the child sitting or lying comfortably and ensure a calm environment. Ensure that the readings are taken in similar positions each time, as a change in either can affect the results. The equipment required is a watch with a second hand, an electronic **thermometer**, an electronic or manual **sphygmomanometer**, and a **stethoscope**.

Follow the manufacturer's guidelines for taking a temperature with an electronic thermometer. Read the result displayed on the LCD screen and then record it in the patient's chart.

The pulse can be recorded in many areas where a surface artery runs over a bone, but the radial artery in the wrist is the most common option. To take the pulse, place the index, middle, and ring fingers over the radial artery that is located above the wrist on the anterior surface of the thumb side of the arm. Apply gentle pressure to avoid obstructing the patient's **blood** flow. The rate, rhythm, strength and tension of the pulse should be noted. If there are no abnormalities detected, the pulsations can be counted for half a minute, and the result doubled. If, however, any irregularities are present, the pulse should be recorded for one full minute to avoid any discrepancies.

Keeping the fingers on the wrist, the frequency of respirations in one minute should be noted. The patient should not be made aware that breathing is being monitored; he or she may consciously modify his or her breathing, thereby affecting the respiratory rate. The pulse and respiration results are noted in the patient's chart.

If the child is old enough, the blood pressure is taken using a cuff that is the correct size. This will provide a more accurate reading.

With an electronic unit, the cuff is placed level with the heart and wrapped around the upper arm. Following the manufacturer's guidelines, the cuff is inflated and then deflated automatically; the nurse records the reading.

If blood pressure is monitored manually, a cuff is placed level with the heart and wrapped around the upper arm. Placing a stethoscope over the brachial artery in front of the elbow with one hand and listening through the earpiece, the cuff is inflated until the artery is occluded and no sound is heard. The cuff is then inflated a further 10 mm Hg above the last audible sound. The valve in the pump is slowly opened no faster than 5mm Hg per second to deflate the pressure in the cuff until a sound is heard over the brachial artery. This point is noted as the systolic pressure. The pressure is further deflated until a soft, muffled sound is heard. That point is noted as the diastolic pressure.

The results are charted: first, the systolic is noted, then the diastolic pressure. It is done in the following manner: xxx/xx (e.g., 120/70).

Aftercare

The child should be made comfortable and give assurance that recording vital signs is part of normal health checks, and that it is necessary to ensure that health is being correctly checked. Electronic temperature monitors have disposable protective guards for hygiene to prevent the spread of infections. Any abnormalities in the vital signs must be reported to the medical staff.

Complications

There is a nationwide initiative to ban the sale of mercury thermometers and mercury devices for monitoring blood pressure. There are concerns among health activists regarding mercury contaminating the environment after its disposal. In fact, several states have banned the use of products containing mercury. Mercury thermometers are no longer sold by many large, commercial retailers. The Environmental Protection Agency recommendation is to use alternatives to mercury products, to avoid the need for increased regulations in the future and to protect human health and wildlife.

Results

The vital signs are recorded and compared with normal ranges for the patient's age and medical condition. With the interpretation of the results, a decision is made regarding the need for any further action.

KEY TERMS

Blood pressure—The tension of the blood in the arteries measured in millimeters of mercury by a sphygmomanometer or by an electronic device.

Respiration—The gaseous exchange between the tissue cells and the atmosphere.

Health care team roles

The nurse can provide counseling on the normal development of children and the prevention of illness and injuries. Alternatively, the nurse can guide the child's caregiver to the patient's doctor.

Resources

PERIODICALS

Board, Michele. "Comparison of disposable and glass mercury thermometers." *Nursing Times* 91, no. 33, pp. 36-37.

ORGANIZATIONS

American Association of Critical Care Nurses. 101 Columbia, Aliso Viejo, CA, 92656.

American Nurses Association. 600 Maryland Avenue, SW, Suite 100 West, Washington, DC 20024. (202) 651-7000.

National Association of Neonatal Nurses. 4700 W Lake Avenue, Glenview, IL 60025. (847) 375-3660 or (800) 451-3795.

National Association of Pediatric Nurse Associates and Practitioners. NAPNAP, 1101 Kings Highway N, Suite 206, Cherry Hill, NJ 08034. (856) 667-1773.

OTHER

Environmental Protection Agency. <http://www.epa.gov/bns/merchealth>.

Margaret A. Stockley, RGN

Vital signs in the aging

Definition

Vital signs are basic health status indicators. They include temperature, pulse, rate of respiration, and **blood pressure**. Several physiologic changes occur in the elderly which may impact the measurement of vital signs by the health care practitioner.

Purpose

Vital signs are measured to obtain basic indicators of a patient's health status. If outside of a normal range of values, they may point to dysfunction or a disease state.

Precautions

There are no significant contraindications to the measurement of vital signs in the aging patient.

Description

Some normal vital sign values may change as a person ages because of normal physiologic processes. The health care practitioner should be aware of these normal changes when assessing vital signs.

Normal body temperature does not significantly change as a person grows older. However, heat regulation may be altered due to physiologic changes that occur as a result of normal aging and from diseases that frequently occur in the elderly. For example, the elderly have a more difficult time maintaining body heat because of a loss of subcutaneous fat and may frequently complain of being too cold. Conversely, an older person, especially one who is obese, may have a harder time keeping cool in warmer weather. The overall ability to perceive temperature decreases, contributing to the problem. The elderly patient may not always be able to mount a **fever** during an **infection**.

Changes in the **heart** may cause the resting heart rate to slow down as a person ages. The pulse may take longer to quicken when exercising and longer to return to normal afterwards. The elderly person who exercises attains a lower maximum heart rate. When assessing heart rate, the pulse should be measured in both arms for a period of 30 seconds and any irregularities noted.

The range of values for normal **blood** pressure does not change with aging. However, arterial stiffness tends to increase, causing blood pressure measurements to sometimes be falsely high. In addition, many older people, especially women, are nervous in the doctor's office, sometimes elevating the blood pressure above the individual's typical values. Proper measurement technique is important. Because occlusive atherosclerotic disease often decreases the systolic pressure in one arm, blood pressure measurements should be taken in both arms. In addition, **blood vessels** tend to respond more slowly to changes in body position as a person ages. For this reason, measurements should be made while the patient is in a sitting

ORGANIZATIONS

Administration on Aging. 330 Independence Avenue SW, Washington, DC, 20201. (202) 619-7501.

Deanna M. Swartout-Corbeil, R.N.

KEY TERMS

Orthostatic hypotension—Hypotension occurring immediately after a person gets up from a sitting or reclining position.

---

or supine (lying down on back) position, then immediately after the patient stands, so that orthostatic hypotension can be detected.

The normal respiratory rate in the older patient may be as high as 16 to 25 breaths per minute. Breathing may appear somewhat shallower than in the younger population. However, even a very elderly person should be able to breathe without effort in the absence of disease. A rate higher than 25 breaths per minute may indicate congestive **heart failure** or a lower respiratory tract infection.

Preparation

The nurse or other health care professional should instruct the patient regarding the rationale for vital sign measurement. The patient should be sitting or lying in a comfortable, relaxed position.

Results

A normal temperature range is 97.5 °F to 99.5 °F (36 °C to 38 °C). The resting heart rate may be lower than the normal 60-100 beats per minute in a younger person. Normal blood pressure is the same as for a younger adult: less than 140 mm Hg (systolic) over less than 90 mm Hg (diastolic). The normal respiratory rate of an older person ranges from 16 to 25 breaths per minute.

Health care team roles

Vital sign readings may be obtained by the physician, the nurse or nursing assistant, and the physical therapist.

Resources

BOOKS

Beers, Mark H., and Robert Berkow, eds. *The Merck Manual of Geriatrics.* Whitehouse Station, NJ: Merck & Co., Inc., 2000.

PERIODICALS

Currey, Chuck. "Biology and Physiology of Aging." *University of Florida PA Program Introduction to Medicine II* (Spring 2001).

Vitamin A

Description

Vitamin A is one of the four fat-soluble **vitamins** necessary for good health. It serves an important role as an antioxidant by helping to prevent free radicals from causing cellular damage. Adequate levels are important for good eyesight, and poor night **vision** may be one of the first symptoms of a deficiency. It is also necessary for proper function of the immune, skeletal, respiratory, reproductive, and integumentary (skin) systems.

General use

An adequate level of vitamin A unquestionably contributes to good health. It is essential for the proper function of the retina, where it can act to prevent night blindness, as well as lower the odds of getting age-related **macular degeneration** (AMD), which is the most common cause of blindness in the elderly. There is also evidence that good levels of vitamin A in the form of carotenoids may decrease the risk of certain cancers, **heart** attacks, and strokes. The **immune system** is also strengthened. It is unclear, however, that supplemental forms have the same benefit as consuming them in natural foods in the case of a person without deficiency. Taking high levels of vitamin A in any supplemental form is not advisable without the counsel of a healthcare professional.

Preparations

Natural sources

There are two basic forms of vitamin A. Retinoids, the active types, are contained in animal sources, including meat, whole milk, and eggs. Liver is particularly rich in vitamin A, since it is one of the storage sites for excess. Precursor forms of the vitamin (carotenoids) are found in orange and leafy green produce such as sweet potatoes, carrots, collard greens, spinach, winter squash, kale, and turnip greens. Very fresh foods have the highest levels, followed by frozen foods. Typically, canned produce has little vitamin A. Preparing vegetables by steaming, baking, or grilling helps them to release the carotenes they contain. Alpha and beta carotene, as well as some of the other lesser-known carotenoids, can be converted to vitamin A in the **small intestine**. This is done by the body on an as-needed basis, so there is no risk of **overdose** as there is with the active form.

Supplemental sources

Supplements may contain either the active or precursor forms of vitamin A. The active form may be more desirable for those who may have some difficulty in converting the carotenoids into the active vitamin. This is more often true in those over age 55 or who have a condition that impairs absorption of fat. There is a water-soluble form of the vitamin, retinyl palmitate, which may be better utilized in the latter case. Carotenes are also available either as oil-based or natural water-based formulas. Be sure to store both away from light and heat, which will destroy them.

Units

There are several units that can express the amount of vitamin A activity in a product. Many supplements are still labeled with the old International Unit (IU), although the more current and most accurate unit is the Retinol Equivalent (RE). The new measurement distinguishes between the differences in absorption of retinol and beta carotene. One RE is equal to one microgram (μg) of retinol, or six μg of beta carotene.

Dose limits

Adults should take no more than 25,000 IU (5,000 RE) per day of vitamin A in its active form, except in the case of women who are pregnant or may become pregnant. The latter group should not exceed 10,000 IU (2,000 RE) per day in order to avoid potential toxic effects to the fetus. The best way to get vitamins is in the natural food form, as the complexities are not always either known or reproducible in a supplement. A diet rich in foods containing carotenoids is optimal, but in the event of nutritional deficiencies, supplements may be needed. Mixed carotenoids are preferable to either large doses of vitamin A or pure beta carotene supplements to avoid toxicity and maximize healthful benefits. Some of the minor carotenoids appear to have beneficial effects that are still being explored. A good mixture will contain alpha and beta carotene, as well as lycopene and xanthophylls. Eating foods high in many carotenoids may confer some benefits—such as lower risk of **cancer**, heart attacks, and strokes—which a supplement may not.

Deficiency

Levels of vitamin A that are low enough to cause symptomatic deficiency are uncommon in people of normal health in industrialized nations. Symptoms of deficiency may include, but are not limited to, loss of appetite, poor immune function causing frequent infections (especially respiratory), hair loss, rashes, dry skin and eyes, visual difficulties including night blindness, poor growth, and fatigue. Generally symptoms are not manifested unless the deficiency has existed for a period of months. Deficiencies are more likely in people who are malnourished, including the chronically ill and those with impaired fat absorption. Those with normal health and nutritional status have a considerable vitamin A reserve.

In countries where nutritional status tends to be poor and deficiency is more common, vitamin A has been found to reduce the mortality rate of children suffering from a number of different viral infections.

Risk factors for deficiency

Taking the RDA level of a nutrient will prevent a deficiency in most people, but under certain circumstances, an individual may require higher doses of vitamin A. Those who consume alcoholic beverages may be more prone to vitamin A deficiency. People taking some medications, including birth control pills, methotrexate, cholestyramine, colestipol, and drugs that act to sequester bile will also need larger amounts. Those who are malnourished, chronically ill, or recovering from surgery or other injuries may also benefit from a higher dose than average. Patients undergoing treatments for cancer, including radiation and **chemotherapy**, typically have compromised immune systems that may be boosted by judicious supplementation with vitamin A. Other conditions that may impair vitamin A balance include chronic **diarrhea**, **cystic fibrosis**, and kidney or liver disease. Diabetics are often deficient in vitamin A, but may also be more susceptible to toxicity. Any supplementation for these conditions should be discussed with a healthcare provider. Supplements are best taken in the form of carotenoids to avoid any potential for toxicity. There is not an established RDA for beta carotene. Recommendations for how much to take vary between six and 30 milligrams a day, but the middle range—around 15mg—is a reasonable average.

Precautions

Overdose can occur when taking megadoses of the active form of this vitamin. Amounts above what is being utilized by the body accumulate in the liver and fatty tissues. Symptoms may include dry lips and skin, bone and joint **pain**, liver and spleen enlargement, diarrhea, vomiting, headaches, blurry or double vision, confusion, irritability, fatigue, and bulging fontanel (soft spot on the head) in infants; these are most often reversible, but a doctor should be contacted if a known overdose occurs. Very high levels of vitamin A may also create deficiencies of vitamins C, E, and K. Symptoms will generally appear within six hours following an acute overdose, and take a few weeks to resolve after ceasing the supplement. Children are more sensitive to high levels of vitamin A than adults are, so instructions on products designed for children should be followed with particular care. Vitamin supplements should always be kept out of reach of children.

It is especially important to avoid overdoses in **pregnancy**, as it may cause **miscarriage** or fetal malformations. Using supplements that provide carotenoids will avoid the potential of overdose. Those with kidney disease are also at higher risk for toxicity due to either vitamin A or beta carotene, and should not take these supplements without professional healthcare advice.

There is some evidence that taking beta carotene supplements puts smokers at higher risk of lung cancers. The CARET (Beta Carotene and Retinol Efficacy Trial) study is one that demonstrated this effect. Clarification through more study is needed, as evidence also exists showing that beta carotene, along with other antioxidants, can be a factor in cancer prevention. Some of the lesser-known carotenoids may be key factors. Whole sources are better obtained from foods than from supplements. Smokers should consult with a healthcare provider before taking supplemental beta carotene.

Side effects

Very high levels of carotenoids (carotenemia) may cause an orange discoloration of the skin, which is harmless and transient.

Interactions

Vitamin A supplements should not be taken in conjunction with any retinoid medications, including isotretinoin (Accutane), a drug used to treat acne. There is a higher risk of toxicity.

A very low fat diet or use of fat substitutes impairs absorption of all the fat-soluble vitamins, including A.

KEY TERMS

Antioxidant—Substance, such as vitamin A, which blocks the destructive action of free radicals.

Carotenoids—Any of a group of over 600 orange or red substances which are found primarily in vegetables, many of which are vitamin A precursors.

Free radical—Highly reactive atoms which are very reactive as a result of having one or more unpaired electrons. They form through exposure to smoke and other environmental pollutants, as well as radiation and other sources. They have great potential to cause cellular damage, and may even be a factor in aging.

Retinoids—Any of the group of substances which comprise active vitamin A, including retinaldehyde, retinol, and retinoic acid.

Mineral oil and aluminum-containing **antacids** may also inhibit absorption, as do the cholesterol-lowering drugs cholestyramine and colestipol. Vitamin A reserves of the body are depleted by a number of substances, including alcohol, barbiturates, **caffeine**, cortisone, tobacco, and very high levels of **vitamin E**. Overuse of alcohol and vitamin A together may increase the possibility of liver damage.

Taking appropriate doses of **vitamin C**, vitamin E, **zinc**, and selenium optimizes absorption and use of vitamin A and carotenoids. As vitamin A is fat-soluble, a small amount of dietary fat is also helpful.

Studies of both children and pregnant women with **iron deficiency anemia** show that this condition is better treated with a combination of **iron** supplements and vitamin A than with iron alone.

Resources

BOOKS

Bratman, Steven, and David Kroll. *Natural Health Bible.* Prima Publishing, 1999.

Feinstein, Alice. *Prevention's Healing with Vitamins.* Rodale Press, 1996.

Griffith, H. Winter. *Vitamins, Herbs, Minerals & Supplements: The Complete Guide.* Fisher Books, 1998.

Jellin, Jeff, Forrest Batz, and Kathy Hitchens. *Pharmacist's Letter/Prescriber's Letter Natural Medicines Comprehensive Database.* Therapeutic Research Faculty, 1999.

Pressman, Alan H., and Sheila Buff. *The Complete Idiot's Guide to Vitamins and Minerals.* Alpha Books, 1997.

Judith Turner

Vitamin B$_{12}$

Description

Cobalamin, also known as B$_{12}$, is a member of the water-soluble family of B **vitamins**. It is a key factor in the body's proper use of **iron** and formation of red **blood** cells. The nervous system also relies on an adequate supply of cobalamin to function appropriately, as it is an essential component in the creation and maintenance of the myelin sheath that lines nerve cells. Other roles of cobalamin include working with pyridoxine (vitamin B$_6$) and **folic acid** to reduce harmful homocysteine levels, participating in the metabolization of food, and keeping the **immune system** operating smoothly.

General use

Very small amounts of cobalamin are needed to maintain good health. The RDA value is 0.3 micrograms (mcg) for infants under six months, 0.5 mcg for those six months to one year old, 0.7 mcg for children one to three years old, 1.0 mcg for children four to six years old, 1.4 mcg for children seven to 10 years old, and 2 mcg for those 11 years of age and older. Requirements are slightly higher for pregnant (2.2 mcg) and lactating (2.6 mcg) women.

The primary conditions that benefit from supplementation with cobalamin are megaloblastic and pernicious anemia. Megaloblastic anemia is a state resulting from an inadequate intake of cobalamin, to which vegans are particularly susceptible because of the lack of animal food sources. Vegans, who do not consume any animal products including meat, dairy, or eggs, should take at least 2 mcg of cobalamin per day in order to prevent this condition. In the case of pernicious anemia, intake may be appropriate but absorption is poor due to a lack of normal **stomach** substance, called intrinsic factor, that facilitates absorption of vitamin B$_{12}$. Large doses are required to treat pernicious anemia, which occurs most commonly in the elderly population as a result of decreased production of intrinsic factor by the stomach. Supplements are generally effective when taken orally in very large amounts (300-1000 mcg/day) even if no intrinsic factor is produced. These supplements require a prescription, and should be administered with the guidance of a health care provider. Injections, instead of the supplements, are often used.

Those who have infections, **burns**, some types of **cancer**, recent surgery, illnesses that cause decay or loss of strength, or high amounts of **stress** may need more than the RDA amount of B$_{12}$ and other B vitamins. A balanced supplement is the best approach.

Male **infertility** can sometimes be resolved through use of cobalamin supplements. Other conditions that may be improved by cobalamin supplementation include: **asthma**, atherosclerosis (hardening of the arteries caused by plaque formation in the arteries), **bursitis** (inflammation of a bodily pouch, especially the shoulder or elbow), **Crohn's disease** (chronic recurrent inflammation of the intestines), depression, diabetes, high cholesterol, **osteoporosis**, and vitiligo (milky-white patches on the skin). There is not enough evidence to judge whether supplementation for these diseases is effective.

Preparations

Natural sources

Usable cobalamin is only found naturally in animal source foods. Fresh food is best, as freezing and exposure to light may destroy some of the vitamin content. Clams and beef liver have very high cobalamin levels. Other good sources include chicken liver, beef, lamb, tuna, flounder, liverwurst, eggs, and dairy products. Some plant foods may contain cobalamin, but it is not in a form that is usable by the body.

Supplemental sources

Cobalamin supplements are available in both oral and injectable formulations. A nasal gel is also made. Generally a balanced B-complex vitamin is preferable to taking high doses of cobalamin unless there is a specific indication for it, such as megaloblastic anemia. Strict vegetarians will need to incorporate a supplemental source of B$_{12}$ in the diet. Cyanocobalamin is the form most commonly available in supplements. Two other, possibly more effective, types are hydro-cobalamin and methyl-cobalamin. As with all supplements, cobalamin should be stored in a cool, dry, dark place and out of the reach of children.

Deficiency

Cobalamin deficiency may be manifested as a variety of symptoms since cobalamin is so widely used in the body. Severe fatigue may occur initially. Effects on the nervous system can be wide-ranging, and include weakness, numbness and tingling of the limbs, **memory** loss, confusion, delusion, poor balance and **reflexes**, **hearing** difficulties, and even **dementia**. Severe deficiency may appear similar to **multiple sclerosis**. Nausea and **diarrhea** are possible gastrointestinal signs. The anemia that results from prolonged deficiency may also be seen as a pallor, especially in mucous membranes such as the gums and the lining of the inner surface of the eye.

Megaloblastic anemia is a common result of inadequate cobalamin. This condition can also result if a person stops secreting enough intrinsic factor in the stomach, a substance essential for the absorption of cobalamin. Inadequate intrinsic factor leads to pernicious anemia, so called because it persists despite iron supplementation. Long-term deficiencies of cobalamin also allow homocysteine levels to build up. Negative effects of large amounts of circulating homocysteine include **heart** disease and possibly **brain** toxicity. Taking high levels of folic acid supplements can mask cobalamin deficiency and prevent the development of megaloblastic anemia, but neurological damage can still occur. This damage may become permanent if the cobalamin deficiency persists for a long period of time.

Risk factors for deficiency

The primary groups at risk for cobalamin deficiency are vegans who are not taking supplements, and the elderly. Older adults are more likely to have both insufficient intrinsic factor secreted by the stomach and low levels of stomach acid, causing cobalamin to be poorly absorbed. Malabsorptive diseases and stomach surgery can also predispose to a deficiency.

Precautions

People who are sensitive to cobalamin or cobalt should not take cobalamin supplements. Symptoms of hypersensitivity may include swelling, itching, and **shock**. Adverse effects resulting from B_{12} supplementation are rare. Cobalamin should also be avoided by those who have a type of hereditary optic nerve atrophy known as Leber's disease.

Side effects

Very high doses of cobalamin may sometimes cause acne.

Interactions

Large amounts of **vitamin C** taken within an hour of vitamin B supplements will destroy the cobalamin component. Absorption of cobalamin is also impaired by deficiencies of folic acid, iron, or **vitamin E**. Improved absorption occurs when it is taken with other B vitamins or **calcium**. Some medications may also cause an increased use or decreased absorption of

---

KEY TERMS

Homocysteine—An amino acid produced from the metabolization of other amino acids. High levels are an independent risk factor for heart disease.

Megaloblastic anemia—A condition caused by cobalamin deficiency, which is characterized by red blood cells which are too few, too fragile, and abnormally large. Also known as macrocytic anemia.

Pernicious anemia—Megaloblastic anemia resulting from a cobalamin deficiency that is the result of poor absorption due to inadequate production of intrinsic factor in the stomach.

Vegan—A person who doesn't eat any animal products, including dairy and eggs.

---

this vitamin. Those on colchicine, **corticosteroids**, methotrexate, metformin, phenformin, oral contraceptives, cholestyramine, colestipol, clofibrate, epoetin, neomycin, or supplemental potassium may need extra cobalamin. Use of nicotine products or excessive alcohol can deplete B_{12}.

Resources

BOOKS

Bratman, Steven, and David Kroll. *Natural Health Bible.* Prima Publishing, 1999.

Feinstein, Alice. *Prevention's Healing with Vitamins.* Rodale Press, 1996.

Griffith, H. Winter. *Vitamins, Herbs, Minerals & Supplements: The Complete Guide.* Fisher Books, 1998.

Jellin, Jeff, Forrest Batz, and Kathy Hitchens. *Pharmacist's Letter/Prescriber's Letter Natural Medicines Comprehensive Database.* Therapeutic Research Faculty, 1999.

Pressman, Alan H., and Sheila Buff. *The Complete Idiot's Guide to Vitamins and Minerals.* Alpha Books, 1997.

Judith Turner

Vitamin B complex

Description

Vitamin B complex is a set of 12 related water-soluble substances. Eight are considered **vitamins**, by

---

virtue of needing to be included in the diet, and four are not, as the body can synthesize them. Since they are water-soluble, most are not stored to any great extent and must be replenished on a daily basis. The eight vitamins have both names and corresponding numbers. They are B_1 (thiamin), B_2 (**riboflavin**), B_3 (**niacin**), B_5 (pantothenic acid), B_6 (pyridoxine), B_7 (**biotin**), B_9 (**folic acid**), and B_{12} (cobalamin). Biotin in particular is not always included in B complex supplements. The numbers that appear to have been skipped were found to be duplicate substances or non-vitamins. The four unnumbered components of B complex that can be synthesized by the body are choline, inositol, PABA, and lipoic acid. As a group, the B vitamins have a broad range of functions. These include maintenance of myelin, which is the covering of nerve cells. A breakdown of myelin can cause a large and devastating variety of neurologic symptoms. B vitamins are also key to producing energy from the nutrients that are consumed. Three members of this group—folic acid, pyridoxine, and cobalamin—work together to keep homocysteine levels low. This is quite important, since high homocysteine levels are associated with **heart** disease. Some B vitamins prevent certain birth defects (like neural tube defects), maintain healthy red **blood** cells, support immune function, regulate cell growth, aid in production of hormones, and may have a role in preventing some types of **cancer**. They also function in maintenance of healthy skin, hair, and nails.

General use

There are many claims for usefulness of various B vitamins. **Thiamine** is thought to be supportive for people with **Alzheimer's disease**. Niacin at very high doses is useful to lower cholesterol, and balance high-density (HDL) and low-density (LDL) lipoproteins. This should be done under medical supervision only. Some evidence shows that niacin may prevent juvenile diabetes (type I insulin dependent) in children at risk. It may also maintain pancreatic excretion of some insulin for a longer time than would occur normally. Niacin has also been used to relieve intermittent claudication and **osteoarthritis**, although the dose used for the latter risks **liver** problems. The frequency of migraines may be significantly reduced, and the severity decreased, by the use of supplemental riboflavin. Pyridoxine is used therapeutically to lower the risk of heart disease, and to relieve nausea associated with morning sickness and to treat premenstrual syndrome (PMS). In conjunction with magnesium, pyridoxine may have some beneficial effects on the behavior of children with autism. Cobalamin supplementation has

been shown to improve male fertility. Folic acid may reduce the odds of cervical or colon cancer in certain at risk groups.

Deficiency

Vitamin B complex is most often used to treat deficiencies that are caused by poor vitamin intake, difficulties with vitamin absorption, or conditions causing increased metabolic rate such as hyperthyroidism that deplete vitamin levels at a higher than normal rate.

Biotin and pantothenic acid are rarely deficient since they are broadly available in food, but often those lacking in one type of B vitamin are lacking in other B components as well. An individual may be symptomatic due to an inadequate level of one vitamin but be suffering from an undetected underlying deficiency as well. One possibility of particular concern is that taking folic acid supplements can cover up symptoms of cobalamin deficiency. This scenario could result in permanent neurologic damage if the cobalamin shortage remains untreated.

Some of the B vitamins have unique functions within the body that allow a particular deficiency to be readily identified. Often, however, they work in concert so symptoms due to various inadequate components may overlap. In general, poor B vitamin levels will cause profound fatigue and an assortment of neurologic manifestations, which may include weakness, poor balance, confusion, irritability, **memory** loss, nervousness, tingling of the limbs, and loss of coordination. Depression may be an early sign of significantly low levels of pyridoxine and possibly other B vitamins. Additional symptoms of vitamin B deficiency are sleep disturbances, nausea, poor appetite, frequent infections, and skin lesions.

A certain type of anemia (megaloblastic) is an effect of inadequate cobalamin. This anemia can also result if a person stops secreting enough intrinsic factor in the **stomach**. Intrinsic factor is essential for the absorption of cobalamin. The result of a lack of intrinsic factor is pernicious anemia, so called because it persists despite **iron** supplementation. Neurologic symptoms often precede anemia when cobalamin is deficient.

A severe and prolonged lack of niacin causes a condition called pellagra. The classic signs of pellagra are dermatitis, **dementia**, and **diarrhea**. It is very rare now, except in alcoholics, strict vegans, and people in areas of the world with very poor **nutrition**.

Thiamine deficiency is similarly rare, save in the severely malnourished and alcoholics. A significant depletion causes a condition known as beriberi, and it can cause weakness, leg spasms, poor appetite, and loss of coordination. Wernicke-Korsakoff syndrome is the most severe form of deficiency, and occurs in conjunction with **alcoholism**. Early stages of neurologic symptoms are reversible, but psychosis and death may occur if the course is not reversed.

Risk factors for deficiency

People are at higher risk for deficiency if they have poor nutritional sources of B vitamins, take medications or have conditions that impair absorption, or are affected by circumstances that increase the need for vitamin B components above the normal level. Since the B vitamins often work in harmony, a deficiency in one type may have broad implications. Poor intake of B vitamins is most often a problem in strict vegetarians and the elderly. People who frequently fast or diet may also benefit from taking B vitamins. Vegans will need to use brewer's yeast or other sources of supplemental cobalamin, since the only natural sources are meats.

Risk factors that may decrease absorption of some B vitamins include smoking, excessive use of alcohol, surgical removal of portions of the digestive tract, and advanced age. Absorption is also impaired by some medications. Some of the drugs that may cause this are **corticosteroids**, colchicine, metformin, phenformin, omeprazol, colestipol, cholestyramine, methotrexate, tricyclic antidepressants, and slow-release potassium.

Need for vitamin B complex may be increased by conditions such as **pregnancy**, breastfeeding, emotional **stress**, and physical stress due to surgery or injury. People who are very physically active require extra riboflavin. Use of birth control pills also increases the need for certain B vitamins.

Preparations

Natural sources

Fresh meats and dairy products are the best sources for most of the B vitamins, although they are prevalent in many foods. Cobalamin is only found naturally in animal source foods. Freezing of food and exposure of food or supplements to light may destroy some of the vitamin content. Dark-green leafy vegetables are an excellent source of folic acid. To make the most of the B vitamins contained in foods, do not overcook them. It is also best to steam rather than boil or simmer vegetables.

Supplemental sources

B vitamins are generally best taken in balanced complement, unless there is a specific deficiency or need of an individual vitamin. An excess of one component may lead to depletion of the others. Injectable and oral forms of supplements are available. The injectable types may be more useful for those with deficiencies due to problems with absorption. B complex products vary as to which components are included, and at what dose level.

Individual components are also available as supplements. These are best used with the advice of a health care professional. Some are valuable when addressing specific problems such as pernicious anemia. Strict vegetarians will need to incorporate a supplemental source of B_{12} in the diet.

Precautions

In many cases, large doses of water-soluble vitamins can be taken with no ill effects since excessive amounts are readily excreted. However, when niacin is taken at daily doses of over 500 mg (and more often at doses six times as high), liver inflammation may occur. It is generally reversible once the supplementation is stopped. Niacin may also cause difficulty in controlling blood sugar in diabetics. It can increase uric acid levels that will aggravate **gout**. Those with ulcers could be adversely affected as niacin increases the production of stomach acid. Niacin also lowers **blood pressure** due to its vasodilatory effect, so should not be taken in conjunction with medications that are used to treat high blood pressure. If the form of niacin known as inositol hexaniacinate is taken instead, problems with flushing, gout, ulcers, and liver inflammation do not occur but beneficial effects on cholesterol are maintained.

High doses of pyridoxine may also cause liver inflammation or permanent nerve damage. Megadoses of this vitamin are not necessary or advisable.

Those on medication for seizures, high blood pressure, and **Parkinson's disease** are at increased risk for interactions. Any person with a chronic health condition or taking other medications should seek the advice of a health professional before beginning any program of supplementation.

Side effects

Niacin in large amounts commonly causes flushing and headache, although this can be circumvented by taking it in the form of inositol hexaniacinate.

KEY TERMS

Homocysteine— An amino acid produced from the metabolization of other amino acids. High levels are an independent risk factor for heart disease.

Macrocytic anemia—A condition caused by cobalamin deficiency, which is characterized by red blood cells that are too few, too fragile, and abnormally large.

Neural tube defect—Incomplete development of the brain, spinal cord, or vertebrae of a fetus, which is sometimes caused by a folic acid deficiency.

Vasodilatory—Causing the veins in the body to dilate, or enlarge.

Vegan—A person who does not eat any animal products, including dairy and eggs.

Large doses of riboflavin make the urine turn very bright yellow.

Interactions

Some medications may be affected by B vitamin supplementation, including those for high blood pressure, Parkinson's disease (such as levodopa, which is inactivated by pantothenic acid) and epileptiform conditions. Folic acid interacts with Dilantin as well as other anticonvulsants. Large amounts of **vitamin C** taken within an hour of vitamin B supplements will destroy the cobalamin component. Niacin may interfere with control of blood sugar in people on **antidiabetic drugs**. Isoniazid, a medication to treat **tuberculosis**, can impair the proper production and utilization of niacin. **Antibiotics** potentially decrease the level of some B vitamins by killing the **bacteria** in the digestive tract that produce them.

Resources

BOOKS

Bratman, Steven, and David Kroll. *Natural Health Bible*. Prima Publishing, 1999.

Feinstein, Alice. *Prevention's Healing with Vitamins*. Rodale Press, 1996.

Griffith, H. Winter. *Vitamins, Herbs, Minerals & Supplements: The Complete Guide*. Fisher Books, 1998.

Janson, Michael. *The Vitamin Revolution in Health Care*. Arcadia Press, 1996.

Jellin, Jeff, Forrest Batz, and Kathy Hitchens. *Pharmacist's Letter/Prescriber's Letter Natural Medicines Comprehensive Database*. Therapeutic Research Faculty, 1999.

Pressman, Alan H., and Sheila Buff. *The Complete Idiot's Guide to Vitamins and Minerals*. Alpha Books, 1997.

Judith Turner

Vitamin C

Description

Vitamin C, or ascorbic acid, is naturally produced in fruits and vegetables. The vitamin, which can be taken in dietary or supplementary form, is absorbed by the intestines. That which the body cannot absorb is excreted in the urine. The body stores a small amount, but daily intake, preferably in dietary form, is recommended for optimum health.

Certain health conditions may cause vitamin C depletion, including diabetes and high **blood pressure**. Individuals who smoke and women who take estrogen may also have lower vitamin C levels. In addition, men are more likely to be vitamin C depleted, as are the elderly. High **stress** levels have also been linked to vitamin C deficiency.

Severe vitamin C deficiency leads to scurvy, a disease common on ships prior to the sixteenth century, due to the lack of fresh fruits and other dietary vitamin C sources. Symptoms of scurvy include weakness, bleeding, tooth loss, bleeding gums, bruising, and joint **pain**. Less serious vitamin C depletion can have more subtle effects such as weight loss, fatigue, weakened **immune system** (as demonstrated by repeated infections and colds), bruises that occur with minor trauma and are slow to heal, and slow healing of other **wounds**.

Low vitamin C levels have also been associated with high **blood** pressure, increased **heart** attack risk, increased risk for developing **cataracts**, and a higher risk for certain types of **cancer** (i.e., prostate, **stomach**, colon, oral, and lung).

General use

Vitamin C is a critical component to both disease prevention and to basic body building processes. The therapeutic effects of vitamin C include:

- Allergy and **asthma** relief. Vitamin C is present in the lung's airway surfaces, and insufficient vitamin C levels have been associated with bronchial constriction and reduced lung function. Some studies have associated vitamin C supplementation with asthmatic symptom relief, but results have been inconclusive and further studies are needed.

- Cancer prevention. Vitamin C is a known antioxidant and has been associated with reduced risk of stomach, lung, colon, oral, and prostate cancer.

- Cataract prevention. Long-term studies on vitamin C supplementation and cataract development have shown that supplementation significantly reduces the risk for cataracts, particularly among women.

- Collagen production. Vitamin C assists the body in the manufacture of collagen, a protein that binds cells together and is the building block of connective tissues throughout the body. Collagen is critical to the formation and ongoing health of the skin, cartilage, ligaments, corneas, and other bodily tissues and structures. Vitamin C is also thought to promote faster healing of wounds and injuries because of its role in collagen production.

- Diabetes control. Vitamin C supplementation may assist diabetics in controlling blood sugar levels and improving **metabolism**.

- **Gallbladder** disease prevention. A study of over 13,000 subjects published in the *Archives in Internal Medicine* found that women who took daily vitamin C supplements were 34% less likely to contract gallbladder disease and gallstones, and that women deficient in ascorbic acid had an increased prevalence of gallbladder disease.

- Immune system booster. Vitamin C increases white blood cell production and is important to immune system balance. Studies have related low vitamin C levels to increased risk for **infection**. Vitamin C is frequently prescribed for HIV-positive individuals to protect their immune system.

- Neurotransmitter and hormone building. Vitamin C is critical to the conversion of certain substances into neurotransmitters, **brain** chemicals that facilitate the transmission of nerve impulses across a synapse (the space between **neurons**, or nerve cells). Neurotransmitters such as serotonin, dopamine, and norepinephrine are responsible for the proper functioning of the **central nervous system**, and a deficiency of neurotransmitters can result in psychiatric illness. Vitamin C also helps the body manufacture adrenal hormones.

Other benefits of vitamin C are less clear cut and have been called into question with conflicting study results. These include vitamin C's role in treating the **common cold**, preventing heart disease, and treating cancer.

Treating the common cold

Doses of vitamin C may reduce the duration and severity of cold symptoms, particularly in those individuals who are vitamin C deficient. The effectiveness of vitamin C therapy on colds seems to be related to the dietary vitamin C intake of the individual and the individual's general health and lifestyle.

Heart disease prevention

Some studies have indicated that vitamin C may prevent heart disease by lowering total blood cholesterol and LDL cholesterol and raising HDL, or good cholesterol, levels. The antioxidant properties of vitamin C have also been associated with protection of the arterial lining in patients with **coronary artery disease**.

However, the results of a recent study conducted at the University of Southern California and released in early 2000 have cast doubt on the heart protective benefits of vitamin C. The study found that daily doses of 500 mg of vitamin C resulted in a thickening of the arteries in study subjects at a rate 2.5 times faster than normal. Thicker arterial walls can cause narrow **blood vessels** and actually increase the risk for heart disease. Study researchers have postulated that the collagen producing effects of vitamin C could be the cause behind the arterial thickening. Further studies will be needed to determine the actual risks and benefits of vitamin C in relation to heart disease and to establish what a beneficial dosage might be, if one exists. For the time being, it is wise for most individuals, particularly those with a history of heart disease, to avoid megadoses over 200 mg because of the risk of arterial thickening.

Blood pressure control

A 1999 study found that daily doses of 500 mg of vitamin C reduced blood pressure in a group of 39 hypertensive individuals. Scientists have hypothesized that vitamin C may improve high blood pressure by aiding the function of nitric oxide, a gas produced by the body that allows blood vessels to dilate and facilitates blood flow. Again, recent findings that vitamin C may promote arterial wall thickening seem to contradict these findings, and further long-term studies are needed to assess the full benefits and risks of vitamin C in relation to blood pressure control.

Cancer treatment

Researchers disagree on the therapeutic use of vitamin C in cancer treatment. On one hand, studies have shown that tumors and cancer cells absorb vitamin C at a faster rate than normal cells because they have lost the ability to transport the vitamin. In addition, radiation and **chemotherapy** work in part by stimulating oxidation and the growth of free radicals in order to stop cancer cell growth. Because vitamin C is an antioxidant, which absorbs free radicals and counteracts the oxidation process, some scientists believe it could be counterproductive to cancer treatments. The exact impact vitamin C has on patients undergoing chemotherapy and other cancer treatments is not fully understood, and for this reason many scientists believe that vitamin C should be avoided by patients undergoing cancer treatment.

On the other side of the debate are researchers who believe that high doses of vitamin C can protect normal cells and inhibit the growth of cancerous ones. In lab-based, *in vitro* studies, cancer cells were killed and/or stopped growing when large doses of vitamin C were administered. Researchers postulate that unlike normal healthy cells, which will take what they need of a vitamin and then discard the rest, cancer cells continue to absorb antioxidant **vitamins** at excessive rates until the cell structure is effected, the cell is killed, or cell growth simply stops. However, it is important to note that there have been no in vivo controlled clinical studies to prove this theory.

Based on the currently available controlled clinical data, cancer patients should avoid taking vitamin C supplementation beyond their recommended daily allowance.

Preparations

The U.S. recommended dietary allowance (RDA) of vitamin C is as follows:

- men: 60 mg
- women: 60 mg
- pregnant women: 70 mg
- lactating women: 95 mg

In April 2000, the National Academy of Sciences recommended changing the RDA for vitamin C to 75 mg for women and 90 mg for men, with an upper limit (UL), or maximum daily dose, of 2,000 mg. Daily values for the vitamin as recommended by the U.S. Food and Drug Administration, the values listed on food and beverage labeling, remain at 60 mg for both men and women age four and older.

Many fruits and vegetables, including citrus fruits and berries, are rich in vitamin C. Foods rich in vitamin C include raw red peppers (174 mg/cup), guava (165 mg/fruit), orange juice (124 mg/cup), and black currants (202 mg/cup). Rose hips, broccoli, tomatoes, strawberries, papaya, lemons, kiwis, and brussels sprouts are also good sources of vitamin C. Eating at least five to nine servings of fruits and vegetables daily should provide adequate vitamin C intake for most people. Fresh, raw fruits and vegetables contain the highest levels of the vitamin. Both heat and light can reduce vitamin C potency in fresh foods, so overcooking and improper storage should be avoided. Sliced and chopped foods have more of their surface exposed to light, so keeping vegetables and fruits whole may also help to maintain full vitamin potency.

Vitamin C supplements are another common source of the vitamin. Individuals at risk for vitamin C depletion such as smokers, women who take birth control pills, and those with unhealthy dietary habits may benefit from a daily supplement. Supplements are available in a variety of different forms including pills, capsules, powders, and liquids. Vitamin C formulas also vary. Common compounds include ascorbic acid, **calcium** ascorbate, sodium ascorbate, and C complex. The C complex compound contains a substance called bioflavonoids, which may enhance the benefits of vitamin C. Vitamin C is also available commercially as one ingredient of a multivitamin formula.

The recommended daily dosage of vitamin C varies by individual need, but an average daily dose might be 200 mg. Some healthcare providers recommend megadoses (up to 40 g) of vitamin C to combat infections. However, the efficacy of these megadoses has not been proven, and in fact, some studies have shown that doses above 200 mg are not absorbed by the body and are instead excreted.

Precautions

Overdoses of vitamin C can cause nausea, **diarrhea**, stomach cramps, skin rashes, and excessive urination.

Because of an increased risk of kidney damage, individuals with a history of kidney disease or **kidney stones** should never take dosages above 200 mg daily, and should consult with their healthcare provider before starting vitamin C supplementation.

A 1998 study linked overdoses (above 500 mg) of vitamin C to cell and DNA damage. However, other studies have contradicted these findings, and further research is needed to establish whether high doses of vitamin C can cause cell damage.

Side effects

Vitamin C can cause diarrhea and nausea. In some cases, side effects may be decreased or eliminated by adjusting the dosage of vitamin C.

Interactions

Vitamin C increases **iron** absorption, and is frequently prescribed with or added to commercial iron supplements for this reason.

Individuals taking anticoagulant, or blood thinning, medications should speak with their doctor before taking vitamin C supplements, as large doses of vitamin C may impact their efficacy.

Large amounts of vitamin C may increase estrogen levels in women taking hormone supplements or birth control medications, especially if both the supplement and the medication are taken simultaneously. Women should speak with their doctor before taking vitamin C if they are taking estrogen-containing medications. Estrogen actually decreases absorption of vitamin C, so larger doses of vitamin C may be necessary. A healthcare provider can recommend proper dosages and the correct administration of medication and supplement.

Individuals who take aspirin, **antibiotics**, and/or steroids should consult with their healthcare provider about adequate dosages of vitamin C. These medications can increase the need for higher vitamin C doses.

Large dosages of vitamin C can cause a false-positive result in tests for diabetes.

Resources

BOOKS

Reavley, Nocola. *The New Encyclopedia of Vitamins, Minerals, Supplements, and Herbs.* New York: M. Evans & Company, 1998.

PERIODICALS

Henderson, C.W."Prevalence Lower in Women with Increased Vitamin C Levels." *Women's Health Weekly* (April 22, 2000): 7.

Leibman, Bonnie."Antioxidants." *Nutrition Action Health Letter* (June 2000):9.

"New Questions About the Safety of Vitamin C Pills." *Tufts University Health & Nutrition Letter* (April 2000): 1.

ORGANIZATIONS

United States Department of Agriculture. Center for Nutrition Policy and Promotion. 1120 20th Street NW,

---

KEY TERMS

Adrenal hormone—The adrenocortical hormones are cortisol and cortisone. They are anti-inflammatory substances that aid in the function of a number of body systems, including the central nervous system, the cardiovascular system, the musculoskeletal system, and the gastrointestinal system.

Antioxidants—Enzymes that bind with free radicals to neutralize their harmful effects.

Bioflavonoids—Plant-derived substances that help to maintain the small blood vessels of the circulatory system.

Free radicals—Reactive molecules created during cell metabolism that can cause tissue and cell damage like that which occurs in aging and with disease processes such as cancer.

In vitro **testing**—A test performed in a lab setting rather than in a human or animal organism. The test may involve living tissue or cells, but takes place out of the body.

In vivo **testing**—A test performed on a living organism, such as a controlled clinical study involving human test subjects. *In vivo* is Latin for "in the living body."

Suite 200, North Lobby, Washington, D.C. 20036. (202) 418–2312. <http://www.usda.gov/cnpp/>. john.webster@usda.gov.

Paula Ford-Martin

Vitamin D

Description

Vitamin D, also known as calciferol, is essential for strong teeth and bones. There are two major forms of vitamin D: D_2 or ergocalciferol and D_3 or cholecalciferol. Vitamin D can be synthesized by the body in the presence of sunlight, as opposed to being required in the diet. It is the only vitamin whose biologically active formula is a hormone. It is fat-soluble, and regulates the body's absorption and use of the **minerals calcium** and **phosphorus**. Vitamin D is important not only to the maintenance of proper bone density, but to the many calcium-driven neurologic and cellular functions, as well as normal growth and development. It also assists the **immune system** by playing a part in the production of a type of white **blood** cell called the monocyte. White blood cells are **infection** fighters. There are many chemical forms of vitamin D, which have varying amounts of biological activity.

General use

The needed amount of vitamin D is expressed as an Adequate Intake (AI) rather than a Required Daily Amount (RDA). This is due to a difficulty in quantifying the amount of the vitamin that is produced by the body with exposure to sunlight. Instead, the AI estimates the amount needed to be eaten in order to maintain normal function. It is measured in International Units (IU) and there are 40 IU in a microgram (mcg). The AI for vitamin D in the form of cholecarciferol or ergocalciferol for everyone under 50 years of age, including pregnant and lactating women, is 200 IU. It goes up to 400 IU for people 51-70 years old, and to 600 IU for those over age 70. A slightly higher dose of vitamin D, even as little as a total of 700 IU for those over age 65, can significantly reduce age-related **fractures** when taken with 500 mg of calcium per day.

One of the major uses of vitamin D is to prevent and treat **osteoporosis**. This disease is essentially the result of depleted calcium, but calcium supplements alone will not prevent it since vitamin D is required to properly absorb and utilize calcium. Taking vitamin D without the calcium is also ineffective. Taking both together may actually increase bone density in postmenopausal women, who are most susceptible to bone loss and complications such as fractures.

Osteomalacia and rickets are also effectively prevented and treated through adequate vitamin D supplementation. Osteomalacia refers to the softening of the bones that occurs in adults that are vitamin D deficient. Rickets is the syndrome that affect deficient children, causing bowed legs, joint deformities, and poor growth and development.

Vitamin D also has a part in **cancer** prevention, at least for colon cancer. A deficiency increases the risk of this type of cancer, but there is no advantage to taking more than the AI level. There may also be a protective effect against breast and **prostate cancer**, but this is not as well established. Studies are in progress to see if it can help to treat leukemia and lymphoma. The action of at least one chemotherapeutic drug, tamoxifen, appears to be improved with small added doses of vitamin D. Tamoxifen is commonly used to treat ovarian, uterine, and breast cancers.

Many older adults are deficient in vitamin D. This can affect **hearing** by causing poor function of the small bones in the ear that transmit sound. If this is the cause of the **hearing loss**, it is possible that supplementation of vitamin D can act to reverse the situation.

Some metabolic diseases are responsive to treatment with specific doses and forms of vitamin D. These include Fanconi syndrome and familial hypophosphatemia, both of which result in low levels of phosphate. For these conditions, the vitamin is given in conjunction with a phosphate supplement to aid in absorption.

A topical form of vitamin D is available, and can be helpful in the treatment of plaque-type psoriasis. It may also be beneficial for those with vitiligo or scleroderma. This cream, in the form of calcitriol, is not thought to affect internal calcium and phosphorus levels. Oral supplements of vitamin D are not effective for psoriasis. The cream is obtainable by prescription only.

Evidence does not support the use of vitamin D to treat **alcoholism**, acne, arthritis, **cystic fibrosis**, or herpes.

Preparations

Natural sources

Exposure to sunlight is the primary method of obtaining vitamin D. In clear summer weather, approximately ten minutes per day in the sun will produce adequate amounts, even when only the face is exposed. In the winter, it may require as much as two hours. Many people do not get that amount of winter exposure, but are able to utilize the vitamin that was stored during extra time in the sun over the summer. Sunscreen blocks the ability of the sun to produce vitamin D, but should be applied as soon as the minimum exposure requirement has passed, in order to reduce the risk of skin cancer. The chemical 7-dehydrocholesterol in the skin is converted to vitamin D_3 by sunlight. Further processing by first the **liver**, and then the **kidneys**, makes D_3 more biologically active. Since it is fat-soluble, extra can be stored in the liver and fatty tissues for future use. Vitamin D is naturally found in fish liver oils, butter, eggs, and fortified milk and cereals in the form of vitamin D_2. Milk products are the main dietary source for most people. Other dairy products are not a good supply of vitamin D, as they are made from unfortified milk. Plant foods are also poor sources of vitamin D.

Supplemental sources

Most oral supplements of vitamin D are in the form of ergocalciferol. It is also available in topical (calcitriol or calcipotriene), intravenous (calcitriol), or intramuscular (ergocalciferol) formulations. Products designed to be given by other than oral routes are by prescription only. As with all supplements, vitamin D should be stored in a cool, dry place, away from direct light, and out of the reach of children.

Deficiency

In adults, a mild deficiency of vitamin D may be manifested as loss of appetite and weight, difficulty sleeping, and **diarrhea**. A more major deficiency causes osteomalacia and muscle spasm. The bones become soft, fragile, and painful as a result of the calcium depletion. This is due to an inability to properly absorb and utilize calcium in the absence of vitamin D. In children, a severe lack of vitamin D causes rickets.

Risk factors for deficiency

The most likely cause of vitamin D deficiency is inadequate exposure to sunlight. This can occur with people who do not go outside much, those in areas of the world where pollution blocks ultraviolet (UV) light or where the weather prohibits spending much time outdoors. Glass filters out the rays necessary for vitamin formation, as does sunscreen. Those with dark skin may also absorb smaller amounts of the UV light necessary to effect conversion of the vitamin. In climates far to the north, the angle of the sun in winter may not allow adequate UV penetration of the atmosphere to create D_3. Getting enough sun in the summer, and a good dietary source, should supply enough vitamin D to last through the winter. Vegans, or anyone who does not consume dairy products in combination with not getting much sun is also at higher risk, as are the elderly, who have a decreased ability to synthesize vitamin D.

Babies are usually born with about a nine-month supply of the vitamin, but breast milk is a poor source. Those born prematurely are at an increased risk for deficiency of vitamin D and calcium, and may be prone to tetany. Infants past around nine months old who are not getting vitamin D fortified milk or adequate sun exposure are at risk of deficiency.

People with certain intestinal, liver and kidney diseases may not be able to convert vitamin D_3 to active forms, and may need at activated type of supplemental vitamin D.

Those taking certain medications may require supplements, including anticonvulsants, **corticosteroids**, or the cholesterol-lowering medications cholestyramine or colestipol. This means that people who are on medication for arthritis, **asthma**, **allergies**, autoimmune conditions, high cholesterol, epilepsy, or other seizure problems should consult with a healthcare practitioner about the advisability of taking supplemental vitamin D. As with some other **vitamins**, the abuse of alcohol also has a negative effect. In the case of vitamin D, the ability to absorb and store it is diminished by chronic overuse of alcohol products.

Populations with poor nutritional status may tend to be low on vitamin D, as well as other vitamins. This can be an effect of poor sun exposure, poor intake, or poor absorption. A decreased ability to absorb oral forms of vitamin D may result from cystic fibrosis or removal of portions of the digestive tract. Other groups who may need higher than average amounts of vitamin D include those who have recently had surgery, major injuries, or **burns**. High levels of **stress** and chronic wasting illnesses also tend to increase vitamin requirements.

Precautions

The body will not make too much vitamin D from overexposure to sun, but since vitamin D is stored in fat, toxicity from supplemental **overdose** is a possibility. Symptoms are largely those of hypercalcemia, and may include high **blood pressure**, headache, weakness, fatigue, **heart** arrhythmia, loss of appetite, nausea, vomiting, diarrhea, constipation, dizziness, irritability, seizures, kidney damage, poor growth, premature hardening of the arteries, and **pain** in the abdomen, muscles, and bones. If the toxicity progresses, itching and symptoms referable to renal disease may develop, such as thirst, frequent urination, proteinuria, and inability to concentrate urine. Overdoses during **pregnancy** may cause fetal abnormalities. Problems in the infant can include tetany, seizures, heart valve malformation, retinal damage, growth suppression, and mental retardation. Pregnant women should not exceed the AI, and all others over one year of age should not exceed a daily dose of 2,000 IU. Infants should not exceed 1,000 IU. These upper level doses should not be used except under the advice and supervision of a healthcare provider due to the potential for toxicity.

Individuals with hypercalcemia, sarcoidosis, or hypoparathyroidism should not use supplemental calciferol. Those with kidney disease, arteriosclerosis, or heart disease should use ergocalciferol only with extreme caution and medical guidance.

KEY TERMS

Osteomalacia—Literally soft bones, a condition seen in adults deficient in vitamin D. The bones are painful and fracture easily.

Scleroderma—A condition causing thickened, hardened skin.

Tetany—Painful muscle spasms and tremors caused by very low calcium levels.

Vegan—A person who does not eat any animal products, including dairy and eggs.

Vitiligo—Patchy loss of skin pigmentation, resulting in lighter areas of skin.

Side effects

Minor side effects may include poor appetite, constipation, dry mouth, increased thirst, metallic **taste**, or fatigue. Other reactions, which should prompt a call to a healthcare provider, can include headache, nausea, vomiting, diarrhea, or confusion.

Interactions

The absorption of vitamin D is improved by calcium, choline, **fats**, phosphorus, and vitamins A and C. Supplements should be taken with a meal to optimize absorption.

There are a number of medications that can interfere with vitamin D levels, absorption, and **metabolism**. Rifampin, H_2 blockers, barbiturates, heparin, isoniazid, colestipol, cholestyramine, carbamazepine, phenytoin, fosphenytoin, and phenobarbital reduce serum levels of vitamin D and increase metabolism of it. Anyone who is on medication for epilepsy or another **seizure disorder** should check with a healthcare provider to see whether it is advisable to take supplements of vitamin D. Overuse of mineral oil, Olestra, and stimulant **laxatives** may also deplete vitamin D. Osteoporosis and hypocalcemia can result from long-term use of corticosteroids. It may be necessary to take supplements of calcium and vitamin D together with this medication. The use of thiazide diuretics in conjunction with vitamin D can cause hypercalcemia in individuals with hypoparathyroidism. Concomitant use of digoxin or other cardiac glycosides with vitamin D supplements may lead to hypercalcemia and heart irregularities. The same caution should be used with herbs containing cardiac glycosides, including black hellebore, Canadian hemp, digitalis, hedge mustard, figwort, lily of the valley, motherwort, oleander, pheasant's eye, pleurisy, squill, and strophanthus.

Resources

BOOKS

Bratman, Steven, and David Kroll. *Natural Health Bible.* Prima Publishing, 1999.

Feinstein, Alice. *Prevention's Healing with Vitamins.* Rodale Press, 1996.

Griffith, H. Winter. *Vitamins, Herbs, Minerals & Supplements: The Complete Guide.* Fisher Books, 1998.

Jellin, Jeff, Forrest Batz, and Kathy Hitchens. *Pharmacist's Letter/Prescriber's Letter Natural Medicines Comprehensive Database.* Therapeutic Research Faculty, 1999.

Pressman, Alan H., and Sheila Buff. *The Complete Idiot's Guide to Vitamins and Minerals.* Alpha Books, 1997.

Judith Turner

Vitamin B_1 *see* **Thiamine**

Vitamin B_2 *see* **Riboflavin**

Vitamin B_3 *see* **Niacin**

Vitamin B_7 *see* **Biotin**

Vitamin E

Description

Vitamin E is an antioxidant responsible for proper functioning of the **immune system** and for maintaining healthy eyes and skin. It is actually a group of fat soluble compounds known as tocopherols (i.e., alpha tocopherol and gamma tocopherol). Gamma tocopherol accounts for approximately 75% of dietary vitamin E. Vitamin E rich foods include nuts, cereals, beans, eggs, cold-pressed oils, and assorted fruits and vegetables. Because vitamin E is a fat soluble vitamin, it requires the presence of fat for proper absorption. Daily dietary intake of the recommended daily allowance (RDA) of vitamin E is recommended for optimum health.

Vitamin E is absorbed by the gastrointestinal system and stored in tissues and organs throughout the body. Certain health conditions may cause vitamin E depletion, including **liver** disease, celiac disease, and **cystic fibrosis**. Patients with end-stage renal disease (kidney failure) who are undergoing chronic dialysis treatment may be at risk for vitamin E deficiency.

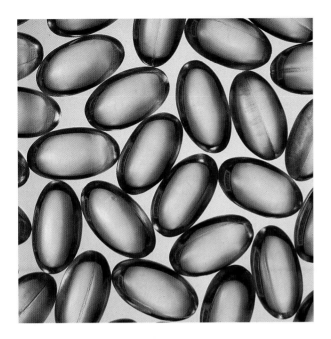

Vitamin E capsules, which are transparent yellow-orange.
(Photograph by David Doody. FPG International Corp. Reproduced by permission.)

These patients frequently receive intravenous infusions of **iron** supplements which can act against vitamin E.

Vitamin E deficiency can cause fatigue, concentration problems, weakened immune system, anemia, and low thyroid levels. It may also cause **vision** problems and irritability. Low serum (or **blood**) levels of vitamin E have also been linked to major depression.

General use

Vitamin E is necessary for optimal immune system functioning, healthy eyes, and cell protection throughout the body. It has also been linked to the prevention of a number of diseases. The therapeutic benefits of vitamin E include:

- **Cancer** prevention. Vitamin E is a known antioxidant, and has been associated with a reduced risk of gastrointestinal, cervical, prostate, lung, and possibly **breast cancer**.

- Immune system protection. Various studies have shown that vitamin E supplementation, particularly in elderly patients, boosts immune system function. Older patients have demonstrated improved **immune response**, increased resistance to infections, and higher antibody production. Vitamin E has also been used with some success to slow disease progression in HIV-positive patients.

- Eye disease prevention. Clinical studies on vitamin E have shown that supplementation significantly reduces the risk for **cataracts** and for **macular degeneration**, particularly among women.

- **Memory** loss prevention. Vitamin E deficiency has been linked to poor performance on memory tests in some elderly individuals.

- **Alzheimer's disease** treatment. In a study performed at Columbia University, researchers found that Alzheimer's patients who took daily supplements of vitamin E maintained normal functioning longer than patients who took a placebo.

- Liver disease treatment. Vitamin E may protect the liver against disease.

- Diabetes treatment. Vitamin E may help diabetic patients process insulin more effectively.

- **Pain** relief. Vitamin E acts as both an anti-inflammatory and analgesic (or pain reliever). Studies have indicated it may be useful for treatment of arthritis pain in some individuals.

- **Parkinson's disease** prevention. High doses of vitamin E intake was associated with a lowered risk of developing Parkinson's disease in one 1997 Dutch study.

- Tardive dyskinesia treatment. Individuals who take neuroleptic drugs for **schizophrenia** or other disorders may suffer from a side effect known as tardive dyskinesia, in which they experience involuntary muscle contractions or twitches. Vitamin E supplementation may lessen or eliminate this side effect in some individuals.

Other benefits of vitamin E are less clear cut, and have been called into question with conflicting study results or because of a lack of controlled studies to support them. These include:

- **Heart** disease prevention. A number of epidemiological studies have indicated that vitamin E may prevent heart disease by lowering total blood cholesterol levels and preventing oxidation of LDL cholesterol. However, a large, controlled study known as the Heart Outcomes Prevention Evaluation (HOPE) published in early 2000 indicates that vitamin E does not have any preventative effects against heart disease. The study followed 9,500 individuals who were considered to be at a high risk for heart disease. Half the individuals were randomly chosen to receive vitamin E supplementation, and the other half of the study population received a placebo. After five years, there was no measurable difference in heart attacks and heart disease between the two patient populations. Still, vitamin E may still hold some hope for heart disease prevention. It is possible that a longer-term study beyond the five years of the HOPE study may demonstrate some heart protective benefits of vitamin E consumption. It is also possible that while the high-risk patient population that was used for the HOPE study did not benefit from vitamin E, an average-risk patient population might still benefit from supplementation. It is also possible that vitamin E needs the presence of another vitamin or nutrient substance to protect against heart disease. Further large, controlled, and long-term clinical studies are necessary to answer these questions.

- Skin care. Vitamin E is thought to increase an individual's tolerance to UV rays when taken as a supplement in conjunction with **vitamin C**. Vitamin E has also been touted as a treatment to promote faster healing of flesh **wounds**. While its anti-inflammatory and analgesic properties may have some benefits in reducing swelling and relieving discomfort in a wound, some dermatologists dispute the claims of faster healing, and there are no large controlled studies to support this claim.

- Hot flashes. In a small study conducted at the Mayo Clinic, researchers found that breast cancer survivors who suffered from hot flashes experienced a decrease in those hot flashes after taking vitamin E supplementation.

- Muscle maintenance and repair. Recent research has demonstrated that the antioxidative properties of vitamin E may prevent damage to tissues caused by heavy endurance exercises. In addition, vitamin E supplementation given prior to surgical procedures on muscle and joint tissues has been shown to limit reperfusion injury (muscle damage which occurs when blood flow is stopped, and then started again to tissues or organs).

- Fertility. Vitamin E has been shown to improve sperm function in animal studies, and may have a similar effect in human males. Further studies are needed to establish the efficacy of vitamin E as a treatment for male infertility.

Preparations

The U.S. recommended dietary allowance (RDA) of the alpha-tocopherol formulation of vitamin E is as follows:

- men: 10 mg or 15 IU

- women: 8 mg or 12 IU

- pregnant women: 10 mg or 15 IU

- lactating women: 12 mg or 18 IU

In April 2000, the National Academy of Sciences recommended changing the RDA for vitamin E to 22 international units (IUs), with an upper limit (UL), or maximum daily dose, of 1,500 IUs. Daily values for the vitamin as recommended by the U.S. Food and Drug Administration, the values listed on food and beverage labeling, remain at 30 IUs for both men and women age four and older.

Many nuts, vegetable-based oils, fruits, and vegetables contain vitamin E. Foods rich in vitamin E include wheat germ oil (26.2 mg/tbsp), wheat germ cereal (19.5 mg/cup), peanuts (6.32 mg/half cup), soy beans (3.19 mg/cup), corn oil (2.87 mg/tbsp), avocado (2.69 mg), and olive oil (1.68 mg/tbsp). Grapes, peaches, broccoli, Brussels sprouts, eggs, tomatoes, and blackberries are also good sources of vitamin E. Fresh, raw foods contain the highest levels of the vitamin. Both heat and light can reduce vitamin and mineral potency in fresh foods, so overcooking and improper storage should be avoided. Sliced and chopped foods have more of their surface exposed to light, therefore keeping vegetables and fruits whole may also help to maintain full vitamin potency.

For individuals considered at risk for vitamin E deficiency, or those with an inadequate dietary intake, vitamin E supplements are available in a variety of different forms, including pills, capsules, powders, and liquids for oral ingestion. For topical use, vitamin E is available in ointments, creams, lotions, and oils. Vitamin E is also available commercially as one ingredient of a multivitamin formula.

The recommended daily dosage of vitamin E varies by individual need and by the amount of polyunsaturated **fats** an individual consumes. The more polyunsaturated fats in the diet, the higher the recommended dose of vitamin E, because vitamin E helps to prevent the oxidizing effects of these fats. Because vitamin E is fat soluble, supplements should always be taken with food.

Supplements are also available in either natural or synthetic formulations. Natural forms are extracted from wheat germ oil and other vitamin E food sources, and synthetic forms are extracted from petroleum oils. Natural formulas can be identified by a d prefix on the name of the vitamin (i.e., d-alpha-tocopherol).

Precautions

Overdoses of vitamin E (over 536 mg) can cause nausea, **diarrhea**, headache, abdominal pain, bleeding, high **blood pressure**, fatigue, and weakened immune system function.

Patients with rheumatic heart disease, **iron deficiency anemia**, **hypertension**, or thyroid dysfunction should consult their healthcare provider before starting vitamin E supplementation, as vitamin E may have a negative impact on these conditions.

Side effects

Vitamin E is well-tolerated, and side effects are rare. However, in some individuals who are **vitamin K** deficient, vitamin E may increase the risk for hemorrhage or bleeding. In some cases, side effects may be decreased or eliminated by adjusting the dosage of vitamin E and vitamin K.

Vitamin E ointments, oils, or creams may trigger an allergic reaction known as contact dermatitis. Individuals who are considering using topical vitamin E preparations for the first time, or who are switching the type of vitamin E product they use, should perform a skin patch test to check for skin sensitivity to the substance. A small, dime sized drop of the product should be applied to a small patch of skin inside the elbow or wrist. The skin patch should be monitored for 24 hours to ensure no excessive redness, irritation, or rash occurs. If a reaction does occur, it may be in response to other ingredients in the topical preparation, and the test can be repeated with a different vitamin E formulation. Individuals who experience a severe reaction to a skin patch test of vitamin E are advised not to use the product topically. A dermatologist or other healthcare professional may be able to recommend a suitable alternative.

Interactions

Individuals who take anticoagulant (blood thinning) or anticonvulsant medications should consult their healthcare provider before starting vitamin E supplementation. Vitamin E can alter the efficacy of these drugs.

Non-heme, inorganic iron supplements destroy vitamin E, so individuals taking iron supplements should space out their doses (e.g., iron in the morning and vitamin E in the evening).

Large doses of **vitamin A** can decrease the absorption of vitamin E, so dosage adjustments may be necessary in individuals supplementing with both **vitamins**.

Alcohol and mineral oil can also reduce vitamin E absorption, and these substances should be avoided if possible in vitamin E deficient individuals.

KEY TERMS

Antioxidants—Enzymes which bind with free radicals to neutralize their harmful effects.

Contact dermatitis—Inflammation, redness, and irritation of the skin caused by an irritating substance.

Epidemiological study—A study which analyzes health events and trends in particular patient populations.

Free radicals—Reactive molecules created during cell metabolism that can cause tissue and cell damage like that which occurs in aging and with disease processes such as cancer.

Macular degeneration—Degeneration, or breakdown, of the retina that can lead to partial or total blindness.

Non-heme iron—Dietary or supplemental iron that is less efficiently absorbed by the body than heme iron (ferrous iron).

Reperfusion—The reintroduction of blood flow to organs or tissues after blood flow has been stopped for surgical procedures.

Vitamin A—An essential vitamin found in liver, orange and yellow vegetables, milk, and eggs that is critical for proper growth and development.

Vitamin K—A fat-soluble vitamin responsible for blood clotting, bone metabolism, and proper kidney function.

Resources

BOOKS

Reavley, Nocola. *The New Encyclopedia of Vitamins, Minerals, Supplements, and Herbs.* New York: M. Evans & Company, 1998.

PERIODICALS

"Vitamin E: E for Exaggerated?" *Harvard Health Letter* 25, no. 5 (March 2000): 6.

ORGANIZATIONS

United States Department of Agriculture. Center for Nutrition Policy and Promotion. 1120 20th Street NW, Suite 200, North Lobby, Washington, D.C. 20036. (202) 418-2312. <http://www.usda.gov/cnpp/>.

Paula Ford-Martin

Vitamin H *see* **Biotin**

Vitamin K

Description

Vitamin K originates from the German term *koajulation*. It is also known as antihemorrhagic factor and is one of the four fat-soluble **vitamins** necessary for good health. The others are vitamins A, D, and E. The primary and best-known purpose of vitamin K is support of the process of **blood** clotting. Prothrombin and other clotting factors are dependent on vitamin K for production. It also plays a role in bone health, and may help to prevent **osteoporosis**. Appropriate growth and development are supported by adequate vitamin K.

There are several forms of the vitamin:

- K_1, or phyiloguinone also known as phytonadione

- K_2, a family of substances called menaquinones

- K_3, or menadione, a synthetic substance

General use

The Required Daily Amount (RDA) of vitamin K is 5 micrograms (mcg) for infants less than six months old, 10 mcg for babies six months to one year old, 15 mcg for children aged one to three years, 20 mcg for those aged four to six years, and 30 mcg for those seven to ten years old. Males require 45 mcg from 11-14 years, 65 mcg from 15-18 years, 70 mcg from 19-24 years, and 80 mcg after the age of 24 years. Females need 45 mcg from 11-14 years, 55 mcg from 15-18 years, 60 mcg from 19-24 years, and 65 mcg after the age of 24, and for pregnant or lactating women. These values are based on an estimate of 1 mcg of vitamin K per kilogram of body weight.

The most common use of vitamin K is to supplement babies at birth, thus preventing hemorrhagic disease of the newborn. Others who may benefit from supplemental vitamin K include those taking medications that interact with it or deplete the supply. It also appears to have some effectiveness in preventing osteoporosis, but the studies done involved patients using a high dietary intake rather than supplements. People taking warfarin, a vitamin K antagonist, are able to use the vitamin as an antidote if the serum level of warfarin is too high, increasing the risk of hemorrhage.

Topical formulations of vitamin K are sometimes touted as being able to reduce spider veins on the face and legs. The creams are quite expensive and the efficacy is questionable at best.

Preparations

Natural sources

Dark green leafy vegetables are among the best food sources of vitamin K in the form of K_1. Seaweed is packed with it, and beef liver, cauliflower, eggs, and strawberries are rich sources as well. Vitamin K is fairly heat stable, but gentle cooking preserves the content of other nutrients that are prone to breaking down when heated. Some of the supply for the body is synthesized as vitamin K_2 by the good **bacteria** in the intestines.

Supplemental sources

Vitamin K is not normally included in daily multivitamins, as deficiency is rare. Oral, topical, and injectable forms are available, but should not be used except under the supervision of a health care provider. Injectable forms are by prescription only. Supplements are generally given in the form of phytonadione since it is the most effective form and has lower risk of toxicity than other types. Synthetic forms of vitamin K are also available for supplemental use.

Deficiency

Deficiency of vitamin K is uncommon in the general population but is of particular concern in neonates, who are born with low levels of vitamin K. Hemorrhagic disease of the newborn can affect infants who do not receive some form of vitamin K at birth. Affected babies tend to have prolonged and excessive bleeding following circumcision or blood draws. In the most serious cases, bleeding into the **brain** may occur. Most commonly an injection of vitamin K is given in the nursery following birth, but a series of oral doses is also occasionally used. The primary sign of a deficiency at any age is bleeding, and poor growth may also be observed in children. Chronically low levels of vitamin K are correlated with higher risk of hip fracture in women.

Risk factors for deficiency

Deficiency is unusual, but may occur in certain populations, including those on the medications mentioned in interactions, alcoholics, and people with diseases of the gastrointestinal tract that impair absorption. Conditions that may be problematic include **Crohn's disease**, chronic **diarrhea**, sprue, and ulcerative colitis. Anything that impairs fat absorption also risks decreasing the absorption of the fat-soluble vitamins. Long term use of broad spectrum **antibiotics**

KEY TERMS

Anticoagulant—Substance which inhibits clotting, used therapeutically for such things as stroke prevention in susceptible people.

Bilirubin—When gathered in large amounts, this water insoluble pigment occures in bile and blood.

Hemolytic anemia—Destruction of red blood cells.

Hemorrhage—Excessive bleeding.

Prothrombin—One protein component of the cascade reaction which results in clot formation.

destroys the bacteria in the intestinal tract that are necessary for the body's production of vitamin K.

Precautions

Allergic reactions to vitamin K supplements can occur, although they are rare. Symptoms may include flushed skin, nausea, rash, and itching. Medical attention should be sought if any of these symptoms occur. Infants receiving vitamin K injections occasionally suffer hemolytic anemia or high bilirubin levels, noticeable from the yellow cast of the skin. Emergency medical treatment is needed for these babies. Liver and brain impairment are possible in severe cases.

Certain types of liver problems necessitate very cautious use of some forms of vitamin K. Menadiol sodium diphosphate, a synthetic form also known as vitamin K_4, may cause problems in people with biliary fistula or obstructive **jaundice**. A particular metabolic disease called G6-PD deficiency also calls for careful use of vitamin K_4. The expertise of a health care professional is called for under these circumstances. Sheldon Saul Hendler, MD, PhD, advises there is no reason to supplement with more than 100mcg daily except in cases of frank vitamin K deficiency.

Side effects

Vitamin K_4 may occasionally irritate the gastrointestinal tract. High doses greater than 500 mcg daily have been reported to cause some allergic-type reactions, such as skin rashes, itching, and flushing.

Interactions

There are numerous medications that can interfere with the proper absorption or function of vitamin K. Long term use of **antacids** may decrease the efficacy of the vitamin, as can certain anticoagulants. Warfarin is an anticoagulant that antagonizes vitamin K. Efficacy of the vitamin is also decreased by dactinomycin and sucralfate. Absorption is decreased by cholestyramine and colestipol, which are drugs used to lower cholesterol. Other drugs that may cause a deficiency include long-term use of mineral oil, quinidine, and sulfa drugs. Primaquine increases the risk of side effects from taking supplements.

Resources

BOOKS

Bratman, Steven, and David Kroll. *Natural Health Bible.* Prima Publishing, 1999.

Feinstein, Alice. *Prevention's Healing with Vitamins.* Rodale Press, 1996.

Griffith, H. Winter. *Vitamins, Herbs, Minerals & Supplements: The Complete Guide.* Fisher Books, 1998.

Jellin, Jeff, Forrest Batz, and Kathy Hitchens. *Pharmacist's Letter/Prescriber's Letter Natural Medicines Comprehensive Database.* Therapeutic Research Faculty, 1999.

Pressman, Alan H., and Sheila Buff. *The Complete Idiot's Guide to Vitamins and Minerals.* Alpha Books, 1997.

Judith Turner

Vitamin poisoning *see* **Vitamin toxicity**

Vitamin tests

Definition

Vitamins are small organic molecules that are necessary for many biochemical reactions in the body. For example, many vitamins participate as cofactors in enzyme reactions within the cells. They must be obtained through diet, microorganisms in the gut or sunlight since humans cannot synthesize them. Vitamin tests measure the levels of certain vitamins in an individual's **blood** which can be correlated to the levels of vitamin in their tissues. They are generally used to aid in the diagnosis of vitamin deficiencies or in detecting toxic amounts of a vitamin in a patient's system.

Purpose

Vitamins are components of food that are needed for growth, reproduction, wound healing, digestion of food, blood clotting, bone **metabolism** and maintaining good health. They can be isolated from plants and organisms or they can be synthesized in the laboratory. The vitamins include **vitamin D**, **vitamin E**, **vitamin A**, and **vitamin K**, which are the fat-soluble vitamins, and folate, **vitamin B$_{12}$**, **biotin** (vitamin H), vitamin B$_6$, **niacin**, thiamine, **riboflavin**, pantothenic acid, and ascorbic acid (**vitamin C**), which are the water-soluble vitamins. Fat soluble vitamins are absorbed and transported differently from the water soluble vitamins. They can remain in the body longer since they can be stored in fat so they are more toxic in high doses.

Vitamins are required in the diet in only tiny amounts, in contrast to sugars, starches, **proteins** and **fats**. However, vitamin requirements can rise after surgery, with **cancer** and other illnesses, and during **infection** and **pregnancy**. Not receiving sufficient quantities of a certain vitamin can be devastating, resulting in vitamin deficiency diseases such as scurvy (vitamin C deficiency), pellagra (niacin deficiency), megaloblastic anemia (vitamin B$_{12}$ or folate deficiency) or rickets (vitamin D deficiency). Less extreme deficiencies can cause a delay in wound healing. Conversely, consuming too much of a certain vitamin, especially the fat soluble ones, can be toxic to a person's system. While most vitamin deficiencies are rare in our society, they can be caused by certain diseases, especially those that affect absorption of food, or can be caused by inborn errors of metabolism, **fad diets**, anorexia, blood loss, **parenteral nutrition** and dialysis. The vitamins that are most commonly measured by doctors are folate, vitamin B$_{12}$, vitamin K, vitamin D, and vitamin A.

Precautions

Most vitamin tests are performed on blood samples collected from a vein in the crease of the arm. The nurse or phlebotomist performing the procedure should observe **universal precautions** for the prevention of transmission of bloodborne pathogens. Some drugs are known to increase or decrease the level of specific vitamins. The physician should obtain a thorough list of the patient's medications when requesting vitamin measurements.

Description

Many of the vitamin tests done today are vitamin status panels, such as megaloblastic anemia panels that measure the concentration of both vitamin B$_{12}$ and folate. A deficiency of either of these vitamins results in anemia associated with enlarged (macrocytic) red blood cells. The actual testing methods take advantage of the compound's chemical composition. Fat soluble vitamins are measured differently from water soluble vitamins. In general, the tests are performed on plasma, although some tests for metabolites of vitamins can be done on urine, as is the case with many of the water soluble vitamins. Each vitamin occurs at extremely small concentrations in the blood and urine when compared to levels of most other molecules. For this reason, a procedure that separates the vitamin from the rest of the compounds in the sample is usually performed immediately prior to conducting the actual test. This isolation is done using filters that allow the vitamin to pass through and leave the bigger molecules behind. Vitamin B$_{12}$ and folate are routinely measured by immunoassay methods, but the most common method to measure other vitamins is high-performance liquid chromatography (HPLC). In HPLC, the vitamin to be measured is extracted from the sample and injected into a stream of solvent that is pumped at high pressure through a column packed with particles to which an organic liquid has been bonded. The molecules separate at different rates depending upon their affinity for the bonded particles. The time at which they elute (i.e., come out of the column) is used to identify the molecules. As the vitamins elute, they flow through a detection cell where they are measured by ultraviolet or infrared light absorption or by fluorescence. In these reactions, the amount of light absorbance or amount of fluorescence is proportional to the amount of vitamin in the sample.

While HPLC and immunoassay are the testing methods used most often, other types of tests exist including biochemical (photometric) tests and microbiological assays. Some tests, such as those for riboflavin, are conducted by giving the patient a riboflavin "load" and looking at metabolites in the urine. Vitamin K defiency, a vitamin crucial in blood clotting, is often evaluated by a surrogate test, the prothrombin time. The prothrombin time is measured routinely on patients before they undergo a surgical procedure since long clotting times can complicate surgeries. The test measures how long it takes for a fibrin clot to form in a plasma sample to which **calcium** and tissue thromboplastin (a clot activator) have been added. Clotting factors II, VII, XI, and X are made from vitamin K. The prothrombin time is prolonged when there is a deficiency of fibrinogen or factors II, V, VII, or X. Therefore, a prolonged prothrombin time can result from an inherited or acquired deficiency of one of these factors or a deficiency of vitamin K.

Other vitamins can be measured by taking advantage of their functions. One example is the measurement of oxidation/reduction reactions to measure vitamins E and C, two major antioxidants. In addition, many of the water soluble vitamins such as vitamin B_6 are measured using microbiological tests. Samples, usually filtered urine, are applied to a culture medium. The medium is inoculated with a standardized concentration of the **bacteria** or yeast that requires the vitamin for growth. The plate is incubated for several days to see if the organism grows. Lack of growth indicates a low concentration of the vitamin and correlates well with vitamin deficiency.

Preparation

Most vitamin tests require no preparation; however, some may require that the patient fast for at least eight hours before giving a blood sample, or stop using some medications.

Results

Levels of vitamins in the body must be interpreted carefully. Many times low levels do not correlate with disease and the patient is asymptomatic. Other times the levels may seem fine, but the patient displays symptoms of a deficiency. Physicians must take into account the patient's dietary history (e.g., is the patient a vegetarian?), medications, and also do a thorough physical exam.

Representative normal ranges for certain vitamins are listed below. Normal ranges vary depending upon the patient's age and method of analysis. Levels of some vitamins will be different in pregnancy. Please note that, by convention, the units used for reporting one vitamin may differ from another. The units picogram/milliliter (pg/mL), nanogram/milliliter (ng/mL), and micrograms per deciliter (micrograms/dL) refer to the weight of vitamin in the specified volume. The units nanomoles/liter (nmol/L) and micromoles/liter (umol/L) refer to the concentration of vitamin in the specified volume.

- folate (**folic acid**): 3.0-20.0 ng/mL in serum, 140-628 ng/ml in red blood cells
- vitamin B_{12}: 200-835 pg/mL
- thiamine: 9-44 nmol/L
- riboflavin: 4-24 micrograms/dL
- vitamin B_6: 5-30 ng/mL
- vitamin C (ascorbic acid): 0.4-1.5 mg/dL
- vitamin A: 30-80 micrograms/dL
- vitamin D (25-hydroxy-vitamin D): 14-60 ng/mL
- vitamin K: 13-1190 pg/mL
- vitamin E: 0.5-1.8 mg/dL

KEY TERMS

Antioxidant—A compound that protects against oxidation, usually by being oxidized itself. Antioxidant vitamins include C and E.

Carotenoids—Pigments found in vegetables and fruits, similar in structure to vitamin A. These compounds act as antioxidants.

Megaloblastic anemia—A disorder caused by a deficiency in vitamin B_{12} and folate. The blood contains immature red blood cells causing a decrease in oxygen carrying capacity and symptoms of fatigue and peripheral neuropathies.

Parenteral nutrition—Also called total parenteral nutrition or TPN. A slang term is "tube feeds." Parenteral nutrition is the taking in of nutrients through any way other than by the gastrointestinal system. TPN can be administered by intravenous, subcutaneous, intramuscular or intramedullary injection. TPN formulations need to be prescribed based on the patient's illness and how long they will be on the feeding regimen.

Pellagra—A disorder caused by a deficiency in niacin. The patient will have dementia, diarrhea and dermatitis.

Peripheral neuropathy—A disorder characterized by tingling and numbness in extremities. This can cause difficulties with walking and using your hands.

RDA—Recommended dietary allowance. The amount of vitamin needed to maintain a healthy level in tissues by a healthy person.

Rickets—A disorder caused by a deficiency in vitamin D. The symptoms are muscle hypotonia (weak muscles) and skeletal deformity. Seen mainly in children.

Scurvy—A disorder caused by a deficiency in ascorbic acid, or vitamin C. The patient will have swollen and bleeding gums, loss of teeth, skin lesions and pain and weakness in lower extremities.

Vitamins—Small compounds required for metabolism that must be supplied by diet, microorganisms in the gut (vitamin K) or sunlight (UV light converts pre-vitamin D to vitamin D).

Health care team roles

Tests for specific vitamins are requested by a physician. Vitamin deficiencies may be suspected by physicians and nurses, and patients who are deficient should be referred to a dietician who can advise them on food choices. In addition, health care providers should be vigilant for hidden deficiencies in those who are pregnant, have malabsorption disorders or chronic illnesses such as **cystic fibrosis**. Blood samples are collected by a nurse or phlebotomist. Vitamin assays are performed by clinical laboratory scientists/medical technologists.

Resources

BOOKS

Burtis, Carl A., and Edward R. Ashwood. *Tietz Textbook of Clinical Chemistry*. Philadelphia: W.B. Saunders Company, 1992.

Kaplan, Lawrence A., and Amadeo J. Pesce. *Clinical Chemistry Theory Analysis and Correlation*. St. Louis: Mosby Publishers, 1996.

Jane E. Phillips, PhD

Vitamin toxicity

Definition

Vitamin toxicity is a condition in which a person develops symptoms as side effects from taking massive doses of **vitamins**. Vitamins vary in the amounts that are required to cause toxicity and in the specific symptoms that result. Vitamin toxicity, which is also called hypervitaminosis or vitamin **poisoning**, is becoming more common in developed countries because of the popularity of vitamin supplements.

Description

Overview

Vitamins are organic molecules in food that are needed in small amounts for growth, reproduction, and the maintenance of good health. Some vitamins can be dissolved in oil or melted fat. These fat-soluble vitamins include **vitamin D**, **vitamin E**, **vitamin A** (retinol), and **vitamin K**. Other vitamins can be dissolved in water. The water-soluble vitamins include folate (**folic acid**), **vitamin B$_{12}$**, biotin, vitamin B$_6$, **niacin**, **thiamine**, **riboflavin**, pantothenic acid, and **vitamin C** (ascorbic acid). Taking too much of any vitamin can produce a toxic effect.

However, megadoses with the fat-soluble vitamins are more likely to become toxic than with water-soluble vitamins because fat-soluble vitamins are often stored in the body while excess water-soluble vitamins are usually excreted in the urine. Vitamins A and D are the most likely to produce hypervitaminosis in large doses, while riboflavin, pantothenic acid, biotin, and vitamin C appear to be the least likely to cause problems.

Vitamins in medical treatment

Vitamin supplements are used for the treatment of various diseases or for reducing the risk of certain diseases. For example, moderate supplements of folic acid appear to reduce the risk for certain birth defects such as neural tube defects, and possibly reduce the risk of **cancer**. Therapy for diseases brings with it the risk for irreversible vitamin toxicity only in the case of vitamin D. This vitamin is toxic at levels that are only moderately greater than the recommended dietary allowance (RDA). Niacin is commonly used as a drug for the treatment of **heart** disease, but niacin is far less toxic than vitamin D. Vitamin toxicity is not a risk with medically supervised therapy using any of the other vitamins.

Vitamin megadoses

With the exception of folic acid supplements, the practice of taking vitamin supplements by healthy individuals has little or no relation to good health. Most adults in the United States can obtain enough vitamins by eating a well-balanced diet. It has, however, become increasingly common for people to take vitamins at levels far greater than the RDA. These high levels are sometimes called vitamin megadoses. Megadoses are harmless for most vitamins. But in the cases of a few of the vitamins—specifically, vitamins D, A, and B$_6$—megadoses can be harmful or fatal. Researchers have also started to look more closely at megadoses of vitamins C and E, since indirect evidence suggests that these two vitamins may reduce the risks of cancer, heart disease, and aging. It is not yet clear whether taking megadoses of either vitamin C or vitamin E has any influence on health. Some experts think that megadoses of vitamin C may protect people from cancer. On the other hand, other researchers have gathered indirect evidence that vitamin C megadoses may cause cancer when combined with smoking.

Causes and symptoms

Fat-soluble vitamins

VITAMIN D. Vitamins D and A are the most toxic of the fat-soluble vitamins. The symptoms of vitamin

D toxicity are nausea, vomiting, **pain** in the joints, and loss of appetite. The patient may experience constipation alternating with **diarrhea**, or have tingling sensations in the mouth. The toxic dose of vitamin D depends on its frequency. In infants, a single dose of 15 milligrams (mg) or greater may be toxic, but it is also the case that daily doses of 1.0 mg over a prolonged period may be toxic. In adults, a daily dose of 1.0 to 2.0 mg of vitamin D is toxic when consumed for a prolonged period. A single dose of about 50 mg or greater is toxic for adults. The immediate effect of an **overdose** of vitamin D is abdominal cramps, nausea, and vomiting. Toxic doses of vitamin D taken over a prolonged period of time can result in irreversible deposits of **calcium** crystals in the soft tissues of the body that may damage the heart, **lungs**, and **kidneys**. The dietary reference intake (DRI) suggests an upper tolerable limit of 25 micrograms (mcg) per day for children and 50 mcg per day for adults. The DRI is between 5 and 15 mcg from childhood to adulthood in the absence of adequate sunlight. Older adults have a requirement on the higher end of the scale due to generally reduced sun exposure.

VITAMIN A. Vitamin A toxicity can occur with long-term consumption of 20 mg of retinol or more per day. The symptoms of vitamin A overdosing include accumulation of water in the **brain** (hydrocephalus), vomiting, tiredness, constipation, bone pain, and severe headaches. The skin may acquire a rough and dry appearance, with hair loss and brittle nails. Vitamin A toxicity is a special issue during **pregnancy**. Expectant mothers who take 10 mg vitamin A or more on a daily basis may have an infant with birth defects. These birth defects include abnormalities of the face, nervous system, heart, and thymus gland. It is possible to take in toxic levels of vitamin A by eating large quantities of certain foods. For example, about 30 grams of beef liver, 500 grams of eggs, or 2,500 grams of mackerel would supply 10 mg of retinol.

VITAMIN E. Megadoses of vitamin E may produce headaches, tiredness, double **vision**, and diarrhea in humans. Studies with animals fed large doses of vitamin E have revealed that this vitamin may interfere with the absorption of other fat-soluble vitamins. The term absorption means the transfer of the vitamin from the gut into the bloodstream. Thus, large doses of vitamin E consumed over many weeks or months might result in deficiencies of vitamin D, vitamin A, and vitamin K. The DRI suggests an upper tolerable limit between 200 and 800 mg per day for children and teenagers, depending on age (younger children have requirements on the lower end of the scale), and 1,000

mg per day for adults. The DRI is 15 mg per day for adults and pregnant women.

VITAMIN K. Prolonged consumption of megadoses of vitamin K (menadione) results in anemia, which is a reduced level of red **blood** cells in the bloodstream. When large doses of menadione are given to infants, they result in the deposit of pigments in the brain, nerve damage, the destruction of red blood cells (hemolysis), and death. A daily injection of 10 mg of menadione into an infant for three days can kill the child. This tragic fact was discovered during the early days of vitamin research, when newborn infants were injected with menadione to prevent a disease known as hemorrhagic disease of the newborn. Today, a different form of vitamin K is used to protect infants against this disease.

Water-soluble vitamins

FOLATE. Folate occurs in various forms in food. There are more than a dozen related forms of folate. The folate in oral vitamin supplements occurs in only one form, however—folic acid. Large doses of folic acid (20 grams/day) can eventually result in kidney damage. Folate is considered, however, to be relatively nontoxic, except in cases where folate supplementation can lead to pernicious anemia. The DRI suggests an upper tolerable limit between 300 and 800 mcg per day for children and teenagers, depending on age (younger children have requirements on the lower end of the scale), and 1,000 mcg per day for adults. The DRI is 400 mcg per day for adults and slightly lower in children; 600 mcg during pregnancy and 500 mcg while lactating.

VITAMIN B$_{12}$. Vitamin B$_{12}$ is important in the treatment of pernicious anemia. Pernicious anemia is more common among middle-aged and older adults; it is usually detected in patients between the ages of 40 and 80. The disease affects about 0.1% of all persons in the general population in the United States, and about 3% of the elderly population. Pernicious anemia is treated with large doses of vitamin B$_{12}$. Typically, 0.1 mg of the vitamin is injected each week until the symptoms of pernicious anemia disappear. Patients then take oral doses of vitamin B$_{12}$ for the rest of their life. Although vitamin B$_{12}$ toxicity is not an issue for patients being treated for pernicious anemia, treatment of these patients with folic acid may cause problems. Specifically, pernicious anemia is often first detected because the patient feels weak or tired. If the anemia is not treated, the patient may suffer irreversible nerve damage. The problem with folic acid supplements is that the folic acid treatment prevents the anemia from developing, but allows the eventual nerve damage to occur.

VITAMIN B₆. Vitamin B_6 is clearly toxic at doses about 1,000 times the RDA. Daily doses of 2–5 grams of one specific form of this vitamin can produce difficulty in walking and tingling sensations in the legs and soles of the feet. Continued megadoses of vitamin B_6 result in further unsteadiness, difficulty in handling small objects, and numbness in the hands. When the high doses are stopped, recovery begins after two months. Complete recovery may take two to three years. The DRI suggests an upper tolerable limit between 30 and 80 mg per day for children and teenagers, depending on age (younger children have requirements on the lower end of the scale), and 100 mg per day for adults. The DRI is between 1.3 and 1.7 mg per day for adults, slightly higher during pregnancy, and lower in children.

VITAMIN C. Large doses of vitamin C are considered to be toxic in persons with a family history of or tendency to form **kidney stones** or **gallbladder** stones. Kidney and gallbladder stones usually consist of calcium oxalate. Oxalate occurs in high concentrations in foods such as cocoa, chocolate, rhubarb, and spinach. A fraction of the vitamin C in the body is normally broken down to produce oxalate. A daily supplement of 3.0 grams of vitamin C has been found to double the level of oxalate that passes through the kidneys and is excreted into the urine. The DRI suggests an upper tolerable limit between 400–1,200 mg per day for children and teenagers, depending on age (younger children have requirements on the lower end of the scale), and 2,000 mg per day for adults.

NIACIN. The DRI for niacin is 14–16 mg per day in adults. Niacin comes in two forms, nicotinic acid and nicotinamide. Either form can satisfy the adult requirement for this vitamin. Nicotinic acid, however, is toxic at levels of 100 times the RDA. It can cause flushing of the skin, nausea, diarrhea, and liver damage. Flushing is an increase in blood passing through the veins in the skin, due to the dilation of arteries passing through deeper parts of the face or other parts of the body. In spite of the side effects, however, large doses of nicotinic acid are often used to lower blood cholesterol in order to prevent heart disease. Nicotinic acid results in a lowering of LDL-cholesterol (so-called bad cholesterol), an increase in HDL-cholesterol (so-called good cholesterol), and a decrease in plasma triglycerides. Treatment involves daily doses of 1.5–4.0 grams of nicotinic acid per day. Flushing of the skin occurs as a side effect when nicotinic acid therapy is started, but may disappear with continued therapy. The DRI suggests an upper tolerable limit between 10–30 mg per day for children and teenagers, depending on age (younger children have requirements on the lower end of the scale), and 35 mg per day for adults. The DRI for vitamin C in adults is between 75 and 90 mg per day, slightly more during pregnancy.

Diagnosis

The diagnosis of vitamin toxicity is usually made on the basis of the patient's dietary or medical history. Questioning the patient about the use of vitamin supplements may shed light on some physical symptoms. The doctor can confirm the diagnosis by ordering blood or urine tests for specific vitamins. When large amounts of the water-soluble vitamins are consumed, a large fraction of the vitamin is absorbed into the bloodstream and promptly excreted into the urine. The fat-soluble vitamins are more likely to be absorbed into the bloodstream and deposited in the fat and other tissues. In the cases of both water-soluble and fat-soluble vitamins, any vitamin not absorbed by the intestines is excreted in the feces. Megadoses of many of the vitamins produce diarrhea, because the non-absorbed nutrient draws water out of the body and into the gut, resulting in the loss of this water from the body.

Treatment

In all cases, treatment of vitamin toxicity requires discontinuing vitamin supplements. Vitamin D toxicity needs additional action to reduce the calcium levels in the bloodstream because it can cause abnormally high levels of plasma calcium (hypercalcemia). Severe hypercalcemia is a medical emergency and is treated by infusing a solution of 0.9% sodium chloride into the patient's bloodstream. The infusion consists of 2.1 to 3.1 qts (2 to 3 L) of salt water given over a period of one to two days.

Prognosis

The prognosis for reversing vitamin toxicity is excellent for most patients. Side effects usually go away as soon as overdoses are stopped. The exceptions are severe vitamin D toxicity, severe vitamin A toxicity, and severe vitamin B_6 toxicity. Too much vitamin D leads to deposits of calcium salts in the soft tissue of the body, which cannot be reversed. Birth defects due to vitamin A toxicity cannot be reversed. Damage to the nervous system caused by megadoses of vitamin B_6

KEY TERMS

Absorption—The transfer of a vitamin from the digestive tract to the bloodstream.

Ascorbic acid—Another name for vitamin C.

Dietary reference intakes (DRI)—These standards explain the daily amounts of energy, protein, minerals, and fat-soluble and water-soluble vitamins needed by healthy males and females, from infancy to old age.

Hypercalcemia—A condition marked by abnormally high levels of calcium in the blood.

Hypervitaminosis—Another name for vitamin toxicity.

Megadose—A very large dose of a vitamin, taken by some people as a form of self-medication.

Menadione—A synthetic form of vitamin K, sometimes called vitamin K_3.

Pernicious anemia—A rare disorder in which the body does not absorb enough vitamin B_{12} from the digestive tract, resulting in an inadequate amount of red blood cells produced.

Recommended dietary allowance (RDA)—The quantities of nutrients in the diet that are needed for good health.

Retinol—Another name for vitamin A.

can be reversed, but complete reversal may require a recovery period of more than a year.

Health care team roles

Health care professionals should familiarize themselves with the symptoms of vitamin toxicities in order to successfully diagnose toxic levels.

Patient education

Health care professionals can direct patients in learning about the recommended requirements for each vitamin so that toxicities do not pose a risk. The DRI can be referred to for information regarding recommended intakes for individuals, estimated average requirements, and upper tolerable limits. The healthiest way to acquire vitamins is through good **nutrition** via food. Following the Dietary Guidelines for Americans, published by the U.S. Department of Agriculture and Health and Human Services, can provide a broad overall view of good nutrition. The Food Guide Pyramid was created by the U.S. Department of Agriculture to help Americans choose foods from each food grouping. The food pyramid, developed by nutritionists, provides a visual guide to healthy eating.

Prevention

Vitamin toxicity can be prevented by minimizing the use of vitamin supplements or by only taking a dose within recommended levels of the DRI or RDA. If vitamin D supplements are being used on a doctor's orders, monitoring the levels of plasma calcium help prevent toxicity. The development of hypercalcemia with vitamin D treatment indicates that the patient is at risk for vitamin D toxicity.

Resources

BOOKS

Food and Nutrition Board. *Recommended Dietary Allowances, 10th ed.* Washington, DC: National Academy Press, 1989.

Institute of Medicine. *Dietary Reference Intakes: Applications in Dietary Assessment.* Washington, DC: National Academy Press, 2001.

Institute of Medicine. *Dietary Reference Intakes: Risk Assessment (Compass Series).* Washington, DC: National Academy Press, 1999.

Larson-Duyff, Roberta. *The American Dietetic Association's Complete Food & Nutrition Guide.* New York: John Wiley & Sons, 1998.

Mahan, L. Kathleen, and Sylvia Escott-Stump. *Krause's Food, Nutrition, & Diet Therapy.* London: W. B. Saunders Co., 2000.

Mindell, Earl, and Hester Mundis. *Earl Mindell's Vitamin Bible for the 21st Century.* London, UK: Warner Books, 1999.

Rodwell-Williams, Sue. *Essentials of Nutrition and Diet Therapy.* London: Mosby-Year Book, 1999.

PERIODICALS

American Dietetics Association. "Women's Health and Nutrition—Position of ADA and Dietitians of Canada." *Journal of the American Dietetic Association* (1999): 99: 738-51.

Azais-Braesco, V., and G. Pascal. "Vitamin A in Pregnancy: Requirements and Safety Limits." *American Journal of Clinical Nutrition* (2000): 71: 1325S-33.

Mills, J. L. "Fortification of Foods with Folic Acid—How Much is Enough?" *New England Journal of Medicine* (2000): 342: 1442-45.

Traber, Maret G. "Vitamin E: Too Much or Not Enough?" *American Journal of Clinical Nutrition* (2001): 73: 997-98.

ORGANIZATIONS

American Dietetic Association. 216 W. Jackson Blvd., Chicago, IL 60606-6995. (312) 899-0040. <http://www.eatright.org/>.

Food and Nutrition Information Center Agricultural Research Service, USDA. National Agricultural Library, Room 304, 10301 Baltimore Avenue, Beltsville, MD 20705-2351. (301) 504-5719. (301) 504-6409. <http://www.nal.usda.gov/fnic>. fnic@nal.usda.gov.

OTHER

Food and Nutrition Professionals Network. <http://nutrition.cos.com>.

Crystal Heather Kaczkowski, M.Sc.

Vitamins

Definition

Vitamins are organic components in food that are needed for growth and for maintaining good health. They include the fat-soluble vitamins, such as **vitamin D**, **vitamin E**, **vitamin A**, and **vitamin K**; and the water-soluble vitamins, such as folate (**folic acid**), **vitamin B₁₂**, **biotin**, vitamin B₆, **niacin**, thiamine, **riboflavin**, pantothenic acid, and **vitamin C** (ascorbic acid). Vitamins are required in the diet in only tiny amounts, in contrast to the energy components (sugars, starches, **fats**, and oils).

Purpose

All of the vitamins serve several important functions in the body and provide many health benefits. Therefore, a lack of a particular vitamin in the diet can cause a corresponding vitamin-deficiency disease.

Vitamin D, which helps to fight **infection**, is available from butter, cream, salmon, egg yolks, and adequate sun exposure. Vitamin D deficiency in children is called rickets, which is a disease of the bones. Symptoms include knocked knees, bowed legs, and protruding chests. Osteomalacia is the adult form of vitamin D deficiency; it is a result of low **calcium** intakes or lack of sun exposure during childhood and the adult years. Vitamin E acts as an antioxidant in the body for cells that are highly exposed to oxygen, and it resists hemolysis of red **blood** cells. Vitamin E is very widespread in food, so a deficiency is rare. However, when vitamin E deficiency does occur, it can cause serious nerve damage. Hemolytic anemia results if there is a vitamin E deficiency. A deficiency in vitamin E usually occurs only in premature babies due to the fact that they are born before the vitamin can be

Essential vitamins	
Vitamin	**What it does for the body**
Vitamin A (Beta Carotene)	Promotes growth and repair of body tissues; reduces susceptibility to infections; aids in bone and teeth formation; maintains smooth skin
Vitamin B-1 (Thiamin)	Promotes growth and muscle tone; aids in the proper functioning of the muscles, heart, and nervous system; assists in digestion of carbohydrates
Vitamin B-2 (Riboflavin)	Maintains good vision and healthy skin, hair, and nails; assists in formation of antibodies and red blood cells; aids in carbohydrate, fat, and protein metabolism
Vitamin B-3 (Niacinamide)	Reduces cholesterol levels in the blood; maintains healthy skin, tongue, and digestive system; improves blood circulation; increases energy
Vitamin B-5	Fortifies white blood cells; helps the body's resistance to stress; builds cells
Vitamin B-6 (Pyridoxine)	Aids in the synthesis and breadown of amino acids and the metabilism of fats and carbohydrates; supports the central nervous system; maintains healthy skin
Vitamin B-12 (Cobalamin)	Promotes growth in children; prevents anemia by regenerating red blood cells; aids in the metabolism of carbohydrates, fats, and proteins; maintains healthy nervous sytem
Biotin	Aids in the metabolism of proteins and fats; promotes healthy skin
Choline	Helps the liver eliminate toxins
Folic Acid (Folate, Folacin)	Promotes the growth and reproduction of body cells; aids in the formation of red blood cells and bone marrow
Vitamin C (Ascorbic Acid)	One of the major antioxidants; essential for healthy teeth, gums, and bones; helps to heal wounds, fractures, and scar tissue; builds resistance to infections; assists in the prevention and treatment of the common cold; prevents scurvy
Vitamin D	Improves the absorption of calcium and phosphorous (essential in the formation of healthy bones and teeth) maintains nervous system
Vitamin E	A major antioxidant; supplies oxygen to blood; provides nourishment to cells; prevents blood clots; slows cellular aging
Vitamin K (Menadione)	Prevents internal bleeding; reduces heavy menstrual flow

transferred to the developing baby during the last few weeks of **pregnancy**.

Vitamin A functions in maintaining **vision**, immune defense, bone development, cell growth, and reproduction. Food sources of vitamin A include fortified milk, spinach, carrots, and sweet potatoes. Vitamin A deficiency is common throughout the poorer parts of the world, and causes night blindness (nyctalopia). Severe vitamin A deficiency can result in xerophthalamia, a disease that, if left untreated, results in total blindness. Dry, scaly skin (hyperkeratosis) also results from vitamin A deficiency. Vitamin

K is a nutrient that is essential for blood clotting; it can be obtained from intestinal **bacteria**. It is also present in dark-green leafy vegetables, cabbage, liver, eggs, cereals, and fruit. Vitamin K deficiency results in spontaneous bleeding. It can be affected by mineral oil, **antibiotics**, and anticoagulants.

Folate, also known as folic acid, is required for the synthesis of new cells in the body. Mild or moderate folate deficiency is common throughout the world, and can result from the failure to eat green leafy vegetables or fruits and fruit juices. Folate deficiency causes megaloblastic anemia, which is characterized by the presence of large abnormal cells, called megaloblasts, in the circulating blood. The symptoms of megaloblastic anemia are tiredness and weakness. Folic-acid deficiency is also associated with neural-tube birth defects such as spina bifida and anencephaly. These serious congenital malformations are the result of inadequate folate intake during pregnancy. Neural-tube defects occur early in pregnancy before most women even know they are pregnant, so it is essential that women of childbearing age receive adequate amounts of folate before they become pregnant, as well as during pregnancy. For this reason, folate fortification of enriched flour, breads, rice, and other grain products was approved by the U.S. Food and Drug Administration (FDA) in 1996. Vitamin B_{12} helps make red blood cells in the body and protect nerve fibers. A deficiency occurs with the failure to consume sufficient meat or milk or other dairy products. Vitamin B_{12} deficiency causes pernicious anemia, which is the result of a lack of the intrinsic factor needed for the absorption of vitamin B_{12}. A deficiency of vitamin B_{12} can be masked by folate deficiency.

The B vitamins niacin, thiamine, and riboflavin each play a role in the energy **metabolism** of cells. Niacin can be found in such foods as tuna, chicken, mushrooms, and baked potatoes. A deficiency of niacin results in the disease known as pellagra, which involves skin rashes, scabs, **diarrhea**, and mental depression. Thiamine is found in pork, ham, green leafy vegetables, legumes, and whole-grain cereals. Thiamine deficiency results in beriberi, a disease resulting in atrophy, weakness of the legs, nerve damage, and **heart failure**. Vitamin C helps protect against infection and enhances the absorption of **iron**. Orange juice, grapefruit, broccoli, green peppers, and brussels sprouts are significant sources of vitamin C. A deficiency results in scurvy, a disease that contributes to the breakdown of collagen, which causes loose teeth, bleeding gums, and swollen wrists and ankles. Specific diseases uniquely associated with deficiencies in vitamin B_6, riboflavin, or pantothenic acid have not been found in humans, though people who have been starving, or consuming poor diets for several months, might be expected to be deficient in most of the nutrients, including vitamin B_6, riboflavin, and pantothenic acid. Homocystinurias, a group of autosomal recessive disorders, are associated with low levels of folate and vitamins B_6 and B_{12}.

Some of the vitamins serve only one function in the body, while other vitamins serve a variety of unrelated functions. Hence, some vitamin deficiencies tend to result in one type of defect, while other deficiencies result in a variety of problems.

Purpose

People are treated with vitamins for three reasons. The primary reason is to relieve a vitamin deficiency when one has been detected. Chemical tests suitable for the detection of all vitamin deficiencies are available. The diagnosis of vitamin deficiency is often aided by visual tests, such as the examination of blood cells with a **microscope**, the x-ray examination of bones, or a visual examination of the eyes or skin.

A second reason for vitamin treatment is to prevent the development of an expected deficiency. In this case, vitamins are administered even with no test for possible deficiency. One example is vitamin K treatment of newborn infants to prevent bleeding. Food supplementation is another form of vitamin treatment. The vitamin D added to foods serves the purpose of preventing the deficiency from occurring in people who may not be exposed much to sunlight and who fail to consume foods that are fortified with vitamin D, such as milk. Niacin supplementation prevents pellagra among people who rely on corn as the main source of food and who do not eat much meat or milk. In general, the U.S. food supply is fortified with niacin.

A third reason for vitamin treatment is to reduce the risk for diseases that may occur even when vitamin deficiency cannot be detected by chemical tests. One example is folate deficiency. The risk for cardiovascular disease can be slightly reduced for a large fraction of the population by folic-acid supplements. These supplements can also sharply reduce the risk for certain birth defects.

Vitamin treatment is important during specific diseases where the body's normal processing of a vitamin is impaired. In these cases, high doses of the needed vitamin can force the body to process or utilize it in the normal manner. One example is pernicious anemia, a disease that tends to occur in middle age or old age; it impairs the absorption of vitamin B_{12}. Surveys have revealed that about 0.1% of the general population, and 2% to 3% of the elderly, may have the disease. If left untreated, pernicious anemia leads to nervous-system damage. The disease can easily be treated with large daily oral doses of vitamin B_{12} (hydroxocobalamin) or with monthly injections of the vitamin.

Vitamin supplements are widely available as over-the-counter products. But whether they work to prevent or curtail certain illnesses, particularly in people with a balanced diet, is a matter of debate and ongoing research. For example, vitamin C is not proven to prevent the **common cold**, yet millions of people take it for that reason.

Precautions

Vitamin A and vitamin D can be toxic in high doses; side effects range from dizziness to kidney failure. High doses of niacin can be toxic to the liver, while excessive intake may occur with vitamin C, especially among the elderly. Doses of vitamin K can have toxic effects in infants. A physician or pharmacist should be consulted about the correct use of a multivitamin supplement that contains these vitamins.

Description

Vitamin treatment is usually done in three ways: by replacing a poor diet with one that supplies the recommended dietary allowance (RDA), by consuming oral supplements, or by injections. Injections are useful for persons with diseases that prevent absorption of fat-soluble vitamins. Oral vitamin supplements are especially useful for people who otherwise cannot or will not consume food that is a good vitamin source, such as meat and dairy products. For example, a vegetarian who will not consume meat may be encouraged to consume oral supplements of vitamin B_{12}.

Treatment of genetic diseases that impair the absorption or utilization of specific vitamins may require megadoses of the vitamin throughout one's lifetime. Megadose means a level of about 10 to 1,000 times greater than the RDA for a particular vitamin. Pernicious anemia, homocystinuria, and biotinidase deficiency are three examples of genetic diseases that are treated with megadoses of vitamins.

Preparation

The diagnosis of a vitamin deficiency usually involves a blood test. An overnight fast is usually

KEY TERMS

Anencephaly—A neural-tube defect that causes lack of brain formation and results in death shortly after birth.

Antioxidant—A compound that prevents other compounds from being damaged by oxygen by reacting with oxygen itself.

Genetic disease—A disease that is passed from one generation to the next but does not necessarily appear in each generation. An example of genetic disease is Down syndrome.

Neural tube defects—A group of birth defects that affect the brain and spinal cord.

Recommended dietary allowance (RDA)—The recommended dietary allowances (RDAs) are quantities of nutrients of the diet that are required to maintain human health. RDAs are established by the Food and Nutrition Board of the National Academy of Sciences and may be revised every few years. A separate RDA value exists for each nutrient. The RDA values refer to the amount of nutrient expected to maintain health in the greatest number of people.

Vitamin status—The state of vitamin sufficiency or deficiency of any person. For example, a test may reveal that a patient's folate status is sufficient, borderline, or severely inadequate.

recommended as preparation prior to the blood test so that vitamin-fortified foods do not affect the test results.

Aftercare

The response to vitamin treatment can be monitored by chemical tests, by an examination of red or white blood cells, or by physiological tests, depending on the exact vitamin deficiency.

Complications

Although there are few complications associated with vitamin treatment, possible risks depend on the vitamin and the reason why it was prescribed. In general, the higher the dose that is taken, the higher the risk of toxicity. It is also important to remember that vitamins are better absorbed from food rather than in concentrated pill form. Physicians or pharmacists should be consulted about how and when to take vitamin supplements, particularly those that have not been prescribed by a physician.

Health care team roles

Dietitians can provide a wide range of information concerning the well-balanced diet that is necessary to receive adequate amounts of all the vitamins. Dietitians also play an important role in educating people about the dangers of consuming too much or too little of a particular vitamin. When a particular vitamin deficiency is present, consulting a dietitian, pharmacist, or physician about how and when to take vitamin supplements is advised.

Resources

BOOKS

Brody, T. *Nutritional Biochemistry*. San Diego: Academic Press, 1998.

Food and Nutrition Board. *Recommended Dietary Allowances, 10th Edition*. Washington, DC: National Academy Press, 1989.

Sizer, F., and E. Whitney. *Nutrition: Concepts and Controversies, 7th Edition*. Belmont, CA: Wadsworth, 1997.

Worthington-Roberts, B. S., and S. Rodwell Williams. *Nutrition Throughout the Life Cycle, 4th Edition*. Boston: McGraw-Hill, 2000.

Lisa Gourley

Voice disorders

Definition

A voice disorder is an abnormality of one or more of the three characteristics of voice: pitch, intensity (loudness), and quality (resonance).

Description

The National Institute on Deafness and Other Communication Disorders estimates that approximately 7.5 million persons in the United States suffer from some sort of voice disorder. The negative impact of a voice disorder is often social, psychological, professional, and economic (as in the case of a singer or actor).

Voice is typically described in terms of three characteristics: pitch, intensity, and quality. Pitch may be described as the relative tone of a person's voice—how high or low it is, how monotonous, or how it demonstrates repeated inappropriate pitch patterns. A disorder may result from pitch being inappropriate for an individual's age and gender. An inability to perceive pitch and pitch patterns may result in a monotonous voice, a high-pitched voice, or inappropriate use of repeated pitch patterns.

Loudness describes the volume or intensity of a person's voice. A person who spends a great deal of time in a noisy location or who is suffering from **hearing loss** may speak with high intensity, or louder than normal. A soft or inaudible voice may be associated with a psychological condition such as shyness or with a structural defect of the vocal cords.

Some disorders of voice quality are related to how the vocal cords function: breathiness is caused by vocal cord vibration that does not have a closed phase, while hoarseness is caused by vocal cords that are closed too tightly, so they cannot vibrate properly. Other disorders are related to how the voice resonates in the oral (mouth), nasal (nose), and pharyngeal (throat) cavities. If the nasal passage becomes blocked such as with a cold, then air is unable to reach the nasal cavity and a voice sounds hyponasal. Hypernasality results when too much air passes through the nasal cavities during phonation or when there is an obstruction in the anterior nasal cavities (pinching the nostrils).

Causes and symptoms

Normal voice production

The larynx is an organ found in the neck that helps to control the flow of air during breathing and to produce sound during speech. The vocal folds, also called the vocal cords, are two folds of muscle covered by a thin membrane that lie inside a framework of cartilage and soft tissue. The tension, position, and shape of the vocal folds are controlled by a number of muscles called intrinsic muscles.

Prior to the production of sound, the vocal folds are brought together by the intrinsic muscles. During exhalation, air pressure builds up beneath the closed vocal folds, causing them to separate. They are brought back together, only to separate again when pressure increases. This cycle repeats itself approximately 200 times per second in order to produce sound.

Abnormal voice production

Some of the most common causes of voice disorders in adults include **infection**, inflammation, vocal misuse or abuse, **cancer**, neuromuscular disorders, and psychological problems. In children, vocal misuse or abuse is the most common cause of voice disorder of quality.

INFECTION. A viral or bacterial infection may directly or indirectly result in voice problems. Upper respiratory infections may cause inflammation of the vocal fold membranes, resulting in changes in voice pitch and/or quality; this condition is called acute viral laryngitis. Recurrent respiratory papillomas (RRP) are wart-like growths caused by infection by the human papilloma virus (HPV); papillomas may grow on the larynx or in the throat, nose, or trachea and cause hoarseness and/or shortness of breath.

INFLAMMATION. A condition called laryngopharyngeal reflux disease (LPRD) has been associated with approximately 55% of voice disorder cases. LPRD is caused by the backflow (reflux) of acidic **stomach** contents into the larynx, causing inflammation. Hoarseness, difficulty swallowing, **pain**, and coughing are some symptoms of LPRD.

Exposure to cigarette smoke has been shown to cause inflammation of the larynx, leading to a negative change in voice quality. Long-term tobacco use has also been associated with the development of LPRD. Reinke's **edema**, a term used to describe very swollen vocal cords, is another condition common in long-term smokers; fluid accumulates under the outer covering of the vocal folds and causes the voice to become low pitched.

VOCAL MISUSE OR ABUSE. Examples of vocal misuse are singing or speaking out of range and producing harsh vocal sounds. Extended screaming and yelling are other examples of vocal abuse. The result of vocal misuse or abuse may be swelling of the vocal folds (edema), followed by the formation of vocal fold nodules (calluses). Consequences may range from vocal fatigue or hoarseness to vocal fold hemorrhage (bleeding).

LARYNGEAL CANCER. Laryngeal cancer accounts for 2–5% of cancers diagnosed in the United States. Chronic tobacco and alcohol use are major risk factors for developing laryngeal cancer. Symptoms include chronic hoarseness, coughing, **sore throat**, difficulty swallowing or breathing, and/or pain that radiates to the neck.

NEUROMUSCULAR DISORDERS. Vocal fold **paralysis** and paresis (partial paralysis) are examples of neuromuscular voice disorders. The cause of vocal fold paralysis is usually due to trauma or to cancer. It may also occur as a result of tumor involvement of the laryngeal nerves. Spasmodic dysphonia (SD) is another neuromuscular disorder and is caused by abnormal contractions of the muscles that control the vocal folds, resulting in a hoarse, shaky, and/or strained or strangled voice. Finally, the causes of neuromuscular disorders include degenerative conditions both of the nervous system and muscle.

PSYCHOLOGICAL CONDITIONS. Voice is often affected by one's emotions; psychological **stress** may cause changes to loudness or pitch. More rarely, voice disorders may be caused by psychological trauma or extreme stress. Aphonia, or a complete loss of voice, may be a result. Often, such voice disorders may be successfully treated with psychological therapy.

Diagnosis

A variety of technologies are available to examine the larynx for abnormalities, including:

- Laryngoscopy: The indirect examination involves holding a small mirror at the back of the throat in order to visualize the larynx. In a direct examination, a flexible (inserted through the nose to the back of the throat) or rigid (held at the back of the mouth) tube-like instrument is used to more clearly visualize the interior of the larynx.

- Video stroboscopy: A strobe light is used in this test to help visualize the rapidly vibrating vocal folds as if they were in slow motion, potentially revealing changes in the vocal folds not readily seen using other methods.

- Electromyography (EMG): A laryngeal EMG is used to examine the electrical activity of the muscles of the larynx as they contract; this may reveal injury to nerves that are important in voice production.

- Double-probe pH monitoring: Special probes are placed in the esophagus and larynx to measure the extent of laryngopharyngeal reflux (LPR) over a 24-hour period. This test is therefore useful in diagnosing LPRD.

Treatment

How a voice disorder is treated depends largely on how it was caused. Often, voice therapy with a certified speech-language pathologist can dramatically improve a person's voice. Voice therapy may include vocal and listening exercises, information on vocal hygiene (appropriate uses of voice), and education regarding proper voice technique. Treatment may also be the medical management of contributing health factors such as **allergies** and, in some cases, surgery. Other than medical treatment, therapy may

KEY TERMS

Botox—A toxin produced by the bacteria *Clostridium botulinum* that can provide temporary relief to people suffering from spasmodic dysphoria.

Neuromuscular—Relating to the muscles and nerves.

Otolaryngologist—A specialist who treats disorders of the ear, nose, and throat.

Trachea—The windpipe.

include modification of the environment and psychological counseling.

A promising treatment for SD is injection with small amounts of a bacterial toxin called botox into the muscles of the larynx. The toxin temporarily weakens the laryngeal muscles, resulting in several months of improved voice quality.

Occasionally, surgery may be required to repair damaged vocal folds or remove cancerous tumors. **Laser surgery** has been used successfully in laryngeal surgery due to its precise cutting beam. Treatment of laryngeal cancer may include **chemotherapy**, radiation therapy, and/or partial or total laryngectomy, in which part, or all, of the larynx is removed. Voice therapy before and after surgery is recommended to provide the patient with a new mode of speech, if necessary.

Health care team roles

Common health care professionals involved with the care of a patient with a voice disorder may include:

- speech-language pathologists
- otolaryngologist, specialists who treat disorders of the ears, nose, and throat
- respiratory therapists
- psychiatrist or psychologist
- oncologists, cancer specialists
- audiologists, **hearing** specialists

Prevention

In order to prevent the development or deterioration of a voice disorder, patients are recommended to:

- Drink six to eight glasses of water a day and minimize intake of alcoholic and caffeinated beverages.
- Decrease exposure to cigarette smoke.
- Avoid unnecessarily coughing or clearing the throat, or speaking or singing out of range.
- Seek medical care if hoarseness or other voice changes persist for longer than 10 days.

Resources

ORGANIZATIONS

American Speech-Language-Hearing Association (ASHA). 10801 Rockville Pike, Rockville, MD 20852. (888) 321-ASHA. <http://www.asha.org>.

National Institute on Deafness and Other Communication Disorders (NIDCD) Information Clearinghouse. 1 Communication Avenue, Bethesda, MD 20892-3456. (800) 241-1044. <http://www.nidcd.nih.gov>.

The Voice Foundation. 1721 Pine Street, Philadelphia, PA 19103. (215) 735-7999. <http://www.voicefoundation.org>.

OTHER

"Frequently Asked Questions Regarding Voice Problems." *University of Pittsburgh Voice Center* 5 July 2001. <http://www.upmc.edu/upmcvoice/faq.htm>.

"The Larynx and Voice: Basic Anatomy and Physiology." *The Johns Hopkins Center for Laryngeal and Voice Disorders* August 1997. <http://www.med.jhu.edu/voice/larynx.html>.

"Questions/Answers about Voice Problems." *American Speech-Language-Hearing Association* 5 July 2001. <http://www.asha.org/speech/disabilities/Voice-problems.cfm>.

"Voice and Laryngeal Disorders." *The Voice Center at Eastern Virginia Medical School* 3 July 2001. <http://www.voice-center.com/dis_index.html>.

"What are Voice Disorders and Who Gets Them?" *Center for Voice Disorders of Wake Forest University* 1 November 1999. <http://www.wfubmc.edu/voice/voice_disorders.html>.

Stéphanie Islane Dionne

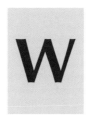

W

Walking pneumonia *see* **Pneumonia**

Water and nutrition

Definition

Water is essential to life and nutritional health. Humans can live for several weeks without food, but we can survive only a few days without water. Water makes up a large percentage of the body, in muscles, fat cells, **blood**, and even bones.

Purpose

Every cell, tissue and organ requires water to function properly. Water transports nutrients and oxygen to the cells, provides a medium for chemical reactions to take place, helps to flush out waste products, aids in maintaining a constant body temperature, and keeps the tissues in the skin, mouth, eyes, and nose moist.

Precautions

The body does not store excess water, unlike it does with other nutrients. With physical exertion, water requirements increase; therefore, fluid replacement during **exercise** is critical. The longer the duration and the more physical exertion athletes put into their exercise, the more fluid they lose during workouts. To keep the body working at its best, it is essential to replenish lost fluid after workouts, and to stay well hydrated during exercise.

The body can accommodate extreme changes in water intake when the **brain** and **kidneys** are functioning normally. It is usually possible for a person to consume enough water to maintain blood volume and **electrolyte balance** in the blood. However, if a person is unable to consume enough water to equal excessive water loss, **dehydration** may result.

Description

Water for sustaining life

The body works to maintain water balance through mechanisms such as the thirst sensation. When the body requires more water, the brain stimulates nerve centers in the brain to encourage a person to drink in order to replenish the water stores.

The kidneys are responsible for maintaining homeostasis of the body water (i.e. water balance) through the elimination of waste products and excess water. Water is primarily absorbed through the gastrointestinal tract and excreted by the kidneys as urine. Water intake can vary widely on a daily basis, influenced by such factors as: access to water, thirst, habit, and cultural factors. The variation in water volume ingested is dependent on the ability of kidneys to dilute and concentrate the urine as needed. There is a reservoir of water outside of the bloodstream that can replace or absorb excess water in the blood when necessary.

For a normal adult, a minimum daily intake between 700-800 ml (0.74-0.84 US quarts) is required to meet water losses and maintain the body's water balance. To protect against dehydration and developing **kidney stones**, greater water consumption (between 1.4-2 L/day or 1.5-2 US quarts/day) is advised. Water losses occur through evaporation in expired air and through the skin. Sweat losses are usually minimal but can be significant in warmer climates or with accompanying **fever**.

The following conditions increase water consumption needs. However, the amount of water necessary depends on body size, age, climate, and exertion level.

Water needs are increased by:

• Exercise. Water is lost through perspiration.

• Hot and humid climates.

- High altitudes. The breathing rate is twice as fast as at sea level. At high altitudes, most water loss is due to respiration rather than perspiration.

- Prescription drugs. If adequate water is not available for proper blood flow, medication can become concentrated in the bloodstream and become less effective.

- Dieting. A reduced carbohydrate intake may have a diuretic effect because **carbohydrates** store water.

- Airplane, bus, or train travel. The re-circulated air causes water to evaporate from skin faster.

- Illness. Fever, **diarrhea** and vomiting lead to increased water losses.

Individuals should not wait until they are thirsty to replenish water stores. By the time the thirst mechanism signals the brain to encourage a person to drink water, already 1–3% of the body fluids are lost and an individual is mildly dehydrated.

Nutrition for optimal health

Not only is water necessary to sustain life, but proper **nutrition** is also required to ensure optimal health. Consumption of wide variety of foods, with adequate vitamin and mineral intake is the basis of a healthy diet. **Vitamins** are compounds that are essential in small amounts for proper body function and growth. Vitamins are either fat soluble: A, D, E, and K; or water soluble: vitamin B and C. The B vitamins include vitamins B_1 (**thiamine**), B_2 (**riboflavin**), and B_6 (pyridoxine), pantothenic acid, **niacin**, **biotin**, **folic acid** (folate), and **vitamin B_{12}** (cobalamin).

Researchers state that no single nutrient is the key to good health, but that optimum nutrition is derived from eating a diverse diet including a variety of fruits and vegetables. Because there are many more nutrients available in foods such as fruits and vegetables than vitamin supplements, food is the best source for acquiring needed vitamins and **minerals**. The mineral nutrients are defined as all the inorganic elements or inorganic molecules that are required for life. As far as human nutrition is concerned, the inorganic nutrients include water, sodium, potassium, chloride, **calcium**, phosphate, sulfate, magnesium, **iron**, **copper**, **zinc**, manganese, iodine, selenium, and molybdenum. Other inorganic nutrients include phosphate, sulfate, and selenium. Inorganic nutrients have a great variety of functions in the body. The electrolytes are affected by **fluid balance** in particular (sodium, potassium, calcium, phosphate, and magnesium etc.). Water, sodium, and potassium deficiencies are most closely associated with abnormal nerve action and cardiac arrhythmias.

Laboratory studies with animals have revealed that severe deficiencies in any one of the inorganic nutrients can result in very specific symptoms, and finally in death, due to the failure of functions associated with that nutrient. In humans, deficiency in one nutrient may occur less often than deficiency in several nutrients. A patient suffering from malnutrition is deficient in a variety of nutrients.

Complications

Sodium deficiency (hyponatremia) and water imbalances (dehydration) are the most serious and widespread deficiencies in the world. These electrolyte deficiencies tend to arise from excessive losses from the body, such as during prolonged and severe diarrhea or vomiting. Diarrheal diseases are a major world health problem, and are responsible for about a quarter of the 10 million infant deaths that occur each year. Nearly all of these deaths occur in impoverished parts of Africa and Asia, where they result from contamination of the water supply by animal and human feces.

Dehydration is a deficit of body water that results when the output of water exceeds intake. Dehydration stimulates the thirst mechanism, instigating water consumption. Sweating and the output of urine both decrease. If water intake continues to fall short of water loss, dehydration worsens.

Causes of dehydration may include:

- vomiting
- diarrhea
- diuretics
- excessive heat
- excessive sweating
- fever
- decreased water intake

Dehydration induces water to move from the reservoir inside cells into the blood. If dehydration progresses, body tissues begin to dry out and the cells start to shrivel and malfunction. The most susceptible cells to dehydration are the brain cells. Mental confusion, one of the most common signs of severe dehydration may result, possibly leading to **coma**. Dehydration can occur when excessive water is lost with diseases such as **diabetes mellitus**, diabetes insipidus, and Addison's disease.

Dehydration is often accompanied by a deficiency of electrolytes, sodium and potassium in particular. Water does not move as rapidly from the reservoir inside of the cells into the blood when electrolyte concentration is decreased. **Blood pressure** can decline due to a lower volume of water circulating in the bloodstream. A drop in blood pressure can cause light-headedness, or a feeling of impending blackout, especially upon standing (orthostatic hypotension). Continued fluid and electrolyte imbalance may further reduce blood pressure, causing **shock** and damage to many internal organs including the brain, kidneys, and **liver**.

Consumption of *plain water* is usually sufficient for mild dehydration. However, when both water and electrolyte losses have occurred after vigorous exercise, electrolytes must be replaced, sodium and potassium in particular. Adding a little salt to drinking water or consuming drinks such as Gatorade during or following exercise can replace lost fluids. Individuals with **heart** or kidneys problems should consult a physician regarding the replacement of fluids after exercise.

Overhydration is an excess of body water that results when water intake exceeds output. Drinking large amounts of water does not typically lead to overhydration if the kidneys, heart, and **pituitary gland** are functioning properly. An adult would have to drink more than 7.6 L per day (2 US gallons/day) to exceed the body's ability to excrete water. Excessive body water causes electrolytes in the blood, including sodium to become overly diluted. Overhydration occurs in individuals whose kidneys do not function normally, primarily in kidney, heart, or liver disease. People with these conditions may have to limit their water and dietary salt intake. Similar to dehydration, the brain is the most sensitive organ to overhydration. The brain cells can adapt to increased fluid volume when overhydration increases slowly, however, when it occurs rapidly, mental confusion, seizures, and coma can result.

Results

Consuming adequate food and fluid before, during, and after exercise can help maintain blood glucose during exercise and also maximize exercise performance. Athletes should be well-hydrated before exercise commencement and should drink enough fluid during and after exercise to maintain homeostasis. The same rules apply to non-athletes who are participating in physical activity or are in conditions that increase dehydration. Careful attention to water intake and urine output should provide the best results.

KEY TERMS

Dehydration—A deficit of body water that results when the output of water exceeds intake.

Diuretic—An agent or drug that eliminates excessive water in the body by increasing the flow of urine.

Electrolyte—A substance such as an acid, bases, or salt. An electrolyte's water solution will conduct an electric current and ionizes. Acids, bases, and salts are electrolytes.

Homeostasis—An organism's regulation of body processes to maintain internal equilibrium in temperature and fluid content.

Overhydration—An excess of body water that results when water intake exceeds output.

Avoiding some beverages such as coffee, tea, alcohol and caffeinated soft drinks may reduce the risk of dehydration. These beverages are all diuretics (substances that increase fluid loss). Water in foods, especially fruits and vegetables, is a great source of fluid. Fruits and vegetables can contain up to 95 percent water, so a well-balanced diet is a good way to stay hydrated.

Health care team roles

All health care professionals should recognize the importance of promoting proper nutrition and hydration. Encouraging patients to follow nutrition guidelines for adequate vitamin and mineral intakes is critical.

Patient education

Patients and individuals can be educated regarding the importance of hydration by nutrition experts and physicians as well as the need for good nutrition. Individuals themselves can become familiar with concepts for healthy eating using a number of resources such as the Food Pyramid, which provides a visual guide to healthy eating. In addition, the U.S. Department of Agriculture and the U.S. Department of Health and Human Services have developed official dietary guidelines that include ten basic recommendations for healthy eating:

- Aim for a healthy weight.

- Be physically active each day.

- Let the Food Pyramid guide your food choices.

- Choose a variety of grains daily, especially whole grains.

- Choose a variety of fruits and vegetables daily.

- Keep food safe to eat.

- Choose a diet low in saturated fat and cholesterol, and moderate in total fat.

- Choose beverages and foods to moderate intake of sugars.

- Choose and prepare foods with less salt.

- If you drink alcoholic beverages, do so in moderation.

Resources

BOOKS

Mindell, Earl and Hester Mundis. *Earl Mindell's Vitamin Bible for the 21st Century*. London: Warner Books, 1999.

Rodwell-Williams, Sue. *Essentials of Nutrition and Diet Therapy (With CD-ROM for Windows and Macintosh)*. London: Mosby-Year Book, 1999.

Speakman, Elizabeth and Weldy, Norma Jean. *Body Fluids and Electrolytes* 8th ed. London: Mosby Incorporated, 2001.

Workman, M. Linda *Introduction to Fluids, Electrolytes and Acid-Base Balance*. London: W B Saunders Co., 2001.

PERIODICALS

Beck, L.H. "The aging kidney. Defending a delicate balance of fluid and electrolytes." *Geriatrics* 55, no. 4 (2000): 26-28, 31-32.

Sawka, M.N. and Montain, S.J. "Fluid and electrolyte supplementation for exercise heat stress." *American Journal of Clinical Nutrition* 72, no. 2 Suppl. (2000): 564S-572S.

ORGANIZATIONS

American Dietetic Association. 216 W. Jackson Blvd. Chicago, IL 60606-6995. (312) 899-0040. <http://www.eatright.org/>.

Food and Nutrition Information Center Agricultural Research Service, USDA. National Agricultural Library, Room 304, 10301 Baltimore Avenue, Beltsville, MD 20705-2351. (301) 504-5719. Fax: (301) 504-6409. <http://www.nal.usda.gov/fnic/>. fnic@nal.usda.gov.

OTHER

Food and Nutrition Professionals Network. <http://nutrition.cos.com/>.

Nr-Space, et al. *Fluids & Electrolytes CD-ROM*. Delmar Publishers, 2001.

Crystal Heather Kaczkowski, MSc.

Water fluoridation

Definition

Water fluoridation is the **public health** practice of altering municipal water supplies to reflect an optimal range of fluoride in drinking water in order to combat **dental caries** (tooth decay).

Description

At the beginning of the 20th century, dental caries were widespread and lead to serious tooth loss. In fact, having sound teeth was so important and such a rarity in the general population that the U.S. military made having a minimum of six opposing teeth a requirement during recruitment for WW I and II.

The first glimmer of an association between fluoride and oral health was observed by Dr. Frederick S. McKay in 1901. Noticing a brown stain on the teeth of his patients, Dr. McKay found that those who had these stains seemed to have fewer caries. In 1909, Dr. F.L. Robertson noticed mottling on the enamel (the hard outer surface) of children's teeth after the digging of a new well—source of the local drinking water. It wasn't until 1930 that the well water was analyzed, and high concentrations of fluoride were found. Fluoride, a naturally occurring fluorine ion, is found in soil, foods, and water.

The brown staining and mottling were characteristic of **fluorosis**, an abnormal condition caused by excessive exposure to fluoride while a child's teeth are forming under the gums. It affects the formation of tooth enamel and can vary from very mild to severe. Very mild fluorosis is manifested as tiny, white spots on 25% of a tooth's surface. Mild fluorosis covers 26% to 50%, and moderate fluorosis compromises all of a tooth's surface. It is most often characterized by brown discoloration of the tooth. Severe fluorosis involves pitting of the enamel and more serious brown staining. Approximately 94% of dental fluorosis today ranges from very mild to mild.

Extensive studies of national water supplies have been conducted. It has been found that dental caries were fewer in cities with more fluoride in the community water supply. A 1945 field study was conducted in four pairs of cities to determine whether a low level of fluoride (between 1.0 ppm and 1.2 ppm) could prevent dental caries. The result was a 50% to 70% reduction in the number of dental caries in communities with fluoridated water; only 10% of the people had mild fluorosis.

In 1962, another study found an optimal fluoride level of 0.7 parts per million (ppm) to 1.2 ppm (warm climates, where water consumption is higher, vs. cooler climates, respectively). This fluoride level range was determined to combat dental caries and pose only a slight risk of mild fluorosis.

Water fluoridation was rapidly adopted in major U.S. cities. About 46% of all public water supplies, however, remain non-fluoridated. Still, there has been a drastic reduction in the incidence of dental caries among children. In 2000, about half of all American children aged five to 17 years had never had a cavity in their permanent teeth. Adults also have experienced a 20% to 40% reduction in dental caries on enamel surfaces, as well as on exposed root caries—a condition peculiar to persons with gingival recession. Some of the earlier studies from the 1980s showed little difference in the reduction rates of dental caries between fluoridated communities and non-fluoridated communities. This may be due to improved **dental hygiene**, and the use of other fluoride products like fluoridated toothpaste and mouth rinses.

Viewpoints

Adding fluoride to drinking water has always been controversial. Though fluoride appears naturally in many water supplies, its purposeful introduction into community water supplies has brought claims of causing **cancer**, **heart** disease, **Down Syndrome**, **osteoporosis**, acquired **immunodeficiency** syndrome (**AIDS**), low intelligence, **Alzheimer's disease**, nephritis, cirrhosis, intracranial lesions, allergic reactions, and hip **fractures**. There has been no credible evidence to link fluoride to these diseases.

Early geographic studies in the 1980s reported a correlation between water fluoridation and bone fractures. However, an October 2000 study of women in four U.S. communities who had a continuous 20-year exposure to fluoride in drinking water found that fluoride was not a factor in increased spinal and hip fractures. In fact, these women exhibited greater bone density in the large bones like the femur, the hip, and the lumbar spine, with a slight decrease in hip and spine fractures. There was, however, a slight increase in the incidence of wrist fractures.

Though claims of increased medical risk when drinking fluoridated water still exist, opponents are finding other issues with platforms from which to fight fluoridation (for example, the fact the individuals do not get to decide whether to fluoridate their own personal drinking water) and whether dental caries are a serious public health problem anymore. These opponents cite studies from the mid-1980s that showed only an 18% difference in dental caries among children living in communities with and without fluoridated water. They claim, and rightly so, that this difference is due to widespread use of fluoridated toothpaste. However, increased use of bottled water, and processed foods that may contain fluoridated water, may also be contributing factors.

Water fluoridation provides inexpensive prevention for at-risk populations in every community. Despite **Medicaid** benefits that cover dental treatment, poor children often have less access than higher income families to dentists and fluoridated dental hygiene products. Children in non-fluoridated communities seek dental treatment in hospital emergency rooms more often than children in fluoridated communities; this increases costs for their dental treatment. The consumption of fluoridated water can reduce these expenses.

Adding fluoride to drinking water is the most cost-effective method for preventing dental caries. The average costs of fluoridation is around $0.50 per person annually, with some communities paying out only $0.12 per person. Smaller areas with fewer than 10,000 people, however, have costs that can run between $3 and $5 a year per person. Still, the cost of fluoridation for a single person over his or her lifetime can be less than the cost of one filling.

Fluoridation has been found to be effective for all citizens within a community regardless of socioeconomic status, and it has been proven safe for every person to use. Fluoridated water has a topical benefit. It provides ambient fluoride, which promotes remineralization of teeth to all ages and populations who consume the treated water. The latest concern, however, centers on over-fluoridation. There are many more ways to ingest fluoride than just in drinking water. Fluoride is added to prepared foods and bottled drinks. Carbonated drinks, juices, and some bottled waters have fluoride in varying amounts. Often, the fluoride in these products is not revealed on the label. Foods high in fluoride are fish with bones, tea, poultry products, cereals, or infant formula, which is made with fluoridated water. Dental products such as mouth rinses, toothpaste, and fluoride supplements all have added fluoride. Some pediatricians prescribe fluoride supplements without determining the fluoride content of the water a child drinks or assessing the amount of fluoride exposure the child has in his or her environment. Parents need to take a proactive role in learning the contents of their children's prescriptions.

KEY TERMS

Dental caries—Tooth decay.

Enamel—The hard, calcified outer surface of a tooth; the hardest known substance in the human body.

Fluoride—A fluorine ion used to treat water or apply directly to tooth surfaces to prevent dental caries.

Fluorosis—Fluorosis is an abnormal condition caused by excessive exposure to fluoride while a child's teeth are forming under the gums. It affects the formation of tooth enamel and can be very mild (a few white spots on a tooth) to severe (etching, pitting, and brown discoloration).

It is of most concern when children ingest large amounts of fluoride, not because of known health risks related to fluoride, but because of the added potential of having fluorosis in children's permanent teeth. Young children under six years of age often use too much fluoride toothpaste and consistently swallow it. This alone has been the biggest cause of excess fluoride ingestion. For that reason, fluoride products should be kept out of the reach of children. Parents should supervise children who are under six years of age as they brush their teeth, ensuring that only a peasized drop of toothpaste is used, and directing them not to swallow toothpaste. Children under six should not use fluoridated mouth rinses.

Professional implications

Water fluoridation has been recognized by more than 90 professional health organizations in the world as the most effective dental caries preventive in the 20th century. Dentists, dental hygienists, pediatricians, nurses, dietitians, and professionals from the United States Centers for Disease Control have endorsed the benefits of fluoridated water. Unfortunately, about half of the population of the United States lives in areas that do not have fluoridated water. Health care professionals need to be aggressive in their efforts to bring fluoride to these areas. Careful monitoring of fluoride present in all environments, and an assessment of the client's fluoride history, need to be carried out by local pediatricians and dentists before fluoride supplements are prescribed. Nurses and other professionals need to take a role in educating parents about fluoride dental products and foods containing fluoride, as well as proper fluoride consumption by children under the age of six.

Resources

BOOKS

Griffen, A.K., ed. *Pediatric Oral Health*. Philadelphia: Saunders, 2000.

PERIODICALS

Author unspecified. "Achievements in Public Health, 1900-1999: Fluoridation of Drinking Water to Prevent Dental Caries." *JAMA, Journal of the American Medical Association* 283, no. 10 (March 8, 2000):1283.

Author unspecified. "Fluoride." *Current Health* 25, no. 5 (January 2, 1999):4.

Author unspecified. "Fluoride in Drinking Water and Hip Fracture." *Journal of the American Dietetic Association* 100, no. 7 (July 2000):851.

Author unspecified. "Position of the American Dietetic Association: The Impact of Fluoride on Health." *Journal of the American Dietetic Association* 101, no. 1 (January 2001):126.

Author unspecified. "Water Fluoridation and Costs of Medicaid Treatment for Dental Decay: Louisiana, 1995-1996." *Morbidity and Mortality Weekly Report* 48, no. 34 (Sept 3, 1999):752.

Featherstone, D.B. "The Science and Practice of Caries Prevention." *Journal of the American Dental Association* 131, no. 7 (July 2000):887.

Heilman, J.R., Kiritsy, M.C., Levy, S.M., and J.S. Wefel. "Assessing Fluoride Levels of Carbonated Soft Drinks." *Journal of the American Dental Association* 130, no. 11 (November 1999):1593.

Larson, Ruth. "Is Fluoride Corrupting 'Precious Bodily Fluids'?" *Insight on the News* 15, no. 28 (August 2, 1999):40.

Lewis, C.W., Grossman, D.C., Domoto, Peter K., and R.A. Deyo. "The Role of the Pediatrician in the Oral Health of Children: a national survey. (Abstract.)" *Pediatrics* 106, no. 6 (December 2000):1475.

Phipps, K.R., Orwoll, E.S., Mason, J.D., and J.A. Cauley. "Community Water Fluoridation, Bone Mineral Density, and Fractures: prospective study of effects in older women." *British Medical Journal* 321, no. 7265 (October 7, 2000):860.

Warren, J.J., Kanellis, M.J., and S.M. Levy. "Fluorosis of the Primary Dentitian: What Does it Mean for Permanent Teeth?" *Journal of the American Dental Association* 130, no. 3 (March 1999):347.

ORGANIZATIONS

American Academy of Pediatrics. 141 Northwest Point Boulevard, Elk Grove Village, IL 60007-1098. (847) 434-4000. <http://www.aap.org>.

American Dental Association. 211 East Chicago Ave., Chicago, IL 60611. (800)947-4746, (312)440-2500. <http://www.ada.org>.

Centers for Disease Control and Prevention. 4770 Buford Highway, NE, Atlanta, GA 30341. (770) 488-6054. <http://www.cdc.gov/nohss>.

National Association of Pediatric Nurse Associates & Practitioners. 1101 Kings Highway, N., Suite 206, Cherry Hill, NJ 08034-1912. <http://www.napnap.org>.

OTHER

"American Dental Association: Oral Health Topics: Fluoridation Facts: Safety Question 18." April 20, 2001. <http://www.ada.org>.

"American Dental Association: Statement on Water Fluoridation Efficacy and Safety." April 20, 2001. <http://www.ada.org>.

Janie F. Franz

Water therapy *see* **Hydrotherapy**

Weber test *see* **Rinne and Weber tests**

Wernicke-Korsakoff disease *see* **Alcoholic paralysis**

Western herbalism *see* **Herbalism, Western**

Wheelchair prescription

Definition

A wheelchair is a mobile chair used by individuals who have impairments that limit their ability to walk. A wheelchair prescription defines the specifications of a chair according to an individual's particular needs.

Purpose

Wheelchairs are used either as primary or secondary means of mobility, depending upon the extent of an individual's functional limitations. When using a wheelchair as a primary means of mobility, an individual may spend the majority of his or her day in the chair and use it for movement within his or her home, work, school or community setting. As a secondary means of mobility, a chair may be used just for longer distances by an individual who has low endurance or tolerance for walking. The wheelchair prescription is used to define the type of wheelchair required, seating needs, and details about necessary components.

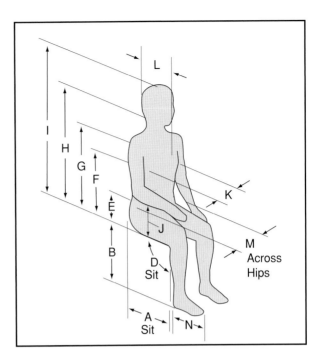

Measurements necessary for a wheelchair prescription.
(Illustration by Argosy. Courtesy of Gale Group.)

Description

Selection of a type of wheelchair, its fit, and included components depends largely on the following factors:

- What are the patient's disability, medical, and management issues? These can include considerations such as level of independence, pressure relief, orthoses, etc.

- What is the patient's size, weight, and posture? Does the patient need a heavy-duty chair? Is there a fixed **scoliosis** or kyphosis that needs to be accommodated?

- What is the individual's functional ability? Sitting balance, ability to transfer oneself and provide pressure relief, upper extremity strength and dexterity, and cognitive level are just a few of the things that must be considered.

- What are the patient and family goals for using the chair? What has been tried already? Will the chair be used as a primary or secondary means of positioning and mobility? Will it be used around the house, at school/work, outside, for sports participation?

- What are the environmental concerns? Access to public and private settings, including work, school, libraries, and transportation, must be considered. Is the individual's own home wheelchair-accessible?

- What are the funding issues? The cost of basic and special features, sources of funding, rental/leasing options, future maintenance, and upgrade costs should all be considered.

The prescription should include the following categories of specifications:

Type of wheelchair

There are standard and heavy-duty adult chairs, in addition to junior, youth, and "growing" frames. In a user assessment study in 2000, ultra lightweight chairs with a high degree of adjustability were shown to be preferred over lightweight chairs for ride comfort and ergonomics in long-term wheelchair use. Chairs for people with hemiplegia include a seat that is lower to accommodate for propulsion with a lower extremity. One-hand drive chairs allow a chair to be propelled with one handrim controlling both wheels. Chairs for people with lower-extremity amputations are designed to widen the base of support, compensating for the loss of anterior weight. Sports wheelchairs are lighter and easier to maneuver, for active individuals. They include a lower back, canted wheels for more efficient propulsion, and small handrims. Reclining and tilt wheelchairs offer individuals the opportunity to either recline, opening up the angle at the hips, or tilt their entire position back. Reclining chairs tend to be used for relief from orthostatic hypotension, while tilt chairs address pressure relief and gravity-assisted positioning. Power wheelchairs may be used by individuals who would have difficulty with operating a manual wheelchair. Dependent bases, which allow only for a caregiver to push the chair, also exist; however, great care must be taken in choosing this option because it does not allow for the user to self-propel the chair in any capacity.

Standard measurements

Measurements should be taken with the individual seated on a firm surface in an erect posture. The individual may require physical support to maintain this position while being measured. If an additional seat cushion or back will be used with the chair, those measurements also must be figured in to the individual measurements.

Specific formulas exist and should be used to determine: seat height, depth and width; back height and armrest height. The size of a standard adult wheelchair is:

- Seat width = 18 in (45 cm).
- Seat depth = 16 in (40 cm).
- Seat height = 20 in (50 cm).

Standard sizes exist for smaller adults and children as well; custom fabrication also is available but can be costly.

Components

Wheel locks are used to prevent movement of the chair while the user is moving into or out of it. The wheels of the chair may have solid rubber, pneumatic or semi-pneumatic tires. Pneumatic tires provide a smoother ride and are easier to maneuver on rough and soft surfaces, but they also create more friction, increasing the energy expenditure required. The caster wheels are the front, smaller wheels that allow turns to occur. The rear wheels are large and include an outer handrim that is used to propel the chair.

Lap and chest belts are used to prevent the user from falling out of the chair. Several types of armrests exist, including fixed, removable, reversible, desk-length, and adjustable. The front rigging supports the lower leg and foot. The leg rest may be swing-away, removable, or elevating. The footplates may be fixed or adjustable, and may include strapping for proper foot positioning. Antitipping devices often are attached to the lower rear support bar to prevent backward tipping of the chair.

All of these components may be included on the chair with various options that must be specified on the wheelchair prescription according to the patient's needs.

Seating

Seating is an important consideration, especially for users who will spend most of their waking day in the chair or for those with pressure relief concerns. Several cushion types exist: planar, contoured, and molded. A planar surface offers the least support and pressure relief, but may be the least expensive and simplest to maintain. A contoured surface may either assume contour with pressure through the use of foam, air, or gel within the cushion, or it may be preformed. It provides more support than the planar surface, but is more adjustable than the molded surface. A molded seat is created from liquid foam that follows the direct contours of the specific user. It offers the most support for an individual with low trunk control and may be formed to accommodate fixed deformities; however, it also is costly and room for growth is limited.

Operation

Operation of a wheelchair varies depending on the type. A user who is going to be active in self-propelling a manual wheelchair must learn the following techniques, if applicable to his or her individual needs:

- Locking brakes, swinging away or removing front riggings, and adjusting or removing armrests.

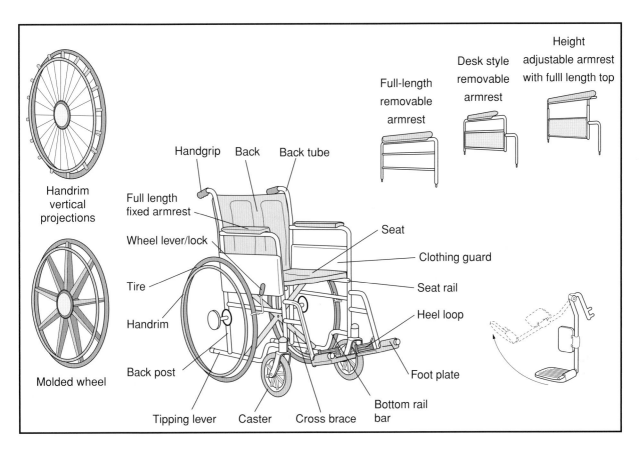

Components of a wheelchair. *(Illustration by Argosy. Courtesy of Gale Group.)*

- Transferring into and out of the chair, which may include transfers to standing, to the floor, to an automobile seat, to various sitting surfaces, or to bed.

- Wheeling the chair, using the handrims, over various types of terrain including smooth tile, carpeting, gravel, sand, asphalt, and/or grass.

- Maneuvering the chair over curbs and ramps.

- Folding or disassembling the chair for transport in a car or for storage.

The user also should be able to educate another individual on how to assist with or perform any of the above activities, in case the user requires assistance at any time. A caregiver should be able to assist with reclining or tilt-in-space functions as well.

A user of a power wheelchair must learn to maneuver the chair using the control interface selected for his or her individual needs. This may be a joystick, sip-and-puff, tongue touch pad, eye gaze, or chin or head control, depending upon the level of disability. Research has found that in individuals with severe disabilities resulting from high-level **spinal cord injury**, nervous system diseases, cognitive impairment or blindness, 10% find it extremely difficult to perform activities of daily living with power wheelchairs, and up to 40% find many steering and maneuvering situations difficult or impossible. New technology using microprocessors and sensors to assist navigation may help to alleviate this problem in the future.

Maintenance

Maintenance, just like operation, depends on the type of wheelchair used. A solidly built manual chair may require minimal maintenance, while a power chair often requires nightly battery charges. Proper function of wheel locks and other components should be monitored frequently and adjusted as necessary by the wheelchair supplier or with his or her explicit instruction.

Health care team roles

A physician, physical therapist, occupational therapist, seating specialist, and assistive technology specialist all may be involved in making recommendations for the wheelchair type and specification of components.

Training

Training is required in order for an individual to successfully operate a wheelchair, regardless of the type. A physical therapist often is the health care team member who works with a patient to learn transferring, propulsion, and maneuvering techniques. The occupational therapist and assistive technology practitioner (who may also be an OT or PT) play key roles as well in training the patient for optimum use of hand, head, mouth, or other controls.

Resources

BOOKS

Minor, Mary Alice Duesterhaus, and Scott Duesterhaus Minor. *Patient Care Skills,* 4th ed. Stamford, CT: Appleton & Lange, 1999.

Pierson, Frank M. *Principles and Techniques of Patient Care.* Philadelphia: W. B. Saunders Company, 1994.

PERIODICALS

Cooper, Rory A. "Wheelchairs and Related Technology for the Millenium." *Journal of Rehabilitation Research and Development* 37 (May/June 2000).

DiGiovine, Michalle M., et al. "User Assessment of Manual Wheelchair Ride Comfort and Ergonomics." *Archives of Physical Medicine and Rehabilitation* 81 (Apr. 2000): 490–3.

Fehr, Linda, et al. "Adequacy of Power Wheelchair Control Interfaces for Persons with Severe Disabilities: A Clinical Survey." *Journal of Rehabilitation Research and Development* 37 (May/June 2000): 353–60.

ORGANIZATIONS

RESNA. 1700 North Moore Street, Suite 1540, Arlington, VA 22209-1903. 703-524-6686. <http://www.resna.org>.

OTHER

Bergen, Adrienne Falk. "Assessment for Seating and Wheeled Mobility Systems." *WheelchairNet.* Apr. 1998. <http://www.wheelchairnet.org>.

"Prioritizing and Making Decisions About Wheelchairs." *WheelchairNet.* <http://www.wheelchairnet.org/ProdServ/Docs>.

Peggy Campbell Torpey

Wheezing

Definition

Wheezing is a high-pitched whistling sound associated with labored breathing.

Description

Wheezing occurs when a child or adult tries to breathe deeply through air passages that are narrowed or filled with mucus as a result of:

- allergy
- infection
- illness
- irritation.

Wheezing is most common when exhaling. It is sometimes accompanied by a mild sensation of tightness in the chest. Anxiety about not being able to breathe easily can cause muscle tension that makes wheezing worse.

Causes and symptoms

Wheezing is the symptom most associated with asthma. It can be brought on by:

- exposure to allergens (food, pollen, and other substances, that cause a person to have an allergic reaction)
- fumes
- ice-cold drinks or very cold air
- medication
- strenuous exercise
- weather changes
- foreign objects trapped in the airway
- cystic fibrosis and other genetic disorders
- illnesses such as pneumonia, bronchitis, congestive heart failure, and emphysema

Diagnosis

A family physician, allergist, or pulmonary specialist takes a medical history that includes questions about illness, allergies or unexplained symptoms that may be the result of allergic reactions. If the pattern of the patient's symptoms suggests the presence of allergy, skin and blood tests can be performed to identify the precise nature of the problem.

A pulmonary function test may be ordered to measure the amount of air moving through the patient's airways. X rays are sometimes indicated for patients whose wheezing seems to be caused by obstruction, chronic bronchitis or emphysema.

In 2004, researchers in Japan discovered a new method for diagnosing asthma in infants by testing for certain antibodies in their sputum (mucus that spits up from the bronchi).

Treatment

Mild wheezing may be relieved by drinking plenty of room temperature or warm juice, water, weak tea, and broth. Cold drinks should be avoided.

A vaporizer can help clear air passages. A steam tent, created by lowering the face toward a sink filled with hot water, placing a towel over the head and sink, and inhaling the steam, can do likewise.

Bronchodilators (medications that help relax and widen narrowed airways) may be prescribed for patients whose wheezing is the result of asthma. Newer asthma medications taken daily can help prevent asthma attacks, as can avoiding asthma and allergy triggers.

Antibiotics are generally used to cure acute bronchitis and other respiratory infections. Expectorants (cough-producing medications that help bring up mucus) or certain bronchodilators are prescribed to remove excess mucus from the airways.

If wheezing is caused by an allergic reaction, antihistamine medications may be prescribed to neutralize body chemicals that react to the allergen.

Medical emergencies

Wheezing can be a sign of a life-threatening medical emergency. Under some conditions wheezing requires immediate medical attention. If the airways are blocked treatment is unsuccessful, and the person dies from lack of oxygen. In cases where the airway is restored after the critical period passes, there may be permanent brain damage. Emergency medical attention is required whenever an individual:

- turns blue or gray or stops breathing
- becomes extremely short of breath and is unable to speak
- coughs up bubbly-pink or white phlegm
- seems to be suffocating
- develops a fever of 101 °F (38.3 °C) or higher and has breathing problems
- wheezes most of the time, and coughs up gray or greenish phlegm.

Alternative treatment

Certain yoga positions (Bridge, Cobra, Pigeon, and Sphinx) may relieve wheezing by improving

breathing control and reducing stress and can be practiced in conjunction with traditional medical treatments. Individuals whose wheezing is related to asthma, chronic bronchitis, or emphysema may benefit from these techniques, but should continue to have their condition monitored by a traditional physician.

Prognosis

Wheezing is a symptom, not a disease. Improvement in wheezing depends on controlling the underlying disease that causes this symptom. Temporary, mild wheezing caused by infection or acute illness usually disappears when the underlying cause is eliminated. Chronic wheezing caused by lung conditions such as chronic obstructive pulmonary disease (COPD) or emphysema may worsen with time depending on the progress of the lung disease. Allergic reactions can cause swelling of the throat tissues. The wheezing that results is a symptom of a medical emergency and can be fatal.

Health care team roles

The health care team involved in treating wheezing depends on the disease or condition causing this symptom. Family physicians, allergists, pediatricians, and pulmonary specialists all may treat diseases that cause symptoms of wheezing. Respiratory therapists may be involved in treating wheezing when the symptom is caused by smoke or chemical inhalation. Emergency medical personnel treat life-threatening wheezing caused by airway obstruction.

Prevention

Stopping smoking can eliminate wheezing. So can reducing or preventing exposure to other substances that cause the problem.

Resources

BOOKS

Fanta, Christopher F., Lynda Christiano, and Kenan Haver. *The Harvard Medical School Guide to Taking Control of Asthma*. New York: Free Press, 2003.

PERIODICALS

"Creola Bodies in Wheezing Infants Predict Asthma Development." *Immunotherapy Weekly* July 7, 2004: 10.

"What's New in: Asthma and Allergic Rhinitis." *Pulse* September 20, 2004: 50.

"Wheezing? Check Your Inhaler." *Prevention* September 2004: 34.

ORGANIZATIONS

Asthma and Allergy Foundation of America. 1233 20th Street, NW, Suite 402, Washington, DC 20036. (800) 727-8462. http://www.aafa.org.

OTHER

"Wheezing" *Medline Plus* August 6, 2004. http://www.nlm.nih.gov/medlineplus/ency/article/003070.htm

Maureen Haggerty
Tish Davidson, A.M.

Whiplash

Definition

Whiplash is the mechanism that causes the neck injury often suffered in a rear-end automobile collision. People also use the same term, whiplash, to mean the resultant neck injury itself. Whiplash produces a wide range of symptoms, but almost all victims experience **pain**. About 1,000,000 whiplash injuries occur in the United States every year.

Description

An occupant of a car struck suddenly from the rear undergoes rapid acceleration and deceleration. The head and neck swing freely while the body remains supported by the seat and seatbelts. The rapid movement of the head causes variable amounts of hyperextension, hyperflexion, stretching, and twisting of neck structures, in a fashion similar to the snapping of a whip.

The structures often affected include muscles, ligaments, nerves, intervertebral disks, and spinal joints. Specific damage may range from minimal strains to complicated tears, hemorrhage, and joint injury, as shown by animal studies and autopsies of accident victims.

Causes and symptoms

Besides motor vehicle accidents, causes of whiplash include sports and other recreational activities, **falls**, and fights. Women tend to have more persistent symptoms than men do, perhaps because women's smaller neck muscles are more vulnerable.

Symptoms following a whiplash injury may begin immediately or any time up to a few days later. Symptoms include variable combinations of:

- pain or stiffness in the neck, jaw, shoulders, arms, or back
- dizziness
- headache
- loss of feeling in the upper extremities
- problems with **vision** or hearing
- problems with concentration
- depression, **anxiety**, or other changes in mood

Symptoms may last for no more than a day or two, or may persist for months or years.

Diagnosis

Many patients with whiplash receive evaluation by **emergency medical technicians** (EMTs) at the scene of an accident, always starting with the ABCs of resuscitation: airway, breathing, and circulation. At the same time, in head or neck trauma, initial care providers always worry about the possibility of dangerous injury to the spine bones or **spinal cord**. Often, the EMTs will immobilize the neck in a stiff brace and strap the patient flat on a board, until a physician determines that it is safe for the neck to move. This minimizes the risk that any serious injury could progress and cause irreversible nerve damage. Unfortunately, this immobilization is usually very uncomfortable for the patient.

When such a patient arrives at the emergency department (ED), the nurse will further assess the patient for stable **vital signs**, proper alertness, and good ability to move and feel the extremities. A patient strapped to a spine immobilization board often demands to remove the neck brace and get up, but the nurse must ensure that the patient remains still until cleared by the physician. The nurse quickly asks the doctor to examine the patient.

Another danger is that a patient may vomit while immobilized. This presents a risk for aspiration of stomach contents, which can threaten breathing. The nurse must be alert to quickly turn the patient on the side, while still immobilized and with the neck brace still in place, to prevent this complication.

The physician obtains the patient's description of the event, then looks for injury to other organs, especially in the head, chest, abdomen, and back. The doctor will check for bony tenderness or limitation of movement, and examine the functions of deep tendon **reflexes** plus motor and sensory nerves. When the physician is confident that no injury threatens the spinal cord the patient is "cleared." The physician will remove the brace and free the patient from the rigid board.

The physician may order x-ray studies to exclude fracture or displacement of bone, but in typical whiplash these tests rarely show any abnormality. When there is severe or persistent pain or numbness, **magnetic resonance imaging** (MRI) may detect more subtle damage.

Treatment

Patients should apply ice in the first 24-48 hours. Physicians prescribe medicines such as ibuprofen (Motrin, Advil) or aspirin, acetaminophen, **muscle relaxants**, or narcotics (codeine, hydrocodone, Vicodin).

Use of soft cervical collars is controversial. Many doctors prescribe them, but some studies have shown that these devices prolong the return to normal activities. **Physical therapy** or exercises may reduce pain or limitation of movement.

Many patients use balms or salves, and seek alternative treatments such as chiropractic manipulation, biofeedback, acupuncture, or **acupressure**. In cases of protracted symptoms, patients may benefit from traction, ultrasound treatments, local injections of cortisone, or use of a nerve stimulator.

Prognosis

The course of an individual whiplash injury is unpredictable. Most people improve within a month, but 20% or more have symptoms that last longer than a year. The risk of greater symptoms increases for an unrestrained victim of a rear-end collision, or for one whose head is turned or tilted at the time of injury.

Controversy surrounds the role that accident-related litigation plays in delaying recovery from whiplash. An April 2000, article in *The New England Journal of Medicine* examined this issue. The authors showed a decreased incidence and improved prognosis

---

KEY TERMS

Aspiration—The inhaling of stomach contents or other unwanted material, potentially leading to a form of pneumonia.

Hyperextension—Overstretching toward the back.

Hyperflexion—Overstretching toward the front.

Intervertebral disk—A cushioning structure between two adjacent spine bones.

---

of whiplash injury when the province of Saskatchewan changed to a new insurance claim system that eliminated payments for pain and suffering. However, other authors downplay the effect of psychosocial factors on recovery from whiplash.

Health care team roles

The EMT performs rescue, assessment, and initial treatment at the scene of an accident. A nurse in the ED or medical office also assesses the patient with whiplash. The nurse carries out physician orders for medication and treatments, monitors the patient throughout the stay, and instructs the patient and caregivers before discharge. The aide assists the nurse.

A radiology technician performs the x-ray or MRI studies. A physical therapist helps with **exercise**, massage, ultrasound, and other treatments. A social worker may coordinate later care.

Prevention

Proper adjustment of the automobile headrest is important to reduce the severity of a whiplash injury, because a headrest that does not come up behind the head offers no protection. Driving habits that reduce the frequency of abrupt stops make it less likely that a driver will suffer a rear-end collision.

Resources

BOOKS

Clark, Charles R., et al, ed. *The Cervical Spine*. Philadelphia: Lippincott-Raven, 1998.

Goetz, Christopher G., and Eric J. Pappert. *Textbook of Clinical Neurology*. Philadelphia: W. B. Saunders, 1999.

PERIODICALS

Cassidy, J. David, et al. "Effect of Eliminating Compensation for Pain and Suffering on the Outcome of Insurance Claims for Whiplash Injury." *New England Journal of Medicine* 342, no. 16 (April 20, 2000): 1179-86.

ORGANIZATIONS

American Academy of Orthopaedic Surgeons. 6300 North River Road, Rosemont, IL 60018-4262. (800) 346-AAOS. <http://www.aaos.org>.

Kenneth J. Berniker, M.D.

Whipple's disease *see* **Malabsorption syndrome**

White blood cell count and differential

Definition

A white **blood** cell (WBC) count determines the concentration of white blood cells in the patient's blood. A differential determines the percentage of each of the five types of mature white blood cells.

Purpose

This test is included in general health examinations and to help investigate a variety of illnesses. An elevated WBC count occurs in **infection**, allergy, systemic illness, inflammation, tissue injury, and leukemia. A low WBC count may occur in some viral infections, **immunodeficiency** states, and bone marrow failure. The WBC count provides clues about certain illnesses, and helps physicians monitor a patient's recovery from others. Abnormal counts that return to normal indicate that the condition is improving, while counts that become more abnormal indicate that the condition is worsening. The differential will reveal which WBC types are affected most. For example, an elevated WBC count with an absolute increase in lymphocytes having an atypical appearance is most often caused by infectious mononucleosis. The differential will also identify early WBCs which may be reactive (e.g. a response to acute infection) or the result of a leukemia.

Precautions

Many medications affect the WBC count. Both prescription and non-prescription drugs including herbal supplements should be noted. Normal values for both the WBC count and differential are age related.

Sources of error in manual WBC counting are largely due to variance in the dilution of the sample and the distribution of cells in the chamber, and the small number of WBCs that are counted. For electronic WBC counts and differentials, interference may be caused by small fibrin clots, nucleated RBCs, platelet clumping, and unlysed RBCs. Immature WBCs and nucleated RBCs may cause interference with the automated differential count. Automated cell counters may not be acceptable for counting white blood cells in other body fluids especially when the number of WBCs is less than 1000/μL or when other nucleated cell types are present.

Description

White cell counts are usually performed using an automated instrument, but may be done manually using a **microscope** and a counting chamber especially when counts are very low, or the person has a condition known to interfere with an automated WBC count. An electronic WBC count is based upon the principle of impedance. The red blood cells are lysed using a detergent in the counting diluent. As the cells move one at a time through a counting aperture, they displace electrolyte in the diluent causing a voltage pulse. The magnitude of the voltage pulse is dependent upon size, which allows the instrument to discriminate between different types of WBCs.

An automated differential may be performed by an electronic cell counter or by an image analysis instrument. The automated electronic cell counter uses a combination of impedence measurement and other means such as radio frequency conductance and angular light scattering to differentiate between closely related WBCs. Image analysis systems use morphometric and densitometric programs to distinguish the cells that are photographed from a stained slide by a digital color camera. When the electronic WBC count is abnormal or a cell population is flagged, meaning that one or more of the results is atypical, a manual differential is performed. The WBC differential is performed manually by microscopic examination of a blood sample that is spread in a thin film on a glass slide. The film is air-dried and stained with Wright stain, a polychromatic stain consisting of buffered solutions of methylene blue and eosin. Acidic structures such as DNA take up the basic methylene blue dye, while basic **proteins**, such as hemoglobin, take up the acidic eosin dye. White blood cells are identified by their size, the shape and texture of the nuclear chromatin, cytoplasmic and nuclear staining, and the presence and color of granules in the cytoplasm.

Causes for abnormalities in the white blood cell (WBC) differential count

Type of WBC and normal differential count	Elevated	Decreased
Neutrophils 55–70%	Neutrophilia Physical or emotional stress Acute suppurative infection Myelocytic leukemia Trauma Cushing's syndrome Inflammatory disorders Metabolic disorders	Neutropenia Aplastic anemia Dietary deficiency Overwhelming bacterial infection Viral infections Radiation therapy Addison's disease Drug therapy: myelotoxic drugs (as in chemotherapy)
Lymphocytes 20–40%	Lymphocytosis Chronic bacterial infection Viral infection Lymphocytic leukemia Multiple myeloma Infectious mononucleosis Radiation Infectious hepatitis	Lymphocytopenia Leukemia Sepsis Immunodeficiency diseases Lupus erythematosus Later stages of HIV infection Drug therapy: adrenocorticosteroids, antineoplastics Radiation therapy
Monocytes 2–8%	Monocytosis Chronic inflammatory disorders Viral infections Tuberculosis Chronic ulcerative colitis Parasites	Monocytopenia Drug therapy: prednisone
Eosinophils 1–4%	Eosinophilia Parasitic infections Allergic reactions Eczema Leukemia Autoimmune diseases	Eosinopenia Increased adrenosteroid production
Basophils 0.5–1.0%	Basophilia Myeloproliferative disease (e.g., myelofibrosis, polycythemia rubra vera) Leukemia	Basopenia Acute allergic reactions Hyperthyroidism Stress reactions

SOURCE: Pagana, K.D. and T.J. Pagana. *Mosby's Diagnostic and Laboratory Test Reference*. 3rd ed. St. Louis: Mosby, 1997.

The manual WBC differential involves a thorough evaluation of a stained blood film. In addition to determining the percentage of each mature white blood cell, the following tests are preformed as part of the differential:

- Evaluation of RBC morphology is performed. This includes grading of the variation in RBC size (aniso-cytosis) and shape (poikioocytosis); reporting the type and number of any abnormal RBCs such as target cells, sickle cells, stippled cells, etc.; reporting the presence of immature RBCs (polychromasia); and counting the number of nucleated RBCs per 100 WBCs.

- An estimate of the WBC count is made and compared to the automated or chamber WBC count. An estimate of the platelet count is made and compared to the automated or chamber platelet count. Abnormal platelets such as clumped platelets or excessively large platelets are noted on the report.

- Any immature white blood cells are included in the differential count of 100 cells, and any inclusions or abnormalities of the WBCs are reported.

WBCs consist of two main subpopulations, the mononuclear cells and the granulocytic cells. Mononuclear cells include lymphocytes and monocytes. Granulocytes include neutropohils (also called polymorphonuclear leukocytes or segmented neutrophils), eosinophils, and basophils. Each cell type is described below:

- Neutrophils are normally the most abundant WBCs. They measure 12-16 µm in diameter. The nucleus stains dark purple-blue, and is divided into several lobes (usually three to four) consisting of dense chromatin. A neutrophil just before the final stage of maturation will have an unsegmented nucleus in the shape of a band. These band neutrophils may be counted along with mature neutrophils or as a separate category. The cytoplasm of a neutrophil contains both primary (azurophilic) and secondary (specific) granules. The secondary granules are lilac in color and are more abundant almost covering the pink cytoplasm. Neutrophils are phagocytic cells and facilitate removal of **bacteria** and antibody-coated antigens. The neutrophilic granules are rich in peroxidase, and aid the cell in destroying bacteria and other ingested cells.

- Eosinophils are 14-16 μm in diameter and contain a blue nucleus that is segmented into two distinct lobes. The cytoplasm is filled with large refractile orange-red granules. The granules contain peroxidase, hydrolases, and basic proteins which aid in the destruction of phagocytized cells. Eosinophils are increased in allergic reactions and parasitic infections.

- Basophils, like eosinophils, are 14-16 μm in diameter and have a blue nucleus that is bilobed. The cytoplasm of the basophil is filled with large dark blue-black granules that may obscure the nucleus. These contain large amounts of histamine, heparin, and acid mucopolysaccharides. Basophils mediate the allergic response by releasing histamine.

- Lymphocytes are the second most abundant WBCs. They may be small (7-9 μm in diameter) or large (12-16 μm in diameter). The nucleus is dark blue and is nearly round or slightly indented and the chromatin is clumped and very dense. The cytoplasm is medium blue and usually agranular. An occasional lymphocyte will have a few azurophilic granules in the cytoplasm. Lymphocytes originate in the lymphoid tissues and are not phagocytic. They are responsible for initiating and regulating the **immune response** by the production of antibodies and cytokines.

- Monocytes are the largest WBCs measuring 14-20 μm in diameter. They have a large irregularly shaped and folded blue nucleus with chromatin that is less dense than other WBCs. The cytoplasm is grey-blue, and is filled with fine dust-like lilac colored granules. Monocytes are phagocytic cells that process and present antigens to lymphocytes, an event required for lymphocyte activation.

Preparation

This test requires a 3.5 mL sample of blood. Venipuncture is usually performed by a nurse or phlebotomist following standard precautions for the prevention of transmission of bloodborne pathogens. There is no restriction on diet or physical activity.

KEY TERMS

Band cell—An immature neutrophil at the stage just preceding a mature cell. The nucleus of a band cell is unsegmented.

Basophil—Segmented white blood cell with large dark blue-black granules that releases histamine in allergic reactions.

Differential—Blood test that determines the percentage of each type of white blood cell in a person's blood.

Eosinophil—Segmented white blood cell with large orange-red granules that increases in response to parasitic infections and allergic reactions.

Lymphocyte—Mononuclear white blood cell that is responsible for humoral (antibody mediated) and cell mediated immunity.

Monocyte—Mononuclear phagocytic white blood cell that removes debris and microorganisms by phagocytosis and processes antigens for recognition by immune lymphocytes.

Neutrophil—Segmented white blood cell normally comprising 50-70% of the total. The cytoplasm contains both primary and secondary granules that take up both acidic and basic dyes of the Wright stain. Neutrophils remove and kill bacteria by phagocytosis.

Phagocytosis—A process by which a white blood cell envelopes and digests debris and microorganisms to remove them from the blood.

Aftercare

Discomfort or bruising may occur at the puncture site. Pressure to the puncture site until the bleeding stops reduces bruising; warm packs relieve discomfort. Some people feel dizzy or faint after blood has been drawn and should be treated accordingly.

Complications

Other than potential bruising at the puncture site, and/or dizziness, there are no complications associated with this test.

Results

Normal values vary with age. White counts are highest in children under one year of age and then decrease somewhat until adulthood. The increase is largely in the lymphocyte population. Adult normal values are shown below.

- WBC count: 4,500-11,000/µL
- polymorphonuclear neutrophils: 1800-7800/µL; (50-70%)
- band neutrophils: 0-700/µL; (0-10%)
- lymphocytes: 1000-4800/µL; (15-45%)
- monocytes: 0-800/µL; (0-10%)
- eosinophils: 0-450/µL; (0-6%)
- basophils: 0-200/µL; (0-2%)

Health care team roles

The WBC count and differential are ordered and interpreted by physicians. The samples may be collected by a nurse, physician assistant, phlebotomist, or technician. Testing is performed by a clinical laboratory scientist CLS(NCA)/medical technologist MT(ASCP) or by a clinical laboratory technician CLT(NCA)/ medical laboratory technician MLT(ASCP).

Resources

BOOKS

Chernecky, Cynthia C., and Barbara J. Berger. *Laboratory Tests and Diagnostic Procedures,* 3rd ed. Philadelphia, PA: W. B. Saunders Company, 2001.

Kee, Joyce LeFever. *Handbook of Laboratory and Diagnostic Tests,* 4th ed. Upper Saddle River, NJ: Prentice Hall, 2001.

Victoria E. DeMoranville

Work activities evaluation and treatment
see Ergonomic **assessment**

Wound care

Definition

A wound is a disruption in the continuity of cells—anything that causes cells that would normally be connected to become separated. Wound healing is the restoration of that continuity. Several effects may result with the occurrence of a wound: immediate loss of all or part of organ functioning, sympathetic **stress** response, hemorrhage and **blood** clotting, bacterial contamination, and death of cells. The most important factor in minimizing these effects and promoting successful care is careful asepsis.

Description

A biological process, wound healing begins with trauma and ends with scar formation. There are two types of tissue injury: full and partial thickness. Partial thickness injury is limited to the epidermis and superficial dermis with no damage to the dermal **blood vessels**. Healing occurs by regeneration of epithelial tissue. Full thickness injury involves loss of the dermis and extends to deeper tissue layers and disrupts dermal blood vessels. Wound healing involves the synthesis of several types of tissue and scar formation.

The three phases of repair are lag, proliferative, and remodeling. Directly after injury, hemostasis is achieved with clot formation. The fibrin clot acts like a highway for the migration of cells into the wound site. Within the first four hours of injury, neutrophils begin to appear. These inflammatory cells kill microbes, and prevent the colonization of the wound. Next the monocyte, or macrophage, appears. Functions of these cells include the killing of microbes, the breakdown of wound debris, and the secretion of cytokines that initiate the proliferative phase of repair. Synthetic cells, or fibroblasts, proliferate and synthesize new connective tissue, replacing the transitional fibrin matrix. At this time, an efficient nutrient supply develops through the arborization (terminal branching) of adjacent blood vessels. This ingrowth of new blood vessels is called angiogenesis. This new very vascularized connective tissue is referred to as granulation tissue.

The first phase of repair is called the lag or inflammatory phase. The inflammatory response is dependent upon the depth and volume of tissue loss from the injury. Characteristics of the lag phase include acute inflammation and the initial appearance and infiltration of neutrophils. Neutrophils protect the host from microorganisms and **infection**. If inflammation is delayed or stopped, the wound becomes susceptible to infection and closure is delayed.

The proliferative phase is the second phase of repair and is anabolic in nature. The lag and remodeling phase are both catabolic processes. The proliferative phase generates granulation tissue. In this process, acute inflammation releases cytokines, promoting fibroblast infiltration of the wound site, then creating a high density of cells. Collagen is the major connective tissue protein produced and released by fibroblasts. The connective tissue physically supports the new blood vessels that form and endothelial cells promote ingrowth of new vessels. These new blood vessels are necessary to meet the nutritional needs of the wound healing process. The mark of wound closure is when a new epidermal cover seals the defect. The process of wound healing continues underneath the new surface. This is the remodeling or maturation phase and is the third phase in healing.

The first principle of wound care is the removal of non-viable tissue including necrotic (dead) tissue, slough, foreign debris, and residual material from dressings. Removal of non-viable tissue is referred to as debridement; removal of foreign matter is referred to as cleansing. Chronic **wounds** are colonized with **bacteria**, but not necessarily infected. A wound is colonized when a limited number of bacteria are present in the wound and are of no consequence in the healing process. A wound is infected when the bacterial burden overwhelms the **immune response** of the host and bacteria grow unchecked. Clinical signs of infection are redness of the skin around the wound, purulent (pus-containing) drainage, foul odor, and **edema**.

The second principle is providing a moist environment. This has been shown to promote re-epitheliazation and healing. Exposing wounds to air dries the surface and may impede the healing process. Gauze dressings provide a moist environment as long as they are kept moist in the wound. These are referred to as wet to dry dressings. Generally a saline soaked gauze dressing is loosely placed into the wound and covered with a dry gauze dressing to prevent drying and contamination. It also supports autolytic debridement (the body's own capacity to lyse and dissolve necrotic tissue), absorbs exudate, and traps bacteria in the gauze, which are removed when the dressing is changed.

Preventing further injury is the third principle of wound care. This involves elimination or reduction of the condition that allowed the wound to develop. Factors that contribute to the development of chronic wounds include losses in mobility, mental status changes, deficits of sensation, and circulatory deficits. Patients must be properly positioned to eliminate continued pressure to the chronic wound. Pressure reducing devices, such as mattresses, cushions, supportive boots, foam wedges, and fitted shoes can be used to keep pressure off wounds.

Providing **nutrition**, specifically protein for healing, is the fourth principle of healing. Protein is essential for wound repair and regeneration. Without essential amino acids, angiogenesis, fibroblast proliferation, collagen synthesis, and scar remodeling will not occur. Amino acids also support the immune response. Adequate amounts of **carbohydrates** and **fats** are needed to prevent the amino acids from being oxidized for caloric needs. Glucose is also needed to meet the energy requirements of the cells

involved in wound repair. Albumin is the most important indicator of malnutrition because it is sacrificed to provide essential amino acids if there is inadequate protein intake.

Preparation

Effective wound care begins with an assessment of the entire patient. This includes obtaining a complete **health history** and a physical assessment. Assessing the patient assists in identifying causes and contributing factors of the wound. When examining the wound, it is important to document its size, location, appearance, and the surrounding skin. The health care professional also examines the wound for exudate, necrotic tissue, signs of infection, and drainage, and documents how long the patient has had the wound. It is also important to know what treatment, if any, the patient has previously received for the wound.

Actual components of wound care include cleaning, dressing, determining frequency of dressing changes, and reeavaluation. Removing dead tissue and debris that impedes healing is the goal of cleaning the wound. When cleaning the wound, protective goggles should be worn and sterile saline solution should be used. Providone iodine, sodium hypochlorite, and hydrogen peroxide should never be used, as they are toxic to cells.

Gentle pressure should be used to clean the wound if there is no necrotic tissue. This can be accomplished by utilizing a 60 cc catheter tip syringe to apply the cleaning solution. If the wound has necrotic tissue, more pressure may be needed. Whirlpools can also be used for wounds having a thick layer of exudate. At times, chemical or surgical debridement may be needed to remove debris.

Dressings are applied to wounds for the following reasons: to provide the proper environment for healing, to absorb drainage, to immobilize the wound, to protect the wound and new tissue growth from mechanical injury and bacterial contamination, to promote hemostasis, and to provide mental/physical patient comfort. There are several types of dressings and most are designed to maintain a moist wound bed:

- Alginate: made of non-woven fibers derived from seaweed, alginate forms a gel as it absorbs exudate. It is used for wounds with moderate to heavy exudate or drainage, and is changed every 12 hours to three days, depending on when the exudate comes through the secondary dressing.

- Composite dressings: combining physically distinct components into a single dressing, composite dressings provide bacterial protection, absorption, and adhesion. The frequency of dressing changes vary.

- Foam: made from polyurethane, foam comes in various thicknesses having different absorption rates. It is used for wounds with moderate to heavy exudate or drainage. Dressing change is every three to seven days.

- Gauze: available in a number of forms including sponges, pads, ropes, strips and rolls, gauze can be impregnated with petroleum, antimicrobials, and saline. Frequent changes are needed because gauze has limited moisture retention properties, and there is little protection from contamination. With removal of a dried dressing, there is a risk of wound damage to the healing skin surrounding the wound. Gauze dressings are changed two to three times a day.

- Hydrocolloid: made of gelatin or pectin, hydrocolloid is available as a wafer, paste, or powder. While absorbing exudate, the dressing forms a gel. Hydrocolloid dressings are used for light to moderate exudate or drainage. This type of dressing is not used for wounds with exposed tendon or bone, or third-degree **burns**, and not in the presence of bacterial, fungal, or viral infection, active cellulitis or vasculitis, because it is almost totally occlusive. Dressings are changed every three to seven days.

- Hydrogel: composed primarily of water, hydrogel dressings are used for wounds with minimal exudate. Some are impregnated in gauze or non-woven sponge. Dressings are changed one or two times a day.

- Transparent film: an adhesive waterproof membrane that keeps contaminants out while allowing oxygen and water vapor to cross through, it is used primarily for wounds with minimal exudate. It is also used as a secondary material to secure non-adhesive gauzes. Dressings are changed every three to five days, if the film is used as a primary dressing.

Complications

- Hematoma: dressings should be inspected for hemorrhage at intervals during the first 24 hours after surgery. A large amount of bleeding is to be reported immediately. Concealed bleeding sometimes occurs in the wound, beneath the skin. If the clot formed is small, it will be absorbed by the body, but if large, the wound bulges and the clot must be removed for healing to continue.

- Infection: the second most frequent nosocomial (hospital acquired) infection in hospitals is surgical wound infections with *Staphylococcus aureus*, *Escherichia coli*, and *Pseudomonas aeruginosa*.

KEY TERMS

Anabolic—Metabolic processes characterized by the conversion of simple substances into more complex compounds.

Catabolic—Metabolic processes characterized by the release of energy through the conversion of complex compounds into simple substances.

Cytokine—A protein that regulates the duration and intensity of the body's immune response.

Dermis—The thick layer of skin below the epidermis.

Epidermis—The outermost layer of the skin.

Exudate—Fluid, cells, or other substances that are slowly discharged by tissue, especially due to injury or inflammation.

Fibrin—The fibrous protein of blood clots.

Fibroblast—An undifferentiated connective tissue cell that is capable of forming collagen fibers.

Neutrophil—A type of white blood cell.

Scar—Scar tissue is the fibrous tissue that replaces normal tissue destroyed by injury or disease.

Prevention is accomplished with meticulous wound management. Cellulitis is a bacterial infection that spreads into tissue planes. Systemic **antibiotics** are usually prescribed. If the infection is in an arm or leg, elevation of the limb reduces dependent edema and heat application promotes blood circulation. **Abscess** is a bacterial infection that is localized and characterized by pus. Treatment consists of surgical drainage or excision with the concurrent administration of antibiotics.

- Dehiscence (disruption of surgical wound) and evisceration (protrusion of wound contents): this condition results from sutures giving way, infection, distention, or cough. **Pain** results and the surgeon is called immediately. Prophylactically, an abdominal binder may be utilized.

- Keloid: refers to excessive growth of scar tissue. Careful wound closure, hemostasis, and pressure support are used to ward off this complication.

Results

The goals of wound care include reducing risks that inhibit wound healing, enhancing the healing process, and lowering the incidence of wound infections.

Health care team roles

Members of the health care team actively work to reduce patients' exposure to infections, as well as to administer prescribed treatments and **patient education**, which includes teaching home wound care.

Resources

PERIODICALS

Brienza, P., and M. Geyer. "Understanding Support Surface Technologies." *Skin & Wound Care* (2000): 237–44.

Ehrlich, H. Paul. "The Physiology of Wound Healing: A Summary of Normal and Abnormal Wound Healing Processes." *Skin & Wound Care* (2000).

"Literature Review." *Dermatology Nursing* 11, no. 1 (February 1999): 64.

Nguyen, H., J. Steinberg, and D. Armstrong. "Assessment of the Diabetic Foot Wound." *Home Healthcare Consultant* 6, no. 9 (June 1999): 34–40.

Salcido, R. "Good Wound Care: What Is It?" *Skin & Wound Care* (September-October 2000).

Thompson, J. "Wounds & Injuries—Treatment; Surgical Dressings." *RN* 63, no. 1 (January 2000): 48.

René A. Jackson, RN

Wound culture

Definition

A wound culture is a diagnostic laboratory test in which microorganisms from an infected wound are grown in the laboratory on media and identified. Wound cultures always include aerobic culture, but direct smear evaluation (**Gram stain**) and anaerobic culture are not performed on every wound. These tests are performed when indicated or requested by the physician.

Purpose

The purpose of a wound culture is to isolate and identify microorganisms causing an **infection** of the wound, and to identify **antibiotics** that will be effective in destroying the organism.

Preparation

A biopsy sample is usually preferred by clinicians, but this is a moderately invasive procedure and may not always be feasible. The patient is prepped by cleansing the area with a sterile solution such as saline. **Antiseptics** such as ethyl alcohol are not recommended since they will kill **bacteria** and results will be negative. The patient is given a local anesthetic and the tissue is removed using a cutting sheath. Pressure is applied to the wound to control bleeding. Needle aspiration is less invasive and is a good technique to use in **wounds** where there is little loss of skin such as puncture wounds. Skin around the wound is cleaned with an antiseptic to kill bacteria on the skin's surface and a small 22 gauge needle is inserted. The clinician should pull back on the plunger and then change the angle of the needle two or three times to remove fluid from different areas of the wound. This procedure may be painful for the patient, so many initial cultures are done with the swab technique. The nurse should clean the wound area with sterile saline and moisten a sterile swab with sterile saline. The tip is inserted into the wound and rotated with pressure applied. The pressure will give a better yield of the fluid that is deeper in the wound. The swab used for anaerobic culture should be oxygen-free. After all three procedures, the wound should be cleaned thoroughly and bandaged.

Tissue specimens collected by biopsy should be placed in a screw capped vial containing a small amount of sterile saline to keep the tissue moist. The anaerobic sample should be placed in a gassed out vial that may contain prereduced medium or a gassed out bag and sealed. Syringes should be tightly capped immediately following aspiration. A common practice for anaerobic culture is to inoculate an anaerobic **blood culture** bottle at the point of care to insure the sample is not exposed to air. Several swabs (at least three) should be collected. One swab is placed in Stuart, Cary-Blair, or Amies transport medium for aerobic culture and another in PRAS transport medium for anaerobic culture. One swab is placed in a clean dry envelope or tube for direct smear examination.

Description

Wounds are injuries to body tissues caused by physical trauma or disease processes including surgery, diabetes, **burns**, punctures, gunshots, lacerations, bites, bed sores and broken bones. Types of wounds include:

- Abraded: Caused by abrasion such as falling on concrete.

- Contused: A bruise or contusion.

- Incised: Caused by a clean cut, as by a sharp instrument.

- Lacerated: Caused by a laceration, tearing of the skin or tissues.

- Nonpenetrating: Injury caused without disruption of the surface of the body. These wounds are usually in the thorax or abdomen and can also be termed blunt trauma wounds.

- Open: A wound in which tissues are exposed to the air.

- Penetrating: Disruption of the body surface and extension into the underlying tissue.

- Perforating: A wound with an exit and an entry, such as a gunshot wound.

- Puncture: A wound formed when something goes through the skin and into the body tissues. This wound has a very small opening but can be very deep.

The chance of a wound becoming infected is dependent upon the nature, size, and depth of the wound; its proximity to and involvement of nonsterile areas such as the skin and gastrointestinal tract; the opportunity for organisms from the environment to enter the wound; and the immunological and general health status of the person. Skin and body compartmentalization prevent many infections. In general, acute wounds are more prone to infection than chronic wounds. Wounds with a large loss of body surface such as abrasions are also easily infected. Puncture wounds may permit the growth of microorganisms since there is a break in the skin with minimal bleeding and they are hard to clean. Deep wounds, closed-off from oxygen, are an ideal environment for an anaerobic infection to develop. Foul-smelling odor, gas, or **gangrene** at the infection site are signs of an infection caused by an anaerobic bacteria. Surgical wounds can cause infection by introducing bacteria from one body compartment into another.

Diagnosing infection in a wound may be difficult. One of the cardinal signs the clinician looks for is slow healing. Within hours of injury, most wounds will display a release of fluid called an exudate. This fluid contains compounds that aid in healing and is normal. It should not be present 48-72 hours after injury. Exudate indicative of infection may be thicker than the initial exudate and may also be purulent (containing pus) and foul smelling. Clinicians will look at color, consistency and the amount of exudate to monitor early infection. In addition, infected wounds may display skin discoloration, swelling, warmth to touch and an increase in **pain**.

Wound infection prevents healing, and the microorganisms can spread from wounds to other body parts, including the **blood**. Infection in the blood is termed septicemia and can be fatal. Symptoms of a systemic infection include a **fever** and rise in white blood cells, along with confusion and mental status changes in the elderly. It is important to treat the infected wound early with a regimen of antibiotics to prevent further complications.

Wound infections often contain multiple organisms including both aerobic and anaerobic gram-positive cocci and gram-negative bacilli and yeast. The most common pathogens isolated from wounds are *Streptococcus* group A, *Staphylococcus aureus*, *Escherichia coli*, *Proteus*, *Klebsiella*, *Pseudomonas*, *Enterobacter*, *Enterococci*, *Bacterioides*, *Clostridium*, *Candida*, *Peptostreptococcus*, *Fusobacterium*, and *Aeromonas*.

A Gram stain is prepared by rolling the smear across the center of a glass slide or dropping a liquid specimen onto the center and allowing it to air dry. The initial Gram stain is used to evaluate the adequacy of the specimen; estimate the amount of any bacteria, yeast, or fungus present; and determine whether a specialized culture medium is required based upon the appearance of the organisms found. For example, the Gram stain may reveal gram positive filamentous bacteria suggestive of *Norcardia* that requires special growth medium.

The tissue used for the tests is obtained by three different methods, tissue biopsy, needle aspiration or the swab technique. The biopsy method involves the removal of tissue from the wound using a cutting sheath. The piece of tissue is transported to the laboratory where it must be liquified. This is done by adding approximately 1 mL of liquid medium and grinding the tissue in a blender or grinder until it forms a thick homogenized liquid. This is vortexed and dispensed onto solid media and into broth with a sterile pipet. Samples aspirated by syringe can be injected directly into broth and dispensed onto solid media. The swab technique is most commonly used but contains the least amount of specimen, and therefore, recovery is lower than with biopsied tissues or aspirates. The swab is pressed against the transport tube and the suspension of transport media is transferred to broth and solid media with a sterile pipet.

Wound specimens are cultured on both nonselective enriched and selective media. Cultures for anaerobes should include anaerobic sheep blood agar supplemented with **vitamin K** and hemin for general isolation; kanomycin-vancomycin laked blood agar for *Bacteroides spp.*; phenylethyl alcohol (PEA) or colistin-nalidixic acid (CNA) anaerobic sheep blood agar to suppress gram-negative bacilli; and thioglycolate broth with hemin and vitamin K for slow growing organisms, especially if tissues or aspirates are being cultured. Anaerobic media are inoculated inside a glove box or in an anaerobic (degassed) holding jar and incubated at 96.8 °F (36 °C) in the absence of oxygen for five to seven days. Aerobic culture should include inoculation of sheep blood agar for general growth; chocolate agar for isolation of *Haemophilus*; MacConkey agar for isolation of enteric gram negative bacilli; CNA or PEA blood agar for gram-positive cocci; and potato dextrose agar with antibiotics for isolation of yeast. Cultures are incubated in humid air at 96.8 °F (36 °C) for 48 hours (except for chocolate agar which is incubated in 5-10% carbon dioxide). Cultures are examined each day for growth and any colonies are Gram stained and subcultured (i.e., transferred) to appropriate media. The subcultured isolates are tested via appropriate biochemical identification panels to identify the species present. Organisms are also tested for antibiotic susceptibility by the microtube broth dilution or Kirby Bauer method. The selection of antibiotics for testing depends upon the organism isolated (i.e., gram-negative versus gram-positive, aerobe versus anaerobe).

Results

The initial Gram stain result is available the same day, or in less than an hour if requested by the physician. An early report, known as a preliminary report, is usually available after one day. After that, preliminary reports will be posted whenever an organism is identified. Cultures showing no growth are signed out after two to three days unless a slow growing mycobacterium or fungus is found. These organisms take several weeks to grow and are held for four to six weeks. The final report includes complete identification, an estimate of the quantity of the microorganisms, and a list of the antibiotics to which each organism is sensitive and resistant.

Complications

The physician may choose to start the person on an antibiotic before the specimen is collected for culture. This may alter results, since antibiotics in the person's system may prevent microorganisms present

---

KEY TERMS

Aerobe—Bacteria that require oxygen to live.

Agar—A gelatinous material extracted from red algae that is not digested by bacteria. It is used as a support for growth in plates.

Anaerobe—Bacteria that live only where there is no oxygen.

Antibiotic—A medicine that can be used topically or taken orally, intramuscularly or intravenously to limit the growth of bacteria.

Antimicrobial—A compound that prevents the growth of microbes which may include bacteria, fungi and viruses.

Antimycotic—A medicine that can be used to kill yeast and fungus.

Antiseptic—A compound that kills all bacteria, also known as a bactericide.

Broth—A growth mixture for bacteria. Different compounds such as sugars or amino acids may be added to increase the growth of certain organisms. Also known as media.

Exudate—Any fluid that has been released by tissue or its capillaries due to injury or inflammation.

Gram stain—A staining technique used in microbiology to identify and classify bacteria. The organisms will stay purple if gram-positive or counterstain pink if gram-negative. The Gram stain result depends upon the chemical composition of the bacterial cell wall.

Normal flora—The mixture of bacteria normally found at specific body sites.

Purulent—Contianing, consisting of or forming pus.

Pus—A fluid that is the product of inflammation and infection containing white blood cells and debris of dead cells and tissue.

---

in the wound from growing in culture. In some cases, the patient may begin antibiotic treatment after the specimen is collected based upon Gram stain results or clinical findings. The antibiotic chosen may or may not be appropriate for one or more organisms recovered by culture.

Nurses must be very careful when finishing a wound culture collection to make sure the wound has been cleaned thoroughly and is bandaged properly. It is important to watch for bleeding and further infection from the procedure. In addition, patients may be in pain from the manipulation so pain killing drugs such as acetaminophen may be advised.

Health care team roles

Wound culture requires the expertise of many clinicians including nurses, doctors and microbiologists. A physician requests the wound culture and is responsible for specimen collection and antibiotic selection. The physician may be assisted by a nurse, nurse practitioner, or physician assistant. Nurses should inform the patient about the testing procedure and what pain to expect. They should clean the wound thoroughly afterwards, bandage it correctly and watch for signs and symptoms of further infection. Doctors should monitor the patient closely for signs of systemic infection and be prepared to repeat the procedure if the patient does not respond to a course of antibiotics. Cultures are performed by clinical laboratory scientists/medical technologists who specialize in clinical microbiology.

Resources

BOOKS

Koneman, Elmer W., et al. *Color Color Atlas and Textbook of Diagnostic Microbiology,* 5th ed. Philadelphia: J. B. Lippincott Company, 1997.

Pagana, Kathleen D., and Timothy J. Pagana. *Manual of Diagnostic and Laboratory Tests.* St. Louis, MO: Mosby, 1998.

Shulman, Standford T., et al., eds. *The Biologic and Clinical Basis of Infectious Diseases,* 5th ed. Philadelphia: W. B. Saunders Company, 1997.

Sussman, Carrie, and Barbara M. Bates-Jensen. *Wound Care.* Gaithersburg, MD: Aspen Publishers, Inc., 1998.

ORGANIZATIONS

The Wound Healing Society. 1550 South Coast Highway, Suite 201, Laguna Beach, CA 92651. (888)434-4234. <http://www.woundhealsoc.org/>.

Jane E. Phillips, PhD

Wounds

Definition

A wound occurs when the integrity of skin is compromised (e.g., skin breaks, **burns**, or bone **fractures**). A wound may be caused by an act, such as a gunshot, fall, or surgical procedure; by an infectious disease; or by an underlying condition.

Description

Types and causes of wounds are wide ranging. They may be chronic, as are pressure ulcers (which are common in persons with diabetes as a result of skin breakdown)—or they may be acute, as in gunshot wounds or an animal bites. Wounds may also be referred to as open, in which the skin has been compromised and underlying tissues are exposed. Alternatively, they may be closed. Here, the skin has not been compromised, but trauma to underlying tissue has occurred (e.g., a bruised rib or cerebral contusion). Emergency personnel generally place acute wounds in one of eight categories:

- Abrasions. Also called scrapes, they occur when the skin is rubbed away by friction against a rough surface (e.g., rope burns and skinned knees).

- Avulsions. Occur when an entire structure or part of it is forcibly pulled away, such as in the loss of a permanent tooth or an ear lobe. Explosions, gunshots, and animal bites may cause avulsions.

- Contusions. Also called bruises, these are the result of a forceful trauma that injures an internal structure without breaking the skin. Blows to the chest, abdomen, or head with a blunt instrument (e.g., a football or a fist) can cause contusions.

- Crush wounds. Occur when a heavy object falls onto a person, splitting the skin and shattering or tearing underlying structures.

- Cuts. These are slicing wounds made with a sharp instrument, leaving even edges, or those made with a dull cutting instrument, which leaves uneven edges. Cuts may be as minimal as those caused by paper (i.e., paper cuts), or as significant as a surgical incisions.

- Lacerations. Also called tears, these are separating wounds that produce ragged edges. They are produced by a tremendous force against the body, either from an internal source, as in **childbirth**, or from an external source, like a punch.

- Missile wounds. Also called velocity wounds, they are caused by an object entering the body at a high speed, typically a bullet.

- Punctures. Deep, narrow wounds produced by sharp objects such as nails, knives, and broken glass.

Causes and symptoms

Acute wounds have a wide range of causes. Often, they are the unintentional results of motor vehicle accidents, falls, mishandling of sharp objects, or sports-related injuries. Wounds may also be the intentional results of violence involving assault with weapons, including fists, knives, and guns.

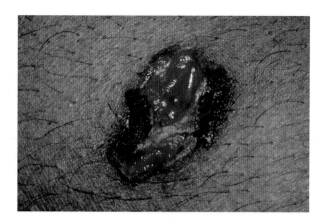

A close-up of a hard-contact gunshot wound with accompanying burn marks on the left and right sides of the wound. *(Custom Medical Stock Photo. Reproduced by permission.)*

The general symptoms of a wound are localized **pain** and bleeding. Descriptions of the appearance of different kinds of wounds are as follows:

- An abrasion usually appears as lines of scraped skin with tiny spots of bleeding.

- An avulsion has heavy, rapid bleeding and a noticeable absence of tissue.

- A contusion may appear as a bruise beneath the skin or may appear only on imaging tests; an internal wound may also generate symptoms such as weakness, perspiration, and pain.

- A crush wound may have irregular margins like a laceration; however, the wound will be deeper, and trauma to muscle and bone may be apparent.

- A cut may have little or profuse bleeding depending on its depth, length, and anatomical site. Its even edges readily line up.

- A laceration, too, may have little or profuse bleeding; the tissue damage is generally greater, and the wound's ragged edges do not readily line up.

- A missile entry wound may be accompanied by an exit wound, and bleeding may be profuse, depending on the nature of the injury.

- A puncture wound will be greater in its length; therefore, there is usually little bleeding around the outside of the wound and more bleeding inside, causing discoloration.

Diagnosis

A diagnosis is made by visual examination and may be confirmed by a report of the causal events.

Health care personnel will also assess the extent of the wound and what effect it has had on the patient's well-being (e.g., profound **blood** loss, damage to the nervous system or **skeletal system**).

Treatment

Treatment of wounds involves stopping any bleeding, then cleaning and dressing the wound to prevent **infection**. Additional medical attention may be required if the effects of the wound have compromised the body's ability to function effectively.

Stopping the bleeding

Most bleeding may be stopped by direct pressure. Direct pressure is applied by placing a clean cloth or dressing over the wound and pressing the palm of the hand over the entire area. This limits local bleeding without disrupting a significant portion of the circulation. The cloth absorbs blood and allows clot formation. The clot should not be disturbed. Therefore, if blood soaks through the original cloth, another one should be placed directly on top of it. The new cloth should not replace the original one.

If the wound is on an arm or a leg that does not appear to have a broken bone, the injured limb should be elevated to a height above the person's **heart**, while direct pressure is applied. Elevating the wound allows gravity to slow the flow of blood to that area.

If severe bleeding cannot be stopped by direct pressure or with elevation, the next step is to apply pressure to the major artery supplying blood to the area of the wound. In the arm, pressure would be applied to the brachial artery by pressing the inside of the upper arm against the bone. In the leg, pressure would be applied to the femoral artery by pressing on the inner crease of the groin, against the pelvic bone.

If the bleeding from an arm or leg is so extreme as to be life threatening, and if it cannot be stopped by any other means, a tourniquet may be required. However, in the process of limiting further blood loss, the tourniquet also drastically deprives the limb tissues of oxygen. As a result, the patient may live, but the limb may die.

Dressing the wound

Once the bleeding has been stopped, cleaning and dressing the wound is important for preventing infection. Although the flowing blood flushes debris from the wound, running water should also be used to rinse away dirt. Embedded particles, such as wood slivers and glass splinters—if not too deep—may be removed

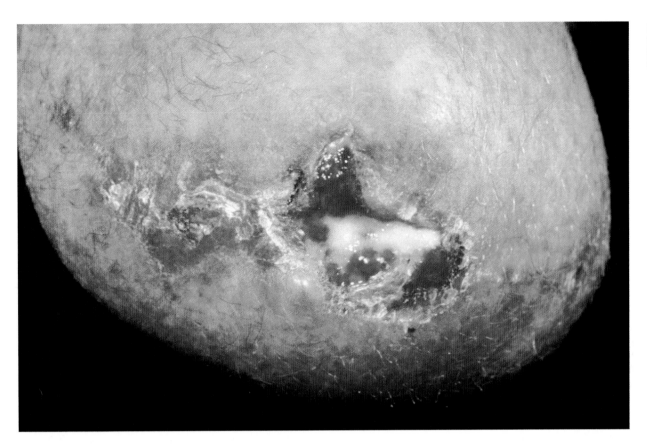

Ulcerated wound on a limb stump. *(Custom Medical Stock Photo. Reproduced by permission.)*

with a needle or pair of tweezers that has been sterilized in rubbing alcohol or in the heat of a flame. Once the wound has been cleared of foreign material and washed, it should be blotted dry gently, with care not to disturb the blood clot. An antibiotic ointment may be applied. The wound should then be covered with a clean dressing and a bandage to hold the dressing in place. Depending on the wound type, dressings can be designed to retain (or absorb) moisture, or to rehydrate desiccated wounds. Dressing materials may include polyurethane films or foams, hydrogels, hydrofibre, **calcium** alginates, and hydrocolloids.

Getting medical assistance

A person who has become impaled on a fixed object, such as a fence post or a stake in the ground, should only be moved by emergency medical personnel. Foreign objects embedded in the eye should only be removed by a physician. Larger penetrating objects, such as a fishhook or an arrow, should only be removed by a doctor, who can prevent further damage as the object is extracted.

In several instances, additional medical attention will be necessary. Wounds that penetrate the muscle beneath the skin should be cleaned and treated by a doctor, and may require stitches to stay closed during healing. Some deep wounds that do not extend to the underlying muscle may only require butterfly bandages. Wounds to the face and neck, even small ones, should always be examined by a physician so that scarring can be minimized and sensory function can be preserved. Deep wounds to the hands and wrists should be examined for nerve and tendon damage. Puncture wounds may require a tetanus shot to prevent serious infection. Animal bites should always be examined and the possibility of rabies infection considered.

Infection

Wounds that develop signs of infection should also be brought to a doctor's attention. Signs of infection are swelling, redness, tenderness, throbbing pain, localized warmth, **fever**, swollen lymph glands, the presence of pus either in the wound or draining from it, and red streaks spreading away from the wound.

Emergency treatment

With as little as one quart of blood lost, a person may lose consciousness and go into traumatic **shock**.

If the person stops breathing, artificial respiration should be administered. In the absence of a pulse, **cardiopulmonary resuscitation (CPR)** must be performed. Once the person is breathing unassisted, one can attend to the bleeding.

In cases of severe blood loss, treatment may include the intravenous replacement of body fluids. This may be infusion with saline or plasma, or with a whole-blood transfusion.

Some alternative therapies may help to support the injured person. Homeopathic remedies include: *Ledum* (*Ledum palustre*) taken internally for puncture wounds, calendula (*Calendula officinalis*) or tea tree oil (*Melaleuca* spp.) used topically as an antiseptic, aloe (*Aloe barbadensis*) applied topically to soothe skin during healing, and St. John's wort (*Hypericum perforatum*) used internally or topically when wounds affect the nerves, especially in the arms and legs. Acupuncture is thought to support the healing process by restoring energy flow in the meridians affected by the wound. In some cases, **vitamin E**, taken orally or applied topically, may speed healing and prevent scarring.

Prognosis

Without the complication of infection, most wounds heal well with time. Depending on the depth and size of the wound, it may or may not leave a visible scar.

Health care team roles

Nurses are extensively involved in the assessment and treatment of wounds. Typical responsibilities include daily cleaning of the wound with disinfectant soap, removal of crusting and loose, non-viable tissue, dressing the wound, and ensuring that a physician is notified of any changes in the wound, especially signs of infection. Other issues to be addressed by nursing staff may include **pain management**, appropriate **nutrition** to promote healing, psychosocial effects of serious or disfiguring wounds, and administration of tetanus toxoid to prevent a systemic infection. It can be very important to determine the cause of wounds, especially those that are chronic—such as leg ulcers.

Prevention

Most actions that result in wounds are preventable. Injuries from motor vehicle accidents may be reduced by advising patients to wear seatbelts and

---

KEY TERMS

Abrasion—Also called a scrape. The rubbing away of the skin surface by friction against another rough surface.

Avulsion—The forcible separation of a piece from the entire structure.

Butterfly bandage—A narrow strip of adhesive with wider flaring ends (shaped like butterfly wings) used to hold the edges of a wound together while it heals.

Cut—Separation of skin or other tissue made by a sharp edge, producing regular edges.

Laceration—Also called a tear. Separation of skin or other tissue by a tremendous force, producing irregular edges.

Plasma—The straw-colored fluid component of blood, without the other blood cells.

Puncture—An injury caused by a sharp, narrow object deeply penetrating the skin.

Tourniquet—A device used to control bleeding, consisting of a constricting band applied tightly around a limb above the wound. It should only be used if the bleeding is life-threatening and cannot be controlled by other means.

Traumatic shock—A condition of depressed body functions as a reaction to injury with loss of body fluids or lack of oxygen. Signs of traumatic shock include weak and rapid pulse, shallow and rapid breathing, and pale, cool, clammy skin.

Whole blood—Blood that contains red blood cells, white blood cells, and platelets in plasma.

---

to place children in size-appropriate car seats in the back seat. Sharp, jagged, or pointed objects or machinery parts should be used according to the manufacturer's instructions and only for their intended purpose. Firearms and explosives should be used only by adults with explicit training; they should also be kept locked and away from children. Persons engaging in sports, games, and recreational activities should wear all proper protective equipment and follow safety rules.

Resources

PERIODICALS

Jull, Andrew. "Decision-Support For Moist Wound Dressings." *New Zealand Nursing Review* (December 2000).

ORGANIZATIONS

American Red Cross. P.O. Box 37243, Washington, D.C. 20013. <http://www.redcross.org>.

OTHER

"Principles of Wound Management." *Critical Care - London Health Sciences Centre*. 2000. <http://critcare.lhsc.on.ca/icu/cctc/procprot/nursing/procedures/wound_mgmt.html> (March 29, 2001).

David Helwig

Writing therapy *see* **Journal therapy**

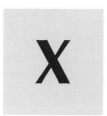

X-ray unit

Definition

An x-ray unit is the equipment used to produce x rays. Because of the risk of over-exposure to x rays, the x-ray unit includes both the machine used for collecting x rays and the protective room within which the x rays are taken and developed.

Purpose

Film radiographs, or x rays, are the most widely used means of medical imaging. Radiographs are used to examine bones for **fractures**, growth abnormalities, and joint dysfunctions. X rays are also used to find abnormal growths in the breasts (**mammography**), other organs and soft tissues; problems in the gastro-intestinal tract; circulatory problems such as clogged arteries and **blood** clots; and a variety of other ail-ments. Additionally, radiation therapy to treat **cancer** is generally performed with x rays.

Description

The production of an x-ray image (radiograph) involves three distinct steps: the generation of an x-ray beam, the interaction of that beam with the structures of the patient to be imaged, and the development of the image.

Generation of an x-ray beam

Visible light is electromagnetic energy that has characteristics that allow it to be seen by humans. There are many other familiar forms of electromag-netic energy that are not visible to humans. These include radio waves, which permit the transmission of radio signals and the operation of cellular phones; microwaves, which are often used to heat food; and x rays. Each of these forms of light has a characteristic size (wavelength) and speed (frequency) range that defines it. An x-ray beam is an invisible form of light that has a wavelength that is much smaller than visible light and a frequency that is much faster than visible light.

Because an x-ray beam is a beam of light, just like visible light, it is generated in a type of light bulb that resembles a camera flash bulb. A flash bulb is used to increase the amount of visible light available for a photograph during the brief time that the camera is actually taking the picture (creating the visual image). An x-ray bulb is used to provide x-ray light during the brief time while the radiograph is being imaged.

The major differences between an x-ray light bulb and a visible flash bulb are the amount of energy required to produce the light and the energy charac-teristics (wavelength and frequency) of the light pro-duced. Also, a flash bulb is not "tunable": a visible light bulb produces light anywhere within the visible light range. An x-ray bulb is "tunable" in that only x rays with the exact wavelength and frequency char-acteristics desired for the production of the radiograph are allowed to contact the patient. An x-ray bulb uses a filter system to produce light only in a specified x-ray range determined either by the filter system being used, or, in more advanced settings, by the x-ray unit operator through a variable control system.

Interaction of the x-ray beam with the patient

When visible light from a flash bulb strikes the skin of a human arm, that light is reflected back to the lens of the camera to which the flash bulb is attached, producing an image of a human arm on the film within the camera. The camera lens and film are designed to be able to image visible light. They generally cannot create an image from light outside the visible range.

Because x rays travel much faster than visible light, and because they have a much smaller wave-length, they have more "penetrating power" than

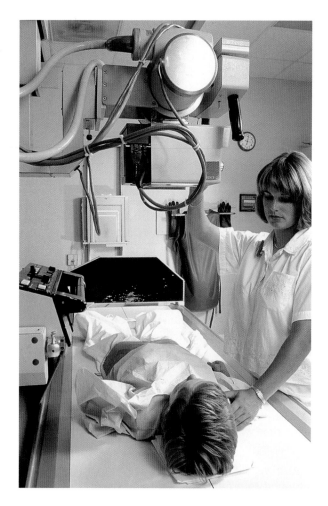

A young boy lying flat on his back is prepared for an x-ray procedure. The radiographer positions the x-ray emitter over the part of the patient's body to be scanned. An x-ray plate with film is fitted beneath the bed to capture the image. Body tissues absorb x rays differently depending on their density. Bones, which are dense, absorb x rays well and appear white on a film; soft tissues do not absorb x rays well and appear dark. *(Bill Bachmann / Photo Researchers, Inc. Reproduced by permission.)*

can often be defined by the particular type of x ray used. For instance, x-ray imaging of the breast (mammography) does not rely on a very large discrepancy in densities between the tissues being imaged and the tissues being ignored. The breast is largely composed of fat tissue and vessels of the circulatory and lymphatic systems, which are relatively dense when compared to skin and other non-fatty tissues. It is possible to tune an x ray to image the fatty tissues, **blood vessels** and lymphatic vessels of the breast in preference to the non-fatty tissues of the breast. Also, because abnormal growths (tumors) in the breast are denser than the typical breast tissue, radiographic mammography is an excellent diagnostic tool for the discovery of such breast abnormalities.

Often it is desirable to selectively image certain structures that are not sufficiently more dense than their surrounding tissue. This may often be accomplished through the use of a tracer, or dye, material that is dense that is administered to the type of tissue that is to be imaged. Examples of this type of x-raying include the use of barium to coat the lower gastrointestinal tract (**barium enema**) and the use of iodine compounds to coat the linings of blood vessels (angiograms). The introduction of barium or iodine tracers makes the gastrointestinal tract or the blood vessels appear to be more dense than the surrounding tissues.

Development of the x-ray image

Only about 1% of the x rays that strike a patient's body emerge from the body to produce the final image. The radiographic image is formed on a radiographic plate that is similar to the film of a camera. The other 99% of the x rays are either absorbed by the body or scattered by the tissues of the body.

Those x rays that are scattered (reflected) by the tissues of the body are generally scattered in a random pattern. If these x rays reach the radiographic plate, they tend to obscure the radiographic image. Therefore, an anti-scatter grid, which is similar to a set of partially closed window blinds, is used to prevent these scattered x rays from reaching the plate. X rays that have passed through the body without being scattered will reach this grid traveling perpendicular to the grid. X rays that have been scattered will reach this grid traveling, for the most part, in directions other than perpendicular. Any x rays that are traveling perpendicular to the grid will pass through and strike the radiographic plate, helping to create the final radiographic image. Those x rays that are not traveling perpendicular to the grid will strike the grid and be absorbed, such that they do not contribute to the final radiographic image.

visible light. This means that when x rays strike the same human arm, they are not stopped (reflected) by the skin and soft tissues, which are composed primarily of liquids. Instead, these x rays continue to travel through the skin and soft tissues until they meet a relatively dense material, such as bone. It is the "penetrating power" of light in the x-ray range that allows an x-ray image to "see inside" the human body.

An x-ray beam passes through sparse materials and only interacts with (becomes reflected by) dense materials. For this reason, x rays are most often thought of as being useful for the observance of dense tissues, such as bone. But, because an x-ray bulb is tunable, what is "sparse" and what is "dense"

After passing through the anti-scatter grid, x rays strike a radiographic plate that works almost identically to a photographic plate, or film in a camera. In recent years, modifications in the development process of radiographic plates have been achieved that allow the necessary clarity of the radiograph with much lower x-ray exposures to the patient.

Those x rays that are absorbed by the body do not reach the radiographic plate. Therefore, they present no difficulty in the production of a clear radiographic image. However, these absorbed x rays have been shown to be a cause of cancer in those individuals who are over-exposed to them, either over time or during periods of intense radiation.

Components of the x-ray unit

To prevent exposure to the operator and to prevent the unnecessary leakage of x-ray radiation to the rest of the facility where x rays are performed, the x-ray unit is generally enclosed in a room that has walls made of, or reinforced with, a dense material (usually lead) that will absorb any x rays that are scattered during the x-ray process.

Additionally, the operator of an x-ray unit generally turns the x-ray equipment on and off from behind a protective wall that is lined with lead. Lead is extremely dense to x rays and even a one-quarter inch thickness of lead will prevent all x rays emitted from current x-ray machines from being able to pass.

A lead-impregnated smock or apron is also provided to patients while they are being x-rayed to prevent unwanted exposure of their bodies to x rays.

Operation

Modern x-ray equipment is automated. An x-ray technician, or other licensed radiographer, properly positions the patient between the x-ray source and the radiographic plate. Then the technician goes into a separate room and pushes a button to turn on the x-ray beam. The reason for leaving the room while x rays are being taken is to prevent harmful effects in the technician that could occur after repeated x-ray exposure. The length of time that the x-ray beam remains on and the intensity level of the beam are based on the part of the body being imaged. In the newest equipment, these times and intensities are controlled by a computer, but may be manually adjusted, within certain safety limits, by the x-ray technician. After exposure, the technician removes the radiographic plate and places it in a fully automated development chamber where the final image is produced.

The skill and training of the technician comes in the proper positioning of the patient and in the examination of the resulting image. The image is ultimately examined for clinical findings by a radiologist and/or by the physician who ordered the x rays. It is the job of the x-ray technician to exam the radiograph to ensure that a clinically useful image has been produced. When an unsuitable image is produced, the x-ray technician will have to retake the x ray. Unsuitable images may be produced when the patient failed to remain still during the x ray exposure, the positioning of the patient was incorrect, there was an alignment or other problem with either the radiographic plate or the x-ray beam, or the exposure time and/or intensity was incorrect for the part of the body being imaged.

Maintenance

X-ray units are large and expensive pieces of equipment. They are generally covered by maintenance contracts provided by their manufacturers. Medical personnel should not attempt to maintain this equipment. Maintenance contracts generally call for routine maintenance every four months to inspect the equipment, replace any aging or wearing parts, check for radiation leakage, and ensure proper operation.

Health care team roles

X rays are generally ordered by primary care, emergency, or other specialized physicians. Most x rays are taken by registered x-ray technologists under the supervision of radiologists. A radiologist is a physician who has completed a minimum of a four-year residency program in radiology after medical school. A registered x-ray technologist is a person who has received a one year certificate, a two year associate degree, or a four year bachelor degree from a training program that is accredited by the Joint Review Committee on Education in **Radiologic Technology** and, if required, has received a license from the state in which he or she practices, to perform radiologic measurements or therapies on the general public.

Training

All people who take x rays of patients or perform radiation therapies in the United States are required to be licensed and/or registered under the Consumer-Patient Radiation Health and Safety Act of 1981. This act was designed to protect the general public from unnecessary exposure to medical and dental radiation by ensuring that operators of radiologic equipment are properly trained in the use of such equipment.

Education and training programs in x-ray technology are offered by hospitals, colleges and universities, the armed forces, and vocational-technical institutes. Formal training is offered in radiography, radiation therapy, mammographic imaging, and diagnostic medical imaging (e.g. ultrasound, CT, and MRI). Programs range in length from 1 to 4 years and lead to a certificate, an associate degree, or a bachelor degree. Associate degrees that require 2 years of training are the most common. One year certificate programs are generally pursued by individuals already trained in another health occupation, such as medical or dental technology, or registered nursing, who want to change fields or expand their skill set within the setting in which they are presently employed; or, by experienced radiographers who want to specialize in radiation therapy or medical imaging.

All x-ray technology programs offer classroom and clinical instruction in anatomy and physiology, **medical terminology**, **medical ethics**, patient care procedures, positioning of patients for appropriate radiologic imaging, radiation physics, radiation protection (of both the patient and the x-ray technician), and radiobiology. In order to retain his or her licensure or registration as an x-ray technician or radiation therapist, a person licensed or registered as such must complete and provide documentation to the licensing or registration board of his or her state of 24 hours of continuing education every two years.

With additional training, available at most major cancer centers, radiation therapy technicians can specialize as medical radiation dosimetrists. A medical radiation dosimetrist works with oncologists (physicians specializing in cancer causes and treatments) and health physicists to develop effective treatment plans for patients who require radiation therapy in the treatment of cancerous tumors.

X-ray technologists who are also able to perform medical imaging are projected to have the best job opportunities, at least through 2006. This is because many hospitals, the main employers of x-ray technologists, are attempting to cut costs by merging their radiologic and nuclear medical imaging (MRI) facilities. The need for independent diagnostic imaging centers that specialize in providing radiographic and other medical imaging techniques to medical clinics and private physician practices is also expected to grow extremely rapidly. Advances in technology that lead to lower cost equipment permit more and more

---

KEY TERMS

Anti-scatter grid—A grid that is placed between the patient and the radiographic plate to prevent x rays that have been reflected from reaching the plate. Without the use of this grid, the resulting x-ray image (radiograph) would be unreadable, or would appear severely "out-of-focus."

Radiograph—An image formed on a radiographic plate (similar to the film in a camera) by x rays. This is the final image produced by an x-ray unit.

Tracer—A chemical that is relatively dense to x rays that is added to the body to make that part of the body imagable with x rays. Examples include barium, used to image the gastrointestinal tract, and iodine, used to image blood vessels. Without the use of a tracer, these structures would be difficult, or impossible, to differentiate from surrounding tissues.

X ray—An invisible form of light that has a wavelength that is much smaller than visible light and a frequency that is much faster than visible light. Because of these properties of x rays, they can be used to image dense structures within the human body.

---

radiographic and medical imaging procedures to be performed outside a hospital environment.

Resources

BOOKS

Wolbarst, Anthony. *Looking Within: How X-ray, CT, MRI, Ultrasound, and Other Medical Images Are Created.* Berkeley: University of California Press, 1999.

ORGANIZATIONS

American Healthcare Radiology Administrators (AHRA). 111 Boston Post Road, Suite 105, Sudbury, MA 01776. 1-800-334-2472 or 978-443-7591. <http://www.ahraonline.org/contact.htm>.

American Society of Radiologic Technologists (ASRT). 15000 Central Avenue, SE, Albuquerque, NM 87213-3917. 505-298-4500. <http://www.asrt.org>.

Radiological Society of North America, Inc. 820 Jorie Boulevard, Oak Brook, IL 60523-2251. 630-571-2670. <http://www.rsna.org/index.html>.

Paul A. Johnson

X-ray technology *see* **Radiologic technology**
X rays of the eye's orbit *see* **X rays of the orbit**

X rays of the orbit

Definition

Orbital x rays are a radiographic study of the area and structures containing the eyes. The orbits are bony cone-shaped cavities that contain and protect the eyes. Each orbit is lined with fatty tissue to cushion the eyeballs. The orbits are thin and easily subjected to **fractures**, particularly blow-out fractures of the orbital floor.

Purpose

Orbital x ray, or orbital radiography, is used to detect problems resulting from injury or trauma to the eye. Seventy percent of all facial fractures involve the orbits in some way. An x ray of the orbits may also be ordered for patients complaining of **pain**, **vision** trouble, or excessive tearing of the eyes. An ophthalmologist may also order orbital x rays when a foreign body cannot be detected with an ophthalmoscope.

Orbital x ray is also used as a screening tool before an MRI is performed, since intraorbital metallic **foreign bodies** are a contraindication for MRI (the magnetic field in the MRI could move the metallic object causing eye injury). Patients scheduled for MRIs are screened for the possible presence of metallic foreign bodies by a questionnaire or interview with the MRI technologist. If there is a suspicion that a metallic foreign body may be present, the patient will have x rays taken of the orbit to ensure that no foreign body is present.

Precautions

Pregnant women and women who could possibly be pregnant should only receive orbital x rays when absolutely necessary. The x-ray technologist will use protective shielding on all women of child-bearing age as well as on children.

Description

Each orbit is formed by the frontal, ethmoid, and sphenoid bones of the **skull** and the lacrimal, palantine, maxillary, and zygomatic bones of the face. Each orbit consists of a medial and lateral wall as well as a roof and floor, therefore a series of views is necessary to see all of the structures well. Both orbits are always imaged so that a comparison can be made of the two sides. A typical routine for the orbits consists of a Water's view, Caldwell and lateral of the affected side. In some cases a basal view may be requested if the patient is able to extend the head backwards.

Projections of the optic canals or Rhese views will be included in some cases.

X rays of the orbits may be done with the patient sitting or lying down. The patient is placed prone (lying horizontally face down) with no rotation of the head. The tube is angled 15° caudad (towards the feet) for the Caldwell position, where the petrous ridges will be in the lower third of the orbits. In the Water's position (occipito-mental) the chin is extended forward at least 37°, centering on the acanthion (the small indentation in the center of the upper lip). This is the best view to see the orbits completely clear of any other structures. The maxillary sinuses are well visualized with the Water's view, so any fluid levels are easily detected. In the lateral position the patient's head is turned onto the affected side if possible, with the interpupillary line perpendicular to the table.

When x rays for a foreign body are requested, a Water's view is done with the patient looking straight ahead. Sometimes two views in the lateral position are done—one with the patient looking up and one with the patient looking down. A soft tissue technique should be used when looking for a foreign body. An ultrasound exam of the eye also will detect any foreign body in the eye.

X rays of the orbits should normally be completed in 15 minutes if the patient is cooperative. The patient must wait until the x rays are developed to ensure that all required structures are well demonstrated with no rotation or movement.

Preparation

There are no special dietary preparations needed prior to an orbital x ray. As with any radiography procedure, the patient should remove dentures, jewelry, or metal objects, which may interfere with obtaining a detailed image.

Aftercare

No aftercare is required following this diagnostic test.

Complications

Radiation exposure is low for this procedure and all certified radiology facilities follow strict personnel and equipment guidelines for radiation protection. Women of child-bearing age and children will be given a protective shielding (lead apron) to cover the genital and/or abdominal areas. Patients who are unable to lie prone can be tested in a supine position (lying horizontally on the back). The lateral view can be done by turning the x-ray tube 90° and placing the film against the affected side. Severe trauma patients will have a CT scan done instead of orbital or facial x rays.

Results

Normal findings show the bones of the orbits are intact, with no fractures, tumors, or cysts that could erode the surrounding bone.

Positive findings from an orbital x ray may show that there has been some injury to the eye. Radiologists look for asymmetry in the facial bones, periorbital or intracranial air as well as fluid in the paranasal sinuses. Tiny fractures in the orbital bones can usually be detected on the radiograph. In a blow-out fracture (one involving the orbital floor), radiographic findings may include overlapping of bone fragments on the orbital floor and opacification of the sinuses (due to hemorrhage).

Indications of differences in size and shape of the various structures in the orbit may be apparent. The orbit may be enlarged, indicating irritation from an injury or foreign body. A number of growing tumors within the eye or **brain** area may also cause orbital enlargement. Destruction of the walls of the orbit may indicate a nearby **infection** or malignancy. Changes in density may also be a sign of bone disease or a **cancer** that has spread to the bone.

Children's orbits are more likely to be enlarged by a fast growing lesion, since their orbital bones have not fully developed, but are less likely to have facial fractures due to the resiliency of their facial skeleton.

Health care team roles

The x-ray technologist works as part of the treatment team to make sure that the patients are radiographed and then returned to the emergency department as soon as possible. If portable (mobile radiography) orbital x rays are ordered the radiography technologist must make sure that all staff members remaining in the room wear proper shielding (lead aprons).

Patient education

Patients are instructed to remain still during the x rays and to allow the x-ray technologist to position the head. Certain positions may be uncomfortable but are necessary to visualize all areas of the orbits. All radiologic technologists must be certified and registered with the American Society of Radiologic Technologists.

KEY TERMS

Blowout fracture—A fracture or break in the orbit that is caused by a sudden and violent impact to the area.

Malignancy—A tumor that is cancerous and growing.

Medial wall—The mid-line bone, or wall, of the eye's orbit. It is generally thicker than the roof and floor walls.

Ophthalmologist—A physician who specializes in the workings, structures, and care of the eyes.

Ophthalmoscope—An instrument routinely used by ophthalmologists to examine the interior of the eye. It consists of a small light, a mirror, and lenses of differing powers that magnify.

Periorbital—The area surrounding the eye.

Radiography—Examination of any part of the body through the use of x rays. The process produces an image of shadows and contrasts on film.

Water's view—A radiographic view of the facial bones invented by Dr. S. Water to see all of the facial bones clearly. The patient is prone with the head straight and the chin extended forward 37°.

X ray—A form of electromagnetic radiation with shorter wavelengths than visible light.

Resources

BOOKS

Ballinger, Frank, et al. *Merrill's Atlas of Radiographic Positioning.* 9th ed. St. Louis, MO: Mosby Yearbook, 1999.

Schull, Patricia, ed. *Illustrated Guide to Diagnostic Tests.* 2nd ed. Springhouse PA: Springhouse Corporation, 1998.

ORGANIZATIONS

American Academy of Ophthalmology. P.O. Box 7424, San Francisco, CA 94120-7424. (415) 561-8500.

National Eye Institute. Building 31, Room 6A32, Bethesda, MD 20892. (301) 496-5248. <http://www.nei.nih.gov>.

Radiological Society of North America. 2021 Spring Rd., Suite 600, Oak Brook, IL 60521-1860. (708) 571-2670. <http://www.rsna.org>.

OTHER

Eye Institute. University of Pennsylvania Health System. <http://www.med.upenn.edu/ophth/patinfo>.

Lorraine K. Ehresman

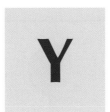

Yeast culture *see* **Fungal culture**

Yoga

Definition

The term *yoga* comes from a Sanskrit word which means yoke or union. Traditionally, yoga is a method joining the individual self with the Divine, Universal Spirit, or Cosmic Consciousness. Physical and mental exercises are designed to help achieve this goal, also called self-transcendence or enlightenment. On the physical level, yoga postures, called *asanas*, are designed to tone, strengthen, and align the body. These postures are performed to make the spine supple and healthy and to promote **blood** flow to all the organs, glands, and tissues, keeping all the bodily systems healthy. On the mental level, yoga uses breathing techniques (*pranayama*) and **meditation** (*dyana*) to quiet, clarify, and discipline the mind. However, experts are quick to point out that yoga is not a religion, but a way of living with health and peace of mind as its aims.

Origins

Yoga originated in ancient India and is one of the longest surviving philosophical systems in the world. Some scholars have estimated that yoga is as old as 5,000 years; artifacts detailing yoga postures have been found in India from over 3000 B.C. Yoga masters (*yogis*) claim that it is a highly developed science of healthy living that has been tested and perfected for all these years. Yoga was first brought to America in the late 1800s when Swami Vivekananda, an Indian teacher and yogi, presented a lecture on meditation in Chicago. Yoga slowly began gaining followers, and flourished during the 1960s when there was a surge of interest in Eastern philosophy. There has since been a vast exchange of yoga knowledge in America, with many students going to India to study and many Indian experts coming here to teach, resulting in the establishment of a wide variety of schools. Today, yoga is thriving, and it has become easy to find teachers and practitioners throughout America. A recent Roper poll, commissioned by *Yoga Journal*, found that 11 million Americans do yoga at least occasionally and 6 million perform it regularly. Yoga stretches are used by physical therapists and professional sports teams, and the benefits of yoga are being touted by movie stars and Fortune 500 executives. Many prestigious schools of medicine have studied and introduced yoga techniques as proven therapies for illness and **stress**. Some medical schools, like UCLA, even offer yoga classes as part of their physician training program.

Benefits

Yoga has been used to alleviate problems associated with high **blood pressure**, high cholesterol, migraine headaches, **asthma**, shallow breathing, backaches, constipation, diabetes, **menopause**, **multiple sclerosis**, **varicose veins**, **carpal tunnel syndrome** and many chronic illnesses. It also has been studied and approved for its ability to promote **relaxation** and reduce stress.

Yoga can also provide the same benefits as any well-designed **exercise** program, increasing general health and stamina, reducing stress, and improving those conditions brought about by sedentary lifestyles. Yoga has the added advantage of being a low-impact activity that uses only gravity as resistance, which makes it an excellent **physical therapy** routine; certain yoga postures can be safely used to strengthen and balance all parts of the body.

Meditation has been much studied and approved for its benefits in reducing stress-related conditions. The landmark book, *The Relaxation Response*, by Harvard cardiologist Herbert Benson, showed that meditation and breathing techniques for relaxation

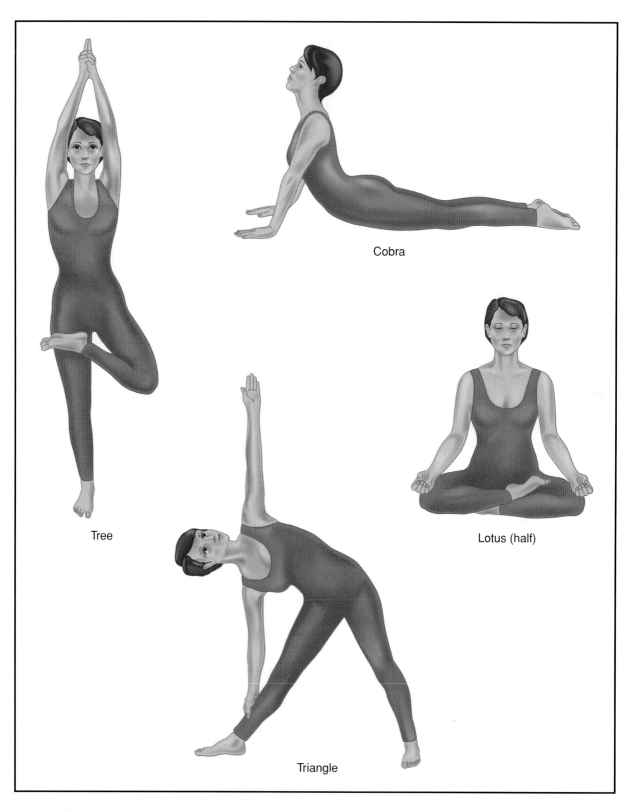

Tree

Cobra

Triangle

Lotus (half)

Demonstrations of the tree, triangle, cobra, and lotus poses. The tree and triangle are good for balance and coordination. Cobra stretches the pelvis and strengthens the back. Lotus is a meditative pose. *(Illustration by Electronic Illustrators Group. The Gale Group.)*

could have the opposite effect of stress, reducing blood pressure and other indicators. Since then, much research has reiterated the benefits of meditation for stress reduction and general health. Currently, the American Medical Association recommends meditation techniques as a first step before medication for borderline **hypertension** cases.

Modern psychological studies have shown that even slight facial expressions can cause changes in the involuntary nervous system; yoga utilizes the mind/body connection. That is, yoga practice contains the central ideas that physical posture and alignment can influence a person's mood and self-esteem, and also that the mind can be used to shape and heal the body. Yoga practitioners claim that the strengthening of mind/body awareness can bring eventual improvements in all facets of a person's life.

Description

Classical yoga is separated into eight limbs, each a part of the complete system for mental, physical and spiritual well-being. Four of the limbs deal with mental and physical exercises designed to bring the mind in tune with the body. The other four deal with different stages of meditation. There are six major types of yoga, all with the same goals of health and harmony but with varying techniques: hatha, raja, karma, bhakti, jnana, and tantra yoga. Hatha yoga is the most commonly practiced branch of yoga in America, and it is a highly developed system of nearly 200 physical postures, movements and breathing techniques designed to tune the body to its optimal health. The yoga philosophy believes the breath to be the most important facet of health, as the breath is the largest source of *prana*, or life force, and hatha yoga utilizes *pranayama*, which literally means the science or control of breathing. Hatha yoga was originally developed as a system to make the body strong and healthy enough to enable mental awareness and spiritual enlightenment.

There are several different schools of hatha yoga in America; the two most prevalent ones are Iyengar and ashtanga yoga. Iyengar yoga was founded by B.K.S. Iyengar, who is widely considered as one of the great living innovators of yoga. Iyengar yoga puts strict emphasis on form and alignment, and uses traditional hatha yoga techniques in new manners and sequences. Iyengar yoga can be good for physical therapy because it allows the use of props like straps and blocks to make it easier for some people to get into the yoga postures. Ashtanga yoga can be a more vigorous routine, using a flowing and dance-like sequence

of hatha postures to generate body heat, which purifies the body through sweating and deep breathing.

The other types of yoga show some of the remaining ideas which permeate yoga. Raja yoga strives to bring about mental clarity and discipline through meditation, simplicity, and non-attachment to worldly things and desires. Karma yoga emphasizes charity, service to others, non-aggression and non-harming as means to awareness and peace. Bhakti yoga is the path of devotion and love of God, or Universal Spirit. Jnana yoga is the practice and development of knowledge and wisdom. Finally, tantra yoga is the path of self-awareness through religious rituals, including awareness of sexuality as sacred and vital.

A typical hatha yoga routine consists of a sequence of physical poses, or asanas, and the sequence is designed to work all parts of the body, with particular emphasis on making the spine supple and healthy and increasing circulation. Hatha yoga asanas utilize three basic movements: forward bends, backward bends, and twisting motions. Each asana is named for a common thing it resembles, like the sun salutation, cobra, locust, plough, bow, eagle, tree, and the head to knee pose, to name a few. Each pose has steps for entering and exiting it, and each posture requires proper form and alignment. A pose is held for some time, depending on its level of difficulty and one's strength and stamina, and the practitioner is also usually aware of when to inhale and exhale at certain points in each posture, as breathing properly is another fundamental aspect of yoga. Breathing should be deep and through the nose. Mental concentration in each position is also very important, which improves awareness, poise and posture. During a yoga routine there is often a position in which to perform meditation, if deep relaxation is one of the goals of the sequence.

Yoga routines can take anywhere from 20 minutes to two or more hours, with one hour being a good time investment to perform a sequence of postures and a meditation. Some yoga routines, depending on the teacher and school, can be as strenuous as the most difficult workout, and some routines merely stretch and align the body while the breath and **heart** rate are kept slow and steady. Yoga achieves its best results when it is practiced as a daily discipline, and yoga can be a life-long exercise routine, offering deeper and more challenging positions as a practitioner becomes more adept. The basic positions can increase a person's strength, flexibility and sense of well-being almost immediately, but it can take years to perfect and deepen them, which is an appealing and stimulating aspect of yoga for many.

Yoga is usually best learned from a yoga teacher or physical therapist, but yoga is simple enough that one can learn the basics from good books on the subject, which are plentiful. Yoga classes are generally inexpensive, averaging around 10 dollars per class, and students can learn basic postures in just a few classes. Many YMCAs, colleges, and community health organizations offer beginning yoga classes as well, often for nominal fees. If yoga is part of a physical therapy program, it can be reimbursed by insurance.

Preparations

Yoga can be performed by those of any age and condition, although not all poses should be attempted by everyone. Yoga is also a very accessible form of exercise; all that is needed is a flat floor surface large enough to stretch out on, a mat or towel, and enough overhead space to fully raise the arms. It is a good activity for those who can't go to gyms, who don't like other forms of exercise, or have very busy schedules. Yoga should be done on an empty **stomach**, and teachers recommend waiting three or more hours after meals. Loose and comfortable clothing should be worn.

Precautions

People with injuries, medical conditions, or spinal problems should consult a doctor before beginning yoga. Those with medical conditions should find a yoga teacher who is familiar with their type of problem and who is willing to give them individual attention. Pregnant women can benefit from yoga, but should always be guided by an experienced teacher. Certain yoga positions should not be performed with a **fever**, or during menstruation.

Beginners should exercise care and concentration when performing yoga postures, and not try to stretch too much too quickly, as injury could result. Some advanced yoga postures, like the headstand and full lotus position, can be difficult and require strength, flexibility, and gradual preparation, so beginners should get the help of a teacher before attempting them.

Yoga is not a competive sport; it does not matter how a person does in comparison with others, but how aware and disciplined one becomes with one's own body and limitations. Proper form and alignment should always be maintained during a stretch or posture, and the stretch or posture should be stopped when there is **pain**, dizziness, or fatigue. The mental component of yoga is just as important as the physical postures. Concentration and awareness of breath

KEY TERMS

Asana—A position or stance in yoga.

Dyana—The yoga term for meditation.

Hatha yoga—Form of yoga using postures, breathing methods and meditation.

Meditation—Technique of concentration for relaxing the mind and body.

Pranayama—Yoga breathing techniques.

Yogi—A trained yoga expert.

should not be neglected. Yoga should be done with an open, gentle, and non-critical mind; when one stretches into a yoga position, it can be thought of accepting and working on one's limits. Impatience, self-criticism and comparing oneself to others will not help in this process of self-knowledge. While performing the yoga of breathing (pranayama) and meditation (dyana), it is best to have an experienced teacher, as these powerful techniques can cause dizziness and discomfort when done improperly.

Side effects

Some people have reported injuries by performing yoga postures without proper form or concentration, or by attempting difficult positions without working up to them gradually or having appropriate supervision. Beginners sometimes report muscle soreness and fatigue after performing yoga, but these side effects diminish with practice.

Research and general acceptance

Although yoga originated in a culture very different from modern America, it has been accepted and its practice has spread relatively quickly. Many yogis are amazed at how rapidly yoga's popularity has spread in America, considering the legend that it was passed down secretly by handfuls of adherents for many centuries.

There can still be found some resistance to yoga, for active and busy Americans sometimes find it hard to believe that an exercise program that requires them to slow down, concentrate, and breathe deeply can be more effective than lifting weights or running. However, on-going research in top medical schools is showing yoga's effectiveness for overall health and for specific problems, making it an increasingly acceptable health practice.

Training and certification

Many different schools of yoga have developed in America, and beginners should experiment with them to find the best-suited routine. Hatha yoga schools emphasize classical yoga postures, and raja yoga schools concentrate on mental discipline and meditation techniques. In America, there are no generally accepted standards for the certification of yoga teachers. Some schools certify teachers in a few intensive days and some require years of study before certifying teachers. Beginners should search for teachers who show respect and are careful in their teaching, and should beware of instructors who push them into poses before they are ready.

Resources

BOOKS

Ansari, Mark, and Lark, Liz. *Yoga for Beginners*. New York: Harper, 1999.

Bodian, Stephan, and Feuerstein, Georg. *Living Yoga*. New York: Putnam, 1993.

Carrico, Mara. *Yoga Journal's Yoga Basics*. New York: Henry Holt, 1997.

Iyengar, B.K.S. *Light on Yoga*. New York: Schocken, 1975.

PERIODICALS

Yoga International Magazine. R.R. 1 Box 407, Honesdale, PA 18431. <http://www.yimag.com>.

Yoga Journal. P.O. Box 469088, Escondido, CA 92046. <http://www.yogajournal.com>.

ORGANIZATIONS

International Association of Yoga Therapists (IAYT). 4150 Tivoli Ave., Los Angeles, CA 90066.

OTHER

Yoga Directory. <http://www.yogadirectory.com>.

Yoga Finder Online. <http://www.yogafinder.com.>.

Douglas Dupler

Z

Z-track injection

Definition

Z-track injection is a method of injecting medication into a large muscle using a needle and syringe. This method seals the medication deeply within the muscle and allows no exit path back into the subcutaneous tissue and skin. This is accomplished by displacing the skin and subcutaneous tissue 1–1.5 inches (2.5–3.75 cm), laterally, prior to injection and releasing the tissue immediately after the injection.

Purpose

The Z-track method of intra-muscular (I.M.) injection is used primarily when giving dark-colored medication solutions, such as **iron** solutions, that can stain the subcutaneous tissue or skin. It is also the method of choice when giving I.M. medications that are very irritating to the tissue, such as haloperidol or vistaril.

Precautions

Precautions taken when giving Z-track injections are all aimed at preventing the medication from leaking into the subcutaneous tissue or skin. These precautions include:

- Do not give a Z-track injection into skin that is lumpy, reddened, irritated, bruised, stained, or hardened.

- Add 0.3–0.5 ml of air into the syringe after drawing up the correct dosage of medication.

- Change the needle after drawing the medication into the syringe.

- Select a long needle (2–3 inches; 5–7.5 cm), depending upon the size of the patient, with a 21- or 22-gauge needle to place the medication deeply within the muscle.

- Give Z-track injections into a large muscle in the buttock (the gluteus medius or gluteus minimus).

- Aspirate on the syringe before injecting the medication to be sure not to hit a **blood** vessel. If blood appears in the syringe, a vein may have been hit. Remove and discard the syringe and medication. Start over with a new syringe, fresh medication, and a new site.

- Caution the patient not to wear restrictive clothing that could put constant pressure on the injection site.

- Rotate the injection sites from one buttock to the other and from site to site.

- Do not place injections into a disabled limb. If there is decreased circulation, the medication absorption will be affected and **abscess** formation can occur.

- Never inject more than 5ml of medication at a time when using the Z-track method. If a larger dose is ordered, divide it and inject it into two separate sites.

Description

To give a Z-track injection, use the non-dominant hand to move and hold the skin and subcutaneous tissue about 1–1 1/2 inches (2.5–3.75 cm) laterally from the injection site. Alert patients when the medication is about to be injected. Ask them to breathe through their mouth and to try to relax the muscle to avoid muscle resistance. Continue holding the displaced skin and tissue until after the needle is removed. Dart the syringe rapidly into the site at a 90° angle. Aspirate on the syringe to be sure that a blood vessel has not been penetrated. Inject the medication slowly into the muscle. Be sure that the syringe is completely empty, including the air, before withdrawing the syringe. Withdraw the syringe and immediately release the skin and subcutaneous tissue.

Preparation

Wash both hands and put on gloves. Check the medication label before giving the medicine to avoid medication errors. Be sure it is the right medicine, the right dose (strength), the right time, the right person, and the right method. Note the expiration date on the label. Do not use outdated medicine. Draw the correct dosage into the syringe including 0.3–0.5 ml of air. Discard the uncapped needle in a needle-box and attach a new sterile needle. Provide privacy and position the patient on the side with the knee slightly bent to relax the buttock muscles. Expose the buttock only, using the patient's clothing or a drape. Use the landmarks defined in the I.M. injection section to identify the desired injection site along the gluteus medius or gluteus minimus muscle. Prepare the site with an alcohol swab by rubbing the swab firmly in a 3-inch (7.5 cm) circle from the center of the site outward to remove **bacteria** from the skin. Allow the skin to air dry.

Aftercare

Apply gentle pressure to the site, using a dry gauze pad, if necessary. Do not rub the site. Continue pressure if bleeding occurs, and apply a bandage, if necessary. Replace the patient's clothing and allow the patient a 5-minute rest period. Then encourage the patient to walk about to enhance absorption of the medication. Discard the used syringe and uncapped needle in a needle-box. Place gloves and used swabs in a plastic trash bag that can be sealed and discarded. Wash both hands when the procedure is complete.

Complications

The complications of a Z-track injection are not common, but include tissue staining, bruising, abscess formation at the injection site, and severe **pain** at the injection site. Notify the physician if any of these conditions are noted.

Results

Medication administered by Z-track injection is absorbed rapidly from the muscle into the bloodstream. The effects are seen over hours to days, depending upon the medication given.

Health care team roles

Medication given intramuscularly, using the Z-track method, is done by an R.N., L.P.N., or a

---

> **KEY TERMS**
>
> **Gluteus medius**—One of the large muscles of the buttock, located above the gluteus maximus that allows the thigh to abduct, rotate, and extend.
>
> **Gluteus minimus**—One of the large muscles of the buttock, located above the gluteus maximus that allows the thigh to abduct, rotate, and extend.
>
> **Laterally**—Toward the side.
>
> **Subcutaneous tissue**—The tissue found immediately below the skin.

physician in the health care setting. Rarely, a physician will ask the nurse to teach a family member or caretaker this injection technique so that Z-track injections can be given correctly in the home. If family members are giving medication in this manner, set up regular follow-up visits with the physician or a **home care** nurse to examine and assess the injection sites.

Resources

BOOKS

"Giving a Z-track Injection". In *Nurse's Clinical Guide* Springhouse: PA: Springhouse Corporation, 2000.

OTHER

"Administering a Z-track I.M. Injection." *Nursing Online*, January 1999. <http://www.findarticles.com/m3231/1_29/53611660/p1/article.jhtml>.

"Giving Injections." *Nurse Minerva Online*, January 2001. <http://www.nurseminerva.co.uk/giving.htm>.

"Haloperidol. Updates." *F.A. Davis Co. Online*, 2000. <http://www.fadavis.com/updates/0483-monographs/haloperidol.htm>.

"Jectofer." *Rx Medical Online*, 1996. <http://www.rxmed.com/monographs/jectofer.html>.

"Locating Sites for Intramuscular Injections. Nursing Interventions and Clinical Skills." *Mosbys Online*, 2000. <http://www.harcourthealth.com/MERLIN/Elkin/Skills/18-05t.html>.

"The Wonderful World of Giving Injections." *Southeastern Nurse Online*, 2001. <http://www.angelfire.com/ns/southeasternnurse/TheWonderfulWorldofGivingInjections3.htm>.

Mary Elizabeth Martelli, R.N., B.S.

ZIFT *see* **Fertility treatments**

Zinc

Description

Zinc is a mineral that is essential for a healthy **immune system**, production of certain hormones, wound healing, bone formation, and clear skin. It is required in very small amounts, and is thus known as a trace mineral. Despite the low requirement, zinc is found in nearly every cell of the body and is a key to the proper function of over 300 enzymes, including superoxide dismutase. Normal growth and development cannot occur without it.

General use

The U.S. Recommended Dietary Allowance (RDA) for zinc is 5 milligrams (mg) for children under one year of age, 10 mg for children aged one to 10 years old, 15 mg for males 11 years or older, 12 mg for females 11 years or older, 15 mg for women who are pregnant, and 16-19 mg for women who are lactating.

Zinc has become a popular remedy for the **common cold**. Evidence shows that it is unlikely to prevent upper respiratory infections, but beginning a supplement promptly when symptoms occur can significantly shorten the duration of the illness. The only form of zinc proven effective for this purpose is the zinc gluconate or zinc acetate lozenge. Formulations of 13-23 mg or more appear to be most effective, and need to be dissolved in the mouth in order to exert antiviral properties. Swallowing or sucking on oral zinc tablets will not work. The lozenges can be used every two hours for up to a week or two at most.

People who are deficient in zinc are prone to getting more frequent and longer lasting infections of various types. Zinc acts as an immune booster, in part due to stimulation of the thymus gland. This gland tends to shrink with age, and consequently produces less of the hormones that boost the production of infection-fighting white **blood** cells. Supplemental zinc, at one to two times RDA amounts, can reverse this tendency and improve immune function.

In another immune stimulant capacity, zinc can offer some relief from chronic infections with *Candida albicans*, or yeast. Most women will experience a vaginal yeast **infection** at some time, and are particularly prone to them during the childbearing years. Some individuals appear to be more susceptible than others. One study showed yeast- fighting benefits for zinc even for those who were not deficient in the mineral to begin with. Other supplements that will complement zinc in combating yeast problems are **vitamin A**, **vitamin C**, and **vitamin E**. Another measure that can help to limit problems with *Candida* is eating yogurt, which is an excellent source of *Lactobacillus*, a friendly **bacteria** that competes with yeast. Limiting sweets in the diet and eating garlic or odor-free garlic supplements may also prove helpful.

People who are going to have surgery are well advised to make sure they are getting the RDA of zinc, vitamin A, and vitamin C in order to optimize wound healing. A deficiency of any of these nutrients can significantly lengthen the time it takes to heal. Adequate levels of these **vitamins** and **minerals** for at least a few weeks before and after surgery can speed healing. The same nutrients are important to minimize the healing time of bedsores, **burns**, and other skin lesions too.

There are two male health problems that can potentially benefit from zinc supplementation. Testosterone is one of the hormones that requires zinc in order to be produced. Men with **infertility** as a result of low testosterone levels may experience improvement from taking a zinc supplement. Another common condition that zinc can be helpful for is benign prostatic hypertrophy, a common cause of abnormally frequent urination in older men. Taking an extra 50 mg a day for three to six months offers symptomatic relief for some men.

Teenagers are often low in zinc, and also tend to experience more acne than the general population. The doses used in studies have been in the high range, requiring medical supervision, but increasing dietary zinc or taking a modest supplement in order to get the RDA amount is low risk and may prove helpful for those suffering from acne. Consult a knowledgeable health care provider before taking large doses of any supplement.

There is some evidence that zinc supplementation may slightly relieve the symptoms of rheumatoid arthritis, but the studies are not yet conclusive. It's possible that those who initially had low zinc levels benefited the most.

Zinc is sometimes promoted as an aid for **memory**. This may be true to the extent that vitamin B_6 and neurotransmitters are not properly utilized without it. However, in the case of people with **Alzheimer's disease**, zinc can cause more harm than good. Some experiments indicate that zinc actually decreases intellectual function of people with this disease. Under these circumstances, it is probably best to stick to the RDA of 15 mg as a maximum daily amount of zinc.

The frequency of sickle-cell crisis in patients with sickle-cell anemia may be decreased by zinc supplementation. The decrease was significant in one study, although the severity of the attacks that occurred was not affected. Use of zinc supplementation or other treatment for sickle- cell anemia, a serious condition, should not be undertaken without the supervision of a health care provider.

Both the retina of the eye, and the cochlea in the inner ear contain large amounts of zinc, which they appear to need in order to function properly. Dr. George E. Shambaugh, Jr., M.D., is a professor emeritus of otolaryngology and head and neck surgery at Northwestern University Medical School in Chicago. In *Prevention's Healing with Vitamins*, he "estimates that about 25% of the people he sees with severe tinnitus are zinc-deficient." He adds that they sometimes have other symptoms of zinc deficiency. Large doses may be used in order to provide relief for this problem. Medical supervision and monitoring are necessary to undertake this course of treatment.

Topical zinc can be useful for some conditions, including cold sores. It is also available in a combination formula with the antibiotic erythromycin for the treatment of acne. Zinc oxide is a commonly used ingredient in the strongest sun block preparations and some creams for the treatment of diaper rash and superficial skin injuries. Men can use topical zinc oxide to speed the healing of **genital herpes** lesions, but it is too drying for women to use in the vaginal area.

There is still not enough information on some of the claims that are made for zinc. A few that may have merit are the prevention or slowing of **macular degeneration**, and relieving psoriasis. Consult a health care provider for these uses.

Deficiency

It is not uncommon to have a mild to moderately low levels of zinc, although serious deficiency is rare. Symptoms can include an increased susceptibility to infection, rashes, hair loss, poor growth in children, delayed healing of **wounds**, rashes, acne, male infertility, poor appetite, decreased sense of **taste** and **smell**, and possibly swelling of the mouth, tongue, and eyelids.

A more serious, chronic deficiency can cause severe growth problems, including dwarfism and poor bone maturation. The spleen and **liver** may become enlarged. Testicular size and function both tend to decrease. **Cataracts** may form in the eyes, the optic nerve can become swollen, and color **vision** is sometimes affected by a profound lack of zinc. **Hearing** is sometimes affected as well.

Since meats are the best sources of zinc, strict vegetarians and vegans are among the groups more likely to be deficient. The absorption of zinc is inhibited by high fiber foods, so people who have diets that are very high in whole grain and fiber need to take supplements separately from the fiber. Zinc is needed in larger amounts for women who are pregnant or breastfeeding. Deficiency during **pregnancy** may lower fetal birthweight, as well as increase maternal risk of toxemia. A good prenatal vitamin is likely to contain an adequate amount. People over age 50 don't absorb zinc as well, nor do they generally have adequate intake, and may require a supplement. Alcoholics generally have poor nutritional status to begin with, and alcohol also depletes stored zinc.

There is an increased need for most vitamins and minerals for people who are chronically under high **stress**. Those who have had surgery, severe burns, wasting illnesses, or poor **nutrition** may require larger amounts of zinc than average.

Some diseases increase the risk of zinc deficiency. Sickle-cell anemia, diabetes, and kidney disease can all affect zinc **metabolism**. People with **Crohn's disease**, sprue, chronic **diarrhea**, or babies with acrodermatitis enteropathica also have an increased need for zinc. Consult a health care provider for appropriate supplementation instructions.

Preparations

Natural sources

Oysters are tremendously high in zinc. Some sources, such as whole grains, beans, and nuts, have good zinc content but the fiber in these foods prevents it from being absorbed well. Foods with zinc that is better utilized include beef, chicken, turkey, milk, cheese, and yogurt. Pure maple syrup also is a good dose of zinc.

Supplemental sources

Zinc supplements are available as oral tablets in various forms, as well as lozenges. Zinc gluconate is the type most commonly used in lozenge form to kill upper respiratory **viruses**. Select brands that do not use citric acid or tartaric acid for flavoring, as these appear to impair the effectiveness. The best-absorbed oral types of zinc may include zinc citrate, zinc acetate, or zinc picolinate. Zinc sulfate is the most likely to cause **stomach** irritation. Topical formulations are used for acne and skin injuries. Oral zinc should not be taken with foods that will reduce its absorption, such as coffee, bran, protein, phytates, **calcium**, or **phosphorus**.

Supplements should be stored in a cool, dry location, away from direct light, and out of the reach of children.

Precautions

Toxicity can occur with excessively large doses of zinc supplements, and produce symptoms, including **fever**, cough, abdominal **pain**, nausea, vomiting, diarrhea, drowsiness, restlessness, and gait abnormalities. If doses greater than 100 mg per day are taken chronically, it can result in anemia, immune insufficiency, **heart** problems, and **copper** deficiency. High doses of zinc can also cause a decrease in high density lipoprotein (HDL), or good, cholesterol.

People who have hemochromatosis, are allergic to zinc, or are infected with HIV should not take supplemental zinc. Ulcers in the stomach or duodenum may be aggravated by supplements as well. Those with **glaucoma** should use caution if using eye drops containing zinc. Overuse of supplemental zinc during pregnancy can increase the risk of premature birth and stillbirth, particularly if the supplement is taken in the third trimester. This increase in adverse outcomes has been documented with zinc dosages of 100 mg taken three times daily.

Side effects

Zinc may cause irritation of the stomach, and is best taken with food in order to avoid nausea. The lozenge form used to treat colds has a strong taste, and can alter the sense of taste and smell for up to a few days.

Interactions

The absorption of vitamin A is improved by zinc supplements, but they may interfere with the absorption of other minerals taken at the same time, including calcium, magnesium, **iron**, and copper. Supplements of calcium, magnesium, and copper should be taken at different times than the zinc. Iron should only be taken if a known deficiency exists. Thiazide and loop diuretic medications, sometimes used for people with high **blood pressure**, congestive **heart failure**, or liver disease, increase the loss of zinc. Levels are also lowered by oral contraceptives. Zinc can decrease the absorption of tetracycline and quinolone class **antibiotics**, **antacids**, soy, or manganese, and should not be taken at the same time of day. Drinking coffee at the same time as taking zinc can reduce the absorption by as much as half. Even moderate amounts of alcohol impair zinc metabolism and increase its excretion. Chelation with EDTA can deplete zinc, so patients undergoing chelation need to supplement with zinc,

---

KEY TERMS

Acrodermatitis enteropathica—Hereditary metabolic problem characterized by dermatitis, diarrhea, and poor immune status. Oral treatment with zinc is curative.

Benign prostatic hypertrophy—Enlargement of the prostate gland, which surrounds the male urethra, causing frequent urination. This condition is very common in older men.

Hemochromatosis—A hereditary condition that results in excessive storage of iron in various tissues of the body.

Macular degeneration—Deterioration of part of the retina, causing progressive loss of vision. This is the most common cause of blindness in the elderly.

Sickle-cell anemia—A genetic malformation of red blood cells that can cause periodic crises in sufferers.

Tinnitus—Perceived ringing, buzzing, whistling, or other noise heard in one or both ears that has no external source. There are a number of conditions that may cause this.

---

according to the instructions of the health care provider.

Resources

BOOKS

Bratman, Steven and David Kroll. *Natural Health Bible.* California: Prima Publishing, 1999.
Feinstein, Alice. *Prevention's Healing with Vitamins.* Pennsylvania: Rodale Press, 1996.
Griffith, H. Winter. *Vitamins, Herbs, Minerals & Supplements: the Complete Guide.* Arizona: Fisher Books, 1998.
Jellin, Jeff, Forrest Batz, and Kathy Hitchens. *Pharmacist's letter/Prescriber's Letter Natural Medicines Comprehensive Database.* California: Therapeutic Research Faculty, 1999.
Pressman, Alan H. and Sheila Buff. *The Complete Idiot's Guide to Vitamins and Minerals.* New York: alpha books, 1997.

Judith Turner

Zinc deficiency *see* **Mineral deficiency**

Zinc protophophyrin test *see* **Trace metal tests**

Zygote intrafallopian transfer *see* **Fertility treatments**

ORGANIZATIONS

The list of organizations is arranged in alphabetical order by topic. Although the list is comprehensive, it is by no means exhaustive. It is a starting point for further information that can be used in conjuction with the Resources section of each entry, as well as other online and print sources. Thomson Gale is not responsible for the accuracy of the addresses or the contents of the websites.

Biomedical Equipment Technology

Association for the Advancement of Medical Instrumentation
1110 North Glebe Road, Ste. 220
Arlington, VA 22201-4795
Tel: (703) 525-4890 or (800) 332-2264
Web: <http://www.aami.org>

North Central Biomedical Association
P.O. Box 484
Elk River, MN 55330
Web: <http://www.ncbiomed.org>

Dental Hygiene

American Dental Association
211 E. Chicago Avenue
Chicago, IL 60611
Tel: (312) 440-2500
Fax: (312) 440-2800
Web: <http://www.ada.org>

American Dental Hygienists' Association
444 N. Michigan Avenue, Ste. 3400
Chicago, IL 60611
Tel: (312) 440-8900
E-mail: mail@adha.net
Web: <http://www.adha.org>

Dietetics

American College of Nutrition
300 S. Duncan Avenue, Ste. 225
Clearwater, FL 33755
Tel: (727) 446-6086
Fax: (727) 446-6202
E-Mail: office@amcollnutr.org
Web: <http://amcollnutr.org>

American Dietetic Association
216 W. Jackson Boulevard

Chicago, IL 60606-6995
Tel: (312) 899-0040
Web: <http://www.eatright.org>

International and American Association of Clinical Nutritionists
15280 Addison Road, Ste. 130
Addison, TX 75001
Tel: (972) 407-9089
Fax: (972) 250-0233
Email: ddc@clinicalnutrition.com
Web: <http://www.iaacn.org>

Healthcare Administration

Accrediting Commission on Education
for Health Services Administration
730 11th Street NW, 4th Floor
Washington, DC 20001
Tel: (202) 638-5131
Fax: (202) 638-3429

American Academy of Medical Administrators
Research and Educational Foundation
701 Lee Street, Ste. 600
Des Plaines, IL 60016-4516
Tel: (847) 759-8601
Fax: (847) 759-8602
E-Mail: info@aameda.org
Web: <http://www.aameda.org>

American College of Health Care Administrators
300 N. Lee Street, Ste. 301
Alexandria, VA 22314
Tel: (703) 739-7900 or (888) 882-2422
Fax: (703) 739-7901
Web: <http://www.achca.org>

American Medical Directors Association
10480 Little Patuxent Parkway, Ste. 760
Columbia, MD 21044

Tel: (410) 740-9743 or
(800) 876-2632
Fax: (410) 740-4572
E-mail: info@amda.com
Web: <http://www.amda.com>

Healthcare Information and Management Systems Society
230 E. Ohio Street, Ste. 500
Chicago, IL 60611-3270
Tel: (312) 664-4467
Fax: (312) 664-6143
Web: <http://www.himss.org>

Healthcare, General

Agency for Healthcare Research and Quality
2101 E. Jefferson Street, Ste. 501
Rockville, MD 20852
Tel: (301) 594-1364
E-mail: info@ahrq.gov
Web: <http://www.ahrq.gov>

American Health Care Association
1201 L Street NW
Washington, DC 20005
Tel: (202) 842-4444
Fax: (202) 842-3860
Web: <http://www.ahca.org>

American Hospital Association
One North Franklin
Chicago, IL 60606-3421
Tel: (312) 422-3000
Fax: (312) 422-4796
Web: <http://www.aha.org>

American Medical Association
515 N. State Street
Chicago, IL 60610
Tel: (312) 464-5000
Web: <http://www.ama-assn.org>

Centers for Disease Control and Prevention
1600 Clifton Road
Atlanta, GA 30333

Tel: (404) 639-3534 or (800) 311-3435
Web: <http://www.cdc.gov>

National Health Council
1730 M Street NW, Ste. 500
Washington, DC 20036
Tel: (202) 785-3910
Fax: (202) 785-5923
E-mail: info@nhcouncil.org
Web: <http://www.
nationalhealthcouncil.org>

New York Biotechnology Association
23 E. Loop Road, Ste. 203
Stony Brook, NY 11790
Tel: (631) 444-8895
Fax: (631) 444-8896
Web: <http://www.nyba.org>

World Health Organization
Avenue Appia 20
1211 Geneva 27
Switzerland
Tel: (+ 00 41 22) 791 2111
Fax: (+ 00 41 22) 791 3111
Web: <http://www.who.int>

Medical Laboratory Science

American Association for Clinical Chemistry
2101 L Street, Ste. 202
Washington, DC 20037-1558
Tel: (202) 857-0717 or (800) 892-1400
Fax: (202) 887-5093
E-mail: info@aacc.org
Web: <http://www.aacc.org>

American Medical Technologists
710 Higgins Road
Park Ridge, IL 60068
Tel: (847) 823-5169 or
(800) 275-1268
Fax: (847) 823-0458
E-mail: amtmail@aol.com
Web: <http://www.amt1.com>

American Society for Clinical Laboratory Science
7910 Woodmont Avenue, Ste. 530
Bethesda, MD 20814
Tel: (301) 657-2768
Fax: (301) 657-2909
E-mail: ascls@ascls.org
Web: <http://www.ascls.org>

Clinical Laboratory Management Association
989 Old Eagle School Road, Ste. 815
Wayne, PA 19087
Tel: (610) 995-9580

Fax: (610) 995-9568
<http://www.clma.org>

National Accrediting Agency for Clinical Laboratory Sciences
8410 W. Bryn Mawr Avenue, Ste. 670
Chicago, IL 60631
Tel: (773) 714-8880
Fax: (773) 714-8886
E-mail: info@naacls.org
Web: <http://www.naacls.org>

Mental Health

Alliance for Psychosocial Nursing
6900 Grove Road
Thorofare, NJ 08086-9447
Tel: (856) 848-1000
Web: <http://www.psychnurse.org>

National Institute of Mental Health
6001 Executive Boulevard
Room 8184, MSC 9663
Bethesda, MD 20892-9663
Tel: (301) 443-4513
Fax: (301) 443-4279
TTY: (301) 443-8431
Web: <http://www.nimh.nih.gov>

National Mental Health Association
1021 Prince Street
Alexandria, VA 22314-2971
Tel: (800) 969-6642
TTY: (800) 433-5959
Web: <http://www.nmha.org>

Substance Abuse and Mental Health Services Administration
Department of Health and Human Services
5600 Fishers Lane
Rockville, MD 20857
E-mail: info@samhsa.gov
Web: <http://www.samhsa.gov>

Nurse Anesthetists

American Association of Nurse Anesthetists
222 S. Prospect Avenue
Park Ridge, IL 60068
Tel: (847) 692-7050
Web: <http://www.aana.com>

American Board of Perianesthesia Nursing Certification
475 Riverside Drive, 6th Floor
New York, NY 10115-0089
Tel: (212) 367-4253 or (800) 622-7262

Fax: (212) 367-4256
Web: <http://www.cpancapa.org>

American Society of Perianesthesia Nurses
10 Melrose Avenue, Ste. 110
Cherry Hill, NJ 08003-3696
Tel: (877) 737-9696
Fax: (856) 616-9601
E-mail: aspan@aspan.org
Web: <http://www.aspan.org>

Nursing, General

Academy of Medical Surgical Nurses
E. Holly Avenue
P.O. Box 56
Pitman, NJ 08071-0056
Tel: (856) 256-2323
Fax: (856) 589-7463
E-mail: amsn@ajj.com
Web: <http://
www.medsurgnurse.org>

The American Assembly for Men in Nursing
c/o NYSNA
11 Cornell Road
Latham, NY 12110-1499
Tel: (518) 782-9400 Ext. 346
E-mail: aamn@aamn.org
Web: <http://www.aamn.org>

American Association of Colleges of Nursing
One Dupont Circle NW, Ste. 530
Washington, DC 20036
Tel: (202) 463-6930
Fax: (202) 785-8320
Web: <http://www.aacn.nche.edu>

American Board of Nursing Specialties
4035 Running Springs
San Antonio, TX 78261
Tel: (830) 438-4897
Web: <http://
www.nursingcertification.org>

American Nurses Association
600 Maryland Avenue SW, Ste. 100
Washington, DC 20024
Tel: (202) 651-7000 or (800) 274-4262
Fax: (202) 651-7001
Web: <http://
www.nursingworld.org>

American Organization of Nurse Executives
One North Franklin
Chicago, IL 60606
Tel: (312) 422-2800

Fax: (312) 422-4503
Web: <http://www.aone.org>

Association of Black Nursing Faculty
5823 Queens Cove
Lisle, IL 60532
Tel: (630) 969-3809
Fax: (630) 969-3895
Web: <http://www.abnfinc.org>

International Council of Nurses
3, Place Jean Marteau
1201 Geneva
Switzerland
Tel: 41-22-908-01-00
Fax: 41-22-908-01-01
E-mail: icn@icn.ch
Web: <http://www.icn.ch>

National Council of State Boards of Nursing
676 N. St. Clair Street, Ste. 550
Chicago, IL 60611-2921
Tel: (312) 787-6555
E-mail: info@ncsbn.org
Web: <http://www.ncsbn.org>

National Federation of Licensed Practical Nurses
893 U.S. Highway 70 West, Ste. 202
Garner, NC 27529
Tel: (919) 779-0046 or (800) 948-2511
Fax: (919) 779-5642
Web: <http://www.nflpn.org>

National Institute of Nursing Research
National Institutes of Health
Bethesda, MD 20892-2178
Tel: (301) 496-0207
E-mail: info@ninr.nih.gov
Web: <http://www.nih.gov/ninr>

National League for Nursing
61 Broadway, 33rd Floor
New York, NY 10006
Tel: (212) 363-5555 or (800) 669-1656
Fax: (212) 812-0393
Web: <http://www.nln.org>

National Organization for Associate Degree Nursing
11250 Roger Bacon Drive, Ste. 8
Reston, VA 20190
Tel: (703) 437-4377
Fax: (703) 435-4390
E-mail: noadn@aol.com
Web: <http://www.noadn.org>

National Student Nurses Association
555 W. 57th Street
New York, NY 10019
Tel: (212) 581-2211
Fax: (212) 581-2368
E-mail: nsna@nsna.org
Web: <http://www.nsna.org>

United Nurses and Allied Professionals
375 Branch Avenue
Providence, RI 02904
Tel: (401) 831-3647
Fax: (401) 831-3677
E-mail: information@unap.org
Web: <http://www.unap.org>

Nurse Midwives

American College of Nurse-Midwives
818 Connecticut Avenue NW, Ste. 900
Washington, DC 20006
Tel: (202) 728-9860
Fax: (202) 728-9897
E-mail: info@acnm.org
Web: <http://www.acnm.org>

Midwifery Today
P.O. Box 2672-350
Eugene, OR 97402
Tel: (541)344-7438
Web: <http://www.
midwiferytoday.com>

Midwives Alliance of North America
4805 Lawrenceville Highway, Ste. 116-279
Lilburn, GA 30047
Tel: (888) 923-6262
E-mail: info@mana.org
Web: <http://www.mana/org>

Nurse Practitioners

American Academy of Nurse Practitioners
P.O. Box 12846
Austin, TX 78711
Tel: (512) 442-4262
Fax: (512) 442-6469
E-mail: webmaster@aanp.org
Web: <http://www.aanp.org>

National Association of Nurse Practitioners
in Women's Health
503 Capitol Court NE, Ste. 300
Washington, DC 20002
Tel: (202) 543-9693
Fax: (202) 543-9858
E-Mail: npwhdc@aol.com
Web: <http://www.npwh.org>

National Association of Pediatric Nurse Practitioners
1101 Kings Highway, Ste. 206

Cherry Hill, NJ 08034-1912
Tel: (856) 667-1773 or (877) 662-7627
Fax: (856) 667-7187
E-mail: info@napnap.org
Web: <http://www.napnap.prg>

National Certification Board of Pediatric
Nurse Practitioners and Nurses
800 S. Frederick Avenue, Ste. 104
Gaithersburg, MD 20877-4150
Tel: (301) 330-2921 or (888) 641-2767
Fax: (301) 330-1504
Web: <http://www.pnpcert.org>

Nurse Practitioner Associates for Continuing Education
5 Militia Drive
Lexington, MA 02421-4740
Tel: (781) 861-0270
Fax: (781) 861-0279
E-mail: npace@npace.org
Web: <http://www.npace.org>

Occupational Therapy

American Occupational Therapy Association
4720 Montgomery Lane
P.O. Box 31220
Bethesda, MD 20824-1220
Tel: (301) 652-2682
TDD: (800) 377-8555
Fax: (301) 652-7711
Web: <http://www.aota.org>

National Board for Certification in Occupational Therapy
800 S. Frederick Avenue, Ste. 200
Gaithersburg, MD 20877-4150
Tel: (301) 990-7979
Fax: (301) 869-8492
Web: <http://www.nbcot.org>

Optometry

American Academy of Optometry
6110 Executive Boulevard, Ste. 506
Rockville, MD 20852 USA
Tel: (301) 984-1441
Fax: (301) 984-4737
Web: <http://www.aaopt.org>

American Optometric Association
243 North Lindbergh Boulevard
St. Louis, MO 63141
Tel: (314) 991-4100
Fax: (314) 991-4101
Web: <http://www.aoanet.org>

Pharmacy Technicians

American Association of Pharmacy Technicians
P.O. Box 1447
Greensboro, NC 27402
Tel: (877) 368-4771
Fax: (336) 275-7222
Web: <http://www.pharmacytechnician.com>

National Pharmacy Technician Association
P.O. Box 683148
Houston, TX 77268-3148
Tel: (888) 247-8700
Fax: (281) 895-7320
E-mail: info@pharmacytechnician.org
Web: <http://www.pharmacytechnician.org>

Physical Therapy

American Physical Therapy Association
1111 N. Fairfax Street
Alexandria, VA 22314-1488
Tel: (703) 684-2782 or (800) 999-2782
TDD: (703) 683-6748
Fax: (703) 684-7343
Web: <http://www.apta.org>

National Rehabilitation Association
633 S. Washington Street
Alexandria, VA 22314
Tel: (703) 836-0850
TDD: (703) 836-0849
Fax: (703) 836-0848
E-mail: info@national rehab.org
Web: <http://www.nationalrehab.org>

Public Health

American Association for Health Education
1900 Association Drive
Reston, VA 20191 USA
Tel: (703) 476-3437 or (800) 213-7193
Fax: (703) 476-6638
E-Mail: aahe@aahperd.org
Web: <http://www.aahperd.org/aahe>

American Public Health Association
800 I Street NW
Washington, DC 20001
Tel: (202) 777-APHA
TTY: (202) 777-2500
Fax: (202) 777-2534
Web: <http://www.apha.org>

Association of Public Health Laboratories
2025 M Street NW, Ste. 550
Washington, DC 20036-3320
Tel: (202) 822-5227
Fax: (202) 887-5098
Web: <http://www.aphl.org>

Association of Schools of Public Health
1101 15th Street NW, Ste. 910
Washington, DC 20005
Tel: (202) 296-1099
Fax: (202) 296-1252
E-Mail: info@asph.org
Web: <http://www.asph.org>

Council on Education for Public Health (CEPH)
800 Eye Street NW, Ste. 202
Washington, DC 20001-3710
Tel: (202) 789-1050
Fax: (202) 789-1895
Web: <http://www.ceph.org>

National Association for Public Health
Statistics and Information Systems
1220 19th Street NW, Ste. 802
Washington, DC 20036
Tel: (202) 463-8851
Fax: (202) 463-4870
E-Mail: hq@napshis.org
Web: <http://www.naphsis.org>

Radiologic Technology

American Registry of Radiologic Technologists
1255 Northland Drive
St. Paul, MN 55120
Tel: (651) 687-0048
Web: <http://www.arrt.org>

American Society of Radiologic Technologists
15000 Central Avenue SE
Albuquerque, NM 87123-3917
Tel: (505) 298-4500 or (800) 444-2778
Fax: (505) 298-5063
Web: <http://www.asrt.org>

International Society for Magnetic Resonance in Medicine
2118 Milvia Street, Ste. 201
Berkeley, CA 94704
Tel: (510) 841-1899
Fax: (510) 841-2340
E-mail: info@ismrm.org
Web: <http://www.ismrm.org>

Radiological Society of North America
820 Jorie Boulevard
Oak Brook, IL 60523-2251
Tel: (630) 571-2670
Fax: (630) 571-7837
Web: <http://www.rsna.org>

Society of Nuclear Medicine
1850 Samuel Morse Drive
Reston, VA 20190-5316
Tel: (703) 708-9000
Fax: (703) 708-9015
Web: <http://www.snm.org>

Respiratory Therapy

American Association for Respiratory Care
11030 Ables Lane
Dallas, TX 75229
Tel: (972) 243-2272
Fax: (972) 484-2720
E-mail: info@aarc.org
Web: <http://www.aarc.org>

National Board for Respiratory Care
8310 Nieman Road
Lenexa, KS 66214-1579
Tel: (913) 599-4200
Fax: (913) 541-0156
E-mail: nbrc-info@nbrc.org
Web: <http://www.nbrc.org>

Respiratory Nursing Society
c/o NYSNA
11 Cornell Rd.
Latham, NY 12110
Tel: (518) 782-9400 Ext. 286
Web: <http://www.respiratorynursingsociety.org>

Speech-Language Pathology

American Institute for Stuttering Treatment
and Professional Training
27 W. 20th Street, Ste. 1203
New York, NY 10011
Tel: (877) 378-8883
Fax: (212) 220-3922
Web: <http://www.stutteringtreatment.org>

American Speech-Language-Hearing
    Association
10801 Rockville Pike
Rockville, MD 20852
Tel/TTY: (800) 638-8255
Web: <http://professional.asha.org>

Surgical Technology

Association of Surgical Technologists
7108-C South Alton Way
Englewood, CO 80112

Tel: (303) 694-9130
Fax: (303) 694-9169
Web: <http://www.ast.org>

INDEX

In the index, references to individual volumes are listed before colons; numbers following a colon refer to specific page numbers within that particular volume. **Boldface** references indicate main topical essays. Illustrations are highlighted with an *italicized* page number; and tables are also indicated with the page number followed by a lowercase, italicized *t*.

A

A-a gradient, 1:342, 344

A-bands, 4:2463

A-linolenic acid, 2:1026

A-mode ultrasonography, 1:3, 5:2768

A-scan ophthalmologic ultrasound, 3:1941, 1942–1943

A549 cells, 4:2557

AABB (American Association of Blood Banks), 4:2032, 5:2756

AABR (Automated auditory brainstem response), 3:1891

AANA (American Association of Nurse Anesthetists), 3:1444, 1907

AAP. *See* American Academy of Periodontology

AARP (American Association of Retired Persons), 1:61

AASECT (American Association of Sexual Educators, Counselors and Therapists), 4:2438

AATA (American Art Therapy Association), 1:216

Abacavir, 1:70

Abatacept, 1:251

Abbreviations, medication, 1:31

ABCD mnemonic (CPR), 1:467

ABCD rule (Skin cancer), 3:1645

Abdominal aortic aneurysm, 1:2, 3, 360

Abdominal artery, 1:470

Abdominal circumference, fetal, 2:1041

Abdominal examination, 4:2104
abdominal sounds in, 4:2569
for acute kidney failure, 1:27

Abdominal mass, 1:1

Abdominal pain
abdominal ultrasound for, 1:1, 3
amylase and lipase tests for, 1:126–128

Abdominal sounds, 4:2569

Abdominal surgery, laparoscopic, 3:1526, 1530

Abdominal ultrasound, 1:**1–5**, *2,* 4:2124

Abdominal wounds
gangrene from, 2:1131
ultrasound of, 1:1

Abdominal x rays, 3:1503–1505

Abdominopelvic cavity, 2:1327

Abducens nerve, 3:1873

Abduction, joint, 2:1326

Abetalipoproteinemia, 3:1566

Ability tests, 4:2266, 2267

Ablation
catheter, 2:938, 939, 4:2006
focused ultrasound, 5:2659

ABMS (American Board of Medical Specialists), 3:1713

ABO blood groups
description of, 1:331, 5:2756
distribution of, 5:2757, 2759*t*
human leukocyte antigen test with, 2:1334–1337
neonatal jaundice and, 3:1861
for parentage testing, 4:2031
prenatal, 4:2208
pretransfusion tests of, 5:*2728,* 2732
typing and screening tests, 5:**2755–2761,** 2755*t*

ABO/NCLE (American Board of Opticianry/National Contact Lens Examiners), 3:1945

Abortion
incomplete, 3:1773
missed, 3:1773
premature infants after, 4:2203
uterine stimulants for, 5:2791
vaginal medications for, 5:2801

ABPTS (American Board of Physical Therapy Specialists), 4:2057

Abrasions, 5:2903, 2905

Abruptio placentae. *See* Placental abruption

Abscess, 1:**5–8,** *6*
from Crohn's disease, 1:673, 674
dental, 2:**731–734,** 785

epidural, 4:2525
ileal, 2:978
from mastitis, 3:1671
pancreatic, 4:2012, 2013
periapical, 2:731–734
periodontal, 2:732–734, 4:2069
wound, 5:2901

Absolute presbyopia, 4:2217

Abstinence, periodic, 1:651, 652, 4:2337

Abstraction impairment, 2:729

Abu Ghraib prison, 3:1695

Abuse. *See* Child abuse; Elder abuse

Acamprosate, 1:91

Acarbose, 1:177–178

Acceptance, five stages of, 2:1320, 1321

Access ports. *See* Vascular access devices

Accessory nerve, 3:1873

Accidents. *See* Motor vehicle accidents

Accolate. *See* Zafirlukast

Accreditation Board for Engineering and Technology, Inc., 1:299

Accreditation Council for Occupational Therapy Education (ACOTE), 3:1937, 1938

Accrediting Bureau of Health Education Schools, 3:1683

Accrediting Commission on Education for Health Services Education, 3:1682

Accupril. *See* Quinapril

Accutane. *See* Isotretinoin

ACE inhibitors. *See* Angiotensin-converting enzyme (ACE) inhibitors

Acebutolol, 1:186–187, 661

Acetabulum, 4:2469

Acetaminophen, 1:133
for burns, 1:411
for cancer pain, 1:432
for carpal tunnel syndrome, 1:477
for cold sores, 1:592
for colposcopy, 1:609

Angiotensin II, 3:1507

Angiotensin receptor antagonists
    for congestive heart failure, 2:1256
    for hypertension, 2:1350
    for myocardial infarction, 3:1826

Angiotensinogen, 4:2132

Angle, Edward H., 1:573

Anhydrous carbonic acid, 1:342, 345

Animal bites, 1:313–318

Anise, 1:140

Anisocytosis, 1:626

Anistreplase, 3:1826

Ankle
    anatomy of, 4:2469
    gait problems from, 2:1120

Ankle-foot orthoses, 3:1590

Ankle injuries
    orthopedic tests, 3:1971
    sports-related, 4:2543
    sprains, 3:1590

Ankylosing spondylitis, 1:249–251
    in gliding joints, 2:1200
    human leukocyte antigen test for,
        2:1334
    in pivot joints, 4:2122

Ankylosis
    in gliding joints, 2:1200
    orthodontic appliances and,
        3:1968
    in pivot joints, 4:2122

Anma, 4:2446

Anodontia, partial, 2:744

Anomia, 1:207

Anorectal manometry, 2:1030

Anorexia
    from chemotherapy, 1:537
    marijuana for, 3:1660, 1661

Anorexia nervosa
    liver failure from, 3:1480
    pituitary hormone tests, 4:2119
    in pregnancy, 4:2213

Anorexiants, 1:512

Anosmia, 4:2497

Anoxia. See Hypoxia

Ansaid. See Flurbiprofen

ANSI (American National Standard
    Institute), 3:1698, 1711

Antabuse. See Disulfiram

Antacids, 1:159–161
    anticoagulants and, 2:876–877
    benzodiazepines and, 1:165
    bisacodyl and, 3:1538
    calcium and, 3:1983
    coagulation tests and, 1:578
    fecal impaction from, 2:1027
    gastric analysis and, 2:1141
    for gastroesophageal reflux,
        2:1148
    hypercalcemia from, 2:919
    iron and, 3:1468
    macular degeneration and, 3:1616

metabolic alkalosis from, 1:347
    phosphorus and, 4:2099
    sucralfate and, 1:197
    vitamin A and, 5:2853
    vitamin K and, 5:2869
    zinc and, 5:2927

Antagonistic muscle pairs, 3:1776

Antagonists, action of, 2:874

Antalgia, 2:1120

Antegrade pyelography, 3:1459

Antenatal care. See Prenatal care

Antepartum testing, 1:161–164

Anterior cruciate ligament (ACL)
    injuries, 3:1971, 4:2543, 2549

Anterior pituitary gland, 4:2111–2112

Anthropometric measurements,
    3:1925, 1926

Anti-diuretic hormone deficiency,
    2:1354–1356

Anti-DNase-B test, 4:2593–2595

Anti-epileptic agents.
    See Anticonvulsants

Anti-HAV/IgG, 2:1282

Anti-HBc (Hepatitis B core
    antibody), 2:1283, 1284–1285,
    3:1585, 5:2758

Anti-HBe (Hepatitis B e-antibody),
    2:1283, 1284–1285

Anti-HBs (Hepatitis B surface
    antibody), 2:1283, 1284–1285,
    5:2758

Anti-HCV, 5:2758

Anti-HIV-1, -2, 5:2758

Anti-human immunoglobin antibodies,
    1:243

Anti-reflective coatings, 2:1010

Anti-seizure drugs.
    See Anticonvulsants

Anti-spasticity drugs, 2:1117

Anti-streptolysin O titer, 4:2593–2595

Antiandrogens, 3:1557

Antianxiety drugs, 1:164–166, 165,
    166t, 203
    for dementia, 2:730
    overdose, 3:1988
    for personality disorders, 4:2087
    for post-traumatic stress disorder,
        4:2167
    for somatoform disorders,
        4:2507

Antibiotic resistance. See Drug
    resistance

Antibiotic susceptibility testing,
    1:339, 4:2445
    skin culture for, 4:2473
    sputum culture for, 4:2558
    stool culture for, 4:2581
    throat culture for, 5:2677, 2678
    for tuberculosis, 1:17

Antibiotics, 1:166–169, 167
    for abscess, 1:7
    antitumor, 1:535
    autoimmune disease tests and,
        1:245
    for bites, 1:316
    broad-spectrum, 1:169, 2:1108
    for burns, 1:412
    for cataracts, 1:483
    coagulation tests and, 1:578
    color blindness from, 1:598
    common cold and, 1:617
    for Crohn's disease, 1:674
    for cross infection, 1:677
    for cystic fibrosis, 1:702
    for dental abscess, 2:733
    for dental trauma, 2:785
    drug resistance to, 1:265, 677
    for emphysema, 2:954
    for endocarditis, 2:957
    for food poisoning, 2:1091
    fungal, 2:1110
    for gangrene, 2:1129
    for gastritis, 2:1144–1145
    immunodeficiency and, 3:1383
    for impacted teeth, 3:1389
    iron supplements and, 2:877
    for kidney stones, 3:1503
    for lymphedema, 3:1612
    in meat, 5:2813
    for meningitis, 3:1740
    overuse of, 1:265, 2:1229
    for periodontal therapy, 3:1898
    for periodontitis, 4:2071
    platelet aggregation test and,
        4:2134
    for pneumonia, 4:2140
    prophylactic, 1:487, 4:2233–2235
    for puerperal infection, 4:2279,
        2280
    for refractive eye surgery, 4:2322
    for septic shock, 4:2430
    for sore throat, 4:2511
    sputum analysis and, 4:2553
    for staphylococcal infections, 4:2563
    for strep throat, 4:2591
    for syphilis, 4:2628
    thiamine and, 5:2668
    for tooth extraction, 5:2704
    for tooth polishing, 5:2706
    topical, 1:365
    toxicity, 3:1397
    tricyclic antidepressants and, 1:175
    vitamin B complex and, 5:2858
    vitamin C and, 5:2861
    for wound care, 5:2901
    for wound infections, 5:2904, 2907
    zinc and, 5:2927

Antibodies
    in acquired immunity, 3:1367
    allergic response and, 1:94, 98
    anti-human immunoglobin, 1:243
    antimitochondrial, 1:244

Carbon dioxide lasers, 2:1219, 3:1535, 1710

Carbon dioxide partial pressure. *See* Partial pressure of carbon dioxide (PCO$_2$)

Carbon dioxide poisoning, 1:343

Carbon disulfide, 1:598, 4:2149

Carbon electrodes, 3:1693

Carbon monoxide detectors, 1:440

Carbon monoxide poisoning, 1:**437–440,** *438*
    color blindness from, 1:598
    hyperbaric oxygen therapy, 1:439, 5:2817–2821
    occupational, 3:1397
    pathophysiology of, 4:2142
    seizures from, 4:2417

Carbonic acid, anhydrous, 1:342, 345

Carbonic anhydrase inhibitors, 2:1196

Carboprost, 5:2792, 2794

Carboxyhemoglobin, 1:345, 437, 439

Carbuncles, 1:6, 364–367

Carcinoembryonic antigen (CEA), 4:2021–2022, 5:2753

Carcinogens, 3:1397, 1398

Carcinoid tumors, 3:1438

Carcinomas, 1:423–424, 3:1577
    basal cell, 3:1428, 1644, 1646
    large-cell undifferentiated, 3:1598
    mixed cell, 3:1578
    in situ, 4:2017
    See also Squamous cell carcinomas

Cardiac catheterization, 1:**440–446,** *442, 443*
    for balloon valvuloplasty, 1:272
    cardiac technologists for, 1:459
    for congestive heart failure, 2:1255–1256, 1257–1258
    for electrophysiology study of the heart, 2:938
    heart-lung machines and, 2:1259
    percutaneous transluminal angioplasty and, 1:157

Cardiac cycle, 1:**446–450,** *447, 448,* 2:1251
    cardiovascular system and, 1:468–469
    disturbances of, 1:448, 450
    dynamic spatial reconstructor for, 2:887–888

Cardiac disorders. *See* Heart diseases

Cardiac electrical conductance
    disturbances of, 1:473
    electrocardiography of, 2:906, 909
    electrophysiology study of the heart for, 2:937–940
    physiology of, 1:*448,* 448–449, 450, 462–463, 470, 2:1251

Cardiac mapping, 2:938

Cardiac marker tests, 1:**450–453**

Cardiac monitors, 1:**453–456,** *454,* 5:2823

Cardiac muscles, 1:462, 468, 3:1812–1816
    contraction of, 3:1797–1800
    function of, 2:1251, 3:1815

Cardiac output, 1:348, 4:2622

Cardiac pressures, 1:444*t,* 445

Cardiac rehabilitation, 1:**456–459,** *457,* 2:1002
    for congestive heart failure, 2:1256
    nurses, 2:1257

Cardiac tamponade, 1:473

Cardiac technology, 1:**459–462**

Cardiac tissue, 1:**462–464**

Cardiogenic shock, 3:1439, 4:2449

Cardiolipin antibody test. *See* Antiphospholipid antibody test

Cardiolipin-lecithin-cholesterol antigen, 4:2627, 2631

Cardiology, invasive, 1:459–462

Cardiomyopathy, 1:472–473, 2:1253
    congestive heart failure from, 2:1254
    dilated, 2:1253
    hypertrophic, 2:899, 1253
    restrictive, 2:1253

Cardioplegia solution, 2:1259

Cardiopulmonary bypass machines, 2:1259–1263

Cardiopulmonary resuscitation (CPR), 1:**464–468,** *465, 467*
    in first aid, 2:1069, 1073
    for near-drowning, 3:1853
    for neonates, 3:1865
    for syncope, 4:2622, 2623

Cardiotomy, 2:1261

Cardiovascular center (Medulla), 1:348

Cardiovascular Credentialing International (CCI), 1:460

Cardiovascular disease
    aerobic/endurance training for, 1:54
    diabetes mellitus and, 2:805
    echocardiography for, 2:898–900
    fetal programming and, 3:1557
    mortality from, 1:359
    risk factors for, 1:359

Cardiovascular fitness testing, 2:968–971

Cardiovascular pharmacology, 4:2089

Cardiovascular system, 1:**468–475,** *469,* 2:1328
    aging and, 2:1187
    anatomy of, 1:468–471
    cardiopulmonary resuscitation and, 1:467
    function of, 1:471–473
    mechanical, 2:1259–1263

    pulmonary, 1:333, 471
    systemic, 1:333–334

Cardiovascular technologists, 1:459–461

Cardioverter-defibrillator, implantable, 3:**1392–1395**

Cardizem. *See* Diltiazem

Care plans
    anesthesia, 3:1906
    documentation of, 3:1688
    for nursing home residents, 3:1918
    patient rights and, 4:2050

Career opportunities. *See* Employment

Caregivers
    for Alzheimer's patients, 1:105–106
    for dementia, 2:730–731
    depression in, 2:730–731

CARET study, 5:2853

Caretakers, child abuse by, 1:550

Caring for the Mind (Hales), 2:792

Carisoprodol, 3:1801

Carotene, 3:1630

Carotenemia, 5:2853

Carotenoids
    aging and, 2:1188
    recommended daily allowances, 5:2852
    sources, 5:2851–2852, 2853

Carotid arteries, 1:470, 475–476

Carotid bodies, 1:399

Carotid duplex sonography, 1:**475–476**

Carpal compression test, 1:477

Carpal tunnel release surgery, 1:476, 477–478

Carpal tunnel syndrome, 1:**476–479**
    orthopedic tests, 3:1971
    ultrasonography, 5:2767

Carpel bones, 4:2469

Carrell, Alexis, 1:462

Carrier testing, 2:1168–1169

Carriers, amalgam, 2:770

Carteolol, 1:187

Cartilage
    in gliding joints, 2:1199
    in osteoarthritis, 3:1975
    in pivot joints, 4:2121–2122
    role of, 4:2466

Cartilage transplantation, 1:646

Cartilaginous joints, 3:1486

Carum carvi. See Caraway

Carvedilol, 1:186

Carvers, dental, 2:771

Cascara, 3:1538

Case management, 2:1228
    for cognitive impairment, 4:2080
    home care and, 2:1314
    managed care plans and, 3:1658

Index

Cleidocranial dysostosis, 5:2698

Clemastine, 1:96

Clenched-fist injuries, 1:314, 315

Cleocin. *See* Clindamycin

Clerc, Laurent, 1:110

CLES (Clinical laboratory equipment specialists), 1:302

CLIA (Clinical Laboratory Improvement Act), 3:1704, 1707

Client-centered therapy, 4:2268

Clindamycin, 1:168
    for boils, 1:365
    for endocarditis prevention, 2:959
    for malaria, 3:1637
    for periodontal therapy, 3:1898
    prophylactic use of, 4:2234
    for puerperal infection, 4:2280
    for strep throat, 4:2591

Clinical chemistry, 3:1701

Clinical chemistry laboratories, 3:1706

Clinical engineering, 1:299

Clinical laboratory equipment specialists (CLES), 1:302

Clinical Laboratory Improvement Act (CLIA), 3:1704, 1707

Clinical managers, 3:1681

Clinical nurse specialists, 1:50–53, **574–576**, 4:2327

Clinical pathology laboratories, 3:1700

Clinical pharmacology, 4:2089

Clinical Test of Sensory Interaction and Balance (CTSIB), 1:268

Clinical trials
    for gene therapy, 2:1153, 1155
    informed consent and, 3:1420
    for marijuana, 3:1661
    pharmacologist and, 4:2090

Clinically significant macular edema (CSME), 4:2371

Clinician-patient relationship. *See* Professional-patient relationship

Clinton, Bill, 2:1290

Clitoral therapy device, 4:2437

Clitoris, 4:2338–2339

Clock, biological, 1:292–293

Clock gene, 1:293

Clofarabine, 3:1544

Clofibrate
    for high cholesterol, 3:1563
    for hypertriglyceridemia, 3:1564
    vitamin B_{12} and, 5:2855

Clolar. *See* Clofarabine

Clomiphene, 4:2431, 2432

Clomipramine, 4:2437

Clonazepam
    for bipolar disorder, 1:307

for nocturnal myoclonus, 4:2489
    for pain, 4:2000
    for seizures, 4:2418

Cloned enzyme donor immunoassay (CEDIA), 2:885, 5:2685

Clonidine, 1:46
    adrenomedullary hormone tests and, 1:46
    for alcoholism, 1:86
    diabetes mellitus from, 2:802
    for hypertension, 2:1350
    overdose, 3:1988

Cloning, 1:290, 2:1163

Cloquet, Hippolyte, 4:2494

Closed-angle glaucoma, 2:1195–1197

Closed-chain exercise, 5:2655

Closed circuit television, 5:2843

Closed head injuries, 2:1223

Clostridium spp., 1:130
    gangrene from, 2:1127
    skin culture for, 4:2472

Clostridium botulinum
    food poisoning from, 2:1087, 1089–1090
    infection with, 1:266

Clostridium difficile culture, 4:2578–2582

Clostridium difficile toxin test, 1:**576–577**

Clostridium perfringens
    diarrhea from, 2:814
    gas gangrene from, 1:264
    infection with, 1:266

Clostridium tetani
    growth requirements of, 1:261
    infection with, 1:266
    tetanus from, 3:1800, 1816, 4:2465
    toxins, 5:2713

Clothing
    protective, 5:2770–2771
    surgical, 1:225

Clotrimazole, 1:179

Clotting, blood. *See* Blood coagulation

Clotting disorders. *See* Bleeding disorders

Clotting factors
    coagulation cascade and, 1:578–579
    coagulation tests and, 1:578
    liver function tests, 3:1584
    pooled factor preparations of, 2:1278
    role of, 1:335
    synthesis of, 3:1572
    See also specific factors

Clozapine, 1:190
    agranulocytosis from, 1:191
    for bipolar disorder, 1:308
    for Parkinson's disease, 4:2040
    for psychosis, 2:730
    for schizophrenia, 4:2398

Clozaril. *See* Clozapine

CMA. *See* Canadian Medical Association

CMBC system, 1:338

CMET (Canadian Early and Mid-trimester Amniocentesis Trial), 1:121

CNA (Colistin-nalidixic acid), 4:2473, 5:2789, 2904

CNS. *See* Central nervous system

CNS stimulants. *See* Central nervous system stimulants

Co-payments, 3:1686

CO_2. *See* Carbon dioxide

Coagulation. *See* Blood coagulation

Coagulation cascade
    in hemophilia, 2:1276
    tests, 1:578–581, 2:1060–1063

Coagulation disorders. *See* Bleeding disorders

Coagulation tests, 1:**578–583**

Coal miners, 3:1397, 1598

Cobalamin. *See* Vitamin B_{12}

Cobalt, 3:1770, 5:2715–2719

Cobalt sensitivity, 5:2855

Cobb angle, 4:2408

Cobrotoxin, 1:498

Cocaine
    abuse of, 4:2607–2610
    anxiety from, 1:201
    bipolar disorder and, 1:306
    depressive disorders from, 2:795
    drug tests, 2:884
    local anesthesia and, 1:147
    overdose, 3:1988, 4:2142
    sleep disorders with, 4:2488
    syncope from, 4:2622

Coccidioides immitis, 2:1111, 4:2556–2557

Coccidioidomycosis, 2:1111

Coccyx, 4:2468, 5:2828, 2829

Cochlea, 5:2926

Cochlear implants, 2:1244, *1244*

Cochrane, Archie, 2:996

Cochrane Centre, 2:996

Code of ethics. *See* Ethical codes and oaths

Code of Federal Regulations, 3:1696

Codeine, 1:133
    for cancer pain, 1:432
    for Crohn's disease, 1:674
    overdose, 3:1988

Codeine phosphates, 2:1031

Codependency, 1:91

Codes, ethical. *See* Ethical codes and oaths

Coding, medical billing, 3:1685

CODIS, 2:862, 4:2033

Codons, 1:503, 2:1166

Coenzyme R. *See* Biotin

Coffee
  caffeine in, 1:417–419
  zinc and, 5:2927

COG (Center of gravity),
  2:1115–1116, 1117–1118

Cogentin. *See* Benztropine

Cognex. *See* Tacrine

Cognitive-behavioral therapy, 4:2269
  for anxiety, 1:203
  for bipolar disorder, 1:307–308
  for personality disorders, 4:2087
  for post-traumatic stress disorder,
    4:2167
  for postpartum depression, 4:2179
  for stress, 4:2597

Cognitive evaluation
  for Alzheimer's disease, 1:104
  geriatric, 2:1184

Cognitive exercise software,
  4:2519–2520

Cognitive impairment
  in Alzheimer's disease, 1:101
  anxiety and, 1:202
  cognitive-perceptual rehabilitation
    for, 1:585–587
  from dementia, 2:728
  gait and balance problems from,
    2:1116
  mild, 4:2078
  neuropsychological assessment
    for, 3:1886–1890
  personal hygiene and,
    4:2078–2080
  with physical impairment, 4:2081
  psychotherapy, 4:2080
  relaxation techniques and, 4:2333
  sexuality and, 4:2440–2441
  wheelchairs for, 5:2891

Cognitive-perceptual rehabilitation,
  1:**585–587**

Cognitive prosthetics, 1:586

Cohen, Bonnie, 3:1785

Cola nidtida. See Kola nuts

Colace. *See* Docusate

Colchicine
  D-xylose test and, 3:1629
  fecal occult blood test and, 2:1032
  for gout, 2:1206
  vitamin B complex and, 5:2857
  vitamin B$_{12}$ and, 5:2855

Cold. *See* Common cold

Cold agglutinins disease, 1:244, 247

Cold agglutinins test, 1:242, 244, 247

Cold antibody autoimmune
  hemolytic anemia, 1:138

Cold bags (Chemical), 1:654

Cold feet, 2:1093

Cold injuries, 1:**587–590**, *588*

Cold laser therapy, 2:945, 947, 4:2100,
  2102

Cold sores, 1:**590–594**
  vs. canker sores, 1:434
  zinc for, 5:2926

Cold therapy. *See* Cooling treatments

Colestid. *See* Colestipol

Colestipol
  for gallstone prevention, 4:2578
  for high cholesterol, 3:1563
  niacin and, 3:1893
  vitamin A and, 5:2852, 2853
  vitamin B complex and, 5:2857
  vitamin B$_{12}$ and, 5:2855
  vitamin D and, 5:2863, 2864
  vitamin K and, 5:2869

Colistin-nalidixic acid (CNA), 4:2473,
  5:2789, 2904

Colitis, 3:1435
  See also Ulcerative colitis

Collagen
  in bone tissue, 4:2465–2466
  copper and, 1:655
  role of, 4:2463
  vitamin C and, 5:2859
  in wound healing, 5:2899–2900

Collagen dressings, 1:274–275

Collapsed lung, 1:545–547

Collars, cervical, 5:2894

College of American Pathologists
  (CAP), 1:16

College of Optometrists and Vision
  Development, 1:284

Collodion, 2:916

Colon. *See* Large intestines

Colon cancer, 1:599–604
  colonoscopy for, 1:594–597
  fecal occult blood test for, 2:1032,
    1033
  folic acid and, 2:1086, 5:2856
  vitamin D and, 5:2862

Colon polyps
  calcium for, 1:420
  colonoscopy for, 1:594–597
  colorectal cancer from, 1:599
  sigmoidoscopy for, 4:2461

Colonic irrigation, 2:974, 1337–1339

Colonoscopy, 1:**594–597**, *595*, 2:965
  barium enema with, 1:277
  for Crohn's disease, 1:673
  for diverticulitis and diverticulosis,
    2:856–857
  for fecal incontinence, 2:1030

Colony-stimulating factors
  for neutropenia, 1:432, 537
  side effects of, 1:433

Color, anxiety and, 1:205

Color blindness, 1:**597–599**, 5:2840,
  2842

Color Doppler ultrasonography,
  2:807
  ophthalmologic, 3:1941, 1942

thyroid, 5:2693–2694
vascular, 5:2806
venous, 5:2816

Color vision, 1:597, 5:2838–2839, 2843

Colorectal cancer, 1:**599–604**, *600,
  602,* 3:1435
  biopsy, 1:601, 4:2459, 2461
  causes, 1:599–601
  colonoscopy, 1:594–597
  colostomy, 1:601, 604–607
  sigmoidoscopy, 1:426, 601,
    602–603, 4:2459–2462
  treatment, 1:601–602
  tumor markers, 5:2753

Colored phototherapy, 4:2102

Colorimetric procedures, 2:923–924

Colostomy, 1:**604–607**
  barium enema, 1:277
  care for, 1:*607,* **607–608**
  for colorectal cancer, 1:601
  for diverticulitis, 2:857

Colostrum, 3:1400, 1514

Colposcopy, 1:**608–610**, *609,* 4:2016

Columnar epithelial tissue, 2:982

Coma, 1:**611–613**

Combining volume, Gay-Lussac's law
  of, 2:1138–1139

Combivir, 1:70

Comfrey
  for burns, 1:412
  for fractures, 2:1100

Comminuted fractures, 2:1098–1099

Commission E (Germany), 2:1290

Commission on Accreditation for
  Dietetics Education (CADE), 2:836

Commission on Accreditation in
  Physical Therapy Education, 3:1881

Commission on Accreditation of
  Allied Health Programs (CAAHP)
  on electrodiagnostic technologists,
    2:916–917
  on electroneurodiagnostic
    technology, 2:929
  on medical assisting, 3:1683
  on respiratory therapy,
    4:2361–2362
  on surgical technology,
    4:2617–2618

Commission on Accreditation of
  Medical Physics Educational
  Programs, 3:1722

Commission on Allied Health
  Personnel in Ophthalmology
  (JCAHPO), 3:1951

Commission on Dental Accreditation,
  2:747, 774

Commission on Dietetic Registration,
  2:836

Commission on Massage Therapy
  Accreditation, 3:1669

D

Dieticians, 2:836–837
    adolescent nutrition and, 1:34
    community nutrition and, 1:619
    diet therapy and, 2:827
    dietary assessment by, 2:830
    dietary counseling by, 2:834–835
    on dietary fats, 2:1027
    geriatric assessment by, 2:1186
    infant nutrition and, 3:1401
    medical nutrition therapy by,
        3:1720–1721
    peritoneal dialysis and, 4:2075
    role of, 2:820
    vitamins and, 5:2879
Differential white blood cell count,
    1:623–629
    cerebrospinal fluid, 1:524, 525
    synovial fluid, 3:1484
Diffusion
    in bioelectricity, 1:287
    in dialysis, 2:809
    of gases, 2:1139–1140
Diffusion impairment, 2:1135
Diffusion tensor magnetic resonance
    imaging, 3:1626
DiGeorge syndrome, 3:1382, 1383
Digestion
    acupressure for, 1:22
    of carbohydrates, 1:435–436,
        3:1632, 4:2010
    cellular, 1:500
    of fats, 2:1122, 3:1610, 1632,
        4:2010, 2013
    hydrochloric acid in, 1:8–9
    large intestine in, 3:1432, 1433
    lymphatic system and, 3:1610
    normal flora for, 1:264
    pancreas and, 4:2009–2011, 2013
    process of, 2:837–840
    of protein, 3:1632, 4:2010,
        2254–2256, 2259
    small intestines in, 3:1435–1436
    stomach in, 4:2571
Digestive enzymes. See Pancreatic
    enzymes
Digestive system, 2:**837–843**, *838,*
    841, 1329
    aging and, 2:1187
    of infants, 3:1399–1400
    normal flora of, 1:264
Digit Span, 3:1888
Digital clubbing, 1:700
Digital hearing aids, 2:1243
Digital radiography, 1:631
Digital rectal examination
    for colorectal cancer, 1:600–601, 602
    for diverticulitis and diverticulosis,
        2:857
    for prostate cancer, 4:2241, 2242
Digital subtraction angiography,
    1:152–153, 2:**843–844**
Digital thermometers, 5:2661, 2662
Digital x rays, bone, 1:376

Digitalis
    antihypertensive drugs and, 2:877
    calcium and, 1:422
    for congestive heart failure, 2:1256
    D-xylose test and, 3:1629
    for edema, 2:902
    NSAIDs and, 3:1897
    vitamin D and, 5:2864
Digoxin
    benzodiazepines and, 1:165
    overdose, 3:1988
    sucralfate and, 1:197
    vitamin D and, 5:2864
Dihematoporphyrin, 3:1710
Dihydroergotamine, 3:1761
Diiodotyrosine (DIT), 5:2687
Dilantin. See Phenytoin
Dilated cardiomyopathy, 1:473,
    2:1253
Dilation, esophageal, 2:892
Dilation and curettage (D&C),
    2:1360, 3:1773
Dilation and evacuation (D&E),
    3:1773
Dilaudid, 1:432
Diltiazem, 1:185
    for coronary artery disease, 1:661
    for hypertension, 2:1350
Dimercaprol, 3:1468
Dimetane. See Brompheniramine
Dimetapp. See Bromephiramine
Dimethicone, 1:159
Dinoprostone, 5:2792
Diode lasers, 3:1617, 1710
Diopter, 5:2842
Dioscorea villosa. See Mexican wild
    yam
Dioscorides, 2:1286
Diovan. See Valsartan
Dioxetane-phosphate, 3:1379
Diphenhydramine, 1:183
    for allergies, 1:96
    for common colds, 1:615
    for hives, 2:1311, 1312
Diphenoxylate overdose, 3:1988
Diphtheria vaccination, 5:2797–2798
Diphyllobothrium latum, 4:2583–2585
Diplegia, 1:518, 4:2023–2024
Diploid cells, 1:493
Diprivan. See Propofol
Dipsticks, 5:2781–2782
Direct antiglobulin tests, 1:180–181,
    182
Direct bilirubin, 3:1583
Direct DNA mutation analysis,
    2:1167–1168, 1170
Direct immunofluorescence assay,
    1:243

Direct laryngoscopy, 3:1532
Direct transmission, 2:849, 4:2565
Disability in America, 2:846
Disabled persons
    Americans with Disabilities Act,
        1:112–116
    definition, 2:845
    demographics, 2:845
    emerging universe, 2:848
    Medicaid for, 3:1678–1679
    models, 2:844–849
    Nagi model, 2:846
    personal hygiene, 4:**2081–2083**
    rehabilitation technology,
        4:2328–2330
    sexuality and, 4:**2439–2442**
    substance abuse, 4:2611–2612
Disablement, models of, 2:**844–849**
Disaccharides, 1:435
Discectomy, 2:1293
Discharge
    documentation, 3:1688
    postpartum care after,
        4:2175–2176
Discitis, 5:2830
Discontinuous capillaries, 1:357–358
Discrimination
    DNA databases and, 2:862–863
    employment, 1:112–116
    visual, 5:2839
Disease
    age-related, 1:61
    Chinese traditional medicine
        on, 1:21
    epidemiology of, 4:2274
    fetal origins of adult disease
        hypothesis, 3:1554
    nutrition and susceptibility to,
        3:1554–1559
Disease-modifying antirheumatic
    drugs (DMARDs), 3:1978, 4:2379
Disease transmission, 2:**849–851,**
    4:2626, 5:2747
    airborne, 1:12, 2:850, 3:1402,
        4:2565, 5:2743
    from autopsy, 1:254
    barriers to, 3:1403
    from blood specimen collection,
        1:354
    from breast feeding, 3:1513
    direct, 2:849, 4:2565
    droplet, 1:12, 2:849–850, 5:2743,
        2747
    infection control for, 3:1404–1407
    of infectious diseases, 3:1402–1403
    of malaria, 2:850, 3:1635–1637,
        1636
    prevention, 5:2836
    skin penetration, 3:1402
    of staphylococcal infections,
        4:2564
    sterilization techniques for,
        4:2565–2566

E

Etidronate
    calcium and, 1:422
    iron and, 3:1468
    for osteoporosis, 3:1981
Etodolac, 3:1895–1896
Etomidate, 1:144
Eucalyptus
    for influenza, 3:1416
    for sore throat, 4:2512
    for strep throat, 4:2592
Eugenic Sterilization Law (1933),
    2:1155
Eugenics, 2:1156–1157
Eukaryotes
    cell membranes of, 1:496
    digestion in, 1:500
    division of, 1:501
    function of, 1:498
    metabolism in, 3:1755
Eupatorium perfoliatum. See Boneset
Euphoric phase, 2:793
Eupsychian management, 3:1663
Europe
    aging in, 1:62–63
    diet in, 2:820
European Atherosclerosis Society,
    2:820
Euthanasia, 1:63, 2:717, **993–996**
Euthanasia Society of America, 2:994
Evaluation
    in evidence-based practice, 2:998
    See also Assessment
Evening primrose oil, 3:1745
Eversions, 1:363
Evidence-based practice, 2:**996–999,**
    4:2056
Evista, 3:1745
Evoked potential studies,
    2:**1000–1001**
    electromyography with, 2:926
    electroneurodiagnostic
        technologists for, 2:928
    for multiple sclerosis, 3:1794
    in neurophysiology, 3:1885
Ewing's sarcoma, 4:2391–2395
Exacta. *See* Ximelagatran
Examinations, certification.
    See Certification and licensing
Excavators, dental, 2:771
Exchange vessels, 1:357–358
Excimer lasers, 3:1710
Excisional biopsy
    breast, 1:*389,* 389–391
    lung, 3:1596–1597, 1600
    for sarcomas, 4:2391
Excretion, drug, 2:874
Executive functions, 2:1184,
    3:1888
Exelderm. *See* Sulconazole
Exelon. *See* Rivastigmine

Exercise, 2:**1002–1005,** *1003*
    after tracheostomy, 5:2723
    aging and, 1:64
    for back and neck pain, 1:258–259
    blood pressure and, 1:348
    cancer risk and, 1:425
    for cardiac rehabilitation,
        1:456–459, *457*
    for carpal tunnel syndrome, 1:477
    for childbirth, 1:557, 560, 561
    closed-chain, 5:2655
    colorectal cancer and, 1:603
    for congestive heart failure, 2:1256
    dehydration and, 5:2885
    for depressive disorders, 2:796
    for dysphagia, 2:892
    eye, 1:284
    for flexibility, 5:2655, 2656
    fluid intake and, 5:2883
    for fracture prevention, 2:1100
    for gait training, 2:1122
    guidelines for, 1:54–55
    heat disorders from, 2:1265
    for herniated disks, 2:1292, 1294
    for injury prevention, 2:984
    isometric, 2:1003
    isotonic, 2:1003–1004
    Kegel, 1:561
    for menopause, 3:1746
    for multiple sclerosis, 3:1794
    for myocardial infarction
        prevention, 3:1828
    nutrition for, 4:2545–2547
    for obesity, 3:1933
    open-chain, 5:2655
    for osteoarthritis, 3:1977
    for osteoporosis, 3:1983
    for pain, 4:2001, 2006
    for Parkinson's disease, 4:2038
    physical therapy and, 4:2106
    for polyneuropathies, 4:2150
    for postpartum depression, 4:2180
    for pulmonary rehabilitation,
        4:2285
    range of motion, 2:1002
    resistance, 5:2654
    respiratory, 4:2172, 2173
    for rheumatoid arthritis, 4:2379
    for sciatica, 4:2404, 2406
    shaping, 1:640, 641
    for sprains and strains, 4:2550
    strengthening, 2:1002–1003
    tension headache from, 5:2647
    therapeutic, 5:**2653–2656**
    thermoregulation and, 5:2664
    trends in, 2:819
    for varicose veins, 5:2803, 2804
    warm-up for, 1:55
    weight-bearing, 2:1301, 5:2655
    for whiplash, 5:2894
    See also Aerobic exercise; Aquatic
        exercises; Breathing exercises
Exercise electrocardiographs.
    See Stress test

Exercise physiologists, 4:2547, 2589
Exercise stress test. *See* Stress test
Exhaustion, heat, 2:1263–1265
Existential anxiety, 1:201
Exocytosis, 1:500
Exogenous biological rhythms, 1:292
Exons, 2:1166
Exoskeletal prosthetics, 3:1592, 5:2778
Exosurf, 4:2346
Exotoxins, 1:265
Expectorants
    for emphysema, 2:954, 955
    for wheezing, 5:2893
Experimentation, human, 3:1398,
    1419
Expert witness, 3:1716
Expiration, 3:1606
Expiratory neurons, 1:399
Explanation of benefits (EOB), 3:1686
Explorers, dental, 2:770, 771
Explosives, 5:2908
Expressive art therapy. *See* Art
    therapy
Expressive language impairments,
    3:1521
Extended family, 2:1023
Extended wear contact lenses, 1:642
Extension, joint, 2:1326
Extensor muscles, 3:1813
External beam radiotherapy, 4:2306
External chest compressions,
    1:464–468, *465*
External ear, 2:1240, 1246
External fetal monitoring.
    See Electronic fetal monitoring
External fixation, fracture, 2:1100
External version, 1:403–404
Extra-temporal resection, 4:2419
Extracapsular cataract extraction,
    1:483
Extracellular fluid (ECF)
    in bicarbonate therapy, 1:346
    calcium in, 4:2026, 2027
    in cellular digestion, 1:500
    electrolyte balance and, 2:918
    in thermoregulation, 5:2664
    thirst and, 2:1076
Extracorporeal circuit (ECC)
    in hemodialysis, 1:25, 569,
        2:808, 812
    in hemofiltration, 1:26
Extracorporeal membrane
    oxygenation (ECMO)
    heart-lung machines for, 2:1259
    in mechanical circulation support,
        3:1672
    specialists for, 2:1262
    venoarterial, 3:1672–1673

F

G

Gamma globulin
immunoelectrophoresis.
See Immunoelectrophoresis

Gamma-glutamyl transferase (GGT),
3:1582–1586

Gamma-linolenic acid (GLA), 4:2379

Gamma rays
medical physics and, 3:1721–1722
in radiotherapy, 4:2305

Gamma tocopherol, 5:2864

Ganciclovir, 1:197–198
for cross infection, 1:677
for cytomegalovirus, 4:2065,
5:2836

Ganglia, autonomic, 3:1868–1870

Gangrene, 2:1127–1131, *1128*
from *Clostridium tetani*, 3:1816
gas, 1:264, 2:1127–1130
wound, 5:2903

Gap junction, 3:1814

Gardnerella vaginalis culture, 2:1175,
4:2443–2444

Gardner's syndrome, 5:2698

Garlic
for diabetes mellitus, 2:805
for genital herpes, 2:1181
for gout, 2:1207
for hypertension, 1:531
for influenza, 3:1416

Gas, intestinal. *See* Flatus

Gas chromatography
for drug tests, 2:883–884
with mass spectrometry, 2:883–884

Gas embolism, 2:720, **1131–1133**

Gas exchange, 2:**1133–1136**, *1134*
blood gas analysis for, 1:341
continuous positive airway
pressure for, 5:2822
respiration for, 3:1604–1605,
1606

Gas gangrene, 1:264, 2:1127–1130

Gas laws, 2:**1136–1139**, 1139–1140

Gas-liquid chromatography, 3:1703

Gas sterilization techniques, 4:2566

Gases
in air, 1:344
blood, 1:**344–347**
medical, 3:**1696–1699**
properties of, 2:1136, **1139–1140**

GasPak system, 1:130

Gastrectomy, 4:2572

Gastric acid. *See* Stomach acid

Gastric acid inhibitors, 1:160

Gastric acid stimulation test,
2:1140–1142

Gastric analysis, 2:**1140–1142**

Gastric bypass surgery, 3:1931

Gastric emptying
delayed, 2:1148
in infants, 3:1399

Gastric juices
in digestion, 2:839
drug tests of, 2:881–887

Gastric lavage
for overdose, 3:1989
for poisoning, 4:2144

Gastric ulcers, 2:840–841, 841
antiulcer drugs for, 1:195–197
prognosis, 2:1145
zinc and, 5:2927

Gastrin, 2:1141, 4:2569–2571

Gastritis, 2:1141, **1143–1147**, 4:2571

Gastroenteritis, 4:2571

Gastroesophageal reflux disease
(GERD), 4:2572
antacids for, 1:160
esophageal function tests, 2:986–989
gastroesophageal reflux scan for,
2:1147–1151
proton pump inhibitors for, 1:196
treatment, 2:892

Gastroesophageal reflux scan,
2:**1147–1151**

Gastrograffin, 1:279

Gastrointestinal bleeding
fecal occult blood test for,
2:1032–2033
iron deficiency anemia from, 3:1470

Gastrointestinal disorders, alcohol-
related, 1:89

Gastrointestinal stromal tumor
(GIST), 3:1438

Gastrointestinal system disorders,
2:840–842
in cystic fibrosis, 1:699
in Down syndrome, 2:868–869
in infants, 2:1333

Gastroscopy, 2:965

Gastrostomy, percutaneous
endoscopic, 5:2741, 2742

Gastrostomy tube, 1:701

Gate control theory, 2:903, 5:2728

Gatorade, 4:2546, 5:2885

Gaucher disease, 2:1155

Gauze dressings, 1:274–275, 5:2900

Gay-Lussac, Joseph Louis,
2:1137, 1138

Gay-Lussac's law, 2:1137, 1138–1139

GBI (Gingival Bleeding Index),
2:767–768

Gel
for electrodes, 2:908, 916, 946
fluoride, 2:1079

Gel packs, 1:654

Gel protein electrophoresis, 4:2252

Gelsemium, 3:1416, 4:2512

Gemfibrozil
for gallstone prevention, 4:2578
for high cholesterol, 3:1563
for hypertriglyceridemia, 3:1564

Gender differences
in aging, 1:62
in alcohol intoxication, 1:84
in autoimmune disorders, 1:248
in bipolar disorder, 1:304
in bites and stings, 1:313
in carpal tunnel syndrome, 1:476
in colorectal cancer, 1:600
in COPD, 1:571
in coronary artery disease, 1:658
in fecal incontinence, 2:1029
in fractures, 2:1099
in genital herpes, 2:1176
in gout, 2:1206
in HIV, 2:1306
in hypertension, 2:1346
in multiple sclerosis, 3:1791
in myocardial infarction, 3:1824
in near-drowning, 3:1852
in oral cancer, 3:1954
in osteoporosis, 3:1979, 1980
in stuttering, 4:2601
in tension headaches, 5:2647

Gender identity, 3:1482

Gene mapping
for dental anomalies, 2:745
for myopia, 3:1830

Gene patents, 1:290

Gene regulation, 2:1155

Gene splicing, 2:1152, 1162–1165

Gene therapy, 2:**1151–1157**, 1163
for brain tumors, 1:386
for cystic fibrosis, 1:703
for dental anomalies, 2:745
for glaucoma, 2:1197
for hemophilia, 2:1278
for malignant melanoma, 3:1646
for muscular dystrophy, 3:1810
for osteoarthritis, 3:1978

General anesthesia, 1:**142–147**,
145, 149
for arthroscopy, 1:222–223
awareness under, 1:145–146,
3:1446, 4:2171
for bronchoscopy, 1:406
for dental prostheses, 2:779
intraoperative care for,
3:1444–1445
for laparoscopy, 3:1526, 1529
nurse anesthetists for, 3:1906

General paresis, 4:2626

Generalized anxiety disorder (GAD),
1:199–200, 202

Generalized seizures, 4:2416–2421

Genes, 2:1166–1167

Genetic counseling, 2:**1157–1162**,
4:2208–2209
for anemia, 1:141
for bleeding disorders, 1:326
for congenital immunodeficiency,
3:1384
for dental anomalies, 2:746
for Down syndrome, 2:869

H

H. pylori. See Helicobacter pylori

H. pylori test, 2:**1215–1216**

H-2 receptor blockers, 1:160

H-bands, 4:2463

H2 receptor blockers. See Histamine H2 receptor blockers

HAART (Highly active antiretroviral therapy), 1:71

Haemophilus ducreyi
   antibiotic susceptibility testing, 4:2445
   culture, 4:2443, 2444

Haemophilus influenzae
   in cystic fibrosis, 1:700
   meningitis from, 3:1738, 1740–1741
   nasopharyngeal culture for, 3:1851–1852
   sputum culture for, 4:2556, 2557
   in synovial fluid, 3:1484
   throat culture for, 5:2676, 2678

Haemophilus influenzae type B vaccination, 5:2797–2798

Hahnemann, Samuel, 2:1287–1288, 1316–1317

Hair
   for fungal cultures, 2:1106
   graying, 1:303

Hair follicles, 3:1427

Hair infections, 3:1509–1511

Hair roots, 3:1427

Hairy leukoplakia, 1:68, 69

Haldol. See Haloperidol

Hales, Dianne, 2:792

Hales, Robert, 2:792

Halitosis, 3:1959–1965

Hallucinations
   in narcolepsy, 4:2487
   somatic, 4:2397

Hallucinogens
   abuse of, 4:2607–2610
   fungi as, 2:1110

Haloalkene, 1:146

Halofantrine, 3:1638

Haloperidol, 1:190
   for bipolar disorder, 1:307
   diabetes mellitus from, 2:802
   Parkinson's disease from, 4:2037
   for personality disorders, 4:2087
   for psychosis, 2:730
   for schizophrenia, 4:2265, 2398
   for stuttering, 4:2602

Halophiles, 1:263

Halothane, 1:144, 146

Halprin, Anna, 3:1783

Hammer (Bone), 2:1241

Hammers, reflex, 4:2317

Hamstring injuries, 4:2550

Hand
   anatomy of, 4:2469
   bionic, 5:2778
   supinated, 1:363

Hand-eye coordination, 2:1066–1067

Hand-foot syndrome, 4:2453

Hand injuries
   constraint-induced movement therapy, 1:640–641
   orthopedic tests, 3:1970–1971

Hand magnifiers, 5:2843

Hand piece, dental, 2:771

Hand prosthetics, 5:2777, 2777–2779

Handwashing
   antiseptics for, 1:194
   aseptic technique for, 1:225, 225
   for cross infection prevention, 1:676, 679
   for diarrhea prevention, 2:816
   for disease transmission prevention, 2:851, 4:2566
   for infection control, 3:1406–1407

Hanna, Thomas, 3:1782

Hansen's disease. See Leprosy

Hanta virus, 5:2834, 2834

Haploid cells, 4:2339

Haptoglobin
   plasma protein tests, 4:2128–2131
   protein electrophoresis for, 4:2250, 2251, 2252–2253

Harelip, 2:744

Harm, to do no, 4:2231

Harnesses, prosthetic, 5:2778

Harper, Susan, 3:1785

Hashimoto's thyroiditis, 1:248–251, 2:1334, 5:2689

Hatching, assisted, 2:1039

Hatha yoga, 5:2919, 2921

Haversian system, 4:2469

Hawthorne, 3:1745

Hay fever. See Allergic rhinitis

Hazardous waste disposal, 2:851

HbA1C test, 2:803, 1201, 1203, 1204

HBeAg (Hepatitis B e-antigen), 2:1283, 1284–1285

HBsAg (Hepatitis B surface antigen), 2:1283, 1284–1285, 3:1585, 5:2758

HBV DNA (Hepatitis B DNA), 2:1283

HCFA. See Health Care Financing Administration

HCG. See Human chorionic gonadotropin

hCG. See Human chorionic gonadotropin

HDF (Human diploid fibroblasts), 4:2473–2474, 2557

HDL. See High-density lipoproteins

Head and neck cancer, 2:**1216–1222**

Head circumference
   fetal, 2:1041
   neonatal, 3:1858

Head examination, 4:2104

Head injuries, 2:1222, **1222–1226**
   Alzheimer's disease and, 1:102
   in children, 4:2548
   coma from, 1:611–613
   concussion from, 1:634–637
   electroencephalography for, 2:912
   first aid for, 2:1070
   sports-related, 4:2548
   taste and, 5:2641
   temporomandibular joint disorders from, 5:2643

Headaches
   acupressure for, 1:22
   from acute kidney failure, 1:25
   lumbar puncture, 1:525
   migraine, 3:**1759–1763**, 1760, 4:2381, 5:2856
   from myelography, 3:1822
   rebound, 5:2647
   spinal, 1:150–151, 4:2174
   tension, 5:**2647–2649**

Headgear
   for orthodontic appliances, 3:1967
   protective, 2:1225

Healing. See Wound healing

Healing Art of Tai Chi (Lee), 5:2635, 2636

Health, diet and, 2:**818–821**

Health assessment. See Assessment

Health care
   computers in, 1:**632–634**, 633
   quality of, 2:**1228–1230**

Health care errors
   computers for, 1:632
   documentation of, 1:32
   ethics and, 3:1695
   Institute of Medicine report on, 4:2048
   malpractice and, 3:1650
   medication, 1:32
   pilot program for, 3:1715

Health care financing, 2:**1226–1228**, 1227

Health Care Financing Administration
   health care financing by, 2:1226
   Medicare and, 3:1727, 1728
   public health and, 4:2275

Health care providers, HIPAA and, 2:1304

Health care services
   adult day, 1:49
   for the aged, 1:63
   utilization of, 2:1229, 4:2229

Health care workers
   drug testing of, 2:880–881
   HIPAA and, 2:1304

Health Eating 2010, 1:620

Immunoglobulin deficiency
syndromes, selective, 3:1382
Immunoglobulin E (IgE), 3:1385
in allergies, 1:94–95
allergy tests, 1:98, 99, 100
anaphylaxis and, 1:134
asthma and, 1:230
protein electrophoresis for, 4:2251
Immunoglobulin G (IgG),
3:1385–1386, 1387
autoimmune disease tests and,
1:244
in autoimmune disorders,
1:250–251
H. pylori test and, 2:1215
immunoelectrophoresis of,
3:1385–1386
immunofixation electrophoresis
of, 3:1386–1388
paraprotein, 4:2253
plasma protein tests, 4:2128–2131
protein electrophoresis for, 4:2251
reference ranges, 3:1386, 1388,
4:2131
TORCH test and, 5:2708, 2709,
2711
Immunoglobulin
immunoelectrophoresis.
See Immunoelectrophoresis
Immunoglobulin M (IgM),
3:1385–1386, 1387
autoimmune disease tests and,
1:244
H. pylori test and, 2:1215
immunoelectrophoresis of,
3:1385–1386
immunofixation electrophoresis
of, 3:1386–1388
plasma protein tests, 4:2128–2131
protein electrophoresis for, 4:2251
reference ranges, 3:1386, 1388,
4:2131
TORCH test and, 5:2708,
2709, 2711
Immunoglobulin O (IgO), 4:2251
Immunoglobulins, 1:325, 327
Immunohematology laboratories,
3:1702
Immunologic disorders, 3:1373–1375
Immunologic therapy.
See Immunotherapy
Immunology laboratories, 3:1702,
1707
Immunonephelometry, 3:1377
for plasma protein tests,
4:2128–2130
for protein electrophoresis, 4:2251
Immunophenotyping, 2:1075
Immunoprecipitation, 1:243,
3:1376–1377
Immunoradiometric assay (IRMA),
3:1377

Immunosuppressive drugs
for autoimmune disorders, 1:251
chronic leukemia from, 3:1548
for Crohn's disease, 1:674
for multiple sclerosis, 3:1794
Immunotherapy, 1:621, 3:1368
for acute leukemia, 3:1545
for allergies, 1:96
for asthma, 1:231
for cancer, 1:428
for chronic leukemia, 3:1549
for malignant melanoma, 3:1646
Imodium AD. *See* Loperamide
Impacted tooth, 3:**1388–1390**, *1389,*
5:2702, 2703
Impairment, defined, 2:846
Impartiality, ethical, 2:992
Impedence counting, 1:627
platelet count, 1:579
white blood cell, 1:624, 5:2896
Impedence phlebography.
See Impedence plethysmography
Impedence plethysmography,
3:**1390–1392**
Impedence test. *See* Impedence
plethysmography
Impetigo, 3:1428
vs. cold sores, 1:592
skin culture for, 4:2472
Implant radiation therapy, 1:385–386
Implantable cardioverter-
defibrillator, 3:**1392–1395**
Implantation (Egg), 1:648, 2:1051
Implanted ports. *See* Vascular access
devices
Implants
biomaterials for, 1:298
breast, 1:396, 3:1655
cochlear, 2:1244, *1244*
contraceptive, 4:2336–2337
dental, 1:665–666, 2:741, 755–756,
773–775, 778–780
for drug-delivery systems, 4:2006
for electroencephalography, 2:911
radioactive, 4:2304, 2306
for temporomandibular joint
disorders, 5:2645
Imprinting disorders, 3:1425
Improvisation (Music therapy), 3:1819
In-the-canal hearing aids,
2:1243–1244
In-the-ear hearing aids, 2:1243, 1248
In vitro allergy tests, 1:99
In vitro fertilization (IVF), 2:1038,
3:1413, 4:2455
In vivo allergy tests, 1:99
Inborn errors of metabolism, 3:1755,
4:2261
Incentive spirometry, 1:543,
4:2357–2358

Incidence, defined, 4:2274
Incipient presbyopia, 4:2217
Incisional biopsy, breast, 1:389–391
Incisors, 2:735
permanent, 5:2697, 2698, 2699
primary, 5:2700–2701
Inclinometry, 5:2656
Income. *See* Salaries
Incompetent cervix, 4:2203
Incomplete abortion, 3:1773
Incontinence
from Alzheimer's disease, 1:105
fecal, 2:**1029–1032**, 4:2529, 2531
personal hygiene for, 4:2081
from spinal cord injuries, 4:2529,
2531
urinary, 3:1794, 4:2081, 2529,
2531, 5:2787, 2788
Incontinence aids, 2:1029
Incubators, 4:2204
Incus, 2:1241
Indapamide, 1:186
Indemnity plans, 4:2228
Independent assortment
(inheritance), 3:1422
Independent lung ventilation (ILV),
5:2825
Inderal. *See* Propranolol
India
aging in, 1:62
medical ethics in, 3:1693
India ink preparation, 2:1104, 4:2557
Indian Health Service, 2:1227
Indices, dental, 2:**765–770,** 766*t*
Indinavir, 1:70, 192
Indirect antiglobulin tests, 1:181, 182
Indirect DNA testing, 2:1168
Indirect immunofluorescence assay,
1:243
Indirect laryngoscopy, 3:1532
Indium scan, 3:**1395–1396**
Individuals with Disabilities
Education Act, 4:2057
Indomethacin
diabetes mellitus from, 2:802
for gout, 2:1206
migraine from, 3:1760
for preterm labor, 4:2224
Induced labor
antepartum testing and, 1:163
oxytocin for, 1:554
uterine stimulants for, 5:2791–2795
Induction therapy
for acute leukemia, 3:1544
for chronic leukemia, 3:1549
Industrial toxicology, 3:**1396–1399**
Indwelling catheterization
female, 1:485–487
male, 1:488–492

Isosorbide mononitrate, 3:1826

Isospora belli, 4:2584

Isotonic dehydration, 2:725

Isotonic exercise, 2:1003–1004

Isotonic fluids, 3:1451

Isotonic muscle contraction, 4:2588

Isotretinoin
    birth defects from, 2:1297
    vitamin A and, 5:2853

Isoxsuprine, 1:185

Isuprel, 5:2696

ISWL (Intracorporeal shock wave
    lithotripsy), 3:1568–1571

Itching
    from acute kidney failure, 1:25
    from chronic kidney failure, 1:568

Itraconazole
    buspirone and, 1:165
    for cross infection, 1:677
    hismanal and, 1:96
    proton pump inhibitors and, 1:197

ITT (Insulin tolerance test), 2:1355,
    1356

IUD. *See* Intrauterine devices

IUGR (Intrauterine growth
    retardation), 3:1557–1558

IV therapy. *See* Intravenous therapy

IVF (In vitro fertilization), 2:1038,
    3:1413, 4:2455

Iyengar, B. K. S., 5:2919

Iyengar yoga, 5:2919

J

J tube insertion, 3:1952–1953

Jacksonian seizures, 4:2417

Jacobson, Edmund, 4:2331

Jacuzzis, 2:1337–1338

Jaffe reaction, 3:1495

Jainism, 5:2811

Jamshidi needles, 1:370, 3:1575

Janov, Arthur, 4:2270

Japan
    diet in, 2:826
    prostate cancer in, 4:2240

Japanese Americans. *See* Asian
    Americans

Jarisch-Herxheimer reaction, 4:2628

Jaundice, 3:**1477–1481**
    neonatal, 3:1478–1479, 1480,
        1856–1857, **1860–1863,** *1861*
    percutaneous transhepatic
        cholangiography for,
        4:2061–2062
    in premature infants, 4:2203
    from sickle cell disease, 4:2454
    urinalysis for, 5:2783

Jawbone, 1:420

Jawbone fractures, 2:784, 785, 4:2478

JCAHO. *See* Joint Commission on
    Accreditation of Healthcare
    Organizations

JCAHPO (Commission on Allied
    Health Personnel in
    Ophthalmology), 3:1951

Jejunostomy, 1:701, 2:976, 977

Jejunum, 3:1436

Jellyfish, 1:315, 317, 318

Jenner, Edward, 3:1368

Jesty, Benjamin, 3:1368

Jet lag, 1:293–294, 4:2487, 2490

Jette, Alan, 2:846–847

Jeune's syndrome, 5:2676

Jews
    acute leukemia in, 3:1543
    burial practices of, 2:718
    chronic leukemia in, 3:1548
    ethical codes and, 2:991–992
    on euthanasia, 2:995
    medical ethics and, 3:1694
    nutrition transition and, 3:1556

Jin Shin Do, 1:21

Jnana yoga, 5:2919

Jobs. *See* Employment

Johnson, Dorothy, 3:1481–1482

Johnson theory of nursing,
    3:**1481–1482**

Joint Commission on Accreditation
    of Healthcare Organizations
    (JCAHO)
    on certification, 3:1713–1714
    on heart-lung machines, 2:1262
    hospital administration and,
        2:1323
    on infection control, 3:1404–1405
    on laboratories, 3:1701
    on malpractice, 3:1651
    on nurse anesthetists, 3:1905
    on nursing homes, 3:1917
    on pain management, 4:2001
    on patient confidentiality, 4:2042
    on patient rights, 4:2050

Joint dislocations. *See* Dislocations

Joint disorders, 3:1487–1488
    arthroscopy for, 1:221–224, *222*
    of hinge joints, 2:1298–1299
    magnetic resonance imaging for,
        1:223, 3:1620
    in sickle cell disease, 4:2454
    tuberculosis, 5:2748
    x rays for, 1:223

Joint fluid. *See* Synovial fluid

Joint fluid analysis, 3:**1483–1485**

Joint hypermobility, 5:2643

Joint integrity and function,
    3:**1485–1488**

Joint mobilization and manipulation,
    3:**1488–1490,** 5:2654, 2775–2776

Joint National Committee on
    Prevention, Detection, Evaluation
    and Treatment of High Blood
    Pressure, 1:348–349, 348*t*

Joint pain, 1:24

Joint play movements, 5:2656

Joint replacement
    hip, 2:1301
    for osteoarthritis, 3:1488

Joint Review Committee on
    Education in Electrodiagnostic
    Technology, 2:916–917

Joint Review Committee on
    Education Programs in Nuclear
    Medicine Technology, 3:1902

Joints, 2:1325–1326
    abduction, 2:1326
    ball and socket, 1:*270,* **270–271,**
        4:2466, 2469
    biaxial, 3:1486
    bleeding into, 2:1277
    cartilaginous, 3:1486
    circumduction, 2:1326
    ellipsoid, 4:2469
    extension, 2:1326
    fibrous, 3:1363–1364, 1486
    flexion, 1:362–363, 2:1326
    function of, 3:1485–1488
    glenohumeral, 4:2386
    gliding, 2:**1199–1200**
    hinge, 2:*1298,* **1298–1299,** 4:2469
    immovable, 3:**1363–1364,** *1364,*
        1486, 1487
    pivot, 4:**2120–2123,** *2121*
    plane, 4:2469
    positioning for x rays, 1:362–363
    pronation, 2:1326
    protraction, 2:1326
    rotation, 2:1326
    saddle, 4:2469
    slightly movable, 4:**2493–2494**
    triaxial, 3:1486–1487
    uniaxial, 3:1486

Journal therapy, 3:**1490–1492**

Judaism. *See* Jews

Judgment, dementia and, 2:729

Judgment of Line Orientation test,
    3:1889

Jung, Carl
    art therapy and, 1:214
    Freud, Sigmund and, 4:2270
    psychotherapy ad, 4:2268

Jungian analysis, 2:714

Justice, 1:584, 2:1160, 4:2231

Justifiability, ethical, 2:992

Juvenile, defined, 2:1330

Juvenile-onset diabetes. *See* Type I
    diabetes

K

K-pads, 2:1352

Kabat-Zinn, Jon, 3:1732, 1733, 4:2508

KAIT (Kaufman Adolescent and Adult Intelligence Test), 3:1888

Kanamycin-vancomycin laked blood agar, 5:2904

Kanax. *See* Alprazolam

Kant, Immanuel, 3:1694

Kaolin, 1:581

Kaposi's sarcoma, 1:68, 69, 3:1644

Karma yoga, 5:2919

Karyotyping
amniotic fluid, 1:122, 124
chorionic villus sampling for, 1:567
in chromosome analysis, 2:1168
spectral, 1:122

Kats, Jack, 1:240

Kaufman Adolescent and Adult Intelligence Test (KAIT), 3:1888

Kava kava, 4:2610

Kay, Neil E., 3:1550

Keflex. *See* Cephalexin

Kegel exercises, 1:561

Kell blood groups, 5:2757

Kellogg, John Harvey, 3:1921

Keloid, 5:2901

Kemadrin. *See* Procyclidine

Keratectomy, photorefractive, 1:234, 3:1832, 4:2321–2325, *2322*

Keratin, 3:1427

Keratinocytes, 3:1427

Keratitis, herpes simplex, 5:2843

Keratoacanthoma, 3:1645

Keratoconus, 1:234, 235, 4:2295

Keratomileusis, laser epithelial, 4:2324
See also Laser-assisted in-situ keratomileusis

Keratoplasty, laser thermal, 2:1345, 4:2321–2325

Keratoscopy, 1:234

Keratotomy, radial, 3:1832, 1833, 4:**2295–2298,** *2296*

Kernicterus, neonatal, 1:311, 3:1862

Keshan disease, 3:1766, 1767

Ketamine, 1:144

Ketoacidosis, 2:801, 802

Ketoconazole, 1:179
alprazolam and, 1:165
for cross infection, 1:677
hismanal and, 1:96
proton pump inhibitors and, 1:197
sucralfate and, 1:197

Ketogenic diet, 4:2419–2420

Ketones, 2:801, 5:2782, 2785

Ketoprofen, 4:2005

Ketorolac, 1:133, 3:1895–1896

Ketosis, 1:436

Kevorkian, Jack, 3:1695

Ki, 4:2447

Kidd blood groups, 5:2757

Kidney, ureter and bladder x rays, 3:**1503–1505**

Kidney angiography, 1:153

Kidney cancer, 5:2788

Kidney dialysis. *See* Dialysis, kidney

Kidney diseases, 3:1507–1508, 5:2787–2788
abdominal ultrasound for, 1:2
antacids and, 1:160
beta-carotenes and, 5:2853
developmental disorders from, 2:1333
fetal programming and, 3:1557
hypertension from, 2:1348
intravenous urography for, 3:1459–1462
reticulocyte count for, 4:2369
sickle cell disease and, 4:2454
tuberculosis and, 5:2748
vitamin C and, 5:2860
zinc and, 5:2926

Kidney failure
acute, 1:**23–29,** 3:1494–1498, 4:2188
chronic, 1:**567–570,** 3:1494–1498, 4:2028–2030, 2072–2077, 2260
dialysis for, 2:808–811
dialysis technology for, 2:812–813
edema from, 2:901
electrolyte tests, 2:922–923
hyperkalemia from, 2:920
hypertension and, 1:349, 2:1347
kidney function tests, 3:1494–1498

Kidney function tests, 3:**1493–1498**

Kidney radionuclide scan, 3:1459, **1498–1500,** *1499*

Kidney scan. *See* Kidney radionuclide scan

Kidney stones, 3:**1500–1503,** *1501,* 1507, 5:2788
analysis of, 4:**2574–2580**
causes, 3:1500–1501, 4:2575–2576
demographics of, 5:2787
diagnosis, 3:1504
lithotripsy for, 3:1502, 1568–1571, 4:2578, 5:2659, 2660
prevention, 3:1503, 4:2578
treatment, 3:1502, 4:2578
types, 3:1501, 4:2576
vitamin C and, 5:2874

Kidney transplantation, 1:569, 570

Kidneys, 3:**1505–1508,** 5:2785–2786
anatomy of, 3:*1505,* 1505–1506, *1506*
blood circulation and, 1:334

fluid balance and, 3:1506, 4:2072–2073, 5:2883
function of, 1:23–24, 3:1400, 1493–1494, 1506–1507
over hydration and, 5:2885

Kineret. *See* Anakinra

Kinesthesia, 4:2428

King, Imogene, 3:1508–1509

King theory of nursing, 3:**1508–1509**

Kinyoun stains, 1:15, 4:2557–2558

Kirby Bauer method, 4:2558, 5:2904

Klebsiella pneumoniae
sputum culture for, 4:2556
stool culture for, 4:2582

Kleihauer-Betke tests, 2:1049–1050

Kleine-Levin syndrome, 4:2487, 2491

Klinefelter syndrome
causes, 1:504
diagnosis, 1:122
genetic testing for, 2:1170

Klonopin. *See* Clonazepam

Klumpke's palsy, 1:311

Knee
arthrography of, 1:219–220
bursitis, 1:414–416
function of, 3:1485–1486
housemaid's, 2:1299
ligaments, 4:2549
phototherapy of, 4:2100–2101

Knee-ankle-foot orthoses, 3:1590

Knee dislocations, 2:853

Knee injuries, 4:2549
continuous passive motion device for, 1:645–648
gait problems from, 2:1120
orthopedic tests, 3:1971
sports-related, 4:2543, 2544

Knee orthoses, 3:1590–1591

Knee prosthetics, 3:1593

Knee replacement
continuous passive motion device for, 1:646
for rheumatoid arthritis, 4:2379

Knives, gingival, 2:771

Koate DVI. *See* Factor VIII

Koch, Robert, 5:2746

Kock pouches, 2:977, 978

Koehler illumination, 3:1757

KOH test, 3:**1509–1511**
for fungal cultures, 2:1103, 1104, 1106, 4:2473
for sputum cultures, 4:2557

Kola nuts, 1:417

Konsil. *See* Psyllium

Koop, C. Everett, 3:1929

Korean ginseng, 3:1467

Korotkoff reading, 4:2187

Korsakoff's syndrome, 1:85, 87, 4:2320

Laser angioplasty
for coronary artery disease, 1:661
for myocardial infarction, 3:1827
Laser-assisted in-situ keratomileusis
(LASIK), 4:2321–2325, *2323*
for astigmatism, 1:234, 235
for myopia, 3:1832–1833
for presbyopia, 4:2218
vs. radial keratotomy, 4:2296
Laser disk decompression, 2:1293
Laser epithelial keratomileusis
(LASEK), 4:2324
Laser nurses, 3:1712
Laser peripheral iridotomy, 2:1197
Laser safety officer, 3:1711–1712
Laser surgery, 3:**1533–1537**, *1534,*
1710–1711
for astigmatism, 1:234
for cervical dysplasia, 1:609
cosmetic, 3:1536, 1710
for dental fillings, 2:762
for head and neck cancer, 2:1219
for human papillomavirus, 4:2066
for macular degeneration, 3:1617
refractive, 3:1947, 1948
for retinopathy, 4:2372
for skin cancer, 3:1646
for voice disorders, 5:2881
Laser therapy, cold, 2:945, 4:2100,
2102
Laser thermal keratoplasty (LTK),
4:2321–2325
for hyperopia, 2:1345
for presbyopia, 4:2218
Lasers, 3:**1709–1712**
alexandrite, 3:1710
argon, 2:1197, 3:1535, 1617, 1710
burns from, 3:1711
carbon dioxide, 2:1219, 3:1535,
1710
cold, 2:945, 947
copper vapor, 3:1710
definition, 3:1533
dental, 2:762
diode, 3:1617, 1710
dye, 3:1710
erbium (Er:YAG), 3:1535, 1710
excimer, 3:1710
holium (Ho:YAG), 3:1535, 1710,
4:2218
krypton, 3:1617
neodymium:yttrium-aluminum-
garnet (Nd:YAG), 3:1535, 1710
potassium-titanyl-phosphate
(KTP), 3:1535
red dye, 3:1710
ruby, 3:1710
safety for, 3:1711–1712
types, 3:1535, 1709, 1710
yttrium aluminum garnet (YAG),
1:483–484, 2:1219
LASIK. *See* Laser-assisted in-situ
keratomileusis

Lasix. *See* Furosemide
Latanoprost, 2:1196
Late-onset breast milk jaundice,
3:1861
Latent syphilis, 4:2625
Lateral decubitus position, 1:362,
5:2669
Lateral pterygoid muscle, 2:737
Latex agglutination assay, 5:2679
Latex allergies
anaphylaxis from, 1:136
from contraceptive devices, 1:650
intraoperative care and, 3:1445
preoperative care and, 4:2214
Latex-free syringes, 4:2633
Latex gloves, 3:1445, 4:2214, 5:2770
Latin, medical terminology and,
3:1725, 1726
Latinos. *See* Hispanics
LATS (Long-acting thyroid
stimulator), 5:2686
Laughing gas. *See* Nitrous oxide
Laurel rocket electrophoresis, 3:1377
Lavender
for alcoholism, 1:91
for boils, 1:366
for seizures, 4:2420
for sore throat, 4:2512
Lavendula officinalis. See Lavender
Law
criminal, 3:1715
Good Samaritan Law, 1:467–468,
2:1071, 3:1651
on informed consent, 3:1419–1420
medical, 3:**1712–1718**
public health, 4:2275, 2276
social work, 4:**2499–2504**
tort, 3:1651, 1714, 4:2501
See also Legal issues; Malpractice
Law of Similars, 2:1317, 3:1464
Law of the Infinitesimal Dose, 2:1317
Laws of motion, 1:295
Laxatives, 3:**1538–1539**
for barium enema preparation,
1:279
for colonoscopy, 1:596
phosphorus and, 4:2099–2100
for retrograde cystography, 4:2375
for sigmoidoscopy, 4:2460
vitamin D and, 5:2864
LC (Lethal concentration), 3:1397
LCR (Ligase chain reaction), 2:1175,
4:2445
LCSW. *See* Licensed clinical social
workers
LD (Lethal dose), 3:1397
LDH. *See* Lactate dehydrogenase
(LDH)
LDL. *See* Low-density lipoproteins
Lead, reference ranges, 5:2718

Lead poisoning, 5:2715, 2717–2718
color blindness from, 1:598
miscarriage from, 3:1772
polyneuropathies from, 4:2149
screening for, 5:2716
seizures from, 4:2417
target organs in, 5:2713
Leadership
for health services administration,
2:1237
in hospital administration, 2:1323
laissez faire, 2:1237
situational, 2:1237
Learned nonuse, 1:640
Learning
distance, 3:1915
observational, 3:1541
Learning disorders
auditory integration training for,
1:240–241
fetal alcohol syndrome with,
2:1044
motor and perceptual disorders
with, 1:585–586
neuropsychological assessment of,
3:1888
personal hygiene and, 4:2079
vision therapy, 3:1948
Learning System, 1:466
Learning theory, 3:**1539–1541**
pediatric physical therapy and,
4:2056
Leber hereditary optic atrophy,
3:1424
Leber's disease, 5:2855
LeBoyer method, 1:557
Lecithin
dietary fats, 2:1026
for hypertension, 1:531
normal values for, 1:124
Ledum, 5:2908
Lee, Martin, 5:2635, 2636
Leech Book of Bald, 2:1286
LEEP (Loop electrosurgical excision),
1:609
Leflunomide, 4:2379
Left lower quadrant (LLQ), 2:1327
Left upper quadrant (LUQ), 2:1327
Leg compression wrapping,
1:275–276
Leg-raising test, 4:2403
Leg vein x ray. *See* Phlebography
Legal blindness, 5:2842, 2844
Legal duty, 3:1651
Legal issues
cybermedicine and, 1:696
forensic medicine and, 3:1716
in home care, 2:1314–1315
hospital administration and,
2:1323
malpractice, 3:1650–1653

health services administration in, 2:1238

nurse midwifes in, 3:1909

optometry assistants and, 3:1950

patient's Bill of Rights and, 4:2049–2050

payment by, 3:1686

professional-patient relationship and, 4:2231–2232

quality of health care and, 2:1229

registered nurses and, 4:2326

social work and, 4:2500

Management
by-walking-around, 2:1323–1324
case, 2:1228
data, 2:1228
eupsychian, 3:1663
financial, 2:1237, 1323
health information, 2:**1233–1235**
health services administration, 2:1236–1239
hospital, 2:1323
by objectives, 2:1237
quality, 2:1228–1229
utilization, 2:1228
See also Administration

Management information systems, 3:1702, 1704

Mandible, 4:2467, 2477

Manganese
trace metals test for, 5:2715–2719
zinc and, 5:2927

Manganese deficiency, 3:1767

Mangled extremity severity score (MESS), 5:2736

Mania, 1:305, 2:793

Manic episodes, 1:305–308

Manipulation, 1:621
for back and neck pain, 1:259
for dislocation and subluxation, 2:854
for herniated disks, 2:1293
joint, 3:**1488–1490**, 5:2654, 2775–2776
precautions for, 1:258
for sciatica, 4:2404

Mannan binding lectin (MBL), 3:1370

Mannitol, 1:528

Manometry, 2:986, 988
anorectal, 2:1030
balloon, 2:1031
esophageal, 2:1149

Mantoux test, 5:2743–2746, 2748–2749

Manual muscle testing, 3:1802–1804, 1804t, 4:2181

Manual therapy, 1:259

Manufacturers' Standardization Society of the Valve and Fittings Industry, 3:1698

MAO (Maximal acid output), 2:1141

MAO inhibitors. *See* Mono-amine oxidase inhibitors

MAOIs. *See* Mono-amine oxidase inhibitors

Maolate. *See* Chlorphenesin

Maple syrup urine disease, 1:117–118, 5:2667

Maprotiline, 1:174

Marcaine. *See* Bupivacaine

Marfan's syndrome
postural evaluation for, 4:2182
scoliosis and, 4:2407

Marijuana, 3:**1659–1661**
abuse of, 4:2607–2610
emphysema from, 2:953
local anesthesia and, 1:147
lung cancer from, 3:1598
for multiple sclerosis, 3:1795
for nausea and vomiting, 1:431–432

Marine animal bites and stings, 1:313–318

Marinol. *See* Dronabinol

Marketing, 2:1237

Marsh mallow
for boils, 1:366
for osteoporosis, 3:1982
for sore throat, 4:2512

Marshall, W., 4:2272

Martial arts training
for post-traumatic stress disorder, 4:2167
Qigong and, 4:2291

Maryland Bridge (Dental), 2:756, 778

MAS (Memory Assessment Scales), 3:1888

Masked face, 4:2038

Masks, 5:2771

Maslow, Abraham, 3:1662–1663

Maslow's hierarchy of needs, 3:*1662,* **1662–1665**

Mass spectrometry
for adrenomedullary hormone tests, 1:45–46
gas chromatography with, 2:883–884

Massage therapy, 3:**1665–1670,** *1666*
acupressure with, 1:*20,* 20–23
brain tumors, 1:386
cancer patients, 4:2394
fibromyalgia, 2:1064
ice, 1:653, 654
menopause, 3:1746
post-traumatic stress disorder, 4:2167
pregnancy, 4:**2196–2198,** *2197*
sciatica, 4:2404
sexual dysfunction, 4:2437
stress, 4:2597
tension headaches, 5:2647–2648
with therapeutic touch, 5:2658

Masseter muscle, 2:737

Mast cell stabilizers, 1:96

Mast cells, 1:134, 3:1371–1372

Mastectomy, 1:393–394, 396

Mastication, 2:837–838

Mastitis, 3:1515, *1670,* **1670–1671,** 4:2176, 2279

Material Safety Data Sheet (MSDS), for mercury, 3:1748

Maternal age
chorionic villus sampling, 1:563
Down syndrome, 2:868, 869
genetic counseling, 2:1159
placental abruption, 4:2126

Maternal-fetal nutrition. *See* Life cycle nutrition

Maternal-fetal transmission, 3:1403
of AIDS, 1:65, 71, 2:1307, 1309
cerebral palsy from, 1:517, 520–521
during childbirth, 1:517
perinatal infection, 4:2062–2069
of syphilis, 4:2626
TORCH test for, 5:2708–2712
vaccination and, 5:2798

Maternal mortality, 1:558, 2:1295–1296

Maternal serum alpha-fetoprotein (MSAFP) screen, 2:869–870
See also Alpha fetoprotein test

Maternal serum screening test. *See* Triple marker screening

Matricaria recultita. See Chamomile

Mattresses, 1:281–282, 2:719

Maxillae, 4:2467, 2477

Maxillary expansion appliance, 3:1967

Maximal acid output (MAO), 2:1141

Maximal voluntary ventilation (MVV), 4:2540–2542

Mayo Clinic, dynamic spatial reconstructor, 2:887

MBL (Mannan binding lectin), 3:1370

MC method, 2:1105

MCH (Mean corpuscular hemoglobin), 1:625, 628, 4:2314–2315

MCHC (Mean corpuscular hemoglobin concentration), 1:626, 628, 4:2314–2315

MCI (Mild cognitive impairment), 4:2078

McKay, Frederick S., 5:2886

MCL (Modified chest lead), 2:909

MCMI (Millon Clinical Multiaxial Inventory), 4:2086, 2489

McRobert's maneuver, 1:311

MCV (Mean corpuscular volume), 1:625, 628, 2:1272, 4:2314–2315

enemas for, 2:971, 973, 974–976
nasal instillation, 1:30,
3:**1839**–**1840**
phonophoresis for, 4:**2096**–**2097**
rectal, 4:**2311**–**2314**
sublingual, 4:**2604**–**2606**
topical, 1:29, 30, 536, 2:895–896,
5:**2707**–**2708**
vaginal, 5:**2800**–**2801**
See also Aerosol drug
administration; Intravenous
medication administration;
Oral medication administration
Medication error documentation,
1:32
Medication orders. *See* Prescriptions
Medication preparation from a vial,
3:**1729**–**1730**
Medicine/Public Health Initiative.
See American Public Health
Association
Medigap, 3:1917, 4:2228
Mediolateral oblique position
(MLO), 3:1655
Medipren. *See* Ibuprofen
Meditation, 3:**1730**–**1734**, *1731*
for anxiety, 1:204, 3:1731, 1734
for brain tumors, 1:386
for hypertension, 5:2919
movement therapy and, 3:1783
for post-traumatic stress disorder,
4:2167
in Qigong, 4:2292
for relaxation, 5:2917, 2919
for seizures, 4:2420
for sexual dysfunction, 4:2437
for sleep disorders, 4:2490
for stress, 4:2597
therapeutic touch and, 5:2657
yoga and, 5:2917, 2920
Mediterranean diet, 2:826, 5:2811
Medium. *See* Culture media
MEDLINE, 1:695
Medorrhinum, 4:2628
Medulla (Cardiovascular center),
1:348
Medulla (Kidney), 3:1505, 5:2785
Medulla oblongata, 1:378, 381, 399
Medullary thyroid cancer, familial,
2:1170
Medulloblastomas, 1:384
Mefloquine, 3:1637, 1638
Megaloblastic anemia, 5:2854, 2855,
2856, 2870
Megapoles Project, 1:62–63
Meglitinides, 1:177–178
Meiosis, 1:492, 493–495
Meiosis disorders, 1:504
Meiotonic contraction, 3:1797
Meissner, Georg, 5:2639

Meissner's corpuscles, 3:1428
Melaleuca. See Tea tree oil
Melanin
copper and, 1:655
in malignant melanoma, 3:1643
role of, 3:1426, 1427
Melanocyte-stimulating hormone,
4:2112
Melanocytes, 3:1427, 1643, 1644
Melanoma. *See* Malignant melanoma
Melatonin
biological rhythms and,
1:293, 294
phototherapy and, 4:2102
role of, 2:961
for sleep disorders, 4:2490
Melissa officinalis. See Lemon balm
Mellaril. *See* Thioridazine
Melzack, Ronald, 2:903
Membrane bone, 4:2466
Membrane oxygenators, 2:1261
Membranes. *See* Cell membranes
Memory, 3:**1734**–**1737**
hypnosis and, 1:638–639
interference theory of forgetting
and, 3:1735
three-box theory of, 3:1735–1736
tolerance-fading, 1:240
traumatic, 3:1491
vision and, 5:2838, 2840
Memory Assessment Scales (MAS),
3:1888
Memory disorders
age-related, 2:728, 1187
in Alzheimer's disease, 1:103
from dementia, 2:729
geriatric assessment of, 2:1184
from head injuries, 2:1225
neuropsychological assessment of,
3:1888
riboflavin for, 4:2381
sleep deprivation and, 4:2483
vitamin E for, 5:2865
zinc for, 5:2925
Men
bone densitometry for, 1:368
urine specimen collection for,
5:2784, 2791
See also entries beginning with
Male
Menadiol sodium diphosphate,
5:2869
Menadione, 5:2868, 2873
Menaquinones, 5:2868
Menarche, 4:2339
Mendel, Gregor, 3:*1421,* 1422
Mendelian inheritance, 1:122,
3:1422
Mendelian traits, 3:1422
Menghini needles, 3:1575

Ménière's disease
hearing loss from, 2:1247
treatment, 2:1117
Meninges
function of, 1:379, 507
spinal cord, 4:2524
Meningiomas, 1:384
Meningitis, 3:**1737**–**1741**, *1738, 1739*
cephalosporins for, 1:167
cerebral palsy from, 1:517
cerebrospinal fluid analysis for,
1:522
Gram stain for, 2:1208
protein electrophoresis for, 4:2251
throat culture for, 5:2676
tubercular, 5:2748
Meningococcal vaccination, 3:1741
Meningovascular syphilis, 4:2626
Meniscal arthroscopy, 1:223
Meniscal tears, 4:2543, 2549
Menkes' disease, 1:655–656, 3:1766
Menopause, 3:**1741**–**1748**, 4:2340
home tests, 4:2117
osteoporosis and, 3:1980
Mensendieck, Bess, 3:1784
Mensendieck system of functional
movement, 3:1784
Menstruation, 4:2339–2340
menopause and, 3:1742
migraines and, 3:1762
Menstruation disorders, 4:2342–2343
Mental health
aging and, 1:60
culture and, 4:2264
vision and, 5:2840
Mental health assistants, 2:797
Mental health information, 4:2043
Mental health technicians.
See Psychiatric assisting
Mental illness
culture and, 4:2264
Freud, Sigmund on, 4:2270
in prisoners, 4:2264
psychiatric rehabilitation for,
4:2264–2266
sexuality and, 4:2440–2441
sleep disorders with, 4:2488
Mental retardation
causes, 1:382
from cytomegalovirus, 5:2910
in Down syndrome, 2:869
from fetal alcohol syndrome,
2:1043
personal hygiene and, 4:2078, 2079
sexuality and, 4:2440–2441
Mental status
assessment of, 2:795, 1069, 1184
changes in, 1:27, 2:1069
Mentax. *See* Butenafine
Mentha piperitas. See Peppermint
Menthol, 4:2592

MHA-TP (Microhemagglutination-*T. pallidium*) test, 4:2627, 2630–2633

MHC (Major histocompatibility complex), 1:250, 3:1372

Micardis. *See* Telmisartan

Micatin. *See* Miconazole

Miconazole, 1:179

Microalbumin test, 5:2780–2781

Microbiological tests
    microscope examination for, 3:1758
    for vitamins, 5:2870–2871

Microbiology laboratories, 3:1701–1702, 1706

Microcytic anemia, 1:626

Microcytotoxicity test, 2:1335–1336

Microdiscetomy, 2:1293

Microdontia, relative, 2:744

Microflora, 3:1369

Microglia, 3:1366

Microhemagglutination-*T. pallidium* (MHA-TP) test, 4:2627, 2630–2633

Microinsemination, 2:1039

Microkeratome procedure, 4:2321, 2323

Microlaparoscopy, 3:1525, 1526, 1528, 1529

Microneurography, 3:1885

Microorganisms
    immune response and, 3:1610
    resident, 3:1406
    sterilization techniques and, 4:2564–2568
    transient, 3:1406

Microscope examination, 3:1756–1759
    of ascites, 4:2021
    for fungal cultures, 2:1105, 1107
    for genital cultures, 2:1175
    Gram stain for, 2:1209
    of liver biopsy tissue, 3:1577
    for malaria, 3:1637
    for Pap test, 4:2016–2017
    for sexually transmitted disease cultures, 4:2443–2444
    of synovial fluid, 3:1484
    for syphilis, 4:2627
    of urine, 5:2783
    uses for, 3:1758
    of viruses, 5:2835

Microscopes, 3:*1756*, **1756–1759**

Microscopically controlled excision, 3:1646

Microsomia, hemifacial, 4:2478

Microsporidia test, 4:2584

Microsporum spp., 1:179
    KOH test for, 3:1510
    skin culture for, 4:2472

Microthermy, 2:945

Microtube broth dilution method, 4:2558, 5:2904

Microvascular surgery, 3:1612

Midazolam, 2:854

Midbrain, 1:378

Middle ear, 2:1240–1241, 1327

Middlebrook 7H10 media, 1:16

Midline catheters, 3:1451

Midstream void method, 5:2784, 2790

Midwifery, nurse, 1:51–53, 558, 3:**1907–1910**, *1908*, 4:2327

Mifepristone, 3:1773

Miglitol, 1:177–178

Migraine headache, 3:**1759–1763**, *1760*, 4:2381, 5:2856

Migration, cell, 1:500–501, 504

Mild cognitive impairment (MCI), 4:2078

Mild hypertension, 1:353

Miliary tuberculosis, 5:2748, 2750

Milieu therapy, 1:213–214

Milk. *See* Cow milk; Dairy products; Human milk

Milk of magnesia. *See* Magnesium hydroxide

Milk thistle
    for alcoholism, 1:91
    for substance abuse, 4:2609

Miller First Step Screening Test for Evaluating preschoolers, 2:798

Millon Clinical Multiaxial Inventory (MCMI), 4:2086, 2489

Milwaukee brace, 4:2408, 2533, 2534, 2535

Mimicry, antigenic, 1:265

Mind-body therapies, 1:215–216, 621–622

Mind exercises, Qigong, 4:2292

Mindfulness training
    for anxiety, 1:204
    meditation for, 3:1732, 1733, 1734

Mineral deficiency, 3:**1763–1769**

Mineral oil
    laxatives, 3:1538
    vitamin A and, 5:2853
    vitamin D and, 5:2864
    vitamin E and, 5:2866

Mineralocorticoids, 1:36–38, 663–665

Minerals, 2:822, 3:**1769–1771**
    in adolescence, 1:33
    aging and, 2:1188
    dietary counseling for, 2:832
    for fractures, 2:1100
    for infants and children, 4:2052
    in nutrition, 3:1920–1921
    in pregnancy, 4:2212
    in sports nutrition, 4:2546
    trace, 3:1770, 1921
    water and, 5:2884

Miners
    coal, 3:1397, 1598
    uranium, 3:1598

Mini-Mental State Examination (MMSE), 1:104

Mini Nutritional Assessment (MNA), 3:1925, 1926

Minimal inhibitory concentration method, 2:1105

Minimally invasive dentistry, 1:295

Minimally invasive surgery, 5:2659

Minipill, 4:2336

Mink encephalopathy, 1:668

Minnesota Multiphasic Personality Inventory (MMPI-2), 3:1888, 4:2086, 2489

Minocin. *See* Minocycline

Minocycline
    for rheumatoid arthritis, 4:2379
    side effects of, 1:168
    for syphilis, 4:2628

Minority groups. *See* Ethnic groups

Minoxidil, 1:185

Miotics, 2:1196

Mirapex. *See* Pramipexole

Mirrors, mouth, 2:770

Mirtazepine, 1:174

Miscarriage, 3:**1771–1774**
    from amniocentesis, 1:123
    causes, 3:1772
    from cell division errors, 1:495
    from chorionic villus sampling, 1:564
    premature infants after, 4:2203
    from prenatal tests, 2:1171

Misfeasance, 3:1714

Misoprostol, 5:2792

Missed abortion, 3:1773

Missile wounds, 5:2905, 2906

Missing teeth
    congenital, 2:744
    dental indices for, 2:768–769
    permanent, 5:2699

MIT (Monoiodotyrosine), 5:2687

Mitochondria, 1:499
    in apoptosis, 1:503
    disorders of, 1:504
    DNA in, 2:860, 861
    in metabolism, 3:1755
    in muscle contraction, 3:1814
    sperm, 4:2343

Mitochondrial diseases, 4:2147

Mitochondrial inheritance, 3:1424

Mitosis, 1:492–493, *493*, 501

Mitoxantrone, 1:511

Mitral valve, 1:470

Mitral valve prolapse, 2:1252

Mitral valve stenosis, 1:271–274, *272*

Mixed cell carcinomas, liver, 3:1578

from cancer therapy, 1:431, 432
colony-stimulating factors for, 1:537
treatment, 1:432
Neutrophil count, 1:524
Neutrophils, 1:329, 626–627
in ascites, 4:2021
in innate immunity, 3:1366, 1371
normal values for, 5:2899
in pleural fluid, 5:2670, 2671
WBC differential for, 5:2897–2898, 2897t
in wound healing, 5:2899
Nevirapine, 1:192
for AIDS, 1:70
for perinatal HIV prevention, 4:2068
New variant Creutzfeldt-Jakob disease, 1:667, 669, 671, 2:1088, 1090
New York City agar, 2:1174, 4:2443
Newman-Bluestein, Donna, 2:715
Newton, Isaac, 1:295
NHLBI. *See* National Heart, Lung, and Blood Institute
NIAAA (National Institute on Alcohol Abuse and Alcoholism), 1:84
Niacin, 3:**1892**–**1893,** 5:2855–2858, 2876–2879
for cataracts, 4:2381
for gallstone prevention, 4:2578
for high cholesterol, 3:1563, 1892
for infants and children, 4:2052
overdose, 5:2857
sources, 3:1892
therapeutic use of, 5:2856
toxicity, 5:2874
Niacin deficiency, 3:1892–1893, 5:2856
Niacinamide, 3:1892, 1893
NIAID (National Institute of Allergy and Infectious Diseases), 2:1176
Niaspan. *See* Niacin
Nicardipine, 1:422
NICHD (National Institute of Child Health and Human Development), 3:1558
Nickel
dietary, 3:1770
inlays, 2:756, 777, 4:2363
reference ranges, 5:2718
toxicity, 5:2717
trace metals test for, 5:2715–2719
Nicobid. *See* Niacin
Nicotinamide, 5:2874
Nicotinamide adenine dinucleotide (NADH), 2:883
Nicotinamide adenine dinucleotide phosphate (NADPH), 3:1751, 1752–1753, 1754

Nicotine
adrenomedullary hormone tests and, 1:46
coagulation tests and, 1:578
transdermal, 3:1893
vitamin B$_{12}$ and, 5:2855
Nicotinic acid
diabetes mellitus from, 2:802
for high cholesterol, 3:1892
toxicity, 5:2874
NIDA (National Institute on Drug Abuse), 2:879
NIDCR (National Institute of Dental and Craniofacial Research), 2:744, 745, 746, 751
Nifedipine, 1:185
for hypertension, 2:1350
migraine from, 3:1760
for preterm labor, 4:2224
Night blindness, 5:2851, 2876
Night guards
for bruxism, 5:2645
for malocclusion, 3:1649
Night shift, 1:294
Night splints, 3:1590
Nightingale, Florence, 1:583, 3:1913
Nightly peritoneal dialysis (NPD), 4:2076
Nightmares, 4:2488
Nigral cells, 4:2038, 2040
NIH. *See* National Institutes of Health
NIMH. *See* National Institute of Mental Health
Nimodipine
for bipolar disorder, 1:308
calcium and, 1:422
Nimotop. *See* Nimodipine
NINDS (National Institute of Neurological Disorders and Stroke), 1:510, 529
NIOSH (National Institute for Occupational Safety and Health), 3:1934
Nipples, sore & inverted, 3:1515
Nissen, Hartwig, 3:1665
Nitrates
for coronary artery disease, 1:660–661
in metabolism, 3:1753
migraine from, 3:1760
for myocardial infarction, 3:1826
urinary, 5:2783, 2785
Nitrofurantoin, 5:2781
Nitrogen
in blood gases, 1:344–347
in decompression sickness, 2:720, 721
as a medical gas, 3:1697
negative balance of, 4:2255–2256

in protein metabolism, 4:2255, 2259
toxicity, 3:1397
Nitroglycerin
adrenomedullary hormone tests and, 1:46
for coronary artery disease, 1:661
for myocardial infarction, 3:1826
sublingual administration of, 4:2605, 2606
syncope from, 4:2622
Nitrosamines, 3:1953
Nitrosourea, 1:385
Nitrostat. *See* Nitroglycerin
Nitrous oxide, 1:144, 3:**1894**–**1895**
for dental fillings, 2:760, 762, 3:1894–1895
for euthanasia, 2:994
liquid, 3:1698
as a medical gas, 3:1697, 1698
Nixon, Richard, 1:20, 3:1934, 4:2337
Nizatidine, 1:195, 196
Nizoral. *See* Ketoconazole
NMES (Neuromuscular electrical stimulation), 2:945–946, 947
NMP22 (Nuclear matrix protein), 5:2754
NMS blood groups, 5:2757
NNCO (National Nephrology Technology Certification Organization), 2:812
NNIS (National Nosocomial Infections Surveillance) System, 3:1406
NOC (Nursing Interventions Classification), 3:1912
Nociception. *See* Pain
Nociceptor reflexes, 4:2318
Nociceptors
in migraines, 3:1759
in pain, 4:1999, 2004
Nocturnal myoclonus, 4:2484, 2487, 2489
Nocturnal presbyopia, 4:2218
Nodes of Ranvier, 3:1883
NOFSW (National Organization of Forensic Social Work), 4:2502
Noise-induced hearing loss, 2:1246t, 1247, 1248
Nolvadex. *See* Tamoxifen
Non-A, non-B hepatitis. *See* Hepatitis C
Non-contact applanation, 2:1196
Non-cycle specific anticancer drugs, 1:170, 432
Non-Hodgkin's lymphoma, 3:1640–1643
causes, 3:1548, 1641
nuclear medicine therapy, 3:1903
Non-inflammatory diarrhea, 2:814

O

O-15, 4:2163, 2164

Oaths. *See* Ethical codes and oaths

Oats
  for menopause, 3:1746
  for osteoporosis, 3:1982

Ober test, 3:1971

Obesity, 3:**1929–1933**, *1930*
  adolescent nutrition and, 1:34
  cancer risk and, 1:425
  central nervous system stimulants for, 1:512
  community nutrition for, 1:619
  coronary artery disease and, 1:659
  diabetes mellitus and, 2:802
  diagnosis, 3:1930, 1932*t*
  gout and, 2:1207
  Heimlich maneuver and, 2:1269
  high-fiber diet for, 3:1921
  hyperplastic, 3:1929–1930
  hypertrophic, 3:1929–1930
  low-fat diet and, 3:1922
  macular degeneration and, 3:1616
  magnetic resonance imaging and, 3:1621
  medical nutrition therapy, 3:1719
  morbid, 1:282
  myocardial infarction and, 3:1825
  nutrition transition and, 3:1556
  pediatric nutrition and, 4:2051, 2053
  prognosis, 3:1932–1933
  risks of, 1:54
  self-reporting and, 2:830
  treatment, 3:1930–1932
  trends in, 2:819

Objectives, management by, 2:1237

Obligate aerobic bacteria, 1:263

Obligate anaerobic bacteria, 1:128, 263

Oblique fractures, 2:1098

Oblique plane, 2:1325

Oblique projection, 1:362

Observation
  for developmental assessment, 2:798
  for pediatric physical therapy, 4:2055

Observational learning, 3:1541

Obsessive-compulsive disorder, 1:203–204, 4:2085–2088

Obstetric ultrasound. *See* Pelvic ultrasound

Obstetricians, 2:1182

Obstructive sleep apnea, 1:562, 563

Oby-Trim. *See* Pheniramine

Occasional commensals, 1:264

Occipital bone, 4:2467, 2476

Occipital lobe, 1:379

Occlusal x rays, 2:786–787

Occlusional bites, 1:314

Occult blood test. *See* Fecal occult blood test

Occupational environment
  anxiety from, 1:201
  in balance and coordination disorders, 1:267
  cancer and, 1:425
  COPD and, 1:571
  hearing loss from, 2:1247, 1248
  herniated disks and, 2:1291
  infertility from, 4:2334
  lung cancer from, 3:1598
  miscarriage from, 3:1772
  modifications to, 4:2329, 2530
  stress from, 4:2597
  traumatic amputation and, 5:2736

Occupational exposure
  to chemicals, 3:1396–1399
  to HIV, 1:65–66, 2:1308–1309
  to metals, 3:1621
  to trace metals, 5:2718

Occupational health nurses, 4:2326

Occupational medicine
  biomechanics and, 1:295–296
  registered nurses in, 4:2326

Occupational outlook.
  See Employment

Occupational Performance History Interview (OPHI), 3:1940

Occupational Safety and Health Act, 3:**1934–1935**

Occupational Safety and Health Administration (OSHA), 3:1934–1935
  on carbon monoxide poisoning, 1:438
  on ergonomics, 2:984
  Ergonomics Rule, 3:1935
  on first aid, 2:1071
  inspections by, 3:1934
  on needle stick injuries, 3:1454
  on universal precautions, 3:1406, 5:2772
  violations of, 3:1934–1934

Occupational therapy, 3:**1936–1939**, *1937*
  activities of daily living evaluation and, 1:19, 3:1936
  for brain tumors, 1:387
  for burns, 1:412
  for carpal tunnel syndrome, 1:478
  for cerebral palsy, 1:519
  for cerebrospinal fluid, 1:529
  developmental assessment and, 2:799–800
  for dysphagia, 2:893
  education and certification for, 3:1936–1938, 4:2329–2329
  Ergonomics Rule and, 3:1935
  for gangrene, 2:1130
  for low vision patients, 5:2844

for multiple sclerosis, 3:1794
  muscle testing for, 3:1805
  for muscular dystrophy, 3:1810
  for paralysis, 4:2025
  personal hygiene and, 4:2082
  for rheumatoid arthritis, 4:2380
  for schizophrenia, 4:2399
  for spinal cord injuries, 4:2530
  for stroke, 1:530
  for upper limb orthoses, 5:2776

Occupational therapy interviews, 3:1939–1941

Ocular dominance, 5:2838

Ocular exam. *See* Eye examination

Ocularists, 3:1945

Oculomotor nerve, 3:1872

Oculomotor system, 2:935–937

Oculopharyngeal muscular dystrophy, 3:1806–1812

Odors. *See* Smell

Oenothera biennis. See Evening primrose oil

Office of Disease Prevention and Health Promotion, 4:2275

Office of National Drug Control Policy, 3:1660

Ofloxacin, 4:2065

OGTT (Oral glucose tolerance test), 2:1202–1203, 1204

OHI (Oral Hygiene Index), 2:767

Oil retention enemas, 2:971, 974–975

Oils (Diet), 3:1922

Ointments, 1:29, 30, 5:2707–2708

Olanzapine, 1:190
  for Alzheimer's disease, 1:105
  for schizophrenia, 4:2398

Old Tuberculin (OT), 5:2743

Older Americans 2000, 1:58, 62

Oleander, 5:2864

Olfactory epithelium, 4:2494, 2496

Olfactory memory, 3:1735

Olfactory nerve, 3:1872

Olfactory neurons, 4:2494

Olfactory receptors, 4:2494–2495

Olfactory sense. *See* Smell

Oligohydramnios polyhydramnios sequence, 3:1789

Oligospermia, 4:2334

Olney, John W., 1:85

Omega-3 fatty acids, 2:1026
  for hearing loss, 2:1248
  in nutrition, 3:1920
  vegan diet and, 5:2810

Omega-6 fatty acids, 3:1920

Omeprazole, 1:195, 196, 5:2857

On-off phenomenon, 1:187

On-the-body hearing aids, 2:1244

PDMS (Peabody Developmental Motor Scales), 2:798–799

PDW (Platelet distribution width), 1:579

Peabody Developmental Motor Scales (PDMS), 2:798–799

Peak acid output (PAO), 2:1141

Peak flow meter
for asthma, 1:230
for pulmonary function tests, 4:2282

Pectoral girdle, 4:2468

Pediatric assessment.
See Developmental assessment

Pediatric dentistry, 2:781–783

Pediatric nutrition, 4:**2051–2054**

Pediatric optometry, 3:1948

Pediatric patients. See Children

Pediatric physical therapy, 4:**2054–2058,** *2055*

PEEP (Positive end expiratory pressure), 4:2204, 5:2819, 2820, 2825

PEG (Percutaneous endoscopic gastrostomy) tube, 5:2741, 2742

Pellagra, 3:1892–1893, 5:2856

Pelvic adhesions
infertility from, 3:1412
treatment, 3:1413

Pelvic examination
prenatal, 4:2208
for preterm labor, 4:2223

Pelvic girdle, 4:2468

Pelvic inflammatory disease, 3:1411, 4:2443, 2444

Pelvic radiation therapy, 3:1743

Pelvic ultrasound, 4:**2058–2061,** *2059*

Pemoline, 3:1795

Pemphigus vulgaris, 1:249–251

Penbutolol, 1:187

Penciclovir, 2:1180

Pencillium notatum, 2:1110

Pendular tracking, 2:936

Penetrating wounds, 2:1223, 1224, 5:2903

Penicillamine, 1:657

Penicillin G, 1:167
for sore throat, 4:2511
for syphilis, 4:2628

Penicillin V, 4:2591

Penicillin VK, 2:733

Penicillinase-resistant penicillins, 1:167

Penicillins, 1:166–167, 168
calcium and, 1:422
for cold injuries, 1:589
discovery of, 2:1110
immune-mediated hemolytic anemia from, 1:180
for mastitis, 3:1671

for meningitis, 3:1740
for pneumonia, 4:2140
prophylactic use of, 4:2234
resistance to, 1:677
for sickle cell disease, 4:2455
for sore throat, 4:2511
for strep throat, 4:2591, 2592
for *Streptococcus,* 4:2066
for syphilis, 4:2066
urinalysis and, 5:2781

Penile cancer, 4:2436

Penile erection. See Erection

Penile prosthetics, 4:2437, 2438

Penis, anatomy of, 4:2344

PENS (Percutaneous electrical nerve stimulation), 2:903–905

Pentagastrin, 2:1141

Pentamidine, 1:69

Pentobarbital
for anxiety, 1:203
calcium and, 1:422

Pepcid, 2:1141

Peppermint
for alcoholism, 1:91
for cold sores, 1:592
for influenza, 3:1416

Pepsin
in digestion, 2:839, 4:2570–2571
in protein metabolism, 4:2255, 2259

Peptic ulcers, 2:840–841, 1215, 4:2571–2572

Peptide-chain synthesis, 4:2258

Peptidoglycan, 1:261

Pepto-Bismol. See Bismuth subsalicylate

Peptostreptococcus spp., 1:130

Perception
definition, 1:585
depth, 5:2838, 2843
of pain, 4:2000, 2003
sensory testing for, 4:2427–2429
subliminal, 1:639

Perceptual impairment
cognitive-perceptual rehabilitation for, 1:585–587
learning disorders and, 1:585–586
visual, 1:586

Percival, Thomas, 3:1694

Perclose, 1:443

Percocet, 1:432

Percodan, 1:432

Percussion
in chest physical therapy, 1:543
in pulmonary rehabilitation, 4:2285

Percutaneous disk excision, 2:1293

Percutaneous electrical nerve stimulation (PENS), 2:903–905

Percutaneous endoscopic gastrostomy (PEG) tube, 5:2741, 2742

Percutaneous liver biopsy. *See* Liver biopsy

Percutaneous transhepatic cholangiography (PTHC), 4:**2061–2062**

Percutaneous transluminal coronary angioplasty (PTCA), 1:157
for coronary artery disease, 1:661
gene therapy with, 2:1155
heart-lung machines for, 2:1259
for myocardial infarction, 3:1826

Perfluorocarbons, 1:330–331

Perforating wounds, 5:2903

Performance-enhancing drugs, 2:878–881

Perfume, 3:1397

Perfusion lung scan. See Lung perfusion scan and ventilation study

Perfusionists, 2:1262–1263

Pergolide, 1:188, 189, 4:2039

Periactin. See Cyproheptadine

Periapical abscess, 2:731–734

Periapical x rays, 2:786–787

Pericardial constriction, 1:473

Pericardial effusion, 1:473

Pericardial fluids, 2:1208

Pericardiocentesis, 5:2669

Pericarditis, 1:473
peritoneal dialysis for, 4:2073
tuberculosis, 5:2748

Pericardium, 2:1250

Perimenopause, 3:1742, 1745

Perimysium, 3:1813

Perinatal infection, 4:**2062–2069**

Perinatal mortality, 1:310

Perinatal teams, 2:1296

Perinatologists, 2:1296

Perineum
anatomy of, 4:2339
postpartum care of, 4:2175, 2176
prostate biopsy through, 4:2238

PerioChip treatment, 3:1898–1899

Period gene, 1:293

Periodic abstinence, 1:651, 652, 4:2337

Periodic acid-Schiff stain, 2:1104

Periodic health examination.
See Physical examination

Periodontal abscess, 2:732–734, 4:2069

Periodontal charting, 2:**739–743,** *740*

Periodontal disease, 2:737–738
calcium for, 1:420
classification of, 2:742
cosmetic dentistry for, 2:782

from cardiac catheterization, 1:442
from chest CT scan, 1:538
chronic leukemia from, 3:1548
from computed radiography, 1:630
from CT scans, 1:686, 689
from dental x rays, 2:787–788
from DEXA, 3:1980
from fluoroscopes, 2:1082
infertility and, 2:1036
injuries from, 4:2298–2300
malignant lymphoma from, 3:1641
from mammography, 3:1655
maximum permissible, 2:787
miscarriage from, 3:1772
from nuclear medicine technology,
    3:1901
from orbital x rays, 5:2915
paralysis from, 4:2024
from phlebography, 4:2094
from secondary radiation,
    2:787–788
skin cancer from, 3:1645
from upper GI exam, 5:2773
from x rays, 1:361
Radiation injuries, 4:**2298–2300**, *2299*
Radiation protection, 1:361
Radiation treatment.
    See Radiotherapy
Radical mastectomy, 1:394
Radical prostatectomy, 4:2242
Radioactive implants, 4:2304, 2306
Radioactive iodine uptake (RAIU),
    5:2691, 2692
Radioactive isotopes.
    See Radiopharmaceuticals
Radioactive positrons.
    See Radiopharmaceuticals
Radioactive tracers.
    See Radiopharmaceuticals
Radioallergosorbent test. *See* RAST
    test
Radiochemists, 4:2165
Radiofrequency systems, 3:1625,
    1721–1722
Radiographs. *See* X rays
Radiography
    computed, 1:**629–630**
    digital, 1:631
Radioimmunoassay (RIA),
    3:1377–1378
    for adrenocortical hormone tests,
        1:39
    for antidiuretic hormone tests,
        4:2118
    for congenital adrenal hyperplasia,
        1:40
    nuclear medicine technology and,
        3:1901
    for pituitary hormone tests,
        4:2115, 2116
    precautions for, 3:1379
    for sex hormone tests, 4:2431

for testosterone, 4:2117
for thyroid function tests, 5:2685
for triple marker screening, 5:2740
Radioimmunoprecipitation assay
(RIPA), 1:77
Radioimmunotherapy, 4:2304, 2306
    for liver cancer, 3:1581
    medical physics and, 3:1722
Radiologic technologists
    certification of, 3:1657, 4:2375
    congestive heart failure imaging
        and, 2:1257
    CT imaging equipment and, 1:686
    education for, 1:686–687, 4:2303
    employment for, 4:2303
    gangrene and, 2:1130
    herniated disk imaging and, 2:1294
Radiologic technology, 1:377,
    4:**2300–2304**, *2301*
    See also specific techniques
Radiological physics
    diagnostic, 3:1721–1722
    therapeutic, 3:1722
Radionuclide scan
    bone, 1:**372–373**, 4:2391, 2537,
        2544
    gallium, 2:**1126–1127**
    gastroesophageal reflux,
        2:**1147–1151**
    indium, 3:**1395–1396**
    kidney, 3:1459, **1498–1500**, *1499*
    liver, 3:**1586–1587**
    lung perfusion, 3:**1603–1604**
    MUGA, 3:**1786–1787**
    salivary, 4:**2389–2390**
    scrotal, 4:**2410–2411**
    thyroid, 5:**2690–2693**
    thyroid gland, 5:2685
Radionuclides.
    See Radiopharmaceuticals
Radiopharmaceuticals
    for bone radionuclide scans, 1:372
    breast feeding and, 3:1513
    for esophageal function tests,
        2:987
    for kidney radionuclide scan,
        3:1498–1499
    medical physics and, 3:1722
    in nuclear medicine technology,
        3:1901
    for nuclear medicine therapy,
        3:1902–1905
    for oral cancer, 3:1955
    for parathyroid scan, 4:2030, 2031
    for positron emission tomography,
        4:2160–2161, 2163, 2164–2165
    radiation injuries from, 4:2299
    for radioimmunoassays, 3:1377
    for salivary gland scan, 4:2389
    for scrotal nuclear medicine scan,
        4:2410
    for technetium heart scans, 5:2642
    for thallium heart scans,
        5:2649–2650

for thyroid radionuclide scans,
    5:2691, 2692
Radiosurgery, stereotactic, 1:386
Radiotherapy, 4:**2302–2303**,
    2304–2308, *2305*
    for acute leukemia, 3:1544
    for brain tumors, 1:385–386
    for breast cancer, 1:*393*, 394
    for cancer, 1:427
    for chronic leukemia, 3:1549
    for colorectal cancer, 1:601–602
    in electrotherapy, 2:945
    for head and neck cancer, 2:1218
    implants, 1:385–386
    for liver cancer, 3:1581
    for lung cancer, 3:1601
    for macular degeneration, 3:1617
    for malignant lymphoma, 3:1642
    menopause from, 3:1743
    pain from, 1:432
    pelvic, 3:1743
    for prostate cancer, 4:2243
    reticulocyte count and, 4:2368
    for sarcomas, 4:2392
    side effects of, 1:387, 4:2307
    stomatitis from, 4:2573, 2574
Radiotracers.
    See Radiopharmaceuticals
Radius, 4:2469
Radon, 3:1598–1599, 4:2299
Raftilin inulin, 1:421
Raftilose oligofructose, 1:421
Rails, side, 1:281
RAIU (Radioactive iodine uptake),
    5:2691, 2692
Raja yoga, 5:2919, 2921
Raloxifene
    for breast cancer, 1:396
    for osteoporosis, 3:1981–1982
Ramazzini, Bernardino, 3:1396
Range of motion
    active, 2:1301
    after spinal cord injuries, 4:2530
    continuous passive motion device
        for, 1:645
    exercise, 2:1002
    falls and, 2:1020
    joint mobilization techniques for,
        5:2654
    measurement of, 5:2656
    music therapy, 3:1818
    orthopedic tests, 3:1970
    passive, 2:1301, 3:1489
Ranitidine, 1:195
Ranson's criteria, 4:2014
Rapid Cosyntropin stimulation test,
    1:42
Rapid cycling, 1:305
Rapid eye movement (REM) sleep,
    4:2482–2483, 2485
    consciousness and, 1:638
    polysomnography of, 4:2154

Index

Scaling and root planing, 3:1898–1899, 1900

Scalpels
dental, 2:772
surgical, 4:2614–2615

Scapegoating, 2:1022

Scarlet fever
from strep throat, 4:2512, 2590
streptococcal antibody tests, 4:2593–2595

Scheuermann's kyphosis, 5:2831

Schiavo, Terri, 4:2048

Schilling test, 3:1630

SCHIP (State Children's Health Insurance Program), 2:1226–1228

Schizoid personality disorder, 4:2085–2088

Schizophrenia, 4:**2395–2400**
antipsychotic drugs for, 1:190, 4:2398, 2399
family therapy, 2:1022
personal hygiene and, 4:2079, 2080
treatment, 4:2265, 2398–2399

Schizotypal personality disorder, 4:2085–2088

Schneider, Kurt, 4:2397

School-based programs
for drug testing, 2:878
for HIV prevention, 2:1309
occupational therapy, 3:1936
pediatric physical therapy, 4:2056
recreation therapy, 4:2311

School nurses, 4:2544–2545

Schoop, Trudi, 2:713

Schoor, Robert, 3:1897

Schwann cells, 4:2146

Sciatic nerve, 4:2401–2403, 2402

Sciatica, 2:1294, 4:**2401–2406**, 2402, 2525

SCID (Severe combined immunodeficiency disease), 3:1382, 1383, 1384

Scientific literature, researching, 2:997, 998

Scintillation camera, 1:373

Scissors
dental, 2:772
surgical, 4:2614–2615

Scleroderma, 1:245, 249–251

Sclerotherapy, 5:2803–2804

SCN (Suprachiasmatic nuclei), 1:293

Scoliosis, 4:**2406–2410**, 2407, 5:2831
braces for, 4:2533–2536, 2534
in cerebral palsy, 1:518, 519
in muscular dystrophy, 3:1809

SCOLP (Speed and Capacity of Language Processing Test), 3:1887

Scooters, 4:2328

Scopolamine, 1:187–188, 3:1987

Scrapie, 1:668

Scratches, cat, 1:314

Screening. See specific screening tests

Scrotal nuclear medicine scan, 4:**2410–2411**

Scrotal ultrasound, 4:**2411–2414**

Scrotum, 4:2343

Scrub, surgical, 1:225

Scrub nurses, 3:1447, 1551, 4:2615

Scuba diving. See Diving (Scuba)

Scurvy
causes, 4:2470, 5:2858, 2877
dental anomalies from, 2:745

Scutellaria lateriflora. See Skullcap

Seal of Acceptance (ADA), 3:1960, 1961, 1963

Sealants (Dental), 2:751, 5:2699, 2701, 2705

Seasonal affective disorder (SAD), 2:793–796
biological rhythms and, 1:294
phototherapy for, 4:2100–2103

Seasons, bipolar disorder and, 1:306

Seating, adaptive, 4:2328

Sebaceous glands, 3:1427–1428

Seborrheic dermatitis, 1:303

Sebum, 3:1428

Seconal drug tests, 2:884

Second-degree burns, 1:409–411, 411

Second impact syndrome, 1:634, 636

Second law of thermodynamics, 3:1751

Secondary prevention, 2:818

Secondary progressive multiple sclerosis, 1:510–511, 3:1793

Secondary protein structure, 4:2257, 2258

Secondary radiation, 2:787–788

Secondhand smoke, 1:571, 3:1602

Sectral. See Acebutolol

Sed rate test. See Sedimentation rate test

Sedation
for airway management, 1:82
for balloon valvuloplasty, 1:272
conscious, 3:1894
inhalation, 3:1894
for mechanical ventilation, 5:2818
nurse anesthetists for, 3:1906
tracheostomy and, 5:2724

Sedative abuse, 4:2607–2610

Sedimentation rate test, 4:**2414–2416**

Segmental resection, colorectal, 1:601

Segregation (inheritance), 3:1422

Seizure disorders, 4:**2416–2422**
causes, 1:382, 4:2417–2418
in cerebral palsy, 1:517, 519
diagnosis, 2:1070, 4:2418
electroencephalography for, 2:913

first aid for, 2:1070, 4:2420
from head injuries, 2:1225
in pregnancy, 4:2187–2189
treatment, 4:2418–2420

Seizures
akinetic, 4:2417
auditory, 4:2416
generalized, 4:2416–2421
Jacksonian, 4:2417
myoclonic, 4:2417–2421
partial, 4:2417–2421
tonic-clonic (grand-mal), 4:2416–2421
visual, 4:2416

Selective dysphonia, 2:889

Selective estrogen receptor modulators (SERMs), 3:1981–1982

Selective IgA deficiency, 3:1382, 1383, 1384

Selective immunoglobulin deficiency syndromes, 3:1382

Selective photothermolysis, 3:1535

Selective reduction, pregnancy, 3:1789

Selective serotonin reuptake inhibitors (SSRIs), 1:174–176
for Alzheimer's disease, 1:105
for anxiety, 1:203
vs. benzodiazepines, 1:164
for bipolar disorder, 1:307
for dementia, 2:730
for depressive disorders, 2:795
MAOIs and, 1:175
for sexual dysfunction, 4:2437

Selegiline, 1:188
for Alzheimer's disease, 1:104
for Parkinson's disease, 3:1780, 4:2038, 2039

Selenium
for colorectal cancer prevention, 1:603
for infants and children, 4:2052
for multiple sclerosis, 3:1795
for osteoarthritis, 3:1978
for Parkinson's disease, 4:2040
recommended daily allowances, 3:1770
reference ranges, 5:2718
sources, 3:1767, 1770
trace metals test for, 5:2715–2719
vitamin A and, 5:2853

Selenium deficiency, 3:1766–1768, 5:2717

Selenium toxicity, 5:2717

Self-actualization, 3:1662

Self-catheterization, 1:489

Self-discovery, 1:214

Self-examination
breast, 1:392, 395
for cancer, 1:426

Self-paced walk test, 2:970

Self-reporting, dietary, 2:830, 833